ml

D0275334

The NMDA Receptor

The NMDA Receptor

Second Edition

Edited by

G. L. COLLINGRIDGE

Department of Pharmacology,
The Medical School,
University of Birmingham,
UK

and

J. C. WATKINS

Department of Pharmacology,
School of Medical Sciences,
University of Bristol,
UK

OXFORD   NEW YORK   TOKYO
OXFORD UNIVERSITY PRESS
1994

Oxford University Press, Walton Street, Oxford OX2 6DP
Oxford   New York
Athens   Auckland   Bangkok   Bombay
Calcutta   Cape Town   Dar es Salaam   Delhi
Florence   Hong Kong   Istanbul   Karachi
Kuala Lumpur   Madras   Madrid   Melbourne
Mexico City   Nairobi   Paris   Singapore
Taipei   Tokyo   Toronto
and associated companies in
Berlin   Ibadan

Oxford is a trade mark of Oxford University Press

Published in the United States
by Oxford University Press Inc., New York

© Oxford University Press, 1994

A catalogue record for this book is available from the British Library

Library of Congress Cataloging in Publication Data
The NMDA receptor/edited by G. L. Collingridge and J. C. Watkins.—2nd ed.
Includes bibliographical references.
1. Methyl aspartate—Receptors—Congresses.   I. Collingridge, G. L.   II. Watkins, J. C.
QP364.7.N63   1994   612.8'042—dc20   94–10163
ISBN 0 19 262371 0 (Hbk)
ISBN 0 19 262502 0 (Pbk)

Typeset by Footnote Graphics, Warminster, Wilts
Printed in Great Britain by Biddles Ltd, Guildford & King's Lynn

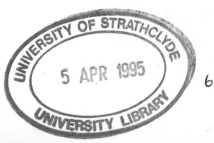

Preface

The last fifteen years or so have witnessed an explosion of interest in excitatory amino acid neurotransmission in the vertebrate central nervous system. This interest was initiated by the pharmacological identification of subtypes of glutamate receptors, now known to comprise two major groups: the metabotropic family of G-protein-coupled receptors and the ionotropic family of receptors, which operate ion channels and which are named after the selective agonists AMPA, kainate and NMDA. This book is about the NMDA receptor.

The acid form of N-methyl-D-aspartate (NMDA) was synthesized in the early 1960s by one of us (JCW) in the laboratory of Sir John Eccles. In a collaborative investigation with David Curtis (Canberra) NMDA was found to be a potent excitant of spinal neurones, such excitation being subsequently ascribed to the activation of a particular subtype of glutamate receptor, to which it gave its name. Fortunately, NMDA has proved to be a highly specific ligand with no known action on any other receptor system. The initial breakthroughs in first recognizing and beginning to characterize the functions of the NMDA receptor occurred in 1977. Firstly, in collaboration with Richard Evans (Bristol) it was shown that magnesium ions potently block activation of the NMDA receptor system. Secondly, the first synthetic specific NMDA antagonists, such as aminoadipate, were developed. This compound was used, in collaborative studies with the late John Davies (London), to provide the first direct evidence that NMDA receptors are involved in synaptic transmission in the nervous system, at the synapse made between excitatory interneurones and Renshaw cells in the spinal cord.

Soon more potent synthetic NMDA antagonists, most notably 2-amino-5-phosphonopentanoate (AP5), were developed and have been used to identify the pivotal role of NMDA receptors in a diverse range of physiological and pathological processes. For example, one of us (GLC), working at the laboratory of Hugh McLennan (Vancouver), found that NMDA receptors are important for the induction of long-term potentiation, a finding which has been expanded to include many other forms of neuronal plasticity including ocular dominance plasticity (Singer, Frankfurt), epileptogenesis (Wilson, Durham) and learning per se (Morris, Edinburgh). In disease, NMDA receptors have been shown to play a crucial role in clinical epilepsy and in neurodegeneration, occurring as a result of ischaemic cell death (Meldrum, London). Important advances in our understanding of the role of NMDA receptors in these pathological states have followed; for example, neurotoxicity is critically associated with NMDA receptor-activated calcium ion flux and the activation of calcium-dependent enzymes, such as nitric oxide synthase (Garthwaite, London).

The NMDA receptor possesses three unique and fundamental features: firstly the blocking action of magnesium ions is highly voltage-dependent; secondly, the NMDA receptor can only be activated by an agonist provided that a co-agonist site is also occupied—this is normally achieved by glycine (Ascher, Paris); thirdly, the NMDA channel has a significant permeability to calcium ions (Mayer, Bethesda). Many substances, most notably the dissociative anaesthetics, ketamine and phencyclidine (Lodge, London) and the related substance MK-801 (Iversen, Harlow) have been identified to act as NMDA receptor channel blockers while others have been found to work via the glycine site. These discoveries have further accelerated the quest for therapeutic agents. At the present time the best therapeutic target for NMDA receptor antagonists seems to be trauma and stroke, where they offer prospects as neuroprotectants; such compounds are currently in phase II clinical trials.

The first edition of The NMDA Receptor appeared in 1989 and was associated with a symposium on this topic held in association with a meeting of the British Pharmacological Society in Bristol in April 1989. Each invited speaker was the leading authority in the field and contributed a chapter to the first edition of the book. These chapters have now been fully updated for this, the second edition. In particular, chapter 2 has been expanded to cover the multiplicity of new NMDA antagonists which have been developed over the last 5 years and to include a range of molecular modelling studies on the NMDA receptor. In addition, a new chapter by Mayer, Benveniste and Patneau provides a kinetic analysis of the action of NMDA receptor agonists and antagonists.

Since 1989 there have been several important advances in the field. Foremost was the cloning of the first NMDA receptor subunit gene and identification of the NMDA receptor subunit family (Nakanishi, Kyoto; Mishina, Niigata and Seeburg, Heidelberg). This rapidly expanding area is covered by a new chapter by Seeburg, Monyer, Sprengel and Burnashev and is also featured in several of the other chapters, notably the studies by Monaghan and Buller on the regional distribution of NMDA receptor subunits and subtypes. In addition, major inroads have been made into the understanding of the kinetic behaviour of NMDA receptor channels. This is reflected by new chapters from Lester, Clements, Tong, Westbrook, and Jahr and from Gibb, Edmonds, Silver, Cull-Candy, and Colquhoun.

Tragically, John Davies died suddenly in September, 1991. He was the principal collaborator for over 20 years of one of us (JCW) and the Ph.D. supervisor of the other (GLC). His pioneering contributions were crucial to the development of the field of NMDA receptor research. Tom Salt has written the new chapter on the role of NMDA receptors in synaptic transmission in the brain and has dedicated the chapter to his memory.

Bristol G.L.C.
August 1994 J.C.W.

Contents

1 The NMDA receptor concept: origins and development   1
J. C. Watkins

2 Agonists and competitive antagonists: structure–
activity and molecular modelling studies   31
D. E. Jane, H. J. Olverman, and J. C. Watkins

3 Non-competitive antagonists of *N*-methyl-D-aspartate   105
David Lodge, Martyn Jones, and Elizabeth Fletcher

4 NMDA receptor agonists and competitive antagonists   132
Mark L. Mayer, Morris Benveniste, and Doris K. Patneau

5 Molecular biology of NMDA receptors   147
P. H. Seeburg, H. Monyer, R. Sprengel, and N. Burnashev

6 Anatomical, pharmacological, and molecular diversity
of native NMDA receptor subtypes   158
Daniel T. Monaghan and Amy L. Buller

7 The NMDA receptor, its channel, and its modulation
by glycine   177
P. Ascher and J. W. Johnson

8 The time course of NMDA receptor-mediated synaptic
currents   206
*Robin A. J. Lester, John D. Clements, Gang Tong,
Gary L. Westbrook, and Craig E. Jahr*

9 Activation of NMDA receptors   219
*A. J. Gibb, B. Edmonds, R. A. Silver, S. G. Cull-Candy,
and D. Colquhoun*

10 NMDA receptors and their interactions with other
excitatory amino acid receptors in synaptic transmission
in the mammalian central nervous system   243
T. E. Salt

11 The importance of NMDA receptors in the processing
of spinal primary afferent input   266
R. H. Evans

Contents

12 The role of NMDA receptors in synaptic integration
and the organization of motor patterns   277
Simon Alford and Lennart Brodin

13 NMDA receptors and long-term potentiation in the
hippocampus   294
Zafar I. Bashir, Nicola Berretta, Zuner A. Bortolotto,
Kath Clark, Ceri H. Davies, Bruno G. Frenguelli,
Jenni Harvey, Brigitte Potier, and Graham L. Collingridge

14 NMDA receptors and developmental plasticity in visual
neocortex   313
Alain Artola and Wolf Singer

15 The role of NMDA receptors in learning and memory   340
R. G. M. Morris and M. Davis

16 Clinical implications of NMDA receptors   376
Paul L. Herrling

17 The NMDA receptor in epilepsy   395
Suzanne Clark, Steven Stasheff, Darrell V. Lewis,
David Martin, and Wilkie A. Wilson

18 NMDA receptors, neuronal development, and
neurodegeneration   428
John Garthwaite

19 Competitive NMDA antagonists as drugs   457
B. S. Meldrum and A. G. Chapman

20 Non-competitive NMDA antagonists as drugs   469
L. L. Iversen and J. A. Kemp

Index   487

Contributors

Simon Alford Department of Physiology, Northwestern University Medical School, 303 E. Chicago Avenue, Chicago, IL 60611, USA.

Alain Artola Department of Neurobiology, ETH-Hönggerberg, CH-8093 Zürich, Switzerland.

P. Ascher Laboratoire de Neurobiologie, Ecole Normale Supérieure, 46 rue d'Ulm, F-75230 Paris Cedex 05, France.

Zafar I. Bashir Department of Pharmacology, The Medical School, The University of Birmingham, Edgbaston, Birmingham B15 2TT, UK.

Morris Benveniste Laboratory of Cellular and Molecular Neurophysiology, Building 49, Room 5A78, NICHD, NIH, Bethesda, MD 20892, USA.

Nicola Berretta Department of Pharmacology, The Medical School, The University of Birmingham, Edgbaston, Birmingham B15 2TT, UK.

Zuner A. Bortolotto Department of Pharmacology, The Medical School, The University of Birmingham, Edgbaston, Birmingham B15 2TT, UK.

Lennart Brodin Nobel Institute for Neurophysiology, Karolinska Institutet, Box 60400, S-104 01, Stockholm, Sweden.

Amy L. Buller Department of Pharmacology, University of Nebraska Medical Center, Omaha, NE 68198-6260, USA.

N. Burnashev Abteilung Zellphysiologie, Max-Planck-Institut für Medizinische Forschung, Jahnstrasse 29, 69120 Heidelberg, Germany.

A. G. Chapman Department of Neurology, Institute of Psychiatry, DeCrespigney Park, London SE5 8AF, UK.

Kath Clark Department of Pharmacology, The Medical School, The University of Birmingham, Edgbaston, Birmingham B15 2TT, UK.

Suzanne Clark Department of Pharmacology, Box 3813, Duke University Medical Center, Durham, NC 27710, USA.

John D. Clements Vollum Institute, Oregon Health Sciences University, Portland, OR 97201, USA.

D. Colquhoun Department of Pharmacology, University College London, Gower Street, London WC1E 6BT, UK.

G. L. Collingridge   Department of Pharmacology, The Medical School, The University of Birmingham, Edgbaston, Birmingham B15 2TT, UK.

S. G. Cull-Candy   Department of Pharmacology, University College London, Gower Street, London WC1E 6BT, UK.

Ceri H. Davies   Department of Pharmacology, The Medical School, The University of Birmingham, Edgbaston, Birmingham B15 2TT, UK.

M. Davis   Department of Psychiatry and Psychology, Yale University, 34 Park Street, New Haven CT 06508, USA.

B. Edmonds   Department of Pharmacology, University College London, Gower Street, London WC1E 6BT, UK.

R. H. Evans   Department of Pharmacology, The School of Medical Sciences, University Walk, Bristol BS8 1TD, UK.

Elizabeth Fletcher   Allelix Biopharmaceuticals, 6850 Goreway Drive, Mississauga, Ontario, Canada L4VIV7.

Bruno G. Frenguelli   Department of Pharmacology, The Medical School, The University of Birmingham, Edgbaston, Birmingham B15 2TT, UK.

John Garthwaite   Wellcome Research Laboratories, Langley Court, South Eden Park Road, Beckenham, Kent BR3 3BS, UK.

A. J. Gibb   Department of Pharmacology, University College London, Gower Street, London WC1E 6BT, UK.

Jenni Harvey   Department of Pharmacology, The Medical School, The University of Birmingham, Edgbaston, Birmingham B15 2TT, UK.

Paul L. Herrling   Sandoz Pharma Ltd, CH4002, Basel, Switzerland.

L. L. Iversen   Merck Sharp and Dohme Research Laboratories, Neuroscience Research Centre, Terlings Park, Eastwick Road, Harlow, Essex CM20 2QR, UK.

Craig E. Jahr   Vollum Institute and Department of Cell Biology and Anatomy, Oregon Health Sciences University, Portland, OR 97201, USA.

D. E. Jane   Department of Pharmacology, School of Medical Sciences, University of Bristol, Bristol BS8 1TD, UK.

J. W. Johnson   Department of Behavioral Neuroscience, University of Pittsburgh, PA 15260, USA.

Martyn Jones   Eli Lilly Research Centre Ltd, Earl Wood Manor, Windlesham, Surrey GU20 6PH, UK.

J. A. Kemp Merck Sharp and Dohme Research Laboratories, Neuroscience Research Centre, Terlings Park, Eastwick Road, Harlow, Essex CM20 2QR, UK.

Robin A. J. Lester Department of Molecular Physiology and Biophysics, Baylor College of Medicine, One Baylor Plaza, Houston, TX 77030, USA.

Darrell V. Lewis Departments of Pediatrics and Neurobiology, Duke University Medical Center, Durham, NC 27710, USA.

David Lodge Eli Lilly Research Centre Ltd, Earl Wood Manor, Windlesham, Surrey GU20 6PH, UK.

David Martin Synergen Inc. 1885 33rd Street, Boulder 80301, CO, USA.

Mark L. Mayer Laboratory of Cellular and Molecular Neurophysiology, Building 49, Room 5A78, NICHD, NIH, Bethesda, MD 20892, USA.

B. S. Meldrum Department of Neurology, Institute of Psychiatry, De Crespigny Park, London SE5 8AF, UK.

Daniel T. Monaghan Department of Pharmacology, University of Nebraska Medical Center, Omaha, NE 68198-6260, USA.

H. Monyer Centre for Molecular Biology (ZMBH), Heidelberg University, INF 282, 69120 Heidelberg, Germany.

R. G. M. Morris Department of Pharmacology, University of Edinburgh, 1 George Square, Edinburgh EH8 9JZ, UK.

H. J. Olverman Department of Pharmacology, University of Edinburgh, 1 George Square, Edinburgh EH8 9JZ, UK.

Doris K. Patneau Laboratory of Cellular and Molecular Neurophysiology, Building 49, Room 5A78, NICHD, NIH, Bethesda, MD 20892, USA.

Brigitte Potier Department of Pharmacology, The Medical School, The University of Birmingham, Edgbaston, Birmingham B15 2TT, UK.

T. E. Salt Department of Visual Science, Institute of Ophthalmology, 11–43 Bath Street, London EC1V 9EL, UK.

P. H. Seeburg Centre for Molecular Biology (ZMBH), Heidelberg University, INF 282, 69120 Heidelberg, Germany.

R. A. Silver Department of Pharmacology, University College London, Gower Street, London WC1E 6BT, UK.

Wolf Singer   Max Planck Institute for Brain Research, Deutschordenstr. 46, D-6000 Frankfurt/Main, Germany.

R. Sprengel   Centre for Molecular Biology (ZMBH), Heidelberg University, INF 282, 69120 Heidelberg, Germany.

Steven Stasheff   Children's Hospital of Philadelphia Department of Pediatrics, PA 19104, USA.

Gang Tong   Vollum Institute and Department of Cell Biology and Anatomy, Oregon Health Sciences University, Portland, OR 97201, USA.

J. C. Watkins   Department of Pharmacology, School of Medical Sciences, University of Bristol, Bristol BS8 1TD, UK.

Gary L. Westbrook   Vollum Institute and Department of Neurology, Oregon Health Sciences University, Portland, OR 97201, USA.

Wilkie A. Wilson   Department of Pharmacology and Medicine, Duke University Medical Center, and Veterans' Administration Medical Center, Durham, NC 27710, PA, USA.

1 The NMDA receptor concept: origins and development

J. C. WATKINS

The progress of research in the excitatory amino acid (EAA) field over the last 40 years is well documented (Curtis and Watkins 1965; Curtis and Johnston 1974; Krnjevic 1974; Watkins and Evans 1981; Foster and Fagg 1984; Watkins 1986; Mayer and Westbrook 1987a; Monaghan *et al.* 1989). The field had its origin in the discovery by Hayashi (1954) of the convulsive effects of L-glutamate and L-aspartate in mammalian brain, and the demonstration later in the decade of the depolarizing and excitatory actions of these amino acids on single central neurones (Curtis *et al.* 1959, 1960). Today L-glutamate is widely accepted as the predominant excitatory transmitter in the mammalian central nervous system (CNS), acting at a range of different receptor types (Watkins and Evans 1981; Monaghan *et al.* 1989; Collingridge and Lester 1989; Lodge and Collingridge 1991). The purpose of this volume is to highlight the particular role of the N-methyl-D-aspartate (NMDA) type of glutamate receptor (Watkins 1978, 1980; Watkins and Evans 1981) in CNS function, with emphasis on the mechanisms underlying synaptic transmission and plasticity and the potential therapeutic value of substances which affect these systems in the treatment of CNS disorders. In this first chapter, historical aspects of the NMDA receptor concept are reviewed.

NMDA as an excitatory amino acid

N-Methyl-D-aspartic acid (Fig. 1.1), the acid form of NMDA, was first synthesized specifically for the study of structure–activity relationships of L-glutamic and L-aspartic acids (Watkins 1962). No marked stereospecificity

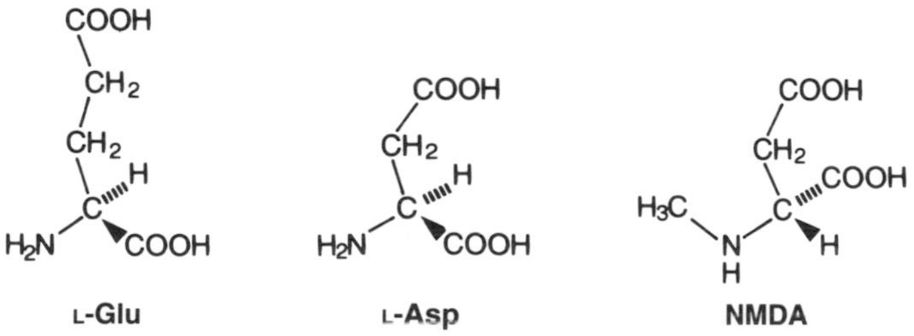

Fig. 1.1 The structures of L-glutamic acid, L-aspartic acid, and N-methyl-D-aspartic acid (NMDA).

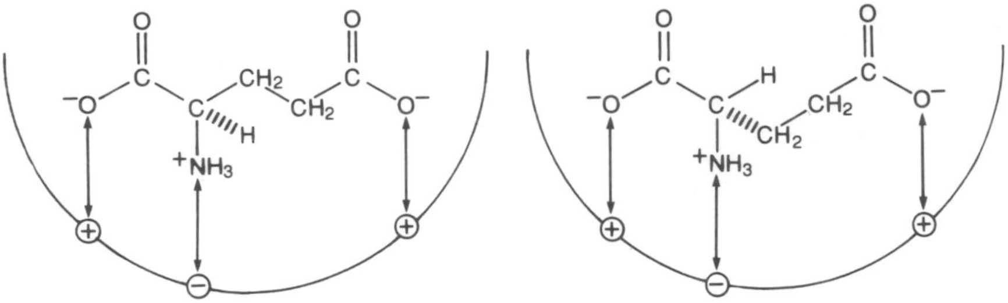

Fig. 1.2 The 'three point receptor' of Curtis and Watkins (1960) showing attachment of both D- and L-glutamate (left and right diagrams, respectively).

of action had been shown by these latter two compounds in the initial iontophoretic experiments performed, the D forms being of similar potency to the natural L forms on cat spinal cord neurones (Curtis and Watkins 1960). This would not have been expected for a receptor-mediated phenomenon. However, it could be explained (Curtis and Watkins 1960) if the receptor contained sufficient space to accommodate substituent groups in both configurations at the asymmetric centre (Fig. 1.2). It seemed less likely that this would also apply to compounds with more bulky substituents at the asymmetric centre. Therefore a series of analogues of the natural and synthetic enantiomers of the two amino acids was prepared, including a range of *N*-alkyl amino acids of both configurations (Watkins 1962). These were mainly new compounds not previously recorded in the chemical literature. The *N*-methyl derivatives were unexpectedly difficult to synthesize due to the tendency of more than one methyl group to be introduced under the usual *N*-methylation conditions. The methods eventually devised (Watkins 1962) still remain the only reported syntheses of NMDA despite the passage of more than 30 years.

Stereoselectivity was indeed demonstrated for these *N*-alkyl derivatives, the D forms being considerably more potent than the L forms (Curtis *et al.* 1961; Curtis and Watkins 1963). NMDA proved to be the most potent of all amino acids tested up to that time, retaining this pre-eminent position throughout the following decade until superseded by the naturally occurring excitants kainic acid (Shinozaki and Konishi 1970; Johnston *et al.* 1974) and (later) quisqualic acid (Shinozaki and Shibuya 1974; Biscoe *et al.* 1976) and the synthetic substance α-amino-3-hydroxy-5-methylisoxazole-4-propionic acid (AMPA) (Krogsgaard-Larsen *et al.* 1980) (Fig. 1.3). However, these amino acids were later shown to act at different receptors from those activated by NMDA (see below). The most potent NMDA receptor agonists now known (approximately 20–50 times more effective than NMDA) include tetrazolylglycine (Lunn *et al.* 1992) and a cyclobutyl analogue of glutamic acid, *trans*-1-aminocyclobutane-1,3-dicarboxylic acid (IUPAC nomenclature) (Allan *et al.* 1990; Lanthorn *et al.* 1990), as well as

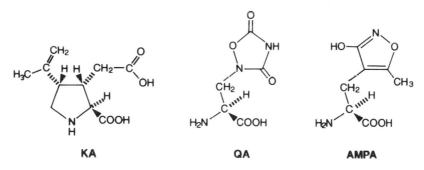

Fig. 1.3 Structures of agonists acting selectively at non-NMDA ionotropic receptors. The structures of antagonists which have the ability to block responses by these agonists are shown in Fig. 1.10.

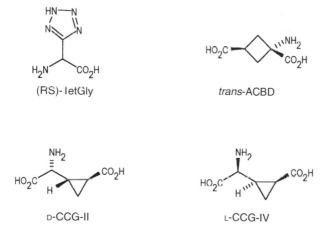

Fig. 1.4 The most potent known NMDA receptor agonists. (RS)-Tetgly, (RS)-α-(tetrazol-5-yl)glycine; trans-ACBD, *trans*-1-aminocyclobutane-1, 3-dicarboxylic acid; CCG, α-(carboxycyclopropyl)glycine. Note: *trans*-1-aminocyclobutane-1,3-dicarboxylic acid (IUPAC nomenclature, where *trans* refers to the senior groups at ring positions 1 and 3, i.e. the amino and carboxyl groups, respectively) also has the trivial name *cis*-methanoglutamate (the term *cis* in this case referring to the relative orientation of the two carboxyl groups).

two cyclopropyl glutamate analogues (Shinozaki *et al.* 1989; Monahan *et al.* 1990; Kawai *et al.* 1992) (Fig. 1.4).

Why was NMDA so much more potent than L-glutamate and like amino acids? It was originally assumed that *N*-methylation had increased the affinity of D-aspartate for the receptor or increased the efficacy of the agonist–receptor interaction in terms of membrane conductance effects. The effect was relatively unique since *N*-methylation of related excitants produced only a slight enhancement of activity (e.g. D-glutamic acid) or, more usually, a marked reduction in potency (e.g. L-glutamic, L-aspartic, D- and L-cysteic and DL-homocysteic acids) (Curtis *et al*. 1961; Curtis and Watkins 1963).

The true explanation of why NMDA is apparently more potent than D-aspartate was first proposed by Balcar and Johnston (1972*a*) following their studies on the ability of a range of amino acid analogues to inhibit high affinity uptake of L-glutamate and L-aspartate into rat brain slices (Balcar and Johnston, 1972*b*). These authors showed that whereas D-aspartate was an excellent substrate for this system, NMDA was relatively inactive. Thus the true potency of D-aspartate at the receptor level could well be much higher than originally thought but masked by the uptake of the amino acid. Such uptake could drastically lower the concentration of D-aspartate at the receptor relative to the concentration administered. In contrast, NMDA was envisaged to reach the receptors without significant loss through uptake, allowing the true potency to be manifested. Uptake would also explain the rapid termination of the action of D-aspartate relative to the much more prolonged offset observed with NMDA (Curtis and Watkins 1963). It was presumed that *N*-methylation of other excitants also reduced uptake, but reduced potency at the receptor as well, this latter effect being the dominant one is most cases. A general decrease in affinity for NMDA receptor sites on *N*-methylation of the parent amino acids (with the exception of D-aspartate) has been confirmed recently in membrane binding studies (Olverman *et al*. 1988*a*).

The existence of multiple EAA receptors

The number of EAAs that are now known runs to well over a hundred. Most have an α-aminomethylcarboxylic acid ('glycine') terminal, with a second (ω) acidic group located at the end of a chain of one to three atoms from the carboxyl group. The ω-acidic group shows wide structural variation (Fig. 1.5). Enantiomeric variation in potency is common (Watkins 1978; Davies *et al*. 1982*b*; Watkins and Olverman 1988; see also Chapter 2), highest activity usually residing in the L isomer, with the notable exception of *N*-alkyl-D-aspartic acids. The first indication of the existence of multiple EAA receptors came from studies on different agonists.

Differential potency of agonists

For the first decade of research in the field, the possible existence of different types of EAA receptors did not figure prominently in the thinking of investigators. However, it was noted by McLennan and colleagues (1968) that L-glutamate showed different potencies relative to other excitants depending on the thalamic region in which they were tested. On the basis of these observations, they proposed that more than one type of receptor may exist for EAAs.

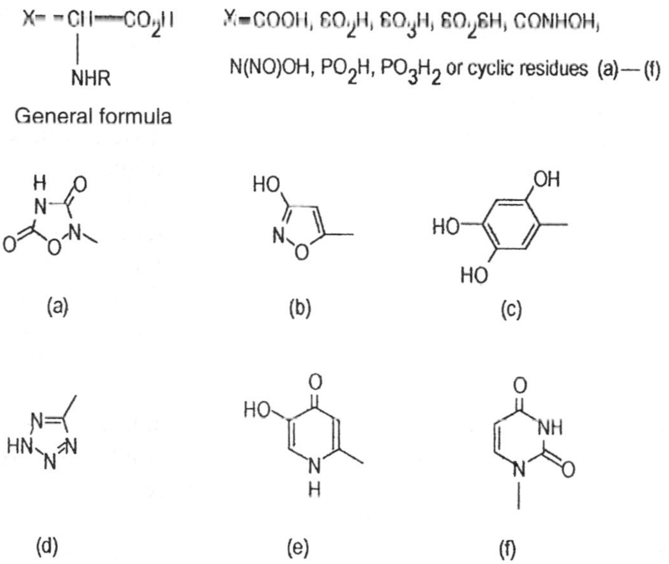

X= -CH—CO₂H   X=COOH, SO₂H, SO₃H, SO₂SH, CONHOH,
     |
     NHR   N(NO)OH, PO₂H, PO₃H₂ or cyclic residues (a)—(f)

General formula

(a)   (b)   (c)

(d)   (e)   (f)

Fig. 1.5 General structure of excitatory amino acids, showing the diversity of the ω-acidic group. Not all excitants have been tested for activity at different receptors, but known agonists at the NMDA receptor include those with ω-carboxy, sulphino, sulphono, thiosulphono, 3-hydroxy-isoxazole, and tetrazolyl groups. For discussion of particular agonists, see Watkins and Olverman (1988) and Chapter 2.

The related observation by Duggan (1974) that L-glutamate and L-aspartate showed small but significant differences in their relative excitatory potencies, depending on the type of spinal neurone on which they were compared, suggested the possibility that these two amino acids may act preferentially at separate types of receptors. Following this observation, Johnston and colleagues (McCulloch *et al.* 1974) surmised that, if such receptor subtypes indeed existed, then substances that were conformationally more restricted than glutamate and/or aspartate might interact with these separate receptors more specifically. On this reasoning, conformationally restricted analogues might show a greater potency differential than the endogenous amino acids on the two types of spinal neurones tested by Duggan. In the case of glutamate, a suitable analogue was kainic acid, recently shown to be a potent excitant and considerably more conformationally restricted than glutamate due to the involvement of part of the chain and the amino nitrogen atom in ring structure (Fig. 1.3). Also, the isopropenyl side chain at ring position 4 could be expected to restrict rotation around the bonds of the side chain at ring position 3. No corresponding aspartate analogues were then available, though quinolinic acid (Stone and Burton 1988) and/or *trans*-2,-3-piperidine dicarboxylic acid (Davies *et al.* 1982*a*), might today be considered suitable for use in

Table 1.1 Excitatory amino acid receptors (mammalian CNS)

		NMDA	Kainate	AMPA	mGluR[4]
Agonists	Specific[1]	N-methyl-D-aspartic acid cis-methanoglutamic acid tetrazolylglycine	kainic acid domoic acid	AMPA 5-fluoro-willardiine	(1S,3R)-ACPD (1S,3S-ACPD) L-CCG-I L-2-Amino-4-phosphonobutyric acid quisqualic acid ibotenic acid
	Other[2]	D-CCG-II L-CCG-IV (1R,3R)-ACPD	5-iodo-willardiine	quisqualic acid	
	Endogenous[3] (mixed actions)	L-glutamate, L-aspartate, L-CSA, L-CA, L-HCSA, L-HCA, Quin			
Antagonists	Potentiators	glycine, D-serine			
	Specific competitive	CPP D-AP5 CGS 19755 CGP 37849		NBQX	(+)-MCPG (S)-CPG (S)-4C3H-PG
	Specific non-competitive	Mg^{2+} MK-801 PCP TCP ketamine		GYKI 52466	L-AP3
	Specific: anti-glycine	5,7-dichloro-Kyn HA-966 (partial agonist)			
	Preferential K/AMPA > NMDA NMDA > K/AMPA	γDGG, Kyn, HDC-QXCA		CNQX, DNQX, pCB-PzDA, pBB-PzDA, GAMS	

Abbreviations: NMDA, *N*-methyl-D-aspartate; K, kainate; AMPA, α-amino-3-hydroxy-5-methylisoxazole-4-propionic acid; mGluR, metabotropic glutamate receptors; ACPD, 1-amino-1,3-cyclopentane dicarboxylic acid; *cis*-methanoglutamic acid, *trans*-1-aminocyclobutane-1,3-dicarboxylic acid (IUPAC nomenclature); CCG, α-(carboxycyclopropyl)-glycine; L-CCG-I, (2S,3S,4S)-CCG, L-CCG-IV, (2S,3R,4S)-CCG; D-CCG-II, (2R,3S,4S)-CCG; HCA, homocysteic acid; CSA, cysteine sulphinic acid; CA, cysteic acid; HCSA, homocysteine sulphinic acid; Quin, quinolinic acid; CPP, 3-[(±)-2-carboxypiperazin-4-yl]propyl-1-phosphonic acid; AP5, 2-amino-5-phosphonopentanoic acid; CGS 19755, *cis*-4-phosphonomethylpiperidine-2-carboxylic acid; CGP 37849, (E)-2-amino-4-methyl-5-phosphono-3-pentenoic acid; MK-801, (+)-5-methyl-10,11-dihydro-5H-dibenzo-[a,d]cyclohepten-5,10-imine maleate; PCP, phencyclidine; TCP, *N*-[1-(2-thienyl)cyclohexyl]-piperidine; 5,7-dichlor-Kyn, 5,7-dichlorokynurenic acid; HA-966, 1-hydroxy-3-aminopyrrolidone-2; NBQX, 6-nitro-7-sulphamoylbenzo(*f*)quinoxaline-2,3-dione; CNQX, 6-cyano-7-nitroquinoxaline-2,3-dione; DNQX, 6,7-dinitroquinoxaline-2,3-dione; *p*CB-PzDA, 1-(*p*-chlorobenzoyl)-piperazine-2,3-dicarboxylic acid; *p*BB-PzDA, 1-(*p*-bromobenzoyl)-piperazine-2,3-dicarboxylic acid; GAMS, γ-D-glutamylaminomethylsulphonic acid; HDC-QXCA, 3-hydroxy-6,7-dichloroquinoxaline-2-carboxylic acid; γDGG, γ-D-glutamylglycine; Kyn, kynurenic acid; MCPG, α-methyl-4-carboxyphenylglycine; 4CPG, 4-carboxyphenylglycine; 4C3H-PG, 4-carboxy-3-hydroxyphenylglycine; GYKI 52466, [1-(4-aminophenyl)-4-methyl-7,8-methylenedioxy-5H-2,3-benzodiazepine HCl]; L-AP3, L-2-amino-5-phosphonopropionic acid.

[1] Not necessarily absolute.
[2] Extent of crossover not fully investigated.
[3] Transmitter candidates; preference for specific receptors not clear.
[4] Subtype specificity under investigation (Nakanishi 1992).

Table 1.2 Summary of functional characteristics and general distribution of excitatory amino acid receptors in the mammalian CNS

NMDA	Widely distributed in mammalian CNS (especially enriched in hippocampus and cerebral cortex). Demonstrated most easily by pharmacological antagonism under Mg-free or depolarized conditions, or in binding experiments (NMDA-sensitive [^{3}H]L-Glu, [^{3}H]D-AP5, [^{3}H]CPP, and other tritiated antagonists). Usually recognized as a slow component in repetitive activity generated primarily by non-NMDA receptors. Important in synaptic plasticity.
AMPA	Widespread in CNS; parallel distribution to NMDA receptors. Involved in the generation of fast component of EPSPs in many central excitatory pathways.
Kainate	Concentrated in a few specific areas of CNS, complementary to NMDA/AMPA receptor distribution (e.g. stratum lucidum region of hippocampus). Difficult to distinguish from AMPA receptors pharmacologically due to lack of sufficiently selective antagonists. However, present specifically (in absence of AMPA receptors) on some dorsal root C fibres and dorsal root ganglion cells.
Metabotropic	A family of receptors linked positively to inositol triphosphate or negatively to cyclic AMP formation. Subtypes differentially activated by L-glutamate, quisqualate, ibotenate, (1S,3R)-1-amino-cyclopentane-1,3-dicarboxylate (ACPD), (1S,3S)-ACPD, (2S,3S,4S)-α-(carboxyxyxlopropyl)glycine, and L-AP4, but not by AMPA, NMDA, or kainate. Not antagonized by NMDA or non-NMDA antagonists but sensitive to pertussis toxin. May be involved in developmental plasticity.

For detailed reviews, see Mayer and Westbrook (1987*a*), Monaghan *et al.* (1989), Lodge and Collingridge (1991), Nakanishi (1992), and Schoepp and Conn (1993).

such experiments; NMDA was selected in view of its potency and the possibility that a bulkier amino group might confer added receptor preference. Another advantage of comparing kainate and NMDA in place of L-glutamate and L-aspartate was that regional differences in rates of uptake—which was considered a possible reason for the regional differences in apparent potency shown by the two endogenous substances (Duggan 1974)—would not be expected to play an important role with the two analogues. Like NMDA, kainate is not a substrate for the high affinity acidic amino acid uptake system (Johnston *et al.* 1979).

When tested on dorsal horn interneurones and ventral horn Renshaw cells, kainate and NMDA showed greater disparity than glutamate and aspartate in their relative potencies on the two types of cell (McCulloch *et al.* 1974) in conformity with the idea that there are two populations of receptors, one showing preference for kainate and the other for NMDA.

Each type of receptor was considered to exist on both dorsal horn and ventral horn neurones, but in different proportions, dorsal horn neurones having a greater proportion of the kainate-preferring type relative to Renshaw cells. The latter neurones had a higher proportion of NMDA-preferring receptors than did dorsal horn neurones.

These original observations were interpreted more in favour of glutamate-preferring and aspartate-preferring types of receptor rather than as kainate- and NMDA-types of glutamate receptor, and were considered to support the possibility that glutamate and aspartate were separate transmitters released from distinct populations of nerve terminals and acting at their own specific receptors. This may indeed be the case, although today it is considered more likely that L-glutamate is the transmitter acting at both kainate- and NMDA-type receptors as well as at other types of EAA receptor (see below).

Results of experiments conducted on other tissues also indicated the existence of different types of EAA receptors. At the crayfish and insect neuromuscular junctions, for example, quisqualate (Fig. 1.3) is a considerably more potent agonist than kainate (Shinozaki and Shibuya 1976; Shinozaki 1978), whereas these compounds are of similar potency in the mammalian CNS (Biscoe *et al.* 1976). On mammalian C fibres, kainate is much more potent than quisqualate (Agrawal and Evans 1986). NMDA is relatively inactive in all these tissues.

Differential activity of the first antagonists

Evidence of differential antagonism of EAAs began to appear in the early 1970s. McLennan and colleagues (Haldeman *et al.* 1972; Haldeman and McLennan 1972) showed that in rat central neurones, responses to L-glutamate were more sensitive to antagonism by L-glutamic acid diethyl ester (GDEE) than were responses to L-aspartate and DL-homocysteate. There was also evidence in the results of Curtis and colleagues (1973) that 3-amino-1-hydroxy-pyrrolidone (HA-966) depressed responses to DL-homocysteate more than responses to L-glutamate. Later in the decade Evans and colleagues (1977a) reported that pentobarbitone suppressed quisqualate more than L-aspartate and L-homocysteate, and that chlorpromazine had the reverse effect. The tricyclic antidepressant amitriptyline had a similar differential effect to chlorpromazine (Evans *et al.* 1977a). While suggestive of the existence of multiple receptors, each contributing to the responses of different agonists in different degree, these observations were not in themselves definitive.

'NMDA-type' and 'non-NMDA-type' EAA receptors

The first clear-cut separation of receptors was obtained with three different types of selective antagonist:

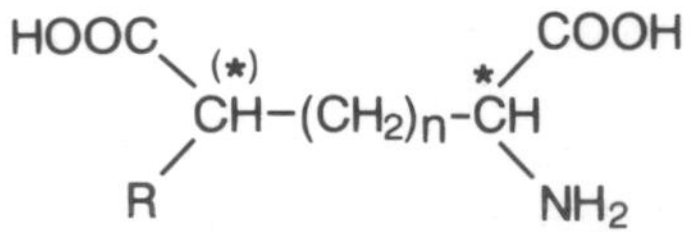

$$\begin{array}{c} \text{HOOC} \diagdown \; {}_{(*)} \qquad\qquad {}_* \diagup \text{COOH} \\ \text{CH-(CH}_2)_n\text{-CH} \\ \diagup \qquad\qquad\qquad\quad \diagdown \\ \text{R} \qquad\qquad\qquad\qquad \text{NH}_2 \end{array}$$

n	R	*	(*)	Compound	Abbreviation
2	H	D	–	D-α-Aminoadipic acid	D-α-AA
3	H	D	–	D-α-Aminopimelic acid	D-α-AP
4	H	D	–	D-α-Aminosuberic acid	D-α-AS
3	NH$_2$	D	D or L	α,ϵ-Diaminopimelic acid	α,ϵ-DAP

Fig. 1.6 'First generation' competitive NMDA antagonists. Abbreviations: D-αAA, D-α-aminoadipic acid; D-αAP, D-α-aminopimelic acid; D-αAS, D-α-aminosuberic acid; DAP, α,ϵ-diaminopimelic acid.

(1) Mg^{2+} (also Co^{2+} and Mn^{2+}) (Davies and Watkins 1977; Evans *et al.* 1977*b*);

(2) longer chain glutamate analogues of the D-configuration (Fig. 1.6), including D-α-aminoadipate (D-αAA) and α,ϵ-diaminopimelate (DAP) (Biscoe *et al.* 1977*a,b*, 1978; Evans and Watkins 1978; Evans *et al.* 1978);

(3) HA-966 (Biscoe *et al.* 1977*a*, 1978; Evans *et al.* 1978) (Fig. 1.9).

The last-mentioned substance had been shown to be an antagonist of L-glutamate- and L-aspartate-induced responses several years earlier (Davies and Watkins 1972, 1973; Curtis *et al.* 1973), but variable signs of differential antagonism in those experiments were not followed up. What distinguished the later experiments and imbued them with greater significance was the use of a particular range of agonists including quisqualate, kainate, and NMDA. Each of the antagonists produced an almost identical pattern of antagonism characterized by potent depression of NMDA-induced responses, with little or no effect on quisqualate- or kainate-induced responses and an intermediate degree of antagonism in the case of other agonists. The ranking order for depression of six 'standard' agonists was NMDA > L-homocysteate > L-aspartate > L-glutamate > kainate $\geqslant$ quisqualate (unaffected). These results were confirmed and extended in subsequent studies (Davies and Watkins, 1979; Davies *et al.* 1979; Evans *et al.* 1979; McLennan and Lodge 1979; Ault *et al.* 1980), leading to the widespread acceptance of 'NMDA'- and 'non-NMDA'-type EAA receptors (Watkins 1978, 1980; Davies *et al.* 1979). Responses to those agonists which were most sensitive to the antagonists were considered to be mediated mainly by NMDA receptors. Conversely, responses to those agonists (e.g. kainate and quisqualate) which were relatively unaffected by the antagonists were considered to be mediated predominantly by non-NMDA receptors.

Since that time the existence of NMDA receptors has been amply confirmed by the development of more potent and selective antagonists of various types (see below) and non-NMDA receptors have been subdivided into 'kainate' and 'AMPA' (formerly 'quisqualate') receptors (Watkins and Evans 1981; Monaghan *et al.* 1989). NMDA, kainate, and AMPA receptors are now categorized as 'ionotropic' receptors since their main function is considered to be the mediation of the ionic fluxes underlying the potential and conductance changes involved in synaptic transmission (Sugiyama *et al.* 1987). Another group of EAA receptors, the so-called 'metabotropic' glutamate receptors (of which at least seven subtypes are known) are considered to play a greater role in longer-term changes due to their linkage to metabolic systems (notably phosphoinositide hydrolysis and cyclic AMP production) involving second messengers (Sugiyama *et al.* 1987; Nakanishi 1992; Tanabe *et al.* 1992; Nakajima *et al.* 1993; Schoepp and Conn 1993). Table 1.1 summarizes some of the main pharmacological features of the various types of EAA receptors.

Special features of the NMDA receptor–ionophore complex

The Mg^{2+} effect

The specific antagonist effect of Mg^{2+} at NMDA receptors was first demonstrated by Evans *et al.* (1977*b*) and Ault *et al.* (1980). In the early 1980s MacDonald and colleagues (MacDonald and Wojtowicz 1980; MacDonald and Porietis 1982) showed that the responses of cultured neurones to a range of amino acids, particularly L-aspartate and NMDA, exhibit a region of negative slope conductance (that is, the conductance induced by the amino acid decreases with increased membrane potential, contrary to Ohm's law). Ascher and colleagues (Nowak *et al.* 1984) and Mayer and Westbrook (1985) showed that this effect occurs only when Mg^{2+} is present in the extracellular medium and is associated specifically with the activation of NMDA receptors. In the presence of Mg^{2+}, and at membrane potentials more negative than about -30 mV, agonists of the NMDA receptor cause less current flow (lower fluxes through the ionic channels that they activate) the higher the level at which the neuronal membrane potential is set under voltage clamp conditions. The effect is not observed in the absence of Mg^{2+} at any potential or in the presence of Mg^{2+} at substantially depolarized levels of membrane potential (see Chapter 7).

Ca^{2+} influx

Activation of NMDA receptors leads to a substantial influx of Ca^{2+} in addition to the Na^+ influx and K^+ efflux seen with all EAA ionotropic receptors (Macdermott *et al.* 1986; Ascher and Nowak 1987; Mayer and Westbrook 1987*b*). Such Ca^{2+} influx has been implicated in a range of physiologic phenomena including synaptic integration (Chapter 12) and plasticity (Chapters 13–15), and in various neuropathologies as discussed further below.

Potentiation by glycine

A relatively recent finding of major importance was that sub-micromolar concentrations of glycine greatly increase the ionic currents induced by NMDA agonists (Johnson and Ascher 1987). Since cerebrospinal fluid (CSF) contains glycine at approximately 10 μM or more (Curtis and Johnston 1974), and since such levels of glycine might be expected also to occur in extracellular fluid, it seems likely that the glycine site of the NMDA receptor is fully saturated under normal physiological conditions, and that the receptor usually exists in this 'glycine-primed' state (Chapter 7). On the other hand, it is possible that glycine is released from presynaptic terminals along with transmitter (probably glutamate), in which case glycine could be regarded as a co-transmitter. No evidence has yet been adduced to support this possibility, however.

NMDA receptor antagonists

Competitive type (acting at the agonist recognition site)

The structures of the longer chain acidic amino acid antagonists suggested a competitive type of antagonism for this type of substance at NMDA receptors. This was consistent with the parallel shift produced by the antagonists in NMDA dose–response curves (Evans *et al.* 1979). D-αAA and like antagonists were not particularly potent, having K_D values, calculated from conventional dose-ratio determinations, of around 20–100 μM (Watkins and Evans 1981). A big advance in the pharmacology of these receptors was the discovery (Davies *et al.* 1980, 1981; Watkins and Evans 1981; Evans *et al.* 1982) that ω-phosphono analogues of D-αAA and its homologues, as well as certain phosphono-dipeptides of similar chain length, had greatly increased potency and selectivity. These compounds (Fig. 1.7) included D-2-amino-5-phosphonopentanoate (D-AP5), originally called D-2-amino-5-phosphonovalerate (D-APV) (Davies *et al.* 1981; Evans and Watkins 1981; Perkins *et al.* 1981; Davies and Watkins 1982; Evans *et al.* 1982), D-2-amino-7-phosphonoheptanoate (D-AP7) (Evans *et al.* 1982; Perkins *et al.* 1982), and β-D-aspartylaminomethylphosphonate (β-D-Asp-AMP) (Jones *et al.* 1984). The most active of these substances had K_D values, estimated from electrophysiological (Evans *et al.* 1982; Jones *et al.* 1984) and binding (Olverman *et al.* 1988*a*) studies, of around 0.5–5 μM (Chapter 2). The fact that they acted competitively at the agonist recognition site was apparent from their linear Schild plots (Evans *et al.* 1982; Harrison

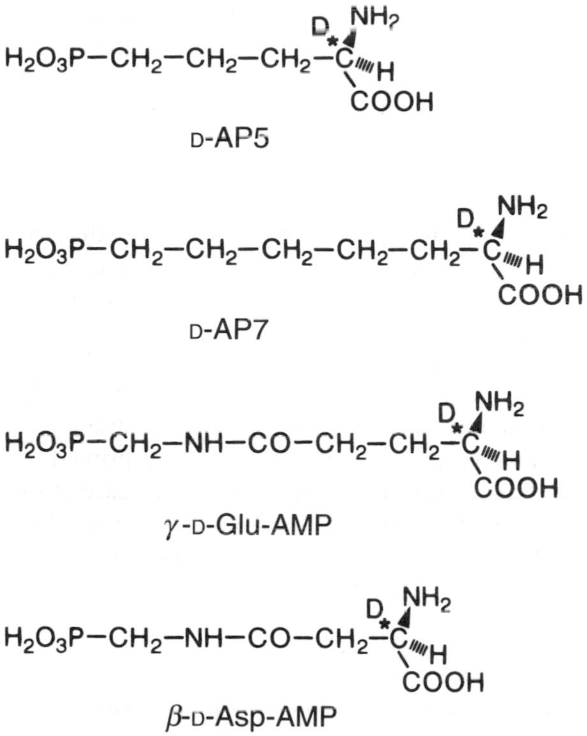

$$H_2O_3P{-}CH_2{-}CH_2{-}CH_2{-}\overset{\overset{\displaystyle NH_2}{\text{D}}}{\underset{\text{COOH}}{C}}{\cdots}H$$

D-AP5

$$H_2O_3P{-}CH_2{-}CH_2{-}CH_2{-}CH_2{-}CH_2{-}\overset{\overset{\displaystyle NH_2}{\text{D}}}{\underset{\text{COOH}}{C}}{\cdots}H$$

D-AP7

$$H_2O_3P{-}CH_2{-}NH{-}CO{-}CH_2{-}CH_2{-}\overset{\overset{\displaystyle NH_2}{\text{D}}}{\underset{\text{COOH}}{C}}{\cdots}H$$

γ-D-Glu-AMP

$$H_2O_3P{-}CH_2{-}NH{-}CO{-}CH_2{-}\overset{\overset{\displaystyle NH_2}{\text{D}}}{\underset{\text{COOH}}{C}}{\cdots}H$$

β-D-Asp-AMP

Fig. 1.7 'Second generation' competitive NMDA antagonists. Abbreviations: D AP5, D-2-amino-5-phosphonopentanoic acid; D-AP7, D 2-amino-7-phosphonoheptanoic acid; γ-D-Glu-AMP, γ-D-glutamylaminomethylphosphonic acid; β-D-Asp-AMP, β-D-aspartylaminomethylphosphonic acid.

and Simmonds 1985) and inhibition of NMDA-sensitive [³H]L-glutamate binding in rat brain membranes (Foster and Fagg 1984; Monaghan and Cotman 1986). The most potent antagonists of this class now include CGP 37849 (Fagg *et al*. 1990) and the cyclic compounds 3-(2-carboxypiperazin-4-yl)propyl-1-phosphonate (CPP) (Davies *et al*. 1986; Harris *et al*. 1986; Murphy *et al*. 1987; Lehmann *et al*. 1988*b*) and the related propene analogue (CPP-ene) (Aebischer *et al*. 1989; Herrling *et al*. 1989), together with 3-(2-carboxypiperidin-4-yl)propyl-1-phosphonate (CPPP) (Lodge *et al*. 1988*c*) and 3-(2-carboxypiperidin-4-yl)methylphosphonate (CGS 19755) (Murphy *et al*. 1987; Lehmann *et al*. 1988*a*; Lodge *et al*. 1988*c*) (Fig. 1.8), with K_D values in the region of one to two orders of magnitude lower than the original phosphonic acid antagonists. As with the latter substances, the pharmacological activity of these cyclic compounds appears to lie mainly in the respective D(−) isomers (Lehmann *et al*. 1988*b*; Aebischer *et al*. 1989; Herrling *et al*. 1989) i.e. in the (R) forms in modern chemical

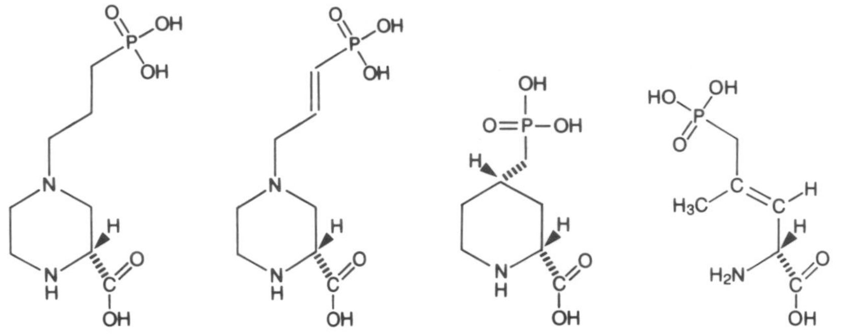

Fig. 1.8 'Third generation' competitive NMDA antagonists. Abbreviations: CPP, 3-(2-carboxypiperazin-4-yl)propyl-1-phosphonic acid; CPP-ene, 3-(2-carboxypiperazin-4-yl)-1-propenyl-1-phosphonic acid; CGS 19755, *cis*-4-phosphonomethylpiperidine-2-carboxylic acid; CGP 37849, (E)-2-amino-4-methyl-5-phosphono-3-pentenoic acid. Note: CPPP (3-(2-carboxypiperidine-4-yl)propyl-1-phosphonic acid) (not shown) is the piperidine analogue of CPP.

notation. However, this is not always the case and highly potent antagonists with the (S) configuration have recently been reported (Ornstein and Klimkowski 1992; Müller *et al.* 1992; see Chapter 2).

Non-competitive (channel blocking) type

Lodge and colleagues (Anis *et al.* 1983; Berry *et al.* 1984; Lodge *et al.* 1988*b*) described a range of substances of the dissociative anaesthetic and sigma opioid type, typified by ketamine and phencyclidine (PCP), which had the same profile of action against a range of EAA agonists as the divalent cations and the competitive NMDA antagonists described above. These substances, which are of quite diverse structure (e.g. Fig. 3.2, Chapter 3), do not inhibit the binding of [^{3}H]D-AP5 (Olverman *et al.* 1988*b*). A series of investigations (Harrison and Simmonds 1985; Wong *et al.* 1986; Honey *et al.* 1988; Lodge *et al.* 1988*b*) indicated that they act by blocking the ion channels opened by the agonist–receptor interaction. The most potent of these agents is MK-801 (Wong *et al.* 1986; Kemp *et al.* 1987). This group of compounds is discussed in detail in Chapters 3 and 20 (see also Wong and Kemp 1991).

'Glycine-site' antagonists

Because of its lower potency (Evans *et al.* 1979) and selectivity (Curtis *et al.* 1973) than other types of NMDA antagonists, HA-966 was somewhat neglected for a number of years, other than being classified as 'non-competitive' since it did not displace labelled agonists or competitive antagonists from rat brain membranes (Watkins and Olverman 1987; Olverman *et al*. 1988*b*). That its action was of a completely novel type was demonstrated by Lodge and colleagues (Lodge *et al*. 1988*a*; Fletcher and Lodge 1988) who showed that HA-966 was an antagonist of the specific agonist-potentiating action of glycine (see Chapter 3). Thus, the depressant action of HA-966 on cortical wedge responses to NMDA is reversed by glycine, and also by D-serine, a glycine-like agonist (Lodge *et al*. 1988*a*; Kemp *et al*. 1988). HA-966 also displaces [³H]glycine from strychnine-insensitive binding sites on rat brain membranes (Singh *et al*. 1990). These binding sites (which are distinct from the strychnine-sensitive inhibitory receptors present mainly in spinal cord and brain stem (Curtis and Johnston 1974) show a remarkably similar autoradiographic distribution to that shown by NMDA-sensitive [³H]glutamate binding sites (Bowery 1987). It has been suggested that bound glycine is an integral part of the NMDA receptor (Kleckner and Dingledine 1988). Apart from HA-966, now considered to be a partial agonist (Kemp and Priestley 1991), a range of other substances, including kynurenic acid (Birch *et al*. 1988; Lodge *et al*. 1988*a*; Singh *et al*. 1990) and (particularly) a range of kynurenic acid derivatives (Kemp *et al*. 1988; Baron *et al*. 1990; Singh *et al*. 1990; Leeson *et al*. 1991, 1992*a*) stemming originally from 7-chlorokynurenic acid (Fig. 1.9), have actions at this site as do the more potent non-NMDA receptor antagonists 6-cyano-7-nitroquinoxaline-2,3-dione (CNQX) and 6,7-dinitroquinoxaline-2,3-dione (DNQX) (Birch *et al*. 1988) (Fig. 1.10). Within the latter group of compounds, 6,8-dinitroquinoxaline-2,3-dione (MNQX) appears to be the most potent and selective at the glycine site (Sheardown *et al*. 1989). Even more potent quinoline-derived and related antagonists have recently been reported (for examples see Carling *et al*. 1992; Leeson *et al*. 1992*b*). It is clear that the pharmacology of this site could have far-reaching consequences for fundamental studies on the NMDA receptor and for potential therapeutic treatments for a variety of neurological disorders (see below and Chapters 16–20).

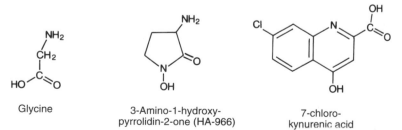

Fig. 1.9 The structure of glycine and two of the original glycine antagonists. (HA-966 is now considered to be a partial agonist.)

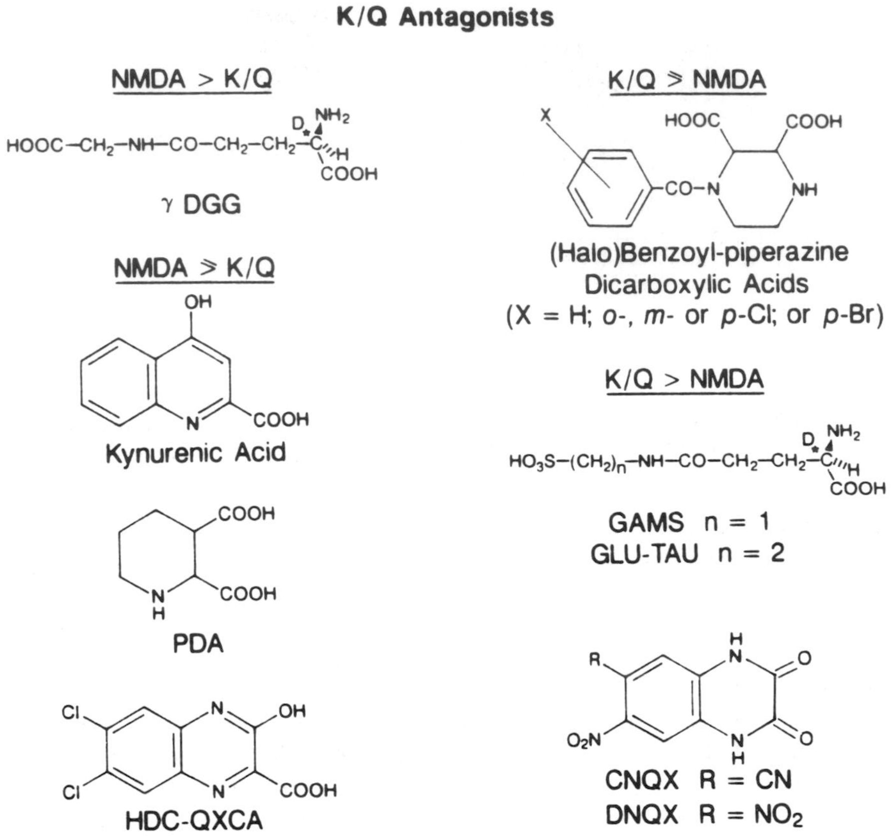

K/Q Antagonists

<u>NMDA > K/Q</u>

$$HOOC-CH_2-NH-CO-CH_2-CH_2-\overset{NH_2}{\underset{COOH}{\overset{D}{C}}_{,,,H}}$$

γ DGG

<u>K/Q ⩾ NMDA</u>

(Halo)Benzoyl-piperazine
Dicarboxylic Acids
(X = H; *o-*, *m-* or *p*-Cl; or *p*-Br)

<u>NMDA ⩾ K/Q</u>

Kynurenic Acid

<u>K/Q > NMDA</u>

$$HO_3S-(CH_2)_n-NH-CO-CH_2-CH_2-\overset{NH_2}{\underset{COOH}{\overset{D}{C}}_{,,,H}}$$

GAMS n = 1
GLU-TAU n = 2

PDA

HDC-QXCA

CNQX R = CN
DNQX R = NO₂

Fig. 1.10 Some early and more recent 'broad-band' EAA antagonists. Abbreviations: γDGG, γ-D-glutamylglycine; PDA, *cis*-2,3-piperidine dicarboxylic acid; GAMS, γ-D-glutamylaminomethylsulphonic acid; Glu-tau, γ-D-glutamyltaurine; CNQX, 6-cyano-7-nitroquinoxaline-2,3-dione; DNQX, 6,7-dinitroquinoxaline-2,3-dione; HDC-QXCA, 3-hydroxy-6,7-dichloroquinoxaline-2-carboxylic acid.

Models of the NMDA receptor–ionophore complex

Much artistry has been brought to bear on schematic models of the NMDA receptor–ionophore complex (e.g. see Wong and Kemp 1991; Bigge 1993). Reduced to the most basic form (Fig. 1.11) such models show an agonist recognition site and a modulatory glycine site, which interact with their respective ligands in a co-operative manner in order to open an ion channel through which the influx of Ca^{2+} and Na^+, and efflux of K^+, take place. Inside the channel are Mg^{2+} and PCP binding sites, which, when occupied, prevent the ionic fluxes occurring. Modulatory sites for zinc and for polyamines have also been proposed (reviewed by Wong and Kemp 1991; Bigge 1993; see also Chapter 3). The receptor channel complex is an

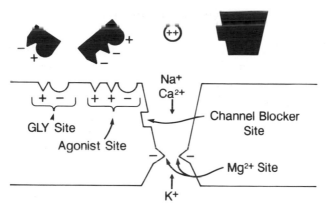

Fig. 1.11 Schematic representation of the NMDA receptor complex. The symbols above the receptor represent (from left) glycine-, glutamate-, Mg^{2+}-, and PCP-like agents.

assembly of subunits, the composition of the assembly determining receptor subtype characteristics (Chapter 5). Irradiation inactivation analysis (Honoré *et al.* 1989) originally suggested, and molecular biology techniques (Moriyoshi *et al.* 1991) have recently confirmed, that agonist, glycine, and PCP binding sites are situated on the same subunit of the receptor–ionophore complex. Occupation of two agonist and two glycine sites (perhaps involving two subunits of the receptor) are probably necessary for activation of the receptor (Williams *et al.* 1988; Benveniste and Mayer 1991). Divalent metal ions may be an integral part of the glutamate and/or glycine recognition sites (Watkins 1992). Competitive antagonists may bridge two subunits (Olverman *et al.* 1988*a*; Honoré *et al.* 1989; see also Chapter 2). However, all these schematic models, as well as the more sophisticated computer-assisted molecular models attempting to map the topography of NMDA receptors (Chapter 2), will probably need to be modified to take account of the various subtypes of NMDA receptor now known to exist (Nakanishi 1992; see also Chapter 5).

NMDA receptors and synaptic activity

The discovery of selective NMDA antagonism by certain divalent metal ions, notably Mg^{2+}, which is present in extracellular fluid, and by longer chain acidic amino acids of D (R) configuration has had great influence on the development of the EAA field. Thus, the organic antagonists allowed the definitive demonstration, for the first time, that EAA receptors participate in synaptic excitation (Biscoe *et al.* 1977*a,b*, 1978; Evans and Watkins 1978; Evans *et al.* 1978, 1979; Davies and Watkins 1979; Davies *et al.* 1979). Although blockade of synaptic excitation by GDEE (Haldeman *et al.* 1972; Haldeman and McLennan 1972) and HA-966 (Davies and Watkins 1973) had been demonstrated previously, neither of these two antagonists were as selective as the D-αAA group of substances as EAA antagonists. Thus, GDEE (Davies and Watkins 1979) and HA-966 (Curtis *et al.* 1973) also affected acetylcholine-induced excitation in some test systems. On the other hand, D-αAA and its congeners were highly specific for EAA-induced excitation; responses to a range of other excitants and depolarizing agents, including acetylcholine and substance P, were unaffected by these antagonists (Evans and Watkins 1978; Watkins and Evans 1981). Hence, the demonstration that D-αAA blocked non-cholinergic excitation of cat Renshaw cells via a polysynaptic pathway activated by primary afferent stimulation, without affecting the cholinergic excitation of the cells evoked by ventral root stimulation (Biscoe *et al.* 1977*b*), greatly reduced the then still-prevailing doubt that EAA receptors indeed played a role in central synaptic excitation. Other pathways in the spinal cord were also found to be sensitive to D-αAA and/or like substances (Biscoe *et al.* 1978; Davies and Watkins 1979; Chapters 10 and 11).

Despite the advent of increasingly potent and selective NMDA antagonists, instances of depression of synaptic excitation by these agents in regions of the CNS other than the spinal cord were slow to accumulate. Many synaptic pathways appeared to be relatively resistant to specific NMDA antagonists, but were nevertheless susceptible to depression by 'broader band' antagonists which depressed responses to kainate and quisqualate in addition to those induced by NMDA. The broader band antagonists, e.g. *cis*-2,3-piperidine dicarboxylic acid (*cis*-2,3-PDA) and γ-D-glutamylglycine (γDGG) (Fig. 1.10), were also specific for EAA-induced responses relative to excitations produced by non-amino acid agonists (Watkins and Evans 1981), hence such observations demonstrated the wide involvement of EAA receptors in synaptic excitation throughout the CNS, and identified the type of EAA receptors primarily mediating transmission in specific pathways under particular modes of stimulation. Since these earlier studies the development of more potent and selective antagonists for both NMDA- (Figs 1.7 and 1.8) and non-NMDA- (Fig. 1.10) type receptors have facilitated and extended knowledge of EAA receptor-mediated synaptic transmission throughout the mammalian CNS. In particular, these days it is considered likely that NMDA receptors, by virtue of their voltage-dependent Mg^{2+} sensitivity, play a modulatory role in many (probably most) synaptic pathways for which AMPA receptors exercise the primary transmitter role (Chapters 10–15). Table 1.2 summarizes some of the main functional features and anatomical distribution of the various types of EAA receptors.

Transmitter acting at NMDA receptors

At the time the concept of the NMDA receptor was first delineated (Watkins 1978, 1980), it seemed likely that the transmitter activating these receptors physiologically was L-aspartate. The evidence for this was three-fold:

1. NMDA was an aspartate analogue considered less able to interact with a receptor specialized to bind L-glutamate than one specialized to bind L-aspartate (McCulloch *et al.* 1974).
2. Specific NMDA antagonists depressed responses induced by L-aspartate to a greater extent than L-glutamate-induced responses (Evans *et al.* 1977*a,b*, 1978, 1979; Biscoe *et al.* 1977*a,b*, 1978; Evans and Watkins 1978; Davies and Watkins 1977, 1979; Davies *et al.* 1979).
3. The excitatory synapses initially found to be sensitive to NMDA antagonists (Biscoe *et al.* 1977*b*; Davies and Watkins 1979) were situated in an area of the spinal cord in which earlier neurochemical evidence favoured L-aspartate as the transmitter over L-glutamate (Davidoff *et al.* 1967).

The assumed preference of the NMDA receptor for L-aspartate was shown to be ill-founded by the observation that L-glutamate had a greater than 10-fold higher affinity for the receptor than L-aspartate in membrane binding studies (Olverman *et al.* 1984, 1988*b*). Other endogenous acidic amino acids have as high or higher affinities for the receptor than L-aspartate, and must also be considered candidates for a transmitter role at NMDA receptors. These include L-cysteine sulphinate, L-homocysteine sulphinate and L-homocysteate (Olverman *et al.* 1984, 1988*b*). L-Homocysteate has been particularly favoured for such a role (Do *et al.* 1988, 1992; Cuenod *et al.* 1990; Ito *et al.* 1991).

Another endogenous amino acid which produces responses that are sensitive to NMDA antagonists is quinolinic acid (Stone and Burton 1988). However, this compound has only low affinity for the NMDA receptor as characterized in membrane binding studies (Olverman *et al.* 1988*b*). While L-glutamate is now the favoured candidate as the transmitter acting at NMDA receptors in most cases, none of the other substances mentioned above, nor an as yet unidentified alternative substance, can be ruled out.

Physiologic and pathologic significance of NMDA receptors

The effect of Mg^{2+} implies that NMDA receptors are virtually blocked in neurones at their resting membrane potential (usually near -70 mV) since the extracellular concentration of Mg^{2+} under normal physiological conditions is believed to be around 1 mM. However, by depolarization-induced relief from the Mg^{2+} block they could become active during synaptic activity in an intensity-dependent manner. Activation would be presumed to be very brief during a single excitatory post-synaptic potential (EPSP), especially when such EPSPs are limited by associated inhibitory post-synaptic potentials (IPSPs), and may not manifest measurably as a component of the response as tested by sensitivity to NMDA antagonists. This probably explains the paucity of synaptic pathways originally shown to be susceptible to depression by NMDA antagonists under the usual single stimulus methods of testing (Watkins and Evans 1981). However, in cases of repetitive synaptic activation, the greater depolarization thus evoked would be expected to result in increased involvement of NMDA receptors. This in turn would lead to greater influx of Ca^{2+} (Macdermott *et al.* 1986; Ascher and Nowak 1987; Mayer and Westbrook 1987*b*). Such recruitment of NMDA receptors in repetitive activity and associated Ca^{2+} influx probably plays a role in synaptic integration (Chapter 12) and is considered to be important in such phenomena as long-term potentiation (LTP) and similar types of synaptic plasticity, discussed in Chapters 13–15. Thus, the NMDA receptor is probably involved in the fine control of co-ordinated movement, behavioural patterns, and memory and learning, as well as in pathologic states including epileptic phenomena (Chapter 17) and neuro-degeneration caused by prolonged depolarization of cells by endogenous or exogenous EAAs (Chapter 18).

NMDA receptors and potential drugs

The advent of ω-phosphono NMDA receptor antagonists not only greatly increased the ease of recognition of NMDA receptors but also heralded an age in which the possibility of manipulating the activity of these receptors has become increasingly prominent in potential therapeutic strategy. The anticonvulsant (Croucher *et al.* 1982), antispastic (Turski *et al.* 1985), and neuroprotective (Simon *et al.* 1984) actions of the first phosphono compounds to be tested paved the way for an intensity of effort towards the synthesis of more potent analogues, particularly those able to cross the blood–brain barrier in effective concentration without excessive systemic doses. The polar character of the phosphono antagonists unfortunately hinders such penetration of the brain. Nevertheless, the range of highly potent 'third generation' phosphonates recently developed (Davies *et al.* 1986; Harris *et al.* 1986; Murphy *et al.* 1987; Lehmann *et al.* 1988*a*; Lodge *et al.* 1988*c*; Aebischer *et al.* 1989; Fagg *et al.* 1989; Herrling *et al.* 1989; Müller *et al.* 1992; Ornstein and Klimkowski, 1992), including D-CPP-ene, CGS 19755, and CGP 37849 (Fig. 1.8), although still passing the blood–brain barrier relatively poorly, nevertheless are sufficiently potent to offer considerable promise as potential drugs (see Chapter 19). The non-competitive antagonists have the advantage that they cross the blood–brain barrier much more readily, but their psychotomimetic side effects (Koek *et al.* 1988) (see also Chapter 16), which may be a problem also with the competitive antagonists (Koek and Woods 1988; Kristensen *et al.* 1992), will need to be carefully assessed. Glycine antagonists constitute a third line of potential drugs currently being comprehensively explored. Clearly the NMDA receptor–ionophore complex offers great scope for novel therapeutic intervention in a range of CNS disorders.

Acknowledgements

I am deeply indebted to all my colleagues and assistants, former and present, whose help and advice have been indispensable during the 35 year period over which I have been associated with this work. I particularly wish to acknowledge the crucial contribution of Dr John Davies over the 20 year period from 1971 to his untimely death in 1991. His *in vivo* studies played a major role in finally and firmly establishing glutamate as the major central excitatory transmitter and elucidating the function of different EAA receptor types in central synaptic transmission. Generous funding by the medical Research Council, The Wellcome Trust, The British Technology Group, and the US Public Health Service (NS 26540) is also gratefully acknowledged.

References

Aebischer, B., Frey, P., Haerter, H. D., Herrling, P. L., Müller, W., Olverman, H. J., and Watkins, J. C. (1989). Synthesis and NMDA antagonist properties of the enantiomers of 4-(3-phosphonopropyl)piperazine-2-carboxylic acid (CPP) and of the unsaturated analogue (E)-4-(3-phosphonopro-2-enyl)piperazine-2-carboxylic acid (CPP-ene). *Helvetica Chimica Acta*, **72**, 1043–51.

Agrawal, S. G. and Evans, R. H. (1986). The primary afferent depolarizing action of kainate in the rat. *British Journal of Pharmacology*, **87**, 345–55.

Allan, R. D., Hanrahan, J. R., Hambley, T. W., Johnston, G. A. R., Mewett, K. N., and Mitrovic, A. D. (1990). Synthesis and activity of a potent N-methyl-D-aspartic acid agonist, *trans*-1-aminocyclobutane-1,3-dicarboxylic acid, and related phosphonic and carboxylic acids. *Journal of Medicinal Chemistry*, **33**, 2905–15.

Anis, N. A., Berry, S. C., Burton, N. R., and Lodge, D. (1983). The dissociative anaesthetics, ketamine and phencyclidine, selectively reduce excitation of central mammalian neurones by N-methyl-D-aspartate. *British Journal of Pharmacology*, **79**, 565–75.

Ascher, P. and Nowak, L. (1987). Electrophysiological studies of NMDA receptors. *Trends in Neuroscience*, **10**, 284–8.

Ault, B., Evans, R. H., Francis, A. A., Oakes, D. J., and Watkins, J. C. (1980). Selective depression of excitatory amino acid induced depolarizations by magnesium ions in isolated spinal cord preparations. *Journal of Physiology* (Lond.), **307**, 413–28.

Balcar, V. J. and Johnston, G. A. R. (1972*a*). Glutamate uptake by brain slices and its relation to the depolarization of neurons by acidic amino acids. *Journal of Neurobiology*, **3**, 295–301.

Balcar, V. J. and Johnston, G. A. R. (1972*b*). The structural specificity of the high affinity uptake of L-glutamate and L-aspartate by rat brain slices. *Journal of Neurochemistry*, **19**, 2657–66.

Baron, B. M., Harrison, B. L., Miller, F. P., McDonald, I. A., Salituro, F. G., Schmidt, C. J., Sorensen, S. M., White, H. S., and Palfreyman, M. G. (1990). Activity of 5,7-dichlorokynurenic acid, a potent antagonist at the N-methyl-D-aspartate receptor-associated glycine binding site. *Molecular Pharmacology*, **38**, 554–61.

Benveniste, M. and Mayer, M. L. (1991). A kinetic analysis of antagonist actions at NMDA receptors. Two binding sites each for glutamate and glycine. *Biophysical Journal*, **59**, 560–72.

Berry, S. C., Dawkins, S. L., and Lodge, D. (1984). Comparison of sigma and kappa-opiate receptor ligands as excitatory amino acid antagonists. *British Journal of Pharmacology*, **83**, 179–85.

Bigge, C. F. (1993). Structural requirements for the development of potent *N*-methyl-D-aspartic acid (NMDA) receptor antagonists. *Biochemical Pharmacology*, **45**, 1547–61.

Birch, P. J., Grossman, C. J., and Hayes, A. G. (1988). Kynurenate and FG 9041 have both competitive and non-competitive antagonist actions at excitatory amino acid receptors. *European Journal of Pharmacology*, **151**, 313–15.

Biscoe, T. J., Evans, R. H., Headley, P. M., Martin, M. R., and Watkins, J. C. (1976). Structure–activity relations of excitatory amino acids on frog and rat spinal neurones. *British Journal of Pharmacology*, **58**, 373–82.

Biscoe, T. J., Davies, J., Dray, J., Evans, R. H., Francis, A. A., Martin, M. R., and Watkins, J. C. (1977a). Depression of synaptic excitation and of amino acid-induced excitatory responses of spinal neurones by D-α-aminoadipate, α,ε-diaminopimelic acid and HA-966. *European Journal of Pharmacology*, **45**, 315–16.

Biscoe, T. J., Evans, R. H., Francis, A. A., Martin, M. R., Watkins, J. C., Davies, J., and Dray, A. (1977b). D-α-Aminoadipate as a selective antagonist of amino acid-induced and synaptic excitation of mammalian spinal neurones. *Nature* (Lond.), **270**, 743–5.

Biscoe, T. J., Davies, J., Dray, A., Evans, R. H., Martin, M. R., and Watkins, J. C. (1978). D-α-Aminoadipate, α, ε-diaminopimelic acid, and HA-966 as antagonists of amino acid-induced and synaptic excitation of mammalian spinal neurones *in vivo*. *Brain Research*, **148**, 543–8.

Bowery, N. G. (1987). Glycine binding sites and NMDA receptors in brain. *Nature* (Lond.), **326**, 338.

Carling, R. W., Leeson, P. D., Mosely, A. M., Baker, R., Foster, A. C., Grimwood, S., Kemp, J. A., and Marshall, G. R. (1992). 2-Carboxytetrahydroquinolines. Conformational and stereochemical requirements for antagonism of the glycine site on the NMDA receptor. *Journal of Medicinal Chemistry*, **35**, 1942–53.

Collingridge, G. L. and Lester, R. A. J. (1989). Excitatory amino acid receptors in the vertebrate central nervous system. *Pharmacological Reviews*, **40**, 143–210.

Croucher, M. J., Collins, J. F., and Meldrum, B. S. (1982). Anticonvulsant action of excitatory amino acid antagonists. *Science*, **216**, 899–901.

Cuenod, M., Do, K. Q., Grandes, P., Morino, P., and Streit, P. (1990). Localisation and release of homocysteic acid, an excitatory sulfur-containing amino acid. *Journal of Histochemistry and Cytochemistry*, **38**, 1713–15.

Curtis, D. R. and Johnston, G. A. R. (1974). Amino acid transmitters in the mammalian CNS. *Ergebnisse der Physiologie*, **69**, 97–188.

Curtis, D. R. and Watkins, J. C. (1960). The excitation and depression of spinal neurones by structurally related amino acids. *Journal of Neurochemistry*, **6**, 117–41.

Curtis, D. R. and Watkins, J. C. (1963). Acidic amino acids with strong excitatory actions on mammalian neurones. *Journal of Physiology* (Lond.), **166**, 1–14.

Curtis, D. R. and Watkins, J. C. (1965). The pharmacology of amino acids related to γ-aminobutyric acid. *Pharmacological Reviews*, **17**, 347–92.

Curtis, D. R., Phillis, J. W., and Watkins, J. C. (1959). Chemical excitation of spinal neurones. *Nature* (Lond.), **183**, 611–12.

Curtis, D. R., Phillis, J. W., and Watkins, J. C. (1960). The chemical excitation of spinal neurones by certain acidic amino acids. *Journal of Physiology* (Lond.), **150**, 656–82.

Curtis, D. R., Phillis, J. W., and Watkins, J. C. (1961). Actions of amino acids on the isolated hemisected spinal cord of the toad. *British Journal of Pharmacology*, **16**, 262–83.

Curtis, D. R., Johnson, G. A. R., Game, G. J. A., and McCulloch, R. M. (1973). Antagonism of neuronal excitation by 1-hydroxy-3-amino-pyrrolidone-2. *Brain Research*, **49**, 467–70.

Davidoff, R. A., Graham, L. T., Jr, Shank, R. P., Werman, R., and Aprison, M. H. (1967). Changes in amino acid concentration associated with loss of spinal interneurons. *Journal of Neurochemistry*, **14**, 1025–31.

Davies, J. and Watkins, J. C. (1972). Is 1-hydroxy-3-aminopyrrolidone-2 (HA-966) a selective excitatory amino acid antagonist? *Nature* (Lond.), **238**, 61–3.

Davies, J. and Watkins, J. C. (1973). Microelectrophoretic studies on the depressant action of HA-966 on chemically and synaptically-excited neurones in the cat cerebral cortex and cuneate nucleus. *Brain Research*, **59**, 311–22.

Davies, J. and Watkins, J. C. (1977). Effect of magnesium ions on the responses of spinal neurones to excitatory amino acids and acetylcholine. *Brain Research*, **130**, 364–8.

Davies, J. and Watkins, J. C. (1979). Selective antagonism of amino acid-induced and synaptic excitation in the cat spinal cord. *Journal of Physiology* (Lond.), **297**, 621–36.

Davies, J. and Watkins, J. C. (1982). Actions of D and L forms of 2-amino-5-phosphonovalerate and 2-amino-4-phosphonobutyrate in the cat spinal cord. *Brain Research*, **235**, 378–86.

Davies, J., Evans, R. H., Francis, A. A., and Watkins, J. C. (1979). Excitatory amino acid receptors and synaptic excitation in the mammalian central nervous system. *Journal of Physiology* (Paris), **75**, 641–5.

Davies, J., Francis, A. A., Jones, A. W., and Watkins, J. C. (1980). 2-Amino-5-phosphonovalerate (2APV), a highly potent and selective antagonist at spinal NMDA receptors. *British Journal of Pharmacology*, **70**, 52–53P.

Davies, J., Francis, A. A., Jones, A. W., and Watkins, J. C. (1981). 2-Amino-5-phosphonovalerate (2APV), a potent and selective antagonist of amino acid-induced and synaptic excitation. *Neuroscience Letters*, **21**, 77–81.

Davies, J., Evans, R. H., Francis, A. A., Jones, A. W., Smith, D. A. S., and Watkins, J. C. (1982a). Conformational aspects of the actions of some piperidine dicarboxylic acids at excitatory amino acid receptors in the mammalian and amphibian spinal cord. *Neurochemistry Research*, **7**, 1119–33.

Davies, J., Evans, R. H., Jones, A. W., Smith, D. A. S., and Watkins, J. C. (1982b). Differential activation and blockade of excitatory amino acid receptors in the mammalian and amphibian central nervous system. *Comparative Biochemistry and Physiology*, **72C**, 211–24.

Davies, J., Evans, R. H., Herrling, P. L., Jones, A. W., Olverman, H. J., Pook, P., and Watkins, J. C. (1986). CPP, a new and selective NMDA antagonist. Depression of central neuron responses, affinity for ^{3}H-D-AP5 binding sites on brain membranes and anticonvulsant activity. *Brain Research*, **382**, 169–73.

Do, K. Q., Herrling, P. L., Streit, P., and Cuenod, M. (1988). Release of neuro-active substances: homocysteic acid as an endogenous agonist of the NMDA receptor. *Journal of Neural Transmission*, **72**, 185–90.

Do, K. Q., Grandes, P., Hansel, C., Jiang, C. H., Klancnik, J., Streit, P., Tschopp, P., Zangerle, L., and Cuenod, M. (1992). Sulphur containing excitatory amino acids: release, activity and localization. *Molecular Neuropharmacology*, **2**, 39–42.

Duggan, A. W. (1974). The differential sensitivity to L-glutamate and L-aspartate of spinal interneurones and Renshaw cells. *Experimental Brain Research*, **19**, 522–8.

Evans, R. H. and Watkins, J. C. (1978). Specific antagonism of excitant amino acids in the isolated spinal cord of the neonatal rat. *European Journal of Pharmacology*, **50**, 123–9.

Evans, R. H. and Watkins, J. C. (1981). Pharmacological antagonists of excitant amino acids. *Life Sciences*, **28**, 1303–8.

Evans, R. H., Francis, A. A., and Watkins, J. C. (1977a). Differential antagonism by chlorpromazine and diazepam of frog motoneurone depolarization induced by glutamate-related amino acids. *European Journal of Pharmacology*, **44**, 325–30.

Evans, R. H., Francis, A. A., and Watkins, J. C. (177b). Selective antagonism by Mg^{2+} of amino acid-induced depolarization of spinal neurones. *Experientia* (Basel), **33**, 489–91.

Evans, R. H., Francis, A. A., and Watkins, J. C. (1978). Mg^{2+}-like selective antagonism of excitatory amino acid-induced responses by α,ε-diaminopimelic acid, D-α-aminoadipate and HA-966 in isolated spinal cord of frog and immature rat. *Brain Research*, **148**, 536–42.

Evans, R. H., Francis, A. A., Hunt, K., Oakes, D. J., and Watkins, J. C. (1979). Antagonism of excitatory amino acid-induced responses and of synaptic excitation in the isolated spinal cord of the frog. *British Journal of Pharmacology*, **67**, 591–603.

Evans, R. H., Francis, A. A., Jones, A. W., Smith, D. A. S., and Watkins, J. C. (1982). The effects of a series of ω-phosphonic α-carboxylic amino acids on electrically evoked and amino acid induced responses in isolated spinal cord preparations. *British Journal of Pharmacology*, **75**, 65–75.

Fagg, G. E., Olpé, H.-H., Pozza, M. F., Baud, J., Steinmann, M., Schmutz, M., Portet, C., Baumann, P., Thedinga, K., Bittiger, H., Allgeier, H., Heckendorn, R., Angst, C., Brundish, D., and Dingwall, J. G. (1990). CGP 37849 and CGP 39551: novel and potent competitive N-methyl-D-aspartate (NMDA) receptor antagonists with oral activity. *British Journal of Pharmacology*, **99**, 791–7.

Fletcher, E. J. and Lodge, D. (1988). Glycine reverses antagonism of N-methyl-D-aspartate (NMDA) by 1-hydroxy-3-aminopyrrolidone-2 (HA-966) but not D-amino-5-phosphonovalerate (D-AP5) on rat cortical slices. *European Journal of Pharmacology*, **151**, 161–2.

Foster, A. C. and Fagg, G. E. (1984). Acidic amino acid binding sites in mammalian neuronal membranes: their characteristics and relationship to synaptic receptors. *Brain Research Review*, **7**, 103–64.

Haldeman, S. and McLennan, H. (1972). The antagonistic action of glutamic acid diethyl ester towards amino acid-induced and synaptic excitations of central neurones. *Brain Research*, **45**, 393–400.

Haldeman, S., Huffman, R. D., Marshall, K. C., and McLennan, H. (1972). The antagonism of the glutamate-induced and synaptic excitations of thalamic neurones. *Brain Research*, **39**, 419–25.

Harris, E. W., Ganong, A. H., Monaghan, D. T., Watkins, J. C., and Cotman, C. W. (1986). Action of 3-([±]-2-carboxypiperazin-4-yl)-propyl-1-phosphonic acid (CPP): a new and highly potent antagonist of N-methyl-D-aspartate receptors in the hippocampus. *Brain Research*, **382**, 174–7.

Harrison, N. L. and Simmonds, M. A. (1985). Quantitative studies on some antagonists of NMDA in slices of rat cerebral cortex. *British Journal of Pharmacology*, **84**, 381–91.

Hayashi, T. (1954). Effects of sodium glutamate on the nervous system. *Keio Journal of Medicine*, **3**, 183–92.

Herrling, P. L., Aebischer, B., Frey, P., Olverman, H. J., and Watkins, J. C. (1989). NMDA-Antagonistic properties of the enantiomers of 3-(2-carboxypiperazin-4-yl)propyl-1-phosphonic acid (CPP) and of its unsaturated analogue 3-(2-carboxypiperazin-4-yl)-1-propenyl-1-phosphonic acid (CPP-ene). *Society for Neuroscience Abstracts*, **16**, 327.

Honey, S. R., Miljkovic, Z., and MacDonald, J. F. (1988). Ketamine and phenylcyclidine cause a voltage dependent block of responses to aspartic acid. *Neuroscience Letters*, **61**, 135–9.

Honoré, T., Drejer, J., Nielsen, E. O., Watkins, J. C., Olverman, H. J., and Nielsen, M. (1989). Molecular target size analyses of the NMDA–receptor complex in rat cortex. *European Journal of Pharmacology*, **172**, 239–47.

Ito, S., Provini, L., and Cherubini, E. (1991). L-Homocysteic acid mediates synaptic excitation at NMDA receptors in the hippocampus. *Neuroscience Letters*, **124**, 157–61.

Johnson, J. W. and Ascher, P. (1987). Glycine potentiates the NMDA response in cultured mouse brain neurons. *Nature* (Lond.), **325**, 529–31.

Johnston, G. A. R., Curtis, D. R., Davies, J., and McCulloch, R. M. (1974). Spinal interneurone excitation by conformationally restricted analogues of L-glutamic acid. *Nature* (Lond.), **248**, 804–5.

Johnston, G. A. R., Kennedy, S. M. E., and Twitchin, B. (1979). Action of the neurotoxin kainic acid on high-affinity uptake of L-glumatic acid in rat brain slices. *Journal of Neurochemistry*, **32**, 121–8.

Jones, A. W., Smith, D. A. S., and Watkins, J. C. (1984). Structure–activity relations of dipeptide antagonists of excitatory amino acids. *Neuroscience*, **13**, 573–81.

Kawai, M., Horikawa, Y., Ishihara, T., Shimamoto, K., and Ohfune, Y. (1992). 2-(Carboxycyclopropyl)glycines: binding, neurotoxicity and induction of intracellular free Ca^{2+} increase. *European Journal of Pharmacology*, **211**, 195–202.

Kemp, J. A. and Priestley, T. (1991). Effects of (+)-HA-966 and 7-chlorokynurenic acid on the kinetics of N-methyl-D-aspartate receptor response in rat cultured cortical cells. *Molecular Pharmacology*, **39**, 666–70.

Kemp, J. A., Foster, A. C., and Wong, E. H. F. (1987). Non-competitive antagonists of excitatory amino acid receptors. *Trends in Neuroscience*, **10**, 294–8.

Kemp, J. A., Priestley, T., and Woodruff, G. N. (1988). Differences in the N-methyl-D-aspartate antagonist profiles of two compounds acting at the glycine modulatory site. *British Journal of Pharmacology*, **95**, 759P.

Kleckner, N. W. and Dingledine, R. (1988). Requirements for glycine in activation of NMDA-receptors expressed in Xenopus oocytes. *Science*, **241**, 835–7.

Koek, W. and Woods, J. H. (1988). N-Methyl-D-aspartate antagonism and phencyclidine-like activity: behavioural studies. In *Frontiers in excitatory amino acid research*, (ed. E. A. Cavalheiro, J. Lehmann, and L. Turski), pp. 535–42. Alan R. Liss, New York.

Koek, W., Woods, J. H., and Winger, G. D. (1988). MK-801, a proposed non-competitive antagonist of excitatory amino acid neurotransmission, produces phencyclidine-like behavioural effects in pigeons, rats and rhesus monkeys. *Journal of Pharmacology and Experimental Therapeutics*, **245**, 969–74.

Kristensen, J. D., Svensson, B., and Gordh, T. (1992). The NMDA-receptor antagonist CPP abolishes neurogenic wind-up pain after intrathecal administration in humans. *Pain*, **51**, 249–53.

Krnjevic, K. (1974). Chemical nature of synaptic transmission in vertebrates. *Physiological Reviews*, **54**, 418–540.

Krogsgaard-Larsen, P., Honoré, T., Hansen, J. J., Curtis, D. R., and Lodge, D. (1980). New class of glutamate agonist structurally related to ibotenic acid. *Nature* (Lond.), **284**, 64–6.

Lanthorn, T. H., Hood, W. F., Watson, G. B., Compton, R. P., Rader, R. K., Gaoni, Y., and Monahan, J. B. (1990). *cis*-2,4-Methanoglutamate is a potent and selective N-methyl-D-aspartate receptor agonist. *European Journal of Pharmacology*, **182**, 397–404.

Leeson, P. D., Baker, R., Carling, R. W., Curtis, N. R., Moore, K. W., Williams, B. J., Foster, A. C., Donald, A. E., Kemp, J. A., and Marshall, G. R. (1991). Kynurenic acid derivatives. Structure–activity relationships for excitatory amino acid antagonism and identification of potent and selective antagonists at the glycine site on the N-methyl-D-aspartate receptor. *Journal of Medicinal Chemistry*, **34**, 1243–52.

Leeson, P. D., Carling, R. W., Williams, B. J., Baker, R., Ladduwahetty, T., Moore, K. W., Rowley, M., Foster, A. C., Kemp, J. A., and Tricklebank, M. D. (1992a). Non-competitive N-methyl-D-aspartate antagonists: structure–activity relationships for compounds acting at the ion-channel and glycine sites. In *Trends in Medicinal Chemistry* (ed. S. Sarel, R. Mechoulam, and I. Agranat), pp. 169–74. Blackwell Scientific Publications, Oxford.

Leeson, P. D., Carling, R. W., Moore, K. W., Moseley, A. M., Smith, J. D., Stevenson, G., Chan, T., Baker, R., Foster, A. C., Grimwood, B., Kemp, J. A., Marshall, G. R., and Hoogsteen, K. (1992b). 4-Amido-2-carboxytetrahydroquinolines. Structure–activity relationships for antagonism at the glycine site of the NMDA receptor. *Journal of Medicinal Chemistry*, **35**, 1954–68.

Lehmann, J., Chapman, A. G., Meldrum, B. S., Hutchison, A., Tsai, C., and Wood, P. L. (1988a). CGS 19755 is a potent and competitive antagonist at NMDA-type receptors. *European Journal of Pharmacology*, **154**, 89–93.

Lehmann, J., Hutchison, A. J., McPherson, S. E., Mondadori, C., Schmultz, M., Sinton, C. M., Tsai, C., Murphy, D. E., Steel, D. J., Williams, M., Cheney, D. L., and Wood, P. L. (1988b). CGS 19755, A selective and competitive N-methyl-D-aspartate-type excitatory amino acid receptor antagonist. *Journal of Pharmacology and Experimental Therapeutics*, **246**, 65–75.

Lodge, D. and Collingridge, G. L. (ed.) (1991). The pharmacology of excitatory amino acids. A special report. *Trends in Pharmacological Sciences*.

Lodge, D., Aram, J. A., and Fletcher, E. J. (1988a). Modulation of N-methylaspartate receptor-channel complexes: an overview. In *Frontiers in excitatory amino acid research*, (ed. E. A. Cavalheiro, J. Lehmann, and L. Turski), pp. 527–34. Alan R. Liss, New York.

Lodge, D., Aram, J. A., Church, J., Davies, S. N., Martin, D., Millar, J., and Zeman, S. (1988b). Sigma opiates and excitatory amino acids. In *Excitatory amino acids in health and disease*, (ed. D. Lodge), pp. 237–59. John Wiley & Sons, Chichester.

Lodge, D., Davies, S. N., Jones, M. G., Millar, J., Manallack, D. T., Ornstein, P. L., Verbenem, A. J. M., Young, N., and Beart, P. M. (1988c). A comparison between the *in vivo* and *in vitro* activity of five potent and competitive NMDA antagonists. *British Journal of Pharmacology*, **95**, 957–65.

Lunn, W. H. W., Schoepp, D. D., Calligaro, D. O., Vasileff, R. T., Heinz, L. J., Salhoff, C. R., and O'Malley, P. J. (1992). DL-Tetrazol-5 ylglycine, a highly potent NMDA agonist—its synthesis and NMDA receptor efficacy. *Journal of Medicinal Chemistry*, **35**, 4608–12.

McCulloch, R. M., Johnston, G. A. R., Game, G. J. A., and Curtis, D. R. (1974). The differential sensitivity of spinal interneurones and Renshaw cells to kainate and NMDA. *Experimental Brain Research*, **21**, 515–18.

Macdermott, A. B., Mayer, M. L., Westbrook, G. L., Smith, S. J., and Barker, J. L. (1986). NMDA-receptor activation increases cytoplasmic calcium concentration in cultured spinal cord neurones. *Nature* (Lond.), **321**, 519–22.

MacDonald, J. F., and Porietis, A. V. (1982). DL-Quisqualic and L-aspartic acids activate separate excitatory conductances in cultured spinal cord neurons. *Brain Research*, **245**, 175–8.

MacDonald, J. F. and Wojtowicz, J. M. (1980). Two conductance mechanisms activated by applications of L-glutamic, L-aspartic, DL-homocysteic, *N*-methyl-D-aspartic and DL-kainic acids to cultured mammalian central neurones. *Canadian Journal of Physiology and Pharmacology*, **58**, 1393–7.

McLennan, H., Huffman, R. D., and Marshall, K. C. (1968). Patterns of excitation of thalamic neurones by amino acids and by acetylcholine. *Nature* (Lond.), **219**, 387–8.

McLennan, H. and Lodge, D. (1979). The antagonism of amino acid-induced excitation of spinal neurones in the cat. *Brain Research*, **169**, 83–90.

Mayer, M. L. and Westbrook, G. L. (1985). The action of *N*-methyl-D-aspartic acid on mouse spinal neurones in culture. *Journal of Physiology* (Lond.), **361**, 65–90.

Mayer, M. L. and Westbrook, G. L. (1987a). The physiology of excitatory amino acids in the vertebrate CNS. *Progress in Neurobiology*, **28**, 197–296.

Mayer, M. L. and Westbrook, G. L. (1987b). Permeation and block of *N*-methyl-D-aspartic acid receptors channels by divalent cations in mouse cultured neurones. *Journal of Physiology* (Lond.), **394**, 501–27.

Monaghan, D. T. and Cotman, C. W. (1986). Anatomical organization of NMDA, kainate and quisqualate receptors. In *Excitatory amino acids*, (ed. P. J. Roberts, J. Storm-Mathisen, and H. F. Bradford), pp. 279–99. Macmillan, London.

Monaghan, D. T., Bridges, R. J., and Cotman, C. W. (1989). The excitatory amino acid receptors: their classes, pharmacology and distinct properties in the function of the central nervous system. *Annual Review of Pharmacology and Toxicology*, **29**, 365–402.

Monahan, J. B., Hood, W. F., Compton, R. P., Cordi, A. A., Snyder, J. P., Pellicciari, R., and Natalina, B. (1990). Characterization of D-3,4-cyclopropyl-glutamates as *N*-methyl-D-aspartate receptor agonists. *Neuroscience Letters*, **112**, 328–32.

Moriyoshi, K., Masu, M., Ishii, T., Shigemoto, R., Mizuno, N., and Nakanishi, S.

(1991). Molecular cloning and characterization of the NMDA receptor. *Nature* (Lond.), **345**, 31–7.

Müller, W., Lowe, D. A., Neijt, H., Urwyler, S., and Herrling, P. L. (1992). Synthesis and *N*-methyl-D-aspartate (NMDA) antagonist properties of the enantiomers of α-amino-5-(phosphonomethyl)[1,1'-biphenyl]-3-propanoic acid. Use of a new chiral glycine derivative. *Helvetica Chimica Acta*, **75**, 855–64.

Murphy, D. E., Schneider, J., Boehm, C., Lehmann, J., and Williams, M. (1987). Binding of [³H]3-(2-carboxypiperazin-4-yl)propyl-1-phosphonic acid to rat brain membranes: A selective high affinity ligand for *N*-methyl-D-aspartate receptors. *Journal of Pharmacology and Experimental Therapeutics*, **240**, 778–84.

Nakajima, Y., Iwakabi, H., Akazawa, C., Nawa, H., Shigemoto, R., Mizuno, N., and Nakanishi, S. (1993). Molecular characterization of a novel retinal metabotropic glutamate receptor mGluR6 with a high agonist selectivity for L-2-amino-4-phosphonobutyrate. *Journal of Biological Chemistry*, **268**, 11868–73.

Nakanishi, S. (1992). Molecular diversity of glutamate receptors and implications for brain function. *Science*, **258**, 597–603.

Nowak, L., Bregestovski, P., Ascher, P., Herbet, A., and Prochiantz, A. (1984). Magnesium gates glutamate-activated channels in mouse central neurones. *Nature* (Lond.), **307**, 462–5.

Olverman, H. J., Jones, A. W., and Watkins, J. C. (1984). L-Glutamate has higher affinity than other amino acids for [³H]-D-AP5 binding sites in rat brain membranes. *Nature* (Lond.), **307**, 460–2.

Olverman, H. J., Jones, A. W., Mewett, K. N., and Watkins, J. C. (1988*a*). Structure/activity relations of NMDA receptor ligands as studied by their inhibition of ³H-D-AP5 binding in rat brain membranes. *Neuroscience*, **26**, 17–31.

Olverman, H. J., Jones, A. W., and Watkins, J. C. (1988*b*). ³H-D-2-Amino-5-phosphonopentanoate (³H-D-AP5) as a ligand for *N*-methyl-D-aspartate in the mammalian central nervous system. *Neuroscience*, **26**, 1–15.

Ornstein, P. L. and Klimkowski, V. J. (1992). Competitive NMDA receptor antagonists. In *Excitatory amino acid receptors: design of agonists and antagonists* (ed. P. Krogsgaard-Larsen and J. J. Hansen), pp. 183–201. Ellis Horwood, Chichester, UK.

Perkins, M. N., Stone, T. W., Collins, J. F., and Curry, K. (1981). Phosphonate analogues of carboxylic acids as amino acid antagonists on rat cortical neurones. *Neuroscience Letters*, **23**, 333–6.

Perkins, M. N., Collins, J. F., and Stone, T. W. (1982). Isomers of 2-amino-7-phosphonoheptanoic acid as antagonists of neuronal excitants. *Neuroscience Letters*, **32**, 65–8.

Schoepp, D. D. and Conn, P. J. (1993). Metabotropic glutamate receptors in brain function and pathology. *Trends in Pharmacological Sciences*, **14**, 13–20.

Sheardown, M. J., Drejer, J., Jensen, L. H., Stidsen, C. E., and Honoré, T. (1989). A potent antagonist of the strychnine insensitive glycine receptor has anticonvulsant properties. *European Journal of Pharmacology*, **174**, 197–204.

Shinozaki, H. (1978). Discovery of novel action of kainic acid and related compounds. In *Kainic acid as a tool in neurobiology*, (ed. E. G. McGeer, J. W. Olney, and P. L. McGeer), pp. 17–35. Raven Press, New York.

Shinozaki, H. and Konishi, S. (1970). Actions of several anthelmintics and insecticides on rat cortical neurones. *Brain Research*, **24**, 368–71.

Shinozaki, H. and Shibuya, I. (1974). A new potent excitant, quisqualic acid: effects on crayfish neuromuscular junction. *Neuropharmacology*, **13**, 665–72.

Shinozaki, II. and Shibuya, I. (1976). Effects of kainic acid analogues on crayfish opener muscle. *Neuropharmacology*, **15**, 145–7.

Shinozaki, H., Ishida, M., Shimamoto, K., and Ohfune, Y. (1989). Potent NMDA-like actions and potentiation of glutamate responses by conformational variants of a glutamate analogue in the rat spinal cord. *British Journal of Pharmacology*, **98**, 1213–24.

Simon, R. P., Swan, J. H., Griffiths, T., and Meldrum, B. S. (1984). Blockade of N-methyl-D-aspartate receptors may protect against ischaemic damage in the brain. *Science*, **226**, 850–2.

Singh, L., Donald, A. E., Foster, A. C., Hutson, P. H., Iversen, L. L., Iversen, S. D., Kemp, J. A., Leeson, P. D., Marshall, G. R., Oles, R. J., Priestley, T., Thorn, L., Tricklebank, M. D., Vass, C. A., and Williams, B. J. (1990). Enantiomers of HA-966 (3-amino-1-hydroxypyrrolid-2-one) exhibit distinct central nervous system effects: (+)-HA 966 is a selective glycine/N-methyl-D-aspartate receptor antagonist, but (−)-HA-966 is a potent γ-butyro-lactone-like sedative. *Proceedings of the National Academy of Science, USA*, **87**, 347–51.

Stone, T. W. and Burton, N. R. (1988). NMDA receptors and ligands in the vertebrate CNS. *Progress in Neurobiology*, **30**, 333–68.

Sugiyama, H., Ito, I., and Hirono, C. (1987). A new type of glutamate receptor linked to inositol phospholipid metabolism. *Nature* (Lond.), **325**, 532–3.

Tanabe, Y., Masu, M., Ishii, T., Shigemoto, R., and Nakanishi, S. (1992). A family of metabotropic glutamate receptors. *Neuron*, **8**, 169–79.

Turski, L., Schwarcz, M., Turski, W. A., Klockgether, T., Sontag, K.-H., and Collins, J. F. (1985). Muscle relaxant action of excitatory amino acid antagonists. *Neuroscience Letters*, **53**, 321–6.

Watkins, J. C. (1962). The synthesis of some acidic amino acids possessing neuropharmacological activity. *Journal of Medicinal and Pharmaceutical Chemistry*, **5**, 1187–99.

Watkins, J. C. (1978). Excitatory amino acids. In *Kainic acid as a tool in neurobiology*, (ed. E. G. McGeer, J. W. Olney, and P. L. McGeer), pp. 37–69. Raven Press, New York.

Watkins, J. C. (1980). NMDA receptors: new light on amino acid-mediated synaptic excitation. *Trends in Neuroscience*, **3**, 61–6.

Watkins, J. C. (1986). Twenty-five years of excitatory amino acid research. In *Excitatory amino acids*, (ed. P. J. Roberts, J. Storm-Mathisen, and H. F. Bradford), pp. 1–39. Macmillan, London.

Watkins, J. C. (1992). NMDA receptors. Agonists and competitive antagonists. In *Trends in medicinal chemistry*, (Proceedings of the XIth International Symposium on Medicinal Chemistry, IUPAC), (ed. S. Shalom, R. Mechoulam, and I. Agranat), pp. 17–29. Blackwell Scientific Publications, Oxford.

Watkins, J. C. and Evans, R. H. (1981). Excitatory amino acid transmitters. *Annual Reviews of Pharmacology and Toxicology*, **21**, 165–204.

Watkins, J. C. and Olverman, H. J. (1987). Agonists and antagonists for excitatory amino acid receptors. *Trends in Neuroscience*, **10**, 265–72.

Watkins, J. C. and Olverman, H. J. (1988). Structural requirements for activation and blockade of EAA receptors. In *Excitatory amino acids in health and disease*, (ed. D. Lodge), pp. 13–45. John Wiley & Sons, Chichester, UK.

Williams, T. L., Smith, D. A. S., Burton, N. R., and Stone, T. W. (1988). Amino acid pharmacology in neocortical slices: evidence for biomolecular actions from an extension of the Hill and Gaddum-Schild equation. *British Journal of Pharmacology*, **95**, 805–10.

Wong, E. H. F. and Kemp, J. A. (1991). Sites for antagonism on the *N*-methyl-D-aspartate receptor channel complex. *Annual Reviews of Pharmacology and Toxicology*, **31**, 401–25.

Wong, E. H. F., Kemp, J. A., Priestley, T., Knight, A. R., Woodruff, G. N., and Iversen, L. L. (1986). The anticonvulsant MK-801 is a potent NMDA antagonist. *Proceedings of the National Academy of Science, USA*, **83**, 7104–8.

2 Agonists and competitive antagonists: structure–activity and molecular modelling studies

D. E. JANE, H. J. OLVERMAN, AND
J. C. WATKINS

Introduction

As described in Chapter 1, it has been known for around 35 years that (S)-glutamate, (S)-aspartate[1], and a variety of closely related structural analogues, both synthetic and naturally occurring substances, can evoke an excitatory response when applied to single cells in the mammalian central nervous system (CNS). Such substances include the synthetic compound N-methyl-(R)-aspartic acid (NMDA), which, under the original test conditions, was up to 100 times more potent than (S)-glutamate (Watkins 1962). In the intervening period numerous other excitants, including α-amino-3-hydroxy-5-methylisoxazole-4-propionic acid (AMPA) and the naturally occurring amino acids kainic acid and quisqualic acid, have been shown to activate glutamate receptors. It is now clear that agonists exert their effect through multiple types of glutamate receptors in the mammalian CNS, of which five distinct types have gained general acceptance. There are three families of ligand-gated or ionotropic receptors, namely NMDA, kainate, and AMPA receptors, and two families of G-protein-coupled metabotropic receptors, the latter including the so-called L-AP4 ((S)-2-amino-4-phosphonobutyrate) receptors originally considered to be a separate unique class (Watkins *et al.* 1991; Nakanishi 1992; Schoepp and Conn 1993). NMDA receptors are defined electrophysiologically by the selectivity of NMDA for particular populations of excitatory amino acid receptors, and more importantly, by the susceptibility of these receptors to blockade by potent and selective antagonists. Historical details of the evolution of the NMDA receptor concept along with the development and actions of early antagonists including Mg^{2+}, 1-hydroxy-3-aminopyrrolidone-2 (HA-966), and (R)-α-aminoadipate are given in Chapter 1.

---

[1] In this chapter, modern stereochemical notation has been used except for some acronyms derived from the older terminology (e.g., NMDA, L-AP4) and for radioligands (e.g. [^{3}H] L glutamate). It should be noted that although for most common amino acids (S) corresponds to L and (R) to D this is not always the case (see footnote 4, Table 2.1).

Competitive antagonists

Because of their obvious potential as therapeutic agents, major advances have been made in the development of high affinity competitive NMDA antagonists, a number of which show potent anticonvulsant and neuro-protective properties when administered peripherally. Two lead compounds in particular provided the pharmacological tools for investigating and identifying the role of NMDA receptors in discrete synaptic pathways in the CNS (Collingridge *et al.* 1983; Harris *et al.* 1984; Morris *et al.* 1986; Mayer and Westbrook 1987; Stone and Burton 1988; Collingridge and Lester 1989) and for showing the potential of NMDA receptor antagonists as antiepileptic and neuroprotective agents for the treatment of cerebral ischaemia (Croucher *et al.* 1982; Simon *et al.* 1984; Meldrum 1985; Wieloch 1985). These were the competitive antagonists 2-amino-5-phosphonopenta-noic acid (AP5) and 2-amino-7-phosphonoheptanoic acid (AP7) (Davies *et al.* 1981; Evans and Watkins 1981; Davies and Watkins 1982; Evans *et al.* 1982*a*; Perkins *et al.* 1982), the (2R) isomer being the active form in both cases. There is now a wide spectrum of competitive NMDA antagonists available and examples of the major series that have provided high affinity compounds are shown in Fig. 2.1. The common feature of the vast majority of these compounds is that they contain the structure of either AP5 or AP7 as the backbone of the molecules, the proximal and distal acid groups being separated by four or six atoms. One major exception to this is the series of substituted quinoxalines (Baudy *et al.* 1993) of which the most potent compounds are based on 2-amino-6-phosphonohexanoic acid (AP6), the higher homologue of AP5. Indeed, α-amino-6,7-dichloro-3-(phosphonomethyl)-2-quinoxalinepropanoic acid is the highest affinity competitive NMDA receptor antagonist yet described, the racemic form having an IC_{50} value of 3.4 nM (Baudy *et al.* 1993; Fig. 2.1, structure II).

One major drawback of the original competitive antagonists is that, since they are highly polar substances, they are poorly absorbed by brain tissue when administered peripherally in contrast to the much more lipophilic MK-801-type non-competitive NMDA antagonists. Therefore the objective of developing new competitive NMDA receptor antagonists has been to make structural alterations to AP5 and AP7 that firstly increase NMDA receptor affinity especially by reducing conformational mobility and promoting inter-action with key sites within the NMDA receptor, and secondly improve penetration into brain tissue, combining to yield agents with an enhanced *in vivo* profile and thus therapeutic potential. This has been achieved by:

(1) incorporation of ring structures linking the α-amino group with the atom in position 3 or 4 of the interacidic group chain such as the 4-substituted piperazine-2-carboxylic acid series (e.g. Fig. 2.1, CPP and CPP-ene) (Aebischer *et al.* 1989), the 3- and 4-substituted piperidine-2-carboxylic

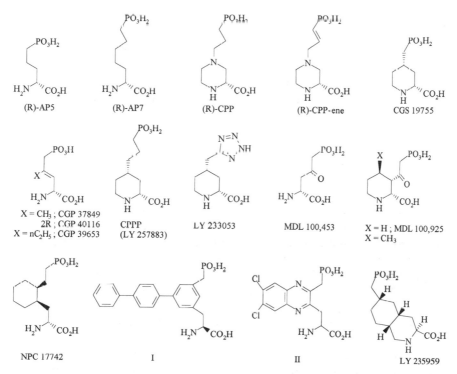

Fig. 2.1 Structures of competitive NMDA antagonists. Abbreviations: (R)-AP5, (2R)-2-amino-5-phosphonopentanoic acid (0.62 μM); (R)-AP7, (2R)-2-amino-7-phosphono-heptanoic acid (1.7 μM); (R)-CPP, (2R)-4-(3-phosphonopropyl)piperazine-2-carboxylic acid (140 nM); (R)-CPP-ene, (2R)-(E)-4-(3-phosphonoprop-2-enyl)piperazine-2-carboxylic acid (44 nM); CGS 19755, (2RS,4SR)-4-phosphonomethyl-2-piperidine carboxylic acid (183 nM); CGP 37849, (RS)-(E)-2-amino-4-methyl-5-phosphono-3-pentenoic acid (35 nM); CGP 40116, (R)-(E)-2-amino-4-methyl-5-phosphono-3-pentenoic acid (19 nM); CGP 39653, (RS)-(E)-2-amino-4-propyl-5-phosphono-3-pentenoic acid (7 nM); CPPP (LY 257883), (2RS,4SR)-4-(3-phosphonopropyl)piperidine-2-carboxylic acid (179 nM); LY 233053, (2RS,4SR)-4-(1H-tetrazol-5-ylmethyl)piperidine-2-carboxylic acid (107 nM); MDL 100,453, (2R)-2-amino-4-oxo-5-phosphonopentanoic acid (109 nM); MDL 100,925, (2R,3S)-3-phosphonoacetylpiperidine-2-carboxylic acid (68 nM); NPC 17742, (2R,4R,5S)-(2-amino-4,5-(1,2-cyclohexyl)-7-phosphonoheptanoic acid (148 nM); structure I, (2S)-2-amino-5-(phosphonomethyl)[1,1′:4′, 1″-terphenyl]-3-propanoic acid (17 nM); structure II, (RS)-α-amino-6,7-dichloro-3-(phosphonomethyl)-2-quinoxalinepropanoic acid (3.4 nM); LY 235959, (3S,4aR,6S,8aR)-6-(phosphono-methyl)-1,2,3,4,4a,5,6,7,8,8a-decahydroisoquinoline-3-carboxylic acid (25 nM; Ornstein and Klimkowski 1992). Source references for the K_i or IC$_{50}$ values quoted in parenthesis can be found in Tables 2.5 and 2.6.

acid series (e.g. Fig. 2.1, MDL 100,925, CGS 19755, CPPP, and LY 233053) (Whitten *et al.* 1991; Lehmann *et al.* 1988; Ornstein *et al.* 1992b; Ornstein and Klimkowski 1992), and isoquinoline derivatives (e.g. Fig. 2.1, LY 235959) (Ornstein *et al.* 1992a; Ornstein and Klimkowski 1992);

(2) incorporation of ring structures in the interacidic group chain alone such as the *m*-substituted phenylalanines, the quinoxaline derivatives, or a cyclohexyl ring (e.g. Fig. 2.1, structures I and II, NPC 17742) (Müller *et al.* 1992; Baudy *et al.* 1993; Ferkany *et al.* 1993*a,b*);

(3) unsaturation of the interacidic group chain (e.g. Fig. 2.1, CGP 40116, CGP 39653, and MDL 100,453) (Fagg *et al.* 1990; Whitten *et al.* 1993*a*);

(4) replacement of the ω-phosphono moiety by an isosteric tetrazole moiety (e.g. Fig. 2.1, LY233053) (Ornstein *et al.* 1992*b*).

A number of the high affinity compounds combine more than one of these features (e.g. Fig. 2.1, CPP-ene and MDL 100,925) and more recently developed agents also contain bulky aromatic ring structures that may interact with an additional hydrophobic pocket within the NMDA receptor thus promoting high affinity (e.g. Fig. 2.1, compounds I and II; see molecular modelling section).

By and large the newer antagonists have the same spectrum of activity as AP5 and AP7, having virtually no effect on any other neurotransmitter receptor studied. Many now show potent *in vivo* activity due to a combination of their higher affinity and ability to penetrate brain tissue. It is worth mentioning that the carboxyethylester of CGP 37849, CGP 39551, has significantly improved oral activity as an anticonvulsant, presumably due to its less polar nature such that it passes the blood–brain barrier more effectively than CGP 37849 (Fagg *et al.* 1990). The potential of both competitive and non-competitive NMDA receptor antagonists as centrally acting antiepileptic drugs and as neuroprotective agents is discussed fully in Chapters 16, 19, and 20.

As has already been described, with the exception of the quinoxaline derivatives (Baudy *et al.* 1993), all potent competitive antagonists are based on the structure of either AP5 or AP7. The quinoxaline derivatives differ from the other compounds in another respect since in addition to being potent competitive antagonists, some, including structure II, display high activity at the NMDA glycine site (Baudy *et al.* 1993). As with AP5 and AP7 the active form of most compounds has been found to reside in the enantiomer having the (R) configuration at the α-carbon. However, here again exceptions have now been found. For the *m*-substituted phenylalanines (e.g. structure I) the isomers having the (S) stereochemistry at the α-carbon are substantially more active than the corresponding (R) isomers (Müller *et al.* 1992). Likewise the (3S) isomer LY 235959 is the active isomer as also in the case of its 6-tetrazolylmethyl analogue, LY 202157 (Ornstein and Klimkowski 1992). Interestingly, however, the (3R) isomer of other epimeric pairs within the decahydroisoquinoline series may be the active form (Ornstein and Klimkowski 1992).

A wealth of information has now been generated, especially from radioligand binding studies, regarding the structural requirements for agonist and antagonist binding to the glutamate recognition site on the NMDA receptor. In combination with a number of molecular modelling studies this has been used to elucidate the three-dimensional topology of the receptor site and thus provide a basis for a rational design of new pharmacological agents with agonist or antagonist action at these sites. This chapter will firstly outline the required structural features for agonist and antagonist binding, and secondly discuss the various molecular modelling studies which have recently been carried out.

Radiolabelled ligands for NMDA receptors

Initial attempts to establish ligand binding assays for the acidic amino acid recognition site on NMDA receptors using radiolabelled compounds such as [3H]NMDA, [3H]DL-AP7, and [3H]DL-AP5 were beset with various problems largely associated with the low affinity of these compounds for the receptor (Foster and Fagg 1987; Fagg and Baud 1988; Olverman *et al.* 1988*b*). Using a microcentrifugation assay, [3H]D-AP5 was the first ligand which was shown to label selectively NMDA receptors (Olverman *et al.* 1984, 1988*a,b*) and allowed routine screening of available compounds. Specific binding using washed membranes prepared from a crude synaptosomal fraction of rat cerebal cortex represented about 40 per cent of total binding and [3H]D-AP5 appeared to label a single population of sites with K_D and B_{max} values of about 0.5 μM and 4 pmol/mg protein respectively. [3H]L-Glutamate labels sites in addition to NMDA receptors. However, at about the same time as [3H]D-AP5 was introduced as an NMDA receptor ligand, it was shown that by using a highly purified membrane preparation, post-synaptic densities, almost all of the specific binding of [3H]L-glutamate was to NMDA receptors (Fagg and Matus 1984; Foster and Fagg 1987; Fagg and Baud 1988). Alternatively, [3H]L-glutamate can still be used successfully to label NMDA receptors in a less purified synaptic plasma membrane fraction where there is a high proportion of binding to non-NMDA receptor sites, by defining and limiting analysis to the NMDA-sensitive component of [3H]L-glutamate binding (Monaghan and Cotman 1986; Monahan and Michel (1987)).

[3H]D-AP5 was used to carry out a detailed investigation of the structural requirements of agonists and antagonists for binding to NMDA receptors (Olverman *et al.* 1988*a*; Watkins and Olverman 1988; Olverman and Watkins 1989). By combining the structure–activity relationship data obtained using [3H]D-AP5 and including some data for [3H]CPP with the known electrophysiological properties of individual compounds, primarily open chain structures, a simple model was postulated to explain the modes of interaction of enantiomeric forms of agonists and antagonists with the NMDA receptor. Based largely on the differences in the preferred ω-acidic group and in the optimum separation of the α- and ω-acidic group for producing high affinity agonists and NMDA receptor antagonists it was suggested that although the α-amino and carboxyl groups of agonists may well interact with the same receptor sites as antagonists, the ω-acidic group of antagonists actually binds to a positive site in the NMDA receptor distinct from that binding to the ω-acidic group of agonists, perhaps even on a separate receptor protein (Olverman *et al.* 1988*a*; Watkins and Olverman 1988; Olverman and Watkins 1989; Watkins 1991). [³H]D-AP5 has been superseded by higher affinity antagonist ligands [³H]CPP (Olverman *et al.* 1986; Murphy *et al.* 1987), an AP7 analogue, and the AP5 analogues [³H]CGS 19755 (Murphy *et al.* 1988) and [³H]CGP 39653 (Sills *et al.* 1991). As with [³H]D-AP5, the suitability of [³H]CPP (K_D = 0.3 μM) as a ligand for NMDA receptors was shown by comparing K_i values of a range of NMDA receptor antagonists measured against [³H]CPP binding with their K_D values derived from dose-ratio measurements for NMDA-induced depolarizations in electrophysiological experiments (Olverman *et al.* 1984, 1986, 1988*b*; Watkins and Olverman 1988; Olverman and Watkins 1989). Substances used included those that were then the most potent and highly selective compounds known (e.g. (RS)-CPP, (R)-AP5, (R)-AP7, (R)-β-aspartylaminomethylphosphonate and (R)-γ-glutamylaminomethylphosphonate). A plot of K_i values, measured against [³H]CPP binding, for some of these substances versus their K_D values for antagonism of NMDA

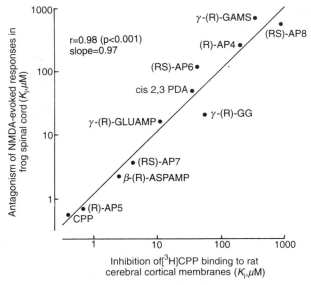

Fig. 2.2 Correlation for excitatory amino acid antagonists of inhibition of [³H]CPP binding and antagonism of NMDA-evoked responses (J. C. Watkins and H. J. Olverman, unpublished observations).

induced depolarizations in electrophysiological experiments (Fig. 2.2) indicates a direct relationship for the potencies of compounds when tested in both systems. These data, together with the lower affinity of (S) isomers of AP5 and AP7 compared with that of the (R) isomers, and the correlation between the activity of the (R) and (S) isomers of CPP and CPP-ene in electrophysiological and binding experiments (Table 2.5, compounds 11/12, 15/16, 59/60, and 161/162; Aebischer *et al.* 1989) thus established [^{3}H]D-AP5 and [^{3}H]CPP as suitable radioligands for NMDA receptors.

A similar pharmacological profile for competitive antagonists was found in other studies using [^{3}H]CPP (Murphy *et al.* 1987), [^{3}H]CGS 19755 (Murphy *et al.* 1988) and [^{3}H]CGP 39653 (Sills *et al.* 1991), and also for [^{3}H]L-glutamate (Fagg and Matus 1984; Monaghan and Cotman 1986; Foster and Fagg 1987; Monahan and Michel, 1987; Fagg and Baud 1988) as ligands for NMDA receptors. The tritiated NMDA antagonists and [^{3}H]L-glutamate have therefore been used to investigate various pharmacological and neurochemical aspects of NMDA receptors in both membrane binding assays and autoradiographic studies (Monaghan *et al.* 1989; Young and Fagg 1991; Kyle *et al.* 1992; Sakurai and Young 1992). Currently, [^{3}H]CPP and [^{3}H]CGS 19755 seem to be the ligands of choice for screening compounds in the search for yet higher affinity antagonists with improved *in vivo* activity. However, with a K_D of 7 nM, [^{3}H]CGP 39653 (Sills *et al.* 1991) appears suitable for use in a standard filtration assay in contrast to the centrifugation assays used for the other two antagonist ligands, thereby increasing sample throughput. An interesting recent modification described for [^{3}H]CGP 39653 and found particularly useful in autoradiographic experiments has been the inclusion of glutamate dehydrogenase to minimize the concentration of free (S)-glutamate during incubations (Jaarsma *et al.* 1993).

Structural requirements for binding to NMDA receptors

Due to the receptor-specific agonist action of even high concentrations of NMDA it has been relatively easy using *in vitro* preparations of CNS tissue to make quantitative measurements of dose-ratios for antagonism of NMDA-induced responses, enabling K_D values of competitive antagonists to be calculated for the NMDA receptor (Watkins and Evans 1981; Evans *et al.*, 1982a; Koerner and Cotman 1982; Jones *et al.*, 1984; Harrison and Simmonds 1985). Comparable data for agonists from electrophysiological studies were not then available. Structure–activity data for antagonists from electrophysiological experiments were therefore available prior to the advent of radioligand binding studies with NMDA receptors. Although this type of work is still used to estimate K_D values for antagonists (Burton *et al.* 1988; Lodge *et al.* 1988; Grimwood *et al.* 1991; Müller *et al.* 1992; Ornstein *et al.* 1993) the more common approach in drug development is first to determine the affinity of agonists and antagonists in membrane binding assays and to combine this with estimates of *in vivo* activity usually using one of a number of convulsant or anticonvulsant models for agonists and antagonists respectively. A full pharmacological characterization may subsequently be carried out.

It should be emphasized that for screening purposes most membrane radioligand binding studies use membranes prepared from rat cerebral cortex or forebrain and therefore the SAR data described relate to the population(s) of NMDA receptors present in those brain areas. It is now clear that there are multiple subtypes of NMDA receptor possibly showing heterogeneity in function. In common with other ligand-gated ion channel receptors, they are heteromeric assemblies comprising possibly five sub-units. In rat brain there are two types of subunit, NMDAR1 and NMDAR2. NMDAR1, which has seven isoforms (1A–1G) generated by alternative splicing, is the principal subunit and seems necessary for a functional NMDA receptor. It is expressed by almost all neurones in the CNS. Four subtypes of NMDAR2 (2A–2D) are encoded by different genes each having a distinct CNS distribution. NMDAR2A is predominantly expressed in cerebral cortex and hippocampus and NMDAR2B in the forebrain whereas NMDAR2C and NMDAR2D predominate in the cerebellum and in the diencephalic and lower brain stem regions respectively (Nakanishi 1992; see also Chapter 5). The subunit composition of native NMDA receptors subtypes is not yet known; however, it seems that the NMDAR2 subunit has a dominant role in determining the pharmacological profile of NMDA receptors present in particular brain areas (Nakanishi 1992).

The original evidence for NMDA receptor heterogeneity was from electrophysiological studies based on regional variation in the CNS of the potency of the NMDA receptor agonist quinolinate (Stone and Burton 1988). This has been confirmed and substantially extended particularly in membrane ligand binding and autoradiographic studies, the variation in pharmacology showing a good correlation with the anatomical localization of individual NMDAR2 subunits (see Chapter 6). Although agonists and antagonists currently vary only in their relative potencies for the different subtypes it might reasonably be expected that NMDA subtype-specific agents will eventually become available with a concomitant therapeutic advantage.

The principal features of the differences between the structural require-ments for agonists and those for antagonists can be most easily demon-strated by considering compounds separately in two groups, firstly com-pounds with the same interacidic chain length as glutamate and aspartate, the majority of these agents being NMDA agonists (Tables 2.1–2.4), and secondly compounds with an interacidic chain length greater than that of glutamate, within which series most of the NMDA antagonists are found (Tables 2.5 and 2.6). The tables give typical values only, designed to illustrate particular structure-activity features, and are not intended to list all values in the literature, some of which are at minor variance with one another. Where possible, values for standard (reference) compounds are given for any set of substances listed in order that comparison can be made between studies from different laboratories.

NMDA receptor agonists

ω-Substituted glutamate and aspartate analogues (Table 2.1)

The first feature to be emphasized for both agonist and antagonist action is that substances lacking the amino or one or both of the acidic groups are inactive (Olverman *et al.* 1988*a*), indicating the necessity for the three ionizable groups, consistent with the 'three point receptor' or pharmacophore of Curtis and Watkins (1960). An α-carboxyl may also be necessary for optimal agonist action since the α-phosphono analogue of glutamate has low NMDA receptor affinity (Table 2.1); however, other modifications of the α-acidic group have not yet been tested.

High affinity NMDA receptor agonists have an optimal separation of the two acidic groups of either two (aspartate length) or three (glutamate length) atoms, although some (S) isomers of longer chain compounds including α-aminoadipate, α-aminopimelate, α-aminosuberate and β-*N*-oxalyl-α,β-diaminopropionate (β-ODAP) (Table 2.5; compounds, 2, 4, 6, and 35) are NMDA receptor agonists with moderate affinity. Of the simple, open chain, unsubstituted agonist amino acids, (S)-glutamate has the highest affinity and (S)- and (R)-glutamate show the widest enantiomeric difference. In addition, (S) isomers of agonist analogues of glutamate chain length are more active than the corresponding analogues of aspartate chain length. Lower enantiomeric differences are shown by the optical isomers of aspartate, and by those of the sulphur-containing analogues of glutamate and aspartate. The rank order for the effectiveness of the ω-acidic group is different for 'aspartate-length' and 'glutamate-length' compounds. For 'aspartate-length' compounds, irrespective of the stereochemistry, the order is: CO_2H and SO_2H > SO_3H > PO_3H_2. For 'glutamate-length' compounds, the order for the stereochemical series corresponding to (S)-glutamate is CO_2H > SO_2H and SO_3H ≫ PO_3H_2, and that for the series corresponding to (R)-glutamate is SO_2H and SO_3H > CO_2H ≫ PO_3H_2[1]. For analogues of (S)-homocysteate at least, a carbon in the chain can be replaced by either sulphur or oxygen with retention of high or moderate activity, respectively. Replacement of carbon by sulphur in (R)-homocysteate was, however, detrimental to activity. Unlike the other short chain compounds, peak activity in the (R) series of α,ω-dicarboxylates is

---

[1] The series corresponding to (S)-glutamate contains the (R)-form of S-sulphocysteine and the series corresponding to (R)-glutamate contains the (S) form of S-sulphocysteine (see footnote 4, Table 2.1).

Table 2.1 Primary open chain glutamate and aspartate analogues: K_i values for NMDA receptors

General formula:

$$\begin{array}{c} H_2N \\ \diagdown \\ CH\text{--}Y\text{--}X \\ \diagup \\ HO_2C \end{array}$$

Compound	Y	$K_i(\mu M)$ (R)	(S)	(RS)
X = H				
Glycine[*,1]	–			
Serine[1]	CH_2O			
X = CO_2H				
Aminomalonate[*]	–			(160)
Aspartate	CH_2	10	11	
Glutamate	$(CH_2)_2$	49	0.9	
Glutamate, α-phosphono analogue[2]	$(CH_2)_2$			>1000
X = SO_2H				
Cysteine sulphinate[4]	CH_2	13	23	
Homocysteine sulphinate	$(CH_2)_2$	6.3	10	
X = SO_3H				
Cysteate[4]	CH_2	120	170	
Homocysteate	$(CH_2)_2$	11	3.9	
S-Sulphocysteine[4]	CH_2S	2.1	86	
O-Sulphoserine	CH_2O		17	
X = PO_2H_2	CH_2			35[3]
	$(CH_2)_2$			8[3]
X = PO_3H_2				
AP3	CH_2			560[b]
AP4	$(CH_2)_2$	250[a]	510	
O-Phosphoserine[1]	CH_2O		>1000	

All compounds have agonist action or little effect in electrophysiological experiments except those indicated with the superscripts a (antagonist) or b (weak agonist/antagonist).

[*] Indicates one form only. Data unless otherwise indicated are for inhibition of [³H]D-AP5 binding taken from Olverman et al. (1988a).

[1] Using [³H]D-AP5 and [³H]CPP binding to rat cerebral cortical membranes in microcentrifugation assays, glycine and (R)-serine inhibited binding of [³H]D-AP5 maximally by 50–60 per cent but whereas (R)-serine had no effect on [³H]CPP binding, glycine potentiated binding by about 20 per cent. EC_{50} values for these effects were about 300 nM for both glycine and (R)-serine and reflect interconversion between 'antagonist preferring' and 'agonist preferring' forms of NMDA receptors mediated through the glycine site (Monaghan et al. 1988; Olverman and Watkins 1989; D. T. Monaghan, C. W. Cotman, H. J. Olverman, and J. C. Watkins, unpublished observations). In contrast, inhibition of [³H]D-AP5 by (R)-O-phosphoserine was biphasic; IC_{50} values for the high (60%) and low (40%) affinity components were about 0.5 μM and 300 μM respectively. (R)-O-Phosphoserine had no effect on [³H]CPP binding at low concentrations but showed monophasic inhibition at higher concentrations (IC_{50} value, 300 μM); inhibition of [³H]CPP binding and the low affinity component of inhibition of [³H]D-AP5 binding may be a direct effect whereas the high affinity component of inhibition of [³H]D-AP5 binding may be mediated via the NMDA glycine site (H. J. Olverman and J. C. Watkins, unpublished observations).

[2] Formula for glutamate, α-phosphono analogue is $H_2O_3P\text{-}CH(NH_2)\text{-}(CH_2)_2\text{-}CO_2H$.

[3] Values are taken or calculated from studies by Fagg and Baud (1988) using [³H]L-glutamate; reference substances are (S)-glutamate ($K_i = 0.2$ μM) and NMDA ($K_i = 5.3$ μM).

[4] For these amino acids the L form in old nomenclature corresponds to the (R) form, and likewise the D form to the (S) form.

Table 2.2 N-Alkylated glutamate and aspartate analogues: K_i values for NMDA receptors

General formula:

$$\underset{HO_2C}{\overset{RNH}{\diagdown}}CH\text{--}CH_2X$$

Compound	R	X	$K_i(\mu M)$ (R)	(S)	(RS)
Aspartate	H	CO_2H	10	11	
N-Methylaspartate	CH_3	CO_2H	11	160	
N-Iminomethylaspartate	$HN{=}CH$	CO_2H	28		
N-Ethylaspartate	C_2H_5	CO_2H	100	710	
N-n-Propylaspartate	$n\text{-}C_3H_7$	CO_2H	180	560	
N-Allylaspartate	$CH_2{=}CH\text{-}CH_2$	CO_2H			140
N-n-Butylaspartate	$n\text{-}C_4H_9$	CO_2H	92		
Cysteine sulphinate[1]	H	SO_2H	13	23	
N-Methylcysteine sulphinate[1]	CH_3	SO_2H	250		140
Cysteate[1]	H	SO_3H	120	170	
N-Methylcysteate[1]	CH_3	SO_3H	630		500
Glutamate	H	CH_2CO_2H	49	0.9	
N-Methylglutamate	CH_3	CH_2CO_2H	800	210	
N-Ethylglutamate	C_2H_5	CH_2CO_2H	>1000	250	
Homocysteate	H	CH_2SO_3H	11	3.9	
N-Methylhomocysteate	CH_3	CH_2SO_3H			890

All compounds have agonist action or little effect in electrophysiological experiments. Data are for inhibition of [³H]D-AP5 binding taken from Olverman *et al.* (1988a).
[1] See foonote 4 Table 2.1.

found with (R)-aspartate, with the first of the two antagonist peaks of activity in its second higher homologue, (R)-α-aminoadipate (Table 2.5, compound 1). Thus the lower activity of (R)-glutamate presumably reflects the transition from the structure necessary to allow the appropriate conformation for agonist action to that required for antagonist action. It would appear that at the ω-terminus a single negative charge is more important than the size of the acidic group for NMDA agonist activity since a homologous series of (RS)-ω-phosphino-α-aminocarboxylates showed a pattern of inhibition of [³H]L-glutamate binding similar to that of the (S)-α,ω-dicarboxylates. The glutamate and aspartate ω-phosphino analogues with about 10-fold lower affinity than glutamate and aspartate (Table 2.1) showed agonist activity in electrophysiological experiments in contrast to the weak NMDA antagonist properties of (RS)-AP3 and (R)-AP4 (Fagg and Baud 1988).

Table 2.3 Chain-substituted glutamate and aspartate analogues: K_i values for NMDA receptors

General formula:

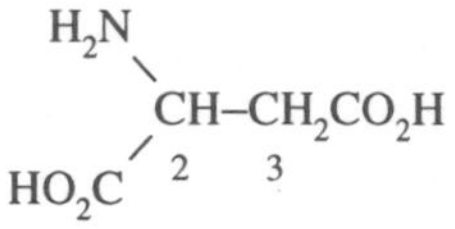

$$H_2N\diagdown$$
$$CH–CH_2CO_2H$$
$$HO_2C\diagup \quad 2 \quad 3$$

Aspartic acid

$$H_2N\diagdown$$
$$CH–CH_2CH_2CO_2H$$
$$HO_2C\diagup \quad 2 \quad 3 \quad 4$$

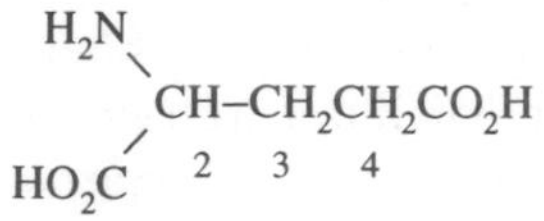

Glutamic acid

Compound	$K_i(\mu M)$		
	(R)	(S)	(RS)
Aspartate	10	11	
2-Methylaspartate			>1000
3-Methylaspartate			42
Threo-3-hydroxyaspartate	44	420	
Glutamate	49	0.9	
2-Methylglutamate			>1000
3-Methylglutamate			810
4-Methylglutamate			7.9
3-Hydroxyglutamate			50
4-Hydroxyglutamate			8.5
4-Methyleneglutamate		2.8	4.7
4-Fluoroglutamate			3.2
4-Aminoglutamate			31
4-Carboxyglutamate			630

All compounds have agonist action in electrophysiological experiments. Data are for inhibition of [^{3}H]D-AP5 binding taken from Olverman *et al.* (1988*a*).

Open chain *N*-alkylated glutamate and aspartate analogues (Table 2.2)

Alkylation of the primary amino group of agonists with a glutamate or aspartate chain length was generally detrimental to the activity of all these compounds except in the case of *N*-methylation of (R)-aspartate, NMDA having the same affinity as the parent compound. The detrimental effect increases in all cases with increase in the size of the *N*-alkyl substituent with moderate activity in addition to NMDA being retained only by *N*-imino-methyl-(R)-aspartate.

Open chain glutamate and aspartate with substituents on the inter-acidic group chain (Table 2.3)

For the majority of the compounds data are available only for unresolved (RS) stereoisomeric mixtures although the activity of (S)-4-methylene-glutamate, compared with that of the (RS) form and of both (R)-and (S)-glutamate, would perhaps indicate that for glutamate analogues the (S) form is the more active isomer. This may not be true for aspartate analogues since, as with *N*-methylation, a 3-hydroxy substitution is less detrimental to activity for (R)-aspartate than for (S)-aspartate. However, it is clear that a 2-methyl group in the case of aspartate or a 2- or 3-methyl group for glutamate is highly detrimental to affinity. 3-Methylaspartate and 4-methylglutamate (where the methyl group has been substituted on the carbon next to the ω-carboxyl) retained high activity, the loss of activity for both compounds relative to unsubstituted aspartate and glutamate being about the same for both substances. For glutamate, other acceptable substitutions on the 4-position were hydroxyl, methylene, fluoro, and amino but not carboxyl.

Cyclic glutamate and aspartate analogues (Table 2.4)

Figure 2.3 shows the structures of a range of cyclic glutamate and aspartate analogues which are potent and selective NMDA receptor agonists. Firstly, the compounds have been used to give valuable information regarding the steric requirements and the spatial orientation of the three ionizable groups which either promote or hinder agonist binding. Secondly, they have been used to deduce the structural features required for agonist action at NMDA rather than non-NMDA receptors when used in conjunction with other structural analogues (Watkins *et al.* 1991; Krogsgaard-Larsen *et al.* 1992; Kyle *et al.* 1992; Shinozaki 1992*a*). As is discussed in detail in a later section, some have also been used to try to determine if high agonist affinity is directly related to excitotoxic action or if other structural features promoting interaction within an 'excitotoxic pocket' of the NMDA receptor are also necessary.

(RS)-TetGly has twice the affinity of (S)-glutamate (Table 2.4, compound 1) for the NMDA receptor and hence is a powerful NMDA agonist with potent convulsant and neurotoxic actions (Schoepp *et al.* 1991*a*; Lunn *et al.* 1992). Although (RS)-TetGly is nominally an aminomalonate analogue, because the negative charge is delocalized throughout the tetrazole ring with the electron density centred on N-2/N-3 (Lunn *et al.* 1992), it probably represents an aspartate analogue (or possibly a folded glutamate analogue), the tetrazole group acting as an isosteric replacement for CH_2-CO_2H (or for a group intermediate in chain length between CH_2-CO_2H and $(CH_2)_2$-CO_2H) rather than a simple ω-carboxyl group. Of the higher homologues, although ω-tetrazole-substituted aspartate and glutamate appear to have lower affinity, somewhat surprisingly only the (S) isomer of the glutamate-substituted compound had agonist activity with about half the potency of NMDA (Table 2.6, compounds 1–4; Ornstein *et al.* 1993). Indeed, the distinct lack of correlation of binding and functional data for these compounds compared with those of reference compounds might suggest that they are either partial agonists or substrates for an amino acid transport mechanism. Highly selective NMDA receptor agonist action is shown by two other aspartate analogues (R)-MNT 950A and (RS)-AMAA,

Table 2.4 Cyclic glutamate and aspartate analogues: binding data for NMDA receptors

No. Acronym	[³H]L-glutamate	[³H]D-AP5	[³H]CGS 19755	[³H]CPP
1 (RS)-TetGly			0.098	
2 *trans*-ACBD[6]	0.11		0.163	
NMDA reference substance			4.15[1]	
(S)-Glu reference substance			0.172[1]	
(S)-Asp reference substance			1.638[1]	
3 (RS)-AMAA	0.79			
4 (RS)-Ibotenate	1.34	16		
5 *trans*-ACPD[6,7]	3.94	13		
6 *cis*-ACBD[6]	8.8			
7 4-HPCA	32			
8 Quinolinate	>100	230		
9 *cis*-ACPD[6,8]	>100			
NMDA reference substance	2.15[2]			
10 (2S,3R,4S)-CCG				0.019
11 (2R,3S,4R)-CCG	0.055			0.215
12 (2R,3S,4S)-CCG	2.8			0.412
NMDA reference substance				15.0[3]
(S)-Glu reference substance	0.036[9]			0.327[3]
13 *trans*-(2RS,3SR)-CPAA[4]				
14 (R)-MNT 950A				8.3
NMDA reference substance				14.0[5]
(S)-Glu reference substance				0.98[5]
15 *trans*-(2RS,3RS)-PDA		30		
16 *cis*-(2RS,3SR)-PDA		46		36
17 *cis*-(2R,3S)-PDA		21		
18 *cis*-(2S,3R)-PDA		>1000		
19 *trans*-(2RS,4RS)-PDA		70		
20 *cis*-(2RS,4SR)-PDA		540		
21 Homoquinolinate		7.1		6.8

Values are Ki or IC$_{50}$ (in μM). For structures of the potent NMDA agonists see Fig. 2.3. Binding data for [³H]D-AP5 ([³H]CPP) for other compounds of interest are: (S)-kainate, 810 μM (280 μM); (S)-quisqualate, 170 μM (81 μM); α-amino-3-hydroxy-5-methylisoxazole-4-propionate (AMPA), 1 mM (1 mM); willardiine, no effect; 5-bromowillardiine, > 1 mM; N-acetyl-α-(S)-aspartyl-(S)-glutamate (NAAG), 410 μM; structures for these compounds are shown in Olverman *et al.* (1988*a*). Data for [³H]D-AP5 and some of the [³H]CPP data are taken from Olverman *et al.* (1988*a*) and H. J. Olverman and J. C. Watkins, unpublished observations.
[1] Refers to studies by Lunn *et al.* (1992); reference substances for compounds 1 and 2.
[2] Refers to studies by Kyle *et al.* (1992); reference substance for compounds 2–9.
[3] Refers to studies by Kawai *et al.* (1992); reference substances for compounds 10–12.
[4] Binding data not available. For agonist-evoked [³H]acetylcholine release from striatal slices, *trans*-(2RS,3SR)-CPAA had an EC$_{50}$ of 45.8 μM compared with 20 μM for NMDA (Tsai *et al.* 1988).
[5] Refers to studies by Iwama *et al.* (1991); reference substances for compound 14.
[6] *cis* and *trans* used according to IUPAC nomenclature; this is opposite to the usage of the terms in most of the pharmacological literature (Schoepp *et al.* 1991*b*).
[7] Equimolecular mixture of (1R,3R) and (1S,3S) isomers.
[8] Equimolecular mixture of (1S,3R) and (1R,3S) isomers.
[9] Refers to studies by Monahan *et al.* (1990); reference substance for compounds 11 and 12.

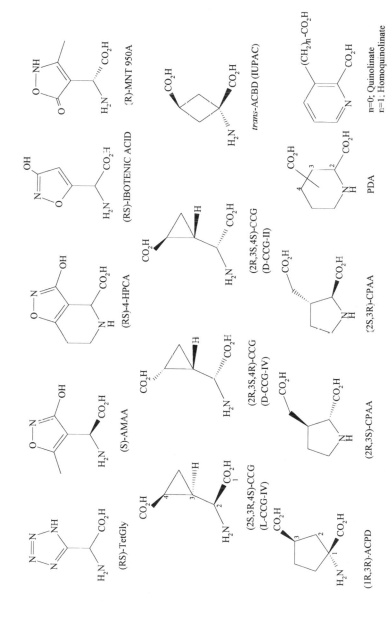

Fig. 2.3 Structures of potent NMDA agonists. Abbreviations: (RS)-TetGly, (RS)-tetrazol-5-ylglycine; (S)-AMAA, (S)-2-amino-2-(3-hydroxy-5-methylisoxazol-4-yl)acetic acid; (RS)-4-HPCA, (RS)-3-hydroxy-4,5,6,7-tetrahydroisoxazol[4,5-c]pyridine-4-carboxylic acid; (R)-MNT 950A, (R)-2-amino-2-(2,5-dihydro-3-methyl-5-oxo-4-isoxazolyl)acetic acid; CCG, 2-(carboxycyclopropyl)glycine; ACPD, 1-aminocyclobutane-1,3-dicarboxylic acid; ACPD, 1-aminocyclopentane-1,3-dicarboxylic acid; CPAA, (2-carboxypyrrolidin-3-yl)acetic acid; PDA, piperidine dicarboxylic acid.

Table 2.5 Structure–activity relations of NMDA receptor antagonists

I. Open chain antagonists

General formula:

$$\underset{HO_2C}{\overset{H_2N}{>}}CH-M-X$$

No.	Acronym	A	M	X	*	K_D^1	$K_i\ (\mu M)^2$			
							Lig1	Lig2	Lig3	Lig4
1	D-αAA		(CH₂)₃	CO₂H	R	42	13			
2	L-αAA		(CH₂)₃	CO₂H	S	ag[3]	89			
3	D-αAP		(CH₂)₄	CO₂H	R	100	84			
4	L-αAP		(CH₂)₄	CO₂H	S	ag	77			
5	D-αAS		(CH₂)₅	CO₂H	R	16	25			
6	L-αAS		(CH₂)₅	CO₂H	S	ag	80			
7	DL-αAO		(CH₂)₆	CO₂H	R,S	>1000				
8	D-AP4		(CH₂)₂	PO₃H₂	R	260	250			
9	L-AP4		(CH₂)₂	PO₃H₂	S	ag	510			
10	DL-AP5		(CH₂)₃	PO₃H₂	R,S	1.4				
11	D-AP5		(CH₂)₃	PO₃H₂	R	0.7	0.62			
12	L-AP5		(CH₂)₃	PO₃H₂	S	22	40			
13	DL-AP6		(CH₂)₄	PO₃H₂	R,S	600	42			
14	DL-AP7		(CH₂)₅	PO₃H₂	R,S	3.1				
15	D-AP7		(CH₂)₅	PO₃H₂	R	1.7				
16	L-AP7		(CH₂)₅	PO₃H₂	S		28			
17	DL-AP7	reference substance	(CH₂)₄CF₂	PO₃H₂	R,S			27		
18	DL-AP8		(CH₂)₆	PO₃H₂	R,S	1000	640	0.8[4a]		
19	DL-AS5		(CH₂)₃	SO₃H	R,S		140			
20	DL-AS6		(CH₂)₄	SO₃H	R,S		950			
21	DL-AS7		(CH₂)₅	SO₃H	R,S		520			
22	DAA		(CH₂)₂-CH(NH₂)	CO₂H	2RS,5RS	420				
23	DAP		(CH₂)₃-CH(NH₂)	CO₂H	2RS,6RS	120				
24	DD-DAP		(CH₂)₃-CH(NH₂)	CO₂H	2R,6R	30				
25	DAS		(CH₂)₄-CH(NH₂)	CO₂H	2RS,7RS	200				

No.	Compound	Bridge	Acid	Config.		
26	β-D-AspGly	CH₂-CO-NH-CH₂	CO_2H	R	29	
27	β-D-Asp-β-Ala	CH₂-CO-NH-(CH₂)₂	CO_2H	R	66	
28	γ-DGG	(CH₂)₂-CO-NH-CH₂	CO_2H	R	19	41
29	γ-LGG	(CH₂)₂-CO-NH-CH₂	CO_2H	S	147	71
30	γ-D-GluSar	(CH₂)₂-CO-N(CH₃)-CH₂	CO_2H	R	5	
31	N-Phe-γ-DGG	(CH₂)₂-CO-N(Ph)-CH₂	CO_2H	R	12	
32	γ-DG-PheGly	(CH₂)₂-CO-NH-CH(Ph)	CO_2H	R	52	
33	β-D-Asp-AMP	CH₂-CO-NH-CH₂	PO_3H_2	R	4.4	2.8
34	γ-D-Glu-AMP	(CH₂)₂-CO-NH-CH₂	PO_3H_2	R	16	25
35	β-L-ODAP	CH₂-NH-CO	CO_2H	S	ag	130
36	β-D-ODAP	CH₂-NH-CO	CO_2H	R	41	
37	γ-L-ODAB	(CH₂)₂-NH-CO	CO_2H	S	7	
38	γ-L-ODAB	(CH₂)₂-NH-CO	CO_2H	S	33	
39	δ-D-Ox-Orn	(CH₂)₃-NH-CO	CO_2H	R	10	
40	ε-D-Ox-Lys	(CH₂)₄-NH-CO	CO_2H	R	20	
41	HSOP	(CH₂)₂-O	PO_3H_2	R,S	250	
42		CH₂-NH-CH₂	PO_3H_2	R,S	4.3[4b]	
43		CH₂-CH(OH)CH₂	PO_3H_2	2RS,4RS	0.13	
44		CH₂-CH(NH₂)CH₂	PO_3H_2	2RS,4RS	1.44	
45		CH₂-CH(NH₂)(CH₂)₃	PO_3H_2	2RS,4RS	2.27	
58	CPP reference substance			R,S	0.028[5]	
46	CGS 19755 reference substance			2RS,4SR	0.02≤[5]	

II. Heterocyclic antagonists

General formula:

No.	Compound	M-X		A	R	Config.		
46	CGS 19755	CH		CH₂	PO_3H_2	2RS,4SR	0.183	0.032
47	trans-19755	CH		CH₂	PO_3H_2	2RS,4RS		0.452
48	N-Me-19755	CH	N-Me	CH₂	PO_3H_2	2RS,4SR		28
49	3-Me-19755	CH	3-Me	CH₂	PO_3H_2	(±)		1.3

Table 2.5 (*contd.*)

II. Heterocyclic antagonists

No.	Acronym	A	M	X	R	*	K_i (µM)[2] Lig1	Lig2	Lig3
50	5-Me-19755	CH	CH_2	PO_3H_2	5-Me	(±)			0.078
51	6-Me-19755	CH	CH_2	PO_3H_2	6-Me	(±)			1.6
52	α-Me-19755	CH	CH(Me)	PO_3H_2		(±)			0.8
53	α,α-DM-19755	CH	$C(Me)_2$	PO_3H_2					1.3
54	cis-CPPP	CH	$(CH_2)_3$	PO_3H_2		2RS,4SR		0.179	0.098
55	trans-CPPP	CH	$(CH_2)_3$	PO_3H_2		2RS,4RS			0.105
56	CPMPz[30]	N	CH_2	PO_3H_2		R,S			
57	CPEPz	N	$(CH_2)_2$	PO_3H_2		R,S		0.32	
58	CPP	N	$(CH_2)_3$	PO_3H_2		R,S	0.48	30	0.22
59	D-CPP	N	$(CH_2)_3$	PO_3H_2		R		0.28	
60	L-CPP	N	$(CH_2)_3$	PO_3H_2		S		0.14	
61	cis-LY 233053	CH	CH_2	tetrazole		2RS,4SR		2.3	0.107[31]
62	trans-LY 233053	CH	CH_2	tetrazole		2RS,4RS			0.777
63	cis	CH	$(CH_2)_2$	tetrazole		2RS,4SR			2.28
64	cis	CH	$(CH_2)_3$	tetrazole		2RS,4SR			5.83
65		CH	CH_2	tetrazole		2R,4S			0.067[31]
66		CH	CH_2	tetrazole		2S,4R			2.39[31]
46	CGS 19755 (reference substance)					2RS,4SR			0.054[32]
67		N	CH_2	CO_2H		R,S		16	
68		N	$(CH_2)_3$	$PO_2(Me)H$		R,S		0.78	
69		N	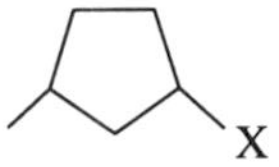 -CH(Ph)	PO_3H_2		(±)		1.6[26]	
70	CGS 19755 (reference substance)	N		PO_3H_2		(±)		5.8	
46	(reference substance)					2RS,4SR		0.065[6]	0.069
71	cis	CH_2			$3\text{-}(CO)CH_2PO_3H_2$	2RS,3SR		0.068[8]	
72	trans	CH_2			$3\text{-}(CO)CH_2PO_3H_2$	2RS,3RS		0.533[8]	
73	cis-MDL100, 925	CH_2			$3\text{-}(CO)CH_2PO_3H_2$	2R,3S		0.040[8]	0.064
74	cis	CH_2			$3\text{-}CH(OH)CH_2PO_3H_2$	(±)			0.106

(Structural formula shown in the M column: a cyclopentane ring bearing an X substituent.)

No.	Name	X / substituent	Stereochem.		
46	CGS 19755	reference substance			
75	SC 48981	5-PO$_3$H$_2$	2RS,4SR R,S	0.82	0.040[7]
76		5-CH$_2$PO$_3$H$_2$	R,S	1.95	
77	PD 134705	5-(CH$_2$)$_2$PO$_3$H$_2$	R,S	0.27	
78	LY 246308	6-CH$_2$PO$_3$H$_2$	R,S	4.08	13.81
79		5-(CH$_2$)$_2$CO$_2$H	R,S	14.5	
80	LY 246811	6-(CH$_2$)[tetrazole]	R,S		26.4
81		7-PO$_3$H$_2$	R,S	1.9	
46	CGS 19755	reference substance			
82	LY 274614	PO$_3$H$_2$	3SR,4aRS,6SR,8aRS	0.055	0.054[9]
83	LY 233536	tetrazole	3SR,4aRS,6SR,8aRS	0.856	
84	LY 285720	CO$_2$H	3SR,4aRS,6SR,8aRS	4.298	
85	LY 266845	PO$_3$H$_2$	3RS,4aSR,6SR,8aSR	0.815	
86	LY 247738	tetrazole	3RS,4aSR,6SR,8aSR	3.38	
87	LY 285719	CO$_2$H	3RS,4aSR,5SR,8aSR	77.92	

Table 2.5 (*contd.*)

II. Heterocyclic antagonists

No.	Acronym	Structure	X	*	K_i $(\mu M)^2$ Lig1	Lig2	Lig3
88	LY 215827		PO$_3$H$_2$	3RS,4aRS,6SR,8aRS		3.557	
89	LY 262294		tetrazole	3RS,4aRS,6SR,8aRS		>10	
90	LY 266506		PO$_3$H$_2$	3SR,4aRS,6SR,8aRS		>10	
91	LY 266505		tetrazole	3SR,4aRS,6SR,8aRS		>10	
92	LY 274827		PO$_3$H$_2$	1SR,4aSR,6RS,8aSR		4.870	
93	LY 209795		tetrazole	1SR,4aSR,6RS,8aSR		2.480	
94	LY 247251		PO$_3$H$_2$	3SR,6SR,8aSR		2.150	
95	LY 202794		tetrazole	3SR,6SR,8aSR		11.470	

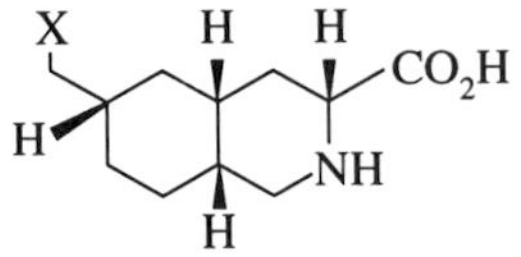

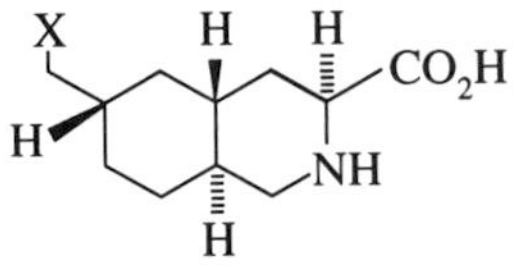

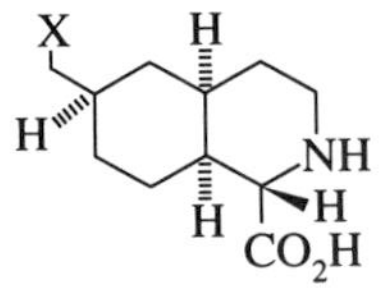

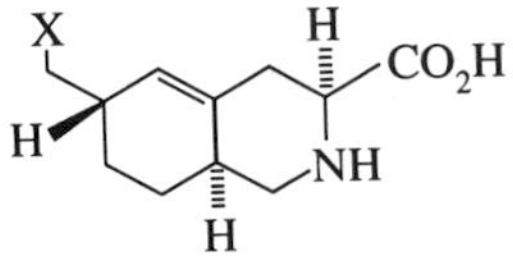

No.	Structure	X	Config.	Activity
96	decahydroisoquinoline-type structure (X, CO$_2$H)	PO$_3$H$_2$	(±)	>10
97		tetrazole	(±)	>10[10]
98	decahydroisoquinoline structure (NH, CO$_2$H, X)	PO$_3$H$_2$	(±)	5.6
99	benzo-fused structure (X, CO$_2$H)	PO$_3$H$_2$	(±)	0.85
100	decahydroquinoline structure (X, CO$_2$H)	CH$_2$PO$_3$H$_2$	(±)	9.2
101		(CH$_2$)$_2$PO$_3$H$_2$	(±)	100
46	CGS 19755 — reference substance		2RS,4SR	0.054[9]
102	pyrimidine structure (X, CO$_2$H)	CH$_2$PO$_3$H$_2$	(±)	5.95
103		(CH$_2$)$_3$PO$_3$H$_2$	(±)	0.42
104	pyridine structure (X, Me, CO$_2$H)	PO$_3$H$_2$		10

Table 2.5 (contd.)

III. Substituted phenylglycine and phenylalanine antagonists

General formula:

No.	Acronym	n	R^1	R^2	R^3	R^4	R^5	*	pA_2[11]	K_i (μM)[2]			
										Lig1	Lig2	Lig3	Lig4
105	m-CPG	0	H	CO_2H	H	H	H	R,S		56			
106	D-m-CPG	0	H	CO_2H	H	H	H	R		25			
107	m-PPG	0	H	PO_3H_2	H	H	H	R,S			17		
108	m-PMPG	0	H	$CH_2PO_3H_2$	H	H	H	R,S			9.3		
109		0	H	$CH_2PO_3H_2$	H	Ph	H	R,S			50[12b]		
110	m-PEPG	0	H	$(CH_2)_2PO_3H_2$	H	H	H	R,S			>100		
111	p-PPG	0	H	H	PO_3H_2	H	H	R,S			>100		
112	PD 129635	0	H	H	$CH_2PO_3H_2$	H	H	R,S			1.0		
113	o-PPG	0	PO_3H_2	H	H	H	H	R,S			>100		
114	NPC451	1	$(CH_2)_2PO_3H_2$	H	H	H	H	R,S			61		
115	m-PPA	1	H	PO_3H_2	H	H	H	R,S			>100		
116	m-PMPA	1	H	$CH_2PO_3H_2$	H	H	H	R,S	4.94		3.3		
117	SDZ EAB515	1	H	$CH_2PO_3H_2$	H	Ph	H	S	6.94				0.2
118		1	H	$CH_2PO_3H_2$	H	Ph	H	R	4.77				15.85
119		1	H	$CH_2PO_3H_2$	H	Ph	H	R,S	6.64				
120		1	H	$CH_2PO_3H_2$	H	4-Cl-Ph	H	R,S	6.76				
121		1	H	$CH_2PO_3H_2$	H	4-F-Ph	H	S	6.94				
122		1	H	$CH_2PO_3H_2$	H	4-F-Ph	H	R	4.90				
123		1	H	$CH_2PO_3H_2$	H	4-(t-Bu)Ph	H	R,S	7.62				
124		1	H	$CH_2PO_3H_2$	H	4-Ph-Ph	H	S	7.77				
125		1	H	$CH_2PO_3H_2$	H	$3-NH_2-Ph$	H	S	6.57				
126	(S)-m-PMPA	1	H	$CH_2PO_3H_2$	H	H	H	S	5.31				3.2
127	(R)-m-PMPA	1	H	$CH_2PO_3H_2$	H	H	H	R	<3.7				79.4

No.	Acronym	n		R	*			config			K_i (μM)[2]	
15	D-AP7	reference substance						R	5.3			0.79[12a]
16	L-AP7	reference substance						S	4.28			2.6[12a]
128	p-PPA	1	H		H	H		R,S	>100			
129	p-PMPA	1	H		H	H		R,S	>100			
14	DL-AP7	reference substance	PO_3H_2					R,S	3.1[13]	0.80[14]		
58	DL-CPP	reference substance	$CH_2PO_3H_2$					R,S	0.48[13]	0.08[14]		
130	NPC 12626 (saturated ring)	1	$(CH_2)_2PO_3H_2$		H	H		(±)	0.172	0.976		
58	DL-CPP	reference substance						R,S	0.15[15a]			
59	D-CPP	reference substance						R	0.116[15b]			

IV. Thiophene and furan antagonists

General formula:

No.	Acronym	X	*	K_i (μM)[2]			
				Lig1	Lig2	Lig3	Lig4
131		S	R,S		0.66[16]		
132		O	R,S		5.9[16]		

V. N-substituted-glycine antagonists

No.	Acronym	Structure	n	m	Substituent	X	R	K_i (μM)[2]			
								Lig1	Lig2	Lig3	Lig4
133		$(CH_2)_m$–PO_3H_2	0	0 (CO_2H)	o				4.0		
134		$(CH_2)_n$–NH–CH_2CO_2H	1	1	m				2.4		
135			2	1	m				13.7		
136			1	1	p				2.3		

Table 2.5 (contd.)

V. N-substituted-glycine antagonists

No.	Acronym	Structure	Substituent	n	m	X	R	K_i (µM)[2]			
								Lig1	Lig2	Lig3	Lig4
137				1	1	CH=CH(E)	H		1.0		
138				1	1	CH=CH(E)	CH$_3$		42.4		
139				2	0	CH=CH(Z,E)	H		2.25		
140									1.2[26]		
10	AP5		reference substance						0.29[17]		
14	AP7		reference substance						0.77[17]		
58	CPP		reference substance						0.079[17]		
46	CGS 19755		reference substance						0.065[17]		

Structure (137–139):

$$X \diagdown (CH_2)_m-PO_3H_2$$
$$X \diagup (CH_2)_n-\underset{H}{N}-\underset{R}{C}HCO_2H$$

Structure (140):

$$\underset{H}{N}\!-\!CH_2\!-\!CO_2H,\ \ CH=CH\!-\!PO_3H_2$$

VI. Cyclopropyl antagonists

General formula:

$$\begin{array}{c} R^1 \diagdown \triangle \diagup R^3 \\ R^2 \diagup \ \ \diagdown R^4 \end{array}$$

No.	Acronym	R^1	R^2	R^3	R^4	Geometry	Stereochemistry	K_i for Lig5 (µM)[2]
141		CH(NH$_2$)CO$_2$H	H	CH$_2$PO$_3$H$_2$	H	cis	(±)	18.9

142	H	CH(NH₂)CO₂H	CH₂PO₃H₂	H	9.5	(±)
143	NH₂	CO₂H	H	(CH₂)₂PO₃H₂	18.7	(±)
144	CO₂H	NH₂	H	(CH₂)₂PO₃H₂	26.7	(±)
145	CH₂CH(NH₂)CO₂H	H	PO₃H₂	H	1.6	2R,4RS,5RS
11	D-AP5	reference substance			0.42[18]	R

VII. Chain-unsaturated antagonists

General formula:

$$H_2N-CH-M-X$$
$$HO_2C$$

No.	Acronym	A	M	X	*	K_i (μM)[2]				
						Lig1	Lig2	Lig3	Lig4	Lig5
146	D-αAA-ene[19]		(E) CH₂-CH=CH	CO₂H	R					0.39
147	trans-APPA[20]		(E) CH=CH-CH₂	PO₃H₂	R,S					
148	AP7-ene[21]		CH₂-CH=CH-(CH₂)₂	PO₃H₂	R,S					
149	CGP 37849		(E) CH=C(CH₃)-CH₂	PO₃H₂	R,S		0.035			
150	CGP 39551		(E) CH=C(CH₃)-CH₂	PO₃H₂	R,S		0.31			
	(α-Carboxyethyl ester of compound 149)[22]									
151	CGP 40116 (D-CGP 37849)				R		0.019			
152	CGP 40117 (L-CGP 37849)				S		3.2			
153	CGP 39653		(E) CH=C(nC₃H₇)-CH₂	PO₃H₂	R,S				0.007	
154			-C≡C-	PO₃H₂	R,S		0.45[26]			
155			CH₂(SO)CH₂	PO₃H₂	R,S		0.14[25]			
156	MDL 100,453		CH₂(CO)CH₂	PO₃H₂	R,S		0.109			
11	D-AP5	reference substance			R					
12	L-AP5	reference substance			S		0.26[22]			
58	DL-CPP	reference substance			R,S	4.3[22]	0.17[22]		0.106[23]	
46	CGS 19755	reference substance			2RS,4SR		0.099[24]			

Table 2.5 (contd.)

VII. Chain-unsaturated antagonists

General formula:

No.	Acronym	A	M	X	*	K_i (μM)[2]			
						Lig1	Lig2	Lig3	Lig4
157	cis-CGS-1-ene[27]	CH	(E) CH=CHCH$_2$	PO$_3$H$_2$	2RS,4SR			0.014	
158	trans-CGS-1-ene[27]	CH	(E) CH=CHCH$_2$	PO$_3$H$_2$	2RS,4RS			0.039	
159	cis-CGS-2-ene[27]	CH	(E) CH$_2$-CH=CH	PO$_3$H$_2$	2RS,4SR			0.072	
160	trans-CGS-2-ene[27]	CH	(E) CH$_2$-CH=CH	PO$_3$H$_2$	2RS,4RS			0.080[27]	
161	D-CPP-ene	N	(E) CH$_2$-CH=CH	PO$_3$H$_2$	R		0.044		
162	L-CPP-ene	N	(E) CH$_2$-CH=CH	PO$_3$H$_2$	S		0.600		
54	cis-CPPP	reference substance			2RS,4SR			0.098[28]	
55	trans-CPPP	reference substance			2RS,4RS			0.105[28]	
59	D-CPP	reference substance			R	0.14[29]			
60	L-CPP	reference substance			S	2.3[29]			

Ligand 1, [³H]D-2-amino-5-phosphonopentanoate ([³H]D-AP5); ligand 2, [³H]3-((±)-2-carboxypiperazin-4-yl)propyl-1-phosphonate ([³H]CPP); ligand 3, [³H]cis-(±)-4-phosphonomethylpiperidine-2-carboxylate ([³H]CGS 19755); ligand 4, [³H](E)-2-amino-4-phosphonomethyl-3-heptenoate ([³H]CGS 39653); ligand 5, [³H]L-glutamic acid. The column headed with an asterisk indicates the stereochemistry at the asymmetric carbon atom(s).

[1] From Evans et al. (1979), Watkins and Evans (1981), Evans et al. (1982a,b), Jones et al. (1984), Aebischer et al. (1989), and P. C.-K. Pook, D. C. Sunter, and J. C. Watkins (unpublished observations).

[2] For many compounds IC$_{50}$s were reported; however, because of the low ligand concentration used, K_i is approximately equal to IC$_{50}$. Ligands 1 and 2: Watkins and Olverman (1987), Olverman et al. (1988a), Olverman and Watkins (1989). Ligand 2: Lodge et al. (1988). Hutchison et al. (1989), Aebischer et al. (1989), Bigge et al. (1989a,b), Fagg et al. (1990), Müller et al. (1985), Hays et al. (1990a,b), Whitten et al. (1991), Hutchison et al. (1986), Herrling and Müller (1988). Ligands 2 and 3: Ortwine et al. (1992), Ferkany et al. (1989). Ligand 3: Hutchison et al. (1989), Ornstein et al. (1990, 1991, 1992b), Ornstein and Klimkowski (1992), Claesson et al. (1992). Ligand 4: Sills et al. (1991), Müller et al. (1992). Ligand 5: Dappen et al. (1991).

[3] ag: Excitatory amino acid agonist activity.

[4a] Refers to studies by Bigge et al. (1989a); reference substance for compound 17.

[4b] Refers to studies by Müller and Herrling (1985).

[5] Refers to studies by Bigge et al. (1992a); reference substances for compounds 43–45, 102, and 103.

[6] Refers to studies by Hays et al. (1990a); reference substance for compounds 56, 67, 68, and 70.

[7] Refers to studies by Claesson et al. (1992); reference substance for compounds 71, 73, 74.

[8] Refers to studies by Whitten et al. (1991); no reference substance for compounds 71, 72, and 73.

[9] Refers to studies by Ortwine et al. (1992); reference substance for compounds 75–81, 98–101, 104, and 140.

[10] Refers to studies by Ornstein and Klimkowski (1992); no reference substance given for compounds 78, 80, and 82–97.

[11] Refers to studies by Müller et al. (1992); pA₂ values for the inhibition of the NMDA-induced depolarization in the rat neocortical slice preparation.

[12a] Refers to studies by Müller et al. (1992); reference substance for compounds 117–127.

[12b] Refers to studies by Herrling and Müller (1988).

[13] Refers to studies by Olverman et al. (1988a); reference substances for compounds 105 and 106.

[14] Refers to studies on phenylglycine and phenylalanine derivatives by Bigge et al. (1989b); reference substances for compounds 107, 108, 110–116, 128, and 129.

[15a] Refers to studies by Ferkany et al. (1989); reference substance for compound 130.

[15b] Refers to studies by Ferkany et al. (1993a); reference substance for compound 130.

[16] Refers to studies by Hays et al. (1990b).

[17] Refers to studies by Bigge et al. (1992b); reference substances for compounds 133–140.

[18] Refers to studies by Dappen et al. (1991); reference substance for compounds 141–145.

[19] No binding data available; potency in electrophysiology studies similar to that of D-α-aminoadipate (compound 1, Allan et al. 1980).

[20] From Fagg et al. (1990), cis-APPA has a K_i of 32 μM ([³H]L-glutamate). The corresponding 4,5-unsaturated compound appears to have considerably lower potency (P. C.-K. Pook, D. C. Sunter, and J. C. Watkins, unpublished observations).

[21] No binding data reported, but Z form cited as equipotent with AP7 (compound 14) and E form as inactive by Hutchison et al. (1989).

[22] Reference substances for compounds 149–152 (Fagg et al. 1990).

[23] Reference substance for compound 153 (Sills et al. 1991).

[24] Reference substance for compound 156 (Whitten et al. 1990).

[25] Refers to studies by Wedler et al. (1992) (value taken from Ortwine et al. 1992).

[26] Taken from Ortwine et al. (1992).

[27] Hutchison et al. (1989); cis and trans refer to relative orientations of the piperidine 2- and 4-substituents, not the double bond.

[28] Reference substances for compounds 157–160 (Hutchison et al. 1989).

[29] Reference substances for compounds 161 and 162 (Olverman and Watkins 1989; Aebischer et al. 1989).

[30] See footnote 6.

[31] Refers to studies by Ornstein et al. (1992b); no reference substance reported.

[32] Reference substance for compounds 61–64 (Ornstein et al. 1991).

Table 2.6 Recently reported potent NMDA antagonists

(A) Straight chain antagonists

General formula:

$$H_2N-\underset{HO_2C}{\overset{}{CH}}-M-X$$

No.	Acronym	M	X	*	IC_{50}^1 (μM)	K_i (μM)^2 Lig1	Lig2	Lig3	Lig4
1		CH_2	tetrazole	S	>100 (antag)^3			0.639	
2		CH_2	tetrazole	R	>100 (antag)^3			0.685	
3		$(CH_2)_2$	tetrazole	S	ag^3			1.601	
4		$(CH_2)_2$	tetrazole	R	31.6 (antag)^3			0.925	
5		$(CH_2)_3$	tetrazole	R,S	antag^3			1.055	
6		$(CH_2)_4$	tetrazole	R,S	antag^3			10.03	
7		$(CH_2)_5$	tetrazole	R,S	>100			>10	
8		$(CH_2)_6$	tetrazole	R,S	>100			>10	
11[14]	AP5	reference substance		R	3.7			0.177^4	
15[14]	AP7	reference substance		R	11.1			0.461^4	
58[14]	CPP	reference substance		R,S	0.6			0.220^4	
46[14]	CGS 19755	reference substance		2RS,4SR	1.6			0.054^4	
61[14]	LY 233053	reference substance		2RS,4SR	4.2			0.107^4	

(B) Straight chain unsaturated antagonists

General formula:

No.	Acronym	R¹	R²	R³	R⁴	R⁵	X	*	K_i (μM)[2] $[^3H]$CFP
9		H	H	H	Me	H	O	R,S	5.0
10		H	H	Me	H	H	O	R	1.8
11		H	Me	H	H	H	O	R,S	7.0
12		H	Me	Me	H	H	O	R,S	<100
13		Me	H	H	H	Me	O	R,S	20.0
14		H	H	H	H	Me	O	R	1.7
15		H	H	H	H	H	N(OH)[5]	R	0.2
16		H	H	H	H	H	N(OCH₃)[5]	R	0.6
17		H	H	H	H	H	N(OCH₂Ph)[5]	R	0.5
156[14]	MDL 100,453	reference substance						R	0.11[e]

Where R¹ = R^1, R² = R^2, R³ = R^3, R⁴ = R^4, R⁵ = R^5.

Table 2.6 Recently reported potent NMDA antagonists

(C) Heterocyclic antagonists

No.	Acronym	Structure	R¹	R²	n	X	*	IC₅₀¹ (μM)	K_i (μM)²			
									Lig1	Lig2	Lig3	Lig4
18		$(CH_2)_n$–X			1	tetrazole	R,S	8.2			1.67	
19					2	tetrazole	R,S	4.7			0.781	
20					3	tetrazole	R,S	16.3			3.150	
21		$(CH_2)_n$–PO_3H_2			4	tetrazole	R,S					
22					2	PO_3H_2	R,S			0.27	>10	
14[14]	AP7	reference substance	Me							0.77[7]		
58[14]	CPP	reference substance	H							0.079[7]		
23				H		PO_3H_2	2RS,3SR			0.32		
24				Me		PO_3H_2	2RS,3SR,4RS			0.015		
25						PO_3H_2	R,S			7.6		

No.		R¹ / substituent	R² / X	stereo	value
26			PO₃H₂	2RS,3SR	3.2
73[14]	*cis*-MDL 100,925	reference substance		2RS,3SR	
27[9]		H		R,S	0.040[8]
28[9]		Ph	H	R,S	
29[9]		H	Ph	R,S	
30		H	H	PO₃H₂	R,S	0.119
31		H	H	PO₃H₂	(−)	0.0293
32		H	H	PO₃H₂	(+)	>1.0
33		H	Cl	PO₃H₂	R,S	0.024
34		Cl	H	PO₃H₂	R,S	0.038
35		Cl	Cl	PO₃H₂	R,S	0.0034
36		Me	Me	PO₃H₂	R,S	0.0223
37		benzo (g)		PO₃H₂	R,S	0.0065
46[14]	CGS 19755	reference substance		2RS,4SR	0.028[10]
58[14]	CPP	reference substance		R,S	0.1126[10]
14[14]	AP7	reference substance		R,S	0.388[10]

Table 2.6 (continued)

(D) Miscellaneous antagonists

No.	Acronym	Structure	n	X	*	K_i (µM)[2] Lig1	Lig2	Lig3	Lig4
38		H_2N ring (squaric acid) $\overset{H}{N}(CH_2)_n X$, two O	2	PO_3H_2	R,S		0.47		
14[14]	AP7	reference substance			R,S		0.39[11]		
39	NPC 12626	$-(CH_2)_n-X$ on cyclohexane	2	PO_3H_2	(±)			0.976	
40	NPC 17742		2	PO_3H_2	2R,4R,5S			0.148	
41		H_2N — CO_2H	2	PO_3H_2	2S,4R,5S			0.264	
42			2	PO_3H_2	2R,4S,5R			0.555	
43			2	PO_3H_2	2S,4S,5R			0.239	
149[14]	CGP 37849	reference substance			R,S			0.018[12]	
59[14]	CPP	reference substance			R			0.086[12]	
44	NPC 12626				(−)-trans			4.05	
45	NPC 12626				(+)-trans			28.00	
58[14]	CPP	reference substance			R,S			0.19[13]	
46[14]	CGS 19755	reference substance			2RS,4SR			0.087[13]	

General formula:

No.	Acronym	X	*	Geometry	K_i $(\mu M)^2$ [^{3}H]CPP
46	CPP-Et-ester	-(CH$_2$)$_3$FO$_3$(Et)H	R,S		8.4
47	CPP-ene Et-ester	-CH$_2$CH=CH-PO$_3$(Et)H	R,S	*trans*	8.9
48	CCP	-(CH$_2$)$_3$-CO$_2$H	R,S		1.
49	CCP-ene	-CH$_2$CH=CH-CO$_2$H	R,S	*trans*	0.56
50	Mal-CCP	-(CO)-CH=CH-CO$_2$H	R,S	*cis*	18
51	Fum-CCP	-(CO)-CH=CH-CO$_2$H	R,S	*trans*	6.
52	Succ-CCP	-(CO)-(CH$_2$)$_2$-CO$_2$H	R,S		11
53	CCE	-(CH$_2$)$_2$-CO$_2$H	R,S		7.9
54	Succ-CCP-yne	-(CO)-C≡C-CO$_2$H	R,S		4.5
55	*iso*-CCE	-CH(Me)-CO$_2$H	R,S		190
56	CCM	-CH$_2$CO$_2$H	R,S		28
57	CSP	-(CH$_2$)$_3$-SO$_3$H	R,S		42
58	CSE	-(CH$_2$)$_2$-SO$_3$H	R,S		63

Table 2.6 (*continued*)
(D) Miscellaneous antagonists
General formula:

No.	n	R¹	R²	R³	R⁴	R⁵	*	K_i (μM)[2] [³H]CPP
59	0	H	CO_2H	H	H	H	R,S	56
60	0	H	CO_2H	H	H	H	R	25
61	0	OH	CO_2H	H	H	H	R,S	35
62	0	H	CO_2H	OH	H	OH	R,S	100
63	0	H	CO_2H	H	H	H	R,S	160
64	0	H	OH	CO_2H	H	H	R,S	7.9
65	0	OH	H	CO_2H	H	H	R,S	40
66	0	OH	OH	H	H	H	R,S	630
67	0	H	H	OH	H	H	R,S	500
68	0	H	CO_2H	OH	H	H	R,S	350
69	0	H	CO_2H	OH	H	H	R	32
70	0	H	CO_2H	H	H	H	S	450
71	1	H	CO_2H	NO_2	H	H	R,S	440
72	1	H	CO_2H	H	H	H	R,S	790
73	1	H	CO_2H	Cl	H	NO_2	R,S	840
74	1	H	CO_2H	NH_2	H	H	R,S	560
75	1	H	CO_2H	H	H	NH_2	R,S	630
76	1	H	CO_2H	CO_2H	H	H	R,S	no effect
77	1	H	H	CO_2H	H	H	R,S	500
78	1	H	OH	CO_2H	H	H	R,S	450
79	1	-CH=CH-CO_2H					R,S	800

59[14]	reference substance	R	0.14[15]
60[14]	reference substance	S	2.3[15]
161[14]	reference substance	R	0.044[15]
162[14]	reference substance	S	0.60[15]

For a definition of ligands 1–4 see Table 2.5.

The column headed by an asterisk indicates the stereochemistry at the asymmetric carbon atom(s).

[1] From Ornstein et al. (1993).

[2] For many compounds IC$_{50}$ values were reported; however, because of the low ligand concentration used, K_i is approximately equal to IC$_{50}$. Ligand 3: Ornstein et al. (1993); Hamilton et al. (1993); Ferkany et al. (1993b). Ligand 2: J. C. Watkins and H. J. Olverman, unpublished observations; Whitten et al. (1993a,b); Bigge et al. (1993); Baudy et al. (1993); Kirney et al. (1992).

[3] ag: excitatory amino acid agonist activity; antag: excitatory amino acid antagonist activity.

[4] Refers to studies by Ornstein et al. (1993); reference substances for compounds 1–8 and 18–21.

[5] Oximes are a mixture of syn and anti isomers.

[6] Refers to studies by Whitten et al. (1993a); reference substances for compounds 9–17.

[7] Refers to studies by Bigge et al. (1993); reference substances for compound 22.

[8] Refers to studies by Whitten et al. (1993b); reference substance for compounds 23–26.

[9] Refers to studies by Shinozaki (1992b): no data given. Compounds 27–29 depress NMDA responses with a potency lower than that of CPP. Compound 27 is reported to be the most potent of this type.

[10] Refers to studies by Baudy et al. (1993); reference substances for compounds 30–37.

[11] Refers to studies by Kinney et al. (1992); reference substances for compound 38.

[12] Refers to studies by Hamilton et al. (1993); reference substances for compounds 39–43, but see also Ferkany et al. (1993a,b).

[13] Refers to studies by Ferkany et al. (1993b); reference substances for compounds 44 and 45.

[14] These compound numbers refer to the main antagonist table (Table 2.5).

[15] Reference substances for compounds 46–79 (J. C. Watkins, H. J. Olverman, A. W. Jones, and D. C. Sunter, unpublished observations).

the aspartate analogue of AMPA (Table 2.4; compounds 3 and 14). Several (R)-aspartate derivatives of the (S)-glutamate analogue TAN950A ((S)-2-amino-3-(2,5-dihydro-5-oxo-4-isoxazolyl)propanoic acid) show increased affinity for NMDA receptors compared with the predominant AMPA/kainate receptor actions of TAN950A (Iwama *et al*. 1991). Within the series, (R)-MNT 950A was a potent and the most selective NMDA receptor agonist, having near equal affinity with NMDA (Table 2.4, compound 14; Iwama *et al*. 1991). (RS)-AMAA is a derivative of the glutamate analogue ibotenate; it has about the same NMDA receptor binding affinity but lacks the AMPA/kainate receptor actions of ibotenate (Table 2.4, compounds 3 and 4; Madsen *et al*. 1990). In contrast to (R)-MNT 950A, the NMDA receptor affinity resides predominantly in the (S) isomer of AMAA (Krogsgaard-Larsen *et al*. 1992). Cyclization of (RS)-AMAA to give (RS)-4-HPCA reduces affinity (Table 2.4, compound 7) as does *N*-methylation (Madsen *et al*. 1990).

Results obtained using cyclic NMDA agonists where part or all of the interacidic carbon chain and in some compounds also the α-amino group are incorporated into the ring system indicate perhaps not too surprisingly that glutamate analogues with a folded rather than an extended conformation have enhanced activity. Of the eight isomers of CCG, one pair of stereoisomers with a folded glutamate conformation, i.e. where the distal carboxyl and the glycine moiety are in the *cis* configuration, (2S,3R,4S)- and (2R,3S,4R)-CCG had the highest affinity (Table 2.4, compounds 10 and 11; Monahan *et al*. 1990; Kawai *et al*. 1992). Indeed, according to published data, it would appear that (2S,3R,4S)-CCG is the highest affinity NMDA agonist so far reported, being 20-fold more active than (S)-glutamate (Kawai *et al*. 1992). Apart from an extended (R)-glutamate analogue, (2R,3S,4S)-CCG, all other CCG analogues had much lower NMDA receptor affinity. The preferred folded glutamate conformation of the proximal and distal carboxyls is also observed with the diastereoisomers of the corresponding cyclobutane and cyclopentane analogues, ACBD and ACPD. The *trans* isomers (IUPAC nomenclature)[1] of the two compounds (with the carboxyls in the *cis* configuration) have substantially higher affinity than the corresponding *cis* isomers (Fig. 2.3; Table 2.4, compounds 2, 6, 5, and 9). For ACPD the (1R,3R) stereoisomer is the most potent and selective agonist (Table 2.4, compound 5, quoted as a mixture of two diastereoisomers; Sunter *et al*. 1991).

The *cis* and *trans* isomers of 2,3- and 2,4-piperidine dicarboxylate (PDA) are included in this section (Table 2.4, compounds 15–20) since these compounds can be regarded as aspartate and glutamate analogues alkylated in both the amino group and the carbon atom next to the ω-carboxyl. Consistent with the effect of *N*-alkylation described previously, the

---

[1] In this chapter IUPAC nomenclature is used throughout. This is of particular importance with *cis* and *trans* nomenclature for certain cyclic glutamate analogues (see editorial comment in article by Schoepp *et al*. 1991*b*).

(2R,3S) isomer of *cis*-2,3-PDA shows activity close to that of (R)-aspartate and it might be anticipated that the (2R,3R) isomer of *trans*-2,3-PDA would also be the active form. Although *cis*- and *trans*-2,3-PDA show similar affinity, the latter compound is a full agonist while the former is a partial agonist with pronounced antagonist action in some systems (Davies *et al*. 1982; Leach *et al*. 1986; Wheatley and Collins 1986) thereby indicating the importance of the spatial orientation of the three ionizable groups of acidic amino acids in determining agonist and antagonist activity. In contrast to the 2,3-PDAs there is considerable *trans*/*cis* differential in the 2,4-PDAs, consistent with electrophysiological data which show *cis*-2,4-PDA to be a weak NMDA antagonist and *trans*-2,4-PDA to be a moderately potent NMDA agonist (Davies *et al*. 1982). ^{1}H-NMR spectroscopy has shown that the *trans* isomers of both 2,3-PDA and 2,4-PDA exist in aqueous solution in both extended and folded conformations whereas the *cis* isomers, particularly *cis*-2,4-PDA, are in single extended conformations (Krogsgaard-Larsen *et al*. 1992). Therefore, allowing for the general lower affinity of the PDAs relative to other compounds discussed previously, the higher affinity of *trans*-2,4-PDA compared with the *cis* isomer remains consistent with a folded glutamate configuration being preferred for NMDA agonist action. In addition (±)-*trans*-CPAA, which in some ways corresponds to a more folded *trans*-2,4-PDA, but where the ring system is more planar, has an EC_{50} of 20 μM, twice as potent as NMDA for evoking [^{3}H]acetylcholine release from striatal slices (Tsai *et al*. 1988).

It can be postulated that *cis*-2,3-PDA exerts both its dual agonist and antagonist effects with the carboxyl at the 3-position interacting with the agonist ω-acidic binding site in the NMDA receptor (Olverman *et al*. 1988a), as would be expected to occur for all the other glutamate and aspartate analogues described. The alternative explanation that this substance exerts the antagonist component of its action by interaction of the C-3 carboxyl with the long-chain antagonist ω-binding site is considered unlikely in view of the short interacidic group chain length present in the compound. In this case, the particular stereochemistry of the molecule must prevent the full manifestation of the agonist action seen with *trans*-2,3-PDA despite the near equal affinity of the two compounds for the receptor (Olverman *et al*. 1988a).

Most of the cyclic compounds described effectively have alkyl substituents or combinations of substituents on positions of glutamate and aspartate which might have been predicted from the corresponding open chain compound substitutions to have reduced receptor affinity. For example, ACBD can be regarded as containing dual substitutions of glutamate at the C-2 and C-4 positions and CCG as substituted at positions C-3 and C-4. The deleterious effects expected for substitutions at these positions is presumably counteracted both by the compact nature of the ring forms and by the favourable orientation they impose on key groups necessary for potent agonist binding.

NMDA receptor antagonists

ω-Substituted open chain compounds

Data derived from binding and some electrophysiological studies for the major structural features of various series of NMDA antagonists are given in Tables 2.5 and 2.6. Data from open chain compounds can be used to deduce a number of general principles which hold for most series of compounds so far investigated.

NMDA antagonists are typically higher homologues of glutamate with peak activity observed where the number of atoms in the chain separating the α-carbon and the ω-acidic group is either three (AP5-length) or five (AP7-length) (e.g. Table 2.5, compounds 1–5 and 11–15) although occasionally peak activity occurs with four atoms (AP6-length) (Table 2.5, compounds 24, 33, and 37). Weak to moderate antagonist activity can still be observed in compounds with a chain length as low as two or as high as six atoms (Table 2.5, compounds 8 and 40; Table 2.6, compound 4). In most compounds which have been resolved the enantiomer with the (R) configuration at the α-terminus has highest affinity, the R/S potency ratio being usually within the range 10–50. Compounds include AP5, AP7, CPP, CPP-ene, LY 233053, CGP 37849, MDL 100,453, MDL 100,925, and 3-carboxy-4-hydroxyphenylglycine (Table 2.5, compounds 11/12, 15/16, 59/60, 161/162, 65/66, 151/152, 156 and 73; Table 2.6, compounds 69/70) and also CGS 19755 (Lehmann *et al.* 1988). The NMDA antagonist activity of (S) isomers was first recognized when it was noted that R/S potency ratios for AP7, CPP, and CPP-ene were much lower than that for AP5, indicating a lower enantiomeric preference of AP7-length compounds for binding to NMDA receptors (Aebischer *et al.* 1989; Olverman and Watkins 1989). Exceptions to the generalization have now been reported with two series of compounds. Firstly, for the decahydroisoquinoline derivatives, LY 274614 and LY 233536 (Table 2.5, compounds 82 and 83), the active enantiomers, LY 235959 and LY 202157, were found to have the (S) configuration at the α-carboxyl terminus. In the C-6 epimer LY 266845, however, activity resided with the (3R) enantiomer LY 288534 (Table 2.5, compounds 82, 83, and 85; Ornstein and Klimkowski 1992). Secondly the (2S) enantiomers of the phenylalanine derivative, SDZ EAB 515, and analogues that have been resolved are about 100-fold more potent as NMDA antagonists than the corresponding (2R) enantiomers (Table 2.5, compounds 117/118, 121/122, and 126/127; Müller *et al.* 1992).

Allowing for one carbon less in the chain length for ω-tetrazole substituted analogues due to the negative charge being delocalized throughout the ring as discussed in the 'agonist' section, where compounds differing only in the ω-acidic terminus have been compared the rank order of potency for NMDA antagonism is PO_3H_2 > tetrazole > CO_2H ≫ SO_3H (e.g. Table 2.5, compounds 1–7, 10–21, 26–28, 33, and 34; Table

2.6, compounds 3–6). This generalization also seems to hold for cyclic antagonists (see Tables 2.5 and 2.6 for various examples). Methylphosphinate also appears to be an effective ω-acidic group (Table 2.5, compound 68) whereas a thio-tetrazole moiety does not (Chenard *et al.* 1990). Esterification of the α- or especially the ω-acidic group reduces affinity (Table 2.5, compound 150; Table 2.6, compounds 9/14 and 46/47), some of the residual activity possibly resulting from hydrolysis to the parent compound, emphasizing the requirement for two functional acidic groups. An α-carboxyl may also be optimal for activity since its replacement with an α-phosphonate group in AP5 is highly detrimental (Monahan and Michel 1987). Although it is not clear if some degree of steric hindrance was also involved, in an attempt to produce a fully ionized ω-phosphonate group the 7,7-difluoro analogue of AP7 was synthesized but was found to have relatively low activity (Table 2.5, compound 17). The α-amino can be either primary or secondary, especially when forming part of a saturated ring structure, where activity is often substantially enhanced relative to the corresponding open chain compound, but a tertiary nitrogen seems unacceptable for activity since *N*-methylation of CGS 19755 was highly detrimental (Table 2.5, compound 48). However, biosteric replacement of the α-amino carboxyl terminal of AP5 at least by the achiral 3,4-diamino-3-cyclobutene-1,2-dione group seems possible without great loss of activity, producing an antagonist with the same affinity as AP7 (Table 2.6, compound 38). Whether the corresponding glutamate analogue, with an IC_{50} of 2.3 μM, was an NMDA agonist or antagonist was not specifically reported (Kinney *et al.* 1992).

For open chain antagonists many compounds have been synthesized that have heteroatoms incorporated within or attached to the interacidic group chain, unsaturated bonds, or a combination of these structural features, and in some cases these modifications lead to high activity. Sulphur in the chain either as a sulphone moiety or as part of a thiophene ring is well tolerated whereas nitrogen or oxygen in the chain of AP5 or oxygen in AP7 as part of a furan ring is detrimental (Table 2.5, compounds 155, 131, 41, 42, and 132). Nitrogen, however, is well tolerated as for example in the (cyclic) piperazine compounds (Table 2.5, compounds 56–60, 161, and 162) or for dipeptide-type substances (Table 2.5, compounds 26–40). These latter compounds can be regarded as also having a chain substituent in the form of an amide-keto group which is slightly detrimental to activity relative to an all-methylene chain (Table 2.5, compounds 1–16 and 18) except for compound 40. Of note is that an *N*-methyl or an *N*-phenyl substituent in the amide group of compound 28 either had no effect or slightly increased activity and the *N*-phenyl analogue was more active than the corresponding compound with the phenyl group on the adjacent carbon (Table 2.5, compounds 28 and 30–32). In another series of compounds (Table 2.5, compounds 133–140) nitrogen forms part of the chain by being

Agonists and competitive antagonists

bonded to the ω-phosphonoalkyl/alkenyl chain. These compounds, considering that some represent open chain analogues of CPPP, were of moderate to low affinity.

ω-Amino substitution of α-amino-alkane-α,ω-dicarboxylic acids and 4-amino substitution of both AP5 and AP7 have weakly detrimental effects on activity (Table 2.5, compounds 22–25, 44, and 45). However, if the substituent on C-4 of AP5 is a keto group (MDL 100,453), a hydroxyl group, or, particularly, a methyl (CGP 37849) or an *n*-propyl (CGP 39653) combined with a 3,4-double bond, NMDA receptor affinity is increased especially for the alkyl-substituted compounds (Table 2.5, compounds 43, 149, 153, and 156). For unsaturated analogues of AP5, activity resides in the (2R) enantiomer having *trans* (E) (Fagg *et al.* 1990) geometry, suggesting that the conformational restriction enforced on the molecule is consistent with the orientation necessary for near optimum interaction with the antagonist binding site. Indeed, among open chain compounds the (R) enantiomer of CGP 37849 and especially CGP 39653 have the highest affinity reported, comparing favourably with the most potent cyclic antagonists. It should be noted, however, that *cis* (Z) geometry appears necessary for the open chain AP7-ene analogues (Table 2.5, compounds 146–153). Further studies with MDL 100,453 have shown firstly that methylation at all positions of the compound reduces affinity and secondly that tautomerism of the keto group is unlikely to explain the increased affinity since a series of corresponding oximes showed almost the same activity (Table 2.6, compounds 9–17). Finally in this section it should be noted that in an attempt to determine the optimal binding conformation of AP5, a series of methano-AP5 compounds was synthesized analogous to the 2-(carboxycyclopropyl)glycine compounds used for agonist studies. Although none of these compounds had higher affinity than (R)-AP5 pure stereoisomers were not tested (Table 2.5, compounds 141–145).

Piperazine and piperidine compounds

Chronologically, CPP and then CGS 19755 were the first compounds reported to have higher affinity than AP5 and AP7 as competitive NMDA antagonists (Davies *et al.* 1986; Harris *et al.* 1986; Lehmann *et al.* 1987, 1988). They can be regarded as cyclic AP7 and AP5 analogues, respectively. Although the most effective interacidic spacing to some extent depends on ring type and ω-acidic terminus, by and large the 4-alkyl substituted piperidine-and piperazine-2-carboxylic acid series of compounds show the same pattern of activity as open chain antagonists. Thus the order of effectiveness for the ω-acidic terminus is $PO_3H_2 >$ tetrazole $> CO_2H \gg SO_3H$ with activity residing in the (2R) enantiomers. For 4-phosphonoalkyl piperidines the AP5-length compound CGS 19755 and AP7-length compound CPPP (LY 257883) have near equal affinity, CGS 19755 showing higher *in vivo* potency, but for ω-tetrazoles the AP5-length compound, LY

233053, shows by far the highest activity In the 4-substituted piperazines, however, peak activity is seen in the AP7-length compounds for ω-phosphonates and ω-carboxylates (CPP and CCP) but in the AP6-length compound for ω-tetrazoles (Table 2.5, compounds 46, 47, 54–67, and 157–160; Table 2.6, compounds 18–21, 48, 53, and 56–58; Lehmann *et al.* 1988; Ornstein and Klimkowski 1992). As discussed for agonists this is probably due to charge delocalization in the tetrazole ring.

Highest activity for the piperidines is shown with a *cis* relationship of the 2-carboxyl and the side chain on C-4, although the differential between *cis* and *trans* forms becomes lower with increasing chain length of the 4-substituent. For AP7-length piperidine and piperazine compounds, side chain unsaturation is well tolerated in the 4-substituent, *trans* (E) geometry of the double bond in most cases increasing NMDA receptor affinity (Table 2.5, compounds 157–162; Table 2.6, compounds 46–52 and 54). However, at least for certain compounds within the piperidine and piperazine series and with the possible exception of compound 103 (Table 2.5), ring unsaturation appears to be highly detrimental (Table 2.5, compounds 102–104, Table 2.6, compounds 25 and 26; Ornstein *et al.* 1989).

In the piperidine series, compounds with an all-methylene phosphonoalkyl group on C-3 of the ring are less active than C-4-substituted compounds (Ornstein *et al.* 1989). However, as with the corresponding open chain AP5-length compound, MDL 100,453, the 3-phosphonoacetyl analogue containing a β-keto moiety has high NMDA receptor affinity, the activity residing in the (2R,3S) enantiomer, i.e. again with *cis* orientation of the two substituents on the piperidine ring (MDL 100,925). Likewise, the β-hydroxy homologue also has high affinity (Table 2.5, compounds 71–74). Methyl substitution of both CGS 19755 and MDL 100,925 at the ring position distal to the ω-phosphono side chain (C-5 and C-4 ring positions respectively) is well tolerated and with *trans* geometry relative to the other two ring substituents actually increases the affinity of MDL 100,925. For both compounds activity is much diminished with methylation at other ring positions and at the α-position of the side chain of CGS 19755 (Table 2.5, compounds 48–53; Table 2.6, compounds 23 and 24). In the case of CPP-type compounds attachment of a ketone group to the carbon of the side chain linked to the piperazine ring is detrimental to activity as is introduction of an alkyl or aryl group on the side chain of any analogues tested (Table 2.5, compounds 69 and 70; Table 2.6, compounds 48–52 and 55).

Isoquinoline compounds

The isoquinoline derivatives can, with a few exceptions, be regarded as CGS 19755 or CPPP analogues where the flexibility of the ω-acidic side chain is further restricted by its incorporation into a second saturated (decahydroisoquinolines) or unsaturated (tetrahydroisoquinolines) ring. For the decahydroisoquinolines since each molecule has four asymmetric carbons, in theory 16 diastereoisomers could be obtained. Ornstein and colleagues have isolated a number of individual stereoisomers and epimeric mixtures of the AP7-length, 6-substituted decahydroisoquinoline-3-carboxylic acids and related compounds (Ornstein and Klimkowski, 1992; Ornstein *et al* 1992a). The most potent NMDA antagonists were the 6-substituted phosphonomethyl (LY 274614) and tetrazolylmethyl (LY 233536) analogues of the diastereoisomers having the 3SR, 4aRS, 6SR, 8aRS stereochemistry, these being substantially more active than the corresponding 6-carboxymethyl compounds. ^{1}H-NMR spectroscopy indicates that the two acidic groups on C-3 and C-6 are in an equatorial orientation (Table 2.5, compounds 82–84; Ornstein *et al.* 1992a). As has already been described, the NMDA receptor affinity resides in the (3S) rather than the (3R) form of both the phosphono (LY 235959) and the tetrazole (LY 202157) analogues with IC_{50} values of 25 nM and 415 nM respectively (Ornstein and Klimkowski 1992), LY 235959 having about the same affinity as CGS 19755. The C-6 and C-3 epimers of the above compounds had lower activity (Table 2.5, compounds 85–89) and at least for the C-6 phosphonomethyl analogue the activity was found in the (3R) stereoisomer (LY 288534) (Ornstein and Klimkowski 1992). Nevertheless, molecular modelling studies have shown that when the α-amino and carboxyl groups are superimposed, there is a close spatial orientation of the phosphono groups of LY 235959 (3S), LY 288534 (3R), and a number of other potent (R)-amino acid antagonists (Ornstein and Klimkowski 1992; see molecular modelling section).

Other 6-substituted isoquinoline analogues, including unsaturated compounds, substances bearing the α-carboxyl at C-1 rather than C-3, and others in which the ring structure is replaced by an octahydroindole structure, all had moderate to low affinity (Table 2.5, compounds 78, 80, 90–98, 100, and 101). Of note is that while the 6-substituted tetrahydro analogues are substantially less active than the corresponding fully saturated compounds (Table 2.5, compounds 78 and 80) the phosphono-octahydro-isoquinoline had higher affinity than its saturated analogue (Table 2.5, compounds 90 and 94). In addition, other tetrahydro and decahydro compounds show moderate and near equal affinity at least when the α-carboxyl and ω-phosphono substituents are in the C-1 and C-7 positions respectively (Table 2.5, compounds 81 and 98).

Of the 5-substituted tetrahydroisoquinolines two show reasonably high NMDA receptor affinity, the AP5-length compound SC 48981 and particularly the AP7-length compound PD 134705 (Table 2.5, compounds 75 and 77) the activity of PD 134705 residing in the (+) enantiomer (Bigge *et al.* 1993). An AP5-length tetrahydroquinoline analogue (Table 2.5, compound 99) with the chain substituent on the ring containing the nitrogen showed affinity close to that of SC 48981 (Table 2.5, compound 75). None of the tetrahydroisoquinolines, however, were as potent as the most active decahydroisoquinolines.

Phenylglycine and phenylalanine derivatives

NMDA receptor antagonists in this section are those where part of the chain linking the two acidic groups is incorporated into a benzene ring system, comprising mainly phenylglycine and phenylalanine derivatives, together with related structures such as the substituted pyran-2-one analogues described by Shinozaki (1992*b*) (Table 2.6, compounds 27–29) but would also include the recently reported quinoxaline derivatives (Baudy *et al*. 1993) (Table 2.6, compounds 30 37).

The AP5-length 3-carboxyphenylglycine (Table 2.5, compounds 105 and 106) showed moderate NMDA receptor affinity as did its 4-carboxy analogue in recent electrophysiological studies (Jones *et al*. 1993). However, highest potency in this group of compounds is shown with the 4-carboxy-3-hydroxyphenylglycine (Table 2.6, compound 64) (Jones *et al*. 1993). The activity of the carboxyphenylglycines resided predominantly in the (R) form (Table 2.6, compounds 60, 69, and 70; see also Jones *et al*. 1993). Hydroxyphenylglycines were virtually inactive as were all carboxyphenylalanine analogues tested (Table 2.6, compounds 66–68 and 71–79).

Generally, where direct comparison is possible, phosphono-substituted phenylglycines and phenylalanines are more potent than the carboxy analogues, as expected. Reasonably high to moderate affinity is found in two AP7-length compounds, *p*-phosphonomethylphenylglycine (PD 129635) and *o*-phosphonoethylphenylalanine (NPC 451) (Table 2.5, compounds 112 and 114). For this latter compound, substantially improved affinity is obtained following ring saturation (NPC 12626). The activity of NPC 12626, a mixture of eight isomers, was found to reside, as in piperidine compounds, with the *cis* diastereoisomer having the (2R,4R,5S) absolute stereochemistry (NPC 17742) (Table 2.6, compounds 39–45; Ferkany *et al*. 1993*a,b*). Highest affinity compounds, however, are found in the AP7-length *m*-phosphonoethylphenylalanine series of compounds, where, importantly, activity of all high affinity compounds resides in the (S) enantiomer, the (R) isomers showing much lower antagonistic effects (Table 2.5, compounds 116–127; Müller *et al*. 1992). Compared with the parent compound, activity was increased 100-fold with a phenyl substituent *meta* to the other two groups (SDZ EAB 515) (Table 2.5, compounds 117–119). While high affinity is maintained by a 4-fluoro, 4-chloro, or 3-amino group on the *m*-phenyl substituent (Table 2.5, compounds 120–122 and 125) a further 10-fold increase in affinity is found when the additional group on the phenyl substituent is a 4-*t*-butyl or a 4-phenyl moiety (Table 2.5, compounds 123 and 124); the K_D value for the (RS) form of the former of the last two compounds is 24 nM and that for the (S) isomer of the latter is 17 nM.

The series of structures related to 3-carboxyphenylalanine, the substituted pyran-2-one analogues, show NMDA receptor antagonist properties. Although quantitative data are not available and the compounds are less potent than CPP, they also contain an additional aryl substituent, the highest activity being found in the 5-naphthalene analogue (Table 2.6, compounds 27–29; Shinozaki 1992*b*). Whether substantially improved affinity would be obtained with phosphono derivatives has yet to be determined.

In the recently reported quinoxaline series of NMDA receptor antagonists, the AP6-length rather than the AP7-length analogue showed highest affinity, with the activity predominantly residing in the (−) isomer (Table 2.6, compounds 30–32; Baudy *et al.* 1993). Affinity was maintained in compounds containing 5,8-dichloro, 6,7-difluoro or 6,7-dimethyl substituents but somewhat reduced with 6,7-dimethoxy substituents (Baudy *et al.* 1993). While a mono-chloro substitution in either C-6 or C-7 increased affinity, a further 10-fold increase was found with the 6,7-dichloro analogue. In addition, the analogue with a phenyl moiety fused at C-6/C-7 also had very high affinity, the racemic forms of these latter two compounds having IC_{50} values of 3.4 nM and 6.5 nM respectively, making them equipotent with the highest affinity NMDA receptor antagonist previously reported, CGP 39653 (Table 2.6, compounds 33–35 and 37). Although they are AP6-length compounds, molecular modelling studies show that the quinoxaline analogues have excellent overlap with the minimum energy conformation of (2R,4S)-CGS 19755 (Baudy *et al.* 1993). In addition to their high affinity for the competitive antagonist site, what makes these compounds particularly interesting is that some also appear to have high affinity for the NMDA receptor glycine site. The 6-chloro and 6,7-dichloro analogues have IC_{50} values as inhibitors of [^{3}H]glycine binding of 1.8 μM and 0.6 μM respectively (Baudy *et al.* 1993); this presumably results from their close structural similarity to the quinoxalinediones and 7-chlorokynurenate. It should, however, be pointed out that while the 7-chloro analogue had low affinity for the glycine site, *in vivo* the 7-chloro and 6,7-dichloro analogues were approximately equipotent but the 6-chloro compound was inactive.

The common feature in the *m*-phosphonoethylphenylalanine analogues (Table 2.5, compounds 116–127), the substituted pyran-2-ones (Table 2.6, compounds 27–29), and the quinoxaline derivatives (Table 2.6, compounds 30–37) is that they all contain bulky aromatic substituents, indicating the existence of a hydrophobic pocket in the receptor to which all of these compounds bind, thereby enhancing their affinity (see molecular modelling section).

Molecular modelling of agonist and competitive phosphono amino acid antagonists acting at the NMDA receptor

In recent years computer-aided molecular modelling has been widely used for investigating the topography of the NMDA receptor agonist and antagonist binding sites. Insights into the spatial orientation of the sites of interaction of the important functional groups with the receptor, as well as the regions of steric tolerance and non-tolerance, are valuable aids in the design of potent new analogues. One problem with this approach, as it has been used so far, is that the existence of receptor subtypes (Chapter 5; see also Nakanishi 1992) has not been taken into account.

Nevertheless, since some of the conclusions of recent molecular modelling studies could well hold true for different subtypes or prove valid for a particular subtype identified in future studies, it is considered valuable to review them here (with reference to Tables 2.4–2.8 and Figs 2.1 and 2.3).

Agonist binding site

O'Callaghan *et al.* (1992) chose a set of conformationally rigid, potent, and selective NMDA receptor agonists in order to model the NMDA receptor agonist binding site (see Table 2.7 for details).

A new program termed INTERVOL was developed to locate possible sites of interaction on the receptor molecule. These sites were limited to the volume described by all points which are a defined distance from the principal atom of an agonist functional group by utilizing the intramolecular distance of the N-H---O-C hydrogen bond (Taylor *et al.* 1984). This volume is known as the volume of possible interaction (VPI). Since the corresponding functional groups of the ligands acting at a given site are assumed to interact with the same receptor recognition site, this site must lie within the VPI of the functional groups of all potent agonists. The structures of the various NMDA receptor agonists studied were superimposed, using a simple RMS (root mean square) fit procedure on the amino nitrogen and carboxyl carbon atoms of the *trans*-ACBD (Table 2.4, compound 2) template. Once all low-energy conformations of the agonists studied had been found and superimposed, INTERVOL was used to discover probable locations for the receptor interaction points. These points were used to build a model for the agonist binding site. Conformations of the agonists studied were checked for energetic accessibility. INTERVOL relies on structural differences between the agonists being compared in order to eliminate sites on the receptor to which not all compounds can interact. Since the amino and α-carboxyl groups can consistently be superimposed for all potent NMDA receptor agonists, the VPI for these functional groups is large and therefore more compounds need to be studied (preferably those of dissimilar structure) in order to locate accurately the points of interaction for these functional groups. The model proposed for the agonist binding site located the interaction point for the distal acidic moiety proximal to the α-carbon atom of the amino acids, on the side of the receptor site (see Fig. 2.4). This allows the receptor to accept compounds of varying chain lengths. O'Callaghan *et al.* (1992) suggest that the optimal chain length seems to be of aspartate (Table 2.1) and *trans*-ACBD length.

A pocket has been located in the receptor which will accommodate

Table 2.7 Compounds and methods used in the agonist modelling studies

Authors	Compounds used in modelling studies[1]	Software	Strategy
O'Callaghan et al. (1992)	(1R,3R)-ACPD (Fig. 2.3); (2S,3R,4S)-CCG (10); (2R,3S,4S)-CCG (12); trans-ACBD (2); (R)-MNT 950A (14); and (R)-AMAA (3)[2]	SYBYL 5.5 (including MAXIMIN2, the Tripos force field (Clark et al. 1989), and SEARCH) MOPAC (AM1 force field (Dewar et al. 1985)) INTERVOL	trans-ACBD used as a template to which all other compounds were fitted
Kyle et al. (1992)	trans-ACBD (2); NMDA (Table 2.2); Quin (8); Homoquin (Fig. 2.3); (S)-Glu (Table 2.1); (2R,3S,4R)-CCG (11); (2S,3R,4S)-CCG (10); (R)-AMAA (3); 4-HPCA (7); (1R,3R)-ACPD (Fig. 2.3); (1S,3R)-ACPD; (1R,3S)-ACPD; (1S,3S)-ACPD; trans-CPAA (13)	MOPAC (AM1 force field used to define the Cartesian coordinates of the trans-ACBD template)	trans-ACBD used as a template
Ortwine et al. (1992)	Quin (8); Homoquin (Fig. 2.3); cis-2,3-PDA (Fig. 2.3); trans-2,3-PDA (Fig. 2.3); trans-2,4-PDA (Fig. 2.3); (S)-Glu (Table 2.1); AMAA (3); ibotenic acid (4); (S)-Asp (Table 2.1); NMDA (Table 2.2); (2S,3R,4S)-CCG (10); (2S,3S,4R)-CCG; (1R,3R)-ACPD (Fig. 2.3)	SYBYL 3.5 (including MAXIMIN and MULTIFIT)	Using MULTIFIT all molecules studied were allowed to fit each other simultaneously; no template molecule was used, resulting in consensus conformation

[1] Figures in parenthesis refer to compound numbers in Table 2.4 unless otherwise stated.
[2] More compounds were added in a later study (O'Callaghan et al. 1993; O'Callaghan (1993)).

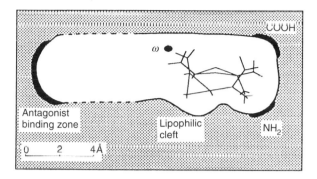

Fig. 2.4 Proposed model for the NMDA agonist site. Three interaction points are illustrated corresponding to the charged functional groups of agonists. A lipophilic pocket is also shown. The interaction point for the *ω*-acidic group (labelled 'ω')lies below the plane of the page. The model is illustrated with the potent agonists *trans*-ACBD and (2S,3R,4S)-carboxycyclopropylglycine. Reproduced with permission from O'Callaghan *et al.* (1992).

uncharged steric bulk, e.g. the cyclopropyl ring of the CCG compounds, and the methyl groups of AMAA (Table 2.4, compound 3) and (R)-MNT 950A (Table 2.4, compound 14), which are co-localized when the distal acidic moiety interacts with the receptor site (Fig. 2.4).

Kyle *et al.* (1992) used the potent and selective agonist *trans*-ACBD (Table 2.4, compound 2) as a template for their molecular modelling studies. Since *trans*-ACBD is an extremely potent agonist, the orientation of its functional groups in space was assumed to be near optimal for binding to the NMDA receptor agonist binding site. In order to determine an optimal geometry for each molecule, several NMDA receptor agonists were superimposed on to the *trans*-ACBD template by overlaying the corresponding functional groups.

(S)-Glutamate (Table 2.1) could be easily fitted to the *trans*-ACBD template but NMDA (Table 2.2) did not fit very well. Quinolinic acid (Table 2.4, compound 8; Fig. 2.3) was found to fit the template to an even lesser extent than NMDA, although homoquinolinic acid (Table 2.4, compound 21; Fig. 2.3) fitted the template with little energy cost (2.42 kcal/mol). Due to the decreased receptor affinities of homoquinolinate and quinolinate relative to (S)-glutamic acid and NMDA respectively, it was concluded that lipophilic bulk in the regions occupied by part of the pyridine ring in these agonists is not well tolerated by the NMDA receptor agonist binding site (this might be especially true for cerebellar NMDA receptors—see Chapter 6). The combination of the excluded volume and the poor fit to the template was used to explain the observed order of agonist potency (quinolinate < homoquinolinate ≈ NMDA < (S)-glutamate). However, many other factors (apart from receptor subtypes) which were not taken into account may be important e.g. planarity, π-interactions (for instance interactions between the highest occupied molecular orbital and the lowest unoccupied molecular orbital), and the charge density on the atoms in the aromatic rings (including basicity of the pyridine N atoms). The region of steric bulk which causes the decrease in affinity for the NMDA receptor was proposed to be responsible for the neurotoxic properties of quinolinate and related compounds. This 'excito-toxic' pocket was defined as the region occupied by the six-membered rings of quinolinate and homoquinolinate and also the methyl group of NMDA.

Both of the cyclopropyl glutamate isomers (2R,3S,4R)-CCG (Table 2.4, compound 11) and (2S,3R,4S)-CCG (Table 2.4, compound 10) were found to be well accommodated by the template. Only a small extension of the surfaces of the cyclopropyl isomers was found relative to the *trans*-ACBD template. These findings are in agreement with the observation that the two cyclopropyl compounds, although they are enantiomers, have similar potencies in binding studies (Monahan *et al.* 1990). It has been reported that (R)-and (S)-aspartate also have similar affinities for the NMDA receptor in binding studies (Olverman *et al.* 1988*a*).

The existence of an 'agonist binding pocket' (distinct from the 'excitotoxic pocket') was proposed on the basis of modelling studies using AMAA (Table 2.4, compound 3). By superimposing the enantiomers of AMAA on to the *trans*-ACBD template, a large extension of the Van der Waals surfaces relative to *trans*-ACBD was found. Since (RS)-AMAA is a potent NMDA receptor agonist, it was concluded that the extended region is well tolerated by the agonist binding site and this extended volume may repre-sent an 'agonist pocket'. On the basis of energy calculations, (R)-AMAA was predicted to be the active enantiomer for NMDA receptor agonist activity (on the basis of better fit to the receptor, ΔRMS = 0.15 Å versus 0.57 Å for (S)-AMAA); however, Krogsgaard-Larsen *et al.* (1992) have reported that the (S)-form is the active enantiomer.

An attempt was made to fit all four diastereoisomers of ACPD (Fig. 2.3 and Table 2.4) to the *trans*-ACBD template. Thus (1S, 3R)-ACPD was found to be the isomer least likely to act as an NMDA receptor agonist since it shows greatest RMS deviation between constrained (to the *trans*-ACBD template) and unconstrained conformations. This is in agreement with the findings of Palmer *et al.* (1989) and Irving *et al.* (1990), who showed that (1S,3R)-ACPD is a selective metabotropic receptor agonist without activity at ionotropic excitatory amino acid receptors. The model predicted that (1R,3R)-ACPD (Fig. 2.3) and (1R,3S)-ACPD would behave similarly to NMDA receptor agonists but would be slightly less potent than (1S,3S)-ACPD. This is not in agreement with the experimental findings of Magnusson *et al.* (1988), Curry *et al.* (1988), or Sunter *et al.* (1991). The very careful study of Sunter *et al.* (1991) with highly purified ACPD stereoisomers showed clearly that only (1R,3R)-ACPD had potent NMDA receptor activity. Clearly the model of Kyle *et al.* (1992) will have to be refined in order to take these observations into account.

From modelling studies involving kainic acid (Table 2.4) it was discovered that apart from the isopropylene moiety (which lies outside the proposed 'agonist pocket'), the remainder of the kainate surface volume shows close correlation with that of *trans*-ACBD. In agreement with the findings of Tsai *et al.* (1988), Kyle *et al.* (1992) concluded that CPAA (Table 2.4, compound 13) should be a potent NMDA receptor agonist (CPAA lacks the isopropylene moiety but is otherwise identical to kainic acid). Indeed, on modelling (2S,3R)-and (2R,3S)-CPAA it was found that both these isomers could be accommodated by the *trans*-ACBD template equally well. It has been reported that (±)-*trans*-CPAA (Table 2.4, compound 13) is a potent NMDA receptor agonist (Tsai *et al.* 1988). However, confirmation of the proposal that the two *trans* enantiomers should have equal affinity as NMDA receptor agonists awaits the preparation of the separate enantiomers.

In order to define a qualitative NMDA receptor agonist pharmacophore, Ortwine *et al.* (1992) undertook a modelling study using a somewhat different set of conformationally restricted selective agonists (see Table 2.7). Initially, it was assumed that NMDA receptor agonists interact at a common receptor site, i.e. that in all cases the amine and the two acidic functional groups were interacting with the same receptor amino acid residues within that site. In order to test this hypothesis a common orientation was sought for the amine, its lone pair, and the two acidic groups amongst a set of conformationally restricted agonists. It was discovered that the only way to superimpose the functional groups of the conformationally restricted agonists was to overlay the α-carboxylic acid, the amine, and the hydroxyl oxygen of the distal acidic group. The ketonic oxygen of the distal carboxylate was found to occupy different areas of space for *cis*-2,3-PDA (Table 2.4, compound 16; the (2R,3S) isomer was used in these modelling studies) and *trans*-2,4-PDA (Table 2.4, compound 19; the (2R,4R) isomer was used). This led the authors to conclude that only the hydroxyl moiety of the distal acidic group is necessary to interact with a common receptor residue (i.e. one O atom only, presumably negatively charged), as was previously proposed on the basis of simpler considerations (Watkins 1981, 1990). It was assumed that acidic groups common to potent agonists would be able to reside in the same planes on the grounds that compounds containing distal phosphonates or sulphonates are either less potent, inactive, or antagonists. However, this is not always true: for example, (S)-homocysteic acid (Table 2.1) and (R)-S-sulphocysteine (Table 2.1) are both more potent NMDA receptor agonists than any of the PDA isomers (Olverman *et al.* 1988*a*).

With a few exceptions, most of the agonists could be fitted with low to moderate energy cost (< 3 kcal/mol). However, (S)-glutamate could only be fitted to the consensus cluster (obtained using MULTIFIT) with a relatively high energy cost. This led the authors to suggest that 'the NMDA receptor agonist activity of (S)-glutamate may be due in part to its inter-action with other sub-sites within the NMDA receptor complex'. This finding contradicts the model proposed by Kyle *et al.* (1992) where (S)-glutamate could readily be fitted to the *trans*-ACBD template (we feel that any model with which (S)-glutamate does not fit may need to be refined; alternatively, it may represent a receptor for which (S)-glutamate is not the physiological transmitter). Two other potent NMDA receptor agonists, AMAA (Table 2.4, compound 3), and ibotenic acid (Table 2.4, compound 4) (modelled as the (R) enantiomers) also gave poor fits to the consensus cluster using the MULTIFIT procedure. This may be due to the fact that since these two ring structures exist as pairs of tautomers, both tautomeric forms need to be modelled.

Ortwine *et al.* (1992) proposed that agonists are in a folded conformation in the pharmacophore model (Fig. 2.5). The planes of the acidic moieties are well defined, thus positioning these groups to interact with com-plementary sites on the receptor protein. The separation distance of the two acidic groups was on average 3.5–4 Å, and their planes were inclined at 60° relative to each other. It was argued that the good superimposition of the hydroxyl group of the distal acidic group, but the varying location of the remainder of the ω-acidic moiety, meant that charge delocalization between the oxygens of the acidic moiety was unlikely. Instead, it was pro-posed that there exists a specific hydrogen bond between the acidic hydroxyl and the receptor (though we feel it equally possible that the charge is fixed on one oxygen by interaction with a cationic site within the receptor).

In summary, both O'Callaghan *et al.* (1992) and Kyle *et al.* (1992) have proposed a pharmacophore for the NMDA receptor agonist binding site using *trans*-ACBD as a template. Ortwine *et al.* (1992), however, used a multifitting routine to obtain a consensus conformation to which most potent NMDA receptor agonists studied fit (with the notable exception of (S)-glutamate). All three models provided information on steric require-ments of the NMDA receptor agonist site. Kyle *et al.* (1992) also defined an 'excitotoxic pocket' which was proposed to account for the excitotoxic

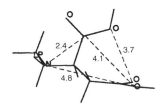

Fig. 2.5 Proposed pharmacophore for the NMDA receptor agonist site. (Distances are in Å.) Reproduced with permission from Ortwine *et al.* (1992).

activity of quinolinate and related compounds. O'Callaghan *et al.* (1993) (see also O'Callaghan 1993) proposed that agonists such as AMAA, (R)-MNT 950A, ibotenic acid, and TetGly (Table 2.4, compound 1) exist as tautomeric pairs in solution and, since it was observed that the energy barrier between the two forms is small (as shown by molecular mechanics calculations), both forms should be included in modelling studies.

The agonist recognition site of the NMDA receptor has been studied less well than the antagonist site. Fewer potent agonists are available for molecular modelling studies. New potent NMDA receptor agonists need to be found and added to these models in order to define more precise steric requirements for the agonist site. Where possible pure enantiomers of all potential and all known agonists need to be studied in order to be sure of which enantiomer is responsible for the activity. In particular, subtype-specific NMDA receptor agonists are required in order to model the binding sites of the subtypes. This could lead to a more accurate topology than the models outlined above which assume that all agonists bind to the same sites.

Competitive NMDA receptor antagonist binding site

Hutchison *et al.* (1989) studied a series of 4-phosphonoalkyl-and 4-phosphonoalkenylpiperidine-2-carboxylic acids using molecular modelling techniques in order to obtain a pharmacophore for the NMDA receptor antagonist binding site. Conformational analysis of CGS 19755 (Table 2.5, compound 46) revealed only three possible bioactive conformations (Fig. 2.6), whereas AP5 (Table 2.5, compound 11) was found to have many conformations that were accessible within 5 kcal/mol above the ground state. Energy calculations indicated that the 4,5-(−)-*gauche* conformation of CGS 19755 corresponded to the ground state, with the 4,5-*anti* conformation approximately equal in energy, and the 4,5-(+)-*gauche* conformation 1 kcal/mol higher in energy. The labels (−)-*gauche* and (+)-*gauche* for the conformations were derived on the basis of either an anticlockwise (−) or clockwise (+) rotation of 120° of the all-*anti* conformer. On energy grounds alone none of these could be ruled out as the bioactive conformation. Various analogues of CGS 19755 with methyl groups substituted on the piperidine ring were analysed in order to resolve this problem. Conformational analysis of 3-methyl-CGS 19755 (Table 2.5, compound 49)

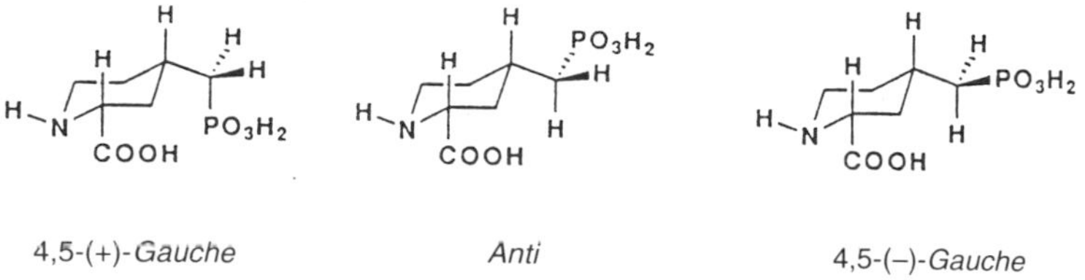

| 4,5-(+)-*Gauche* | *Anti* | 4,5-(−)-*Gauche* |

Fig. 2.6 Low energy conformations of CGS 19755.

revealed that the 4,5-(+)-*gauche* conformation was energetically inaccessible whereas the *anti* was favoured over the 4,5-(−)-*gauche* conformation. An analysis of 5-methyl-CGS 19755 (Table 2.5, compound 50) proved that again the 4,5-(+)-*gauche* conformation was energetically inaccessible whereas the 4,5-(−)-*gauche* conformation was favoured over the *anti*. Since 5-methyl-CGS 19755 is known to be much more potent ($IC_{50} = 78$ nM) than 3-methyl-CGS 19755 ($IC_{50} = 1.3$ μM), the bioactive conformer of CGS 19755 could be the 4,5-(−)-*gauche*. However, another interpretation of these results is that the 3-methyl group cannot be accommodated by the receptor as easily as the 5-methyl group. Hutchison *et al.* (1989) favour the 4,5-(−)-*gauche* conformation and independent studies on acyclic AP5 analogues support this hypothesis.

Hutchison *et al.* (1989) made qualitative observations about the active conformation of AP7-like antagonists based on their experimental observations. Their proposal that the bioactive rotamer for C(6)–C(7) in CPP (Table 2.5, compound 59) and *cis*-CPPP (Table 2.5, compound 54) is the *anti* conformer was based on the observed potent activity of CGS-2-ene (Table 2.5, compound 159). Thus the double bond in CGS-2-ene freezes the C(6)–C(7) bond into the *anti* conformation. Their proposed bioactive conformation of *cis*-CPPP is shown in Fig. 2.7. The potent activity of CGS-1-ene (Table 2.5, compound 157; $IC_{50} = 14$ nM versus [^{3}H]CGS 19755) supports the view that the bond C(5)–C(6) is *anti* in the bioactive conformation of *cis*-CPPP. In the bioactive conformation of *cis*-CPPP the C(4)–C(5) bond was proposed to be (−)-*gauche* because this conformation allows for the possibility that the phosphonate groups of both AP5- and AP7-like molecules interact with the same basic group on the receptor. Studies on chain unsaturated acyclic AP7 analogues support this hypothesis. Also, the global minimum energy conformation of CPP was found to have the *gauche* conformation around the C(4)–C(5) bond.

The methyl-substituted analogues of CGS 19755 were used to find exclusion volumes for the sites of interaction at the receptor. Steric bulk on the carbon α to the phosphonic acid, and that around the basic nitrogen, is poorly tolerated in most cases. Also around position 6 of the piperidine ring there is a highly space-limited contact point. Only at position 5 of the piperidine ring is steric bulk tolerated and potent activity retained.

The isomers of CGS 19755, CPPP, CGS-1-ene, and CGS-2-ene possess-

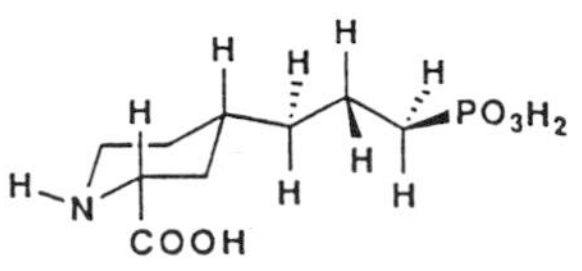

4,5-(−)-*Gauche*

Fig. 2.7 Proposed bioactive conformation of *cis*-CPPP.

ing a *trans* orientation of the C2 and C4 substituents retain some of the potency of the corresponding *cis* isomers (some being almost equipotent). Their potency was explained by the *trans* forms adopting a relatively low energy twist-boat conformation (within 3–5 kcal/mol of the chair ground state). Modelling by Hutchison *et al.* (1989) demonstrates that the *trans* forms in a twist-boat conformation can be superimposed on to the corresponding *cis* isomers (which are locked in a chair conformation) in the proposed bioactive conformations. Their proposed receptor model (Fig. 2.8) suggests that there is a basic group at the ligand binding site that allows for the phosphonate groups of both AP5- and AP7-like molecules to bind from two different directions, i.e. there is only one basic group at the binding site but for AP5 and AP7 analogues the phosphonate groups occupy two different areas of space when they interact with this group (the phosphorus atoms of the phosphonate groups of AP5 and AP7 analogues cannot be overlaid).

In apparent contradiction to the conclusions of Hutchison *et al.* (1989), Whitten *et al.* (1992) suggested that the phosphonate groups of both AP5 and AP7 analogues can be overlaid, and therefore that there is no need to invoke two separate positions in space for these groups. In order to validate this theory, conformations were sought which were common to potent antagonists but to which weakly active antagonists would not fit. This was achieved by generating as many conformations as possible for each molecule using conformational searching (SEARCH) and flexible fitting (with energy minimization using MULTIFIT) routines. Since some of these molecules are very flexible, restrictive Van der Waals non-bonding interactions were included to exclude high energy conformations. It was found that AP5 (Table 2.5, compound 11), AP7 (Table 2.5, compound 15), *cis*-CGS 19755 (Table 2.5, compound 46), and CGS-1-ene (Table 2.5, compound 157) could adopt similar conformations whereas AP6 (Table 2.5,

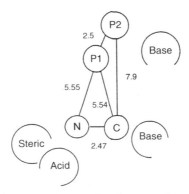

Fig. 2.8 Proposed NMDA receptor antagonist pharmacophore model (distances are in Å). Reproduced with permission from Hutchison *et al.* (1989).

compound 13) (a weakly active analogue) could not. Common conformations were sought using vector maps of AP5, AP7, CGS 19755, and
CGS-1-ene. One common conformation for each of the four molecules was
identified; each of these was further minimized using MULTIFIT. The
result clearly confirmed the proposal that a single pharmacophore can be
used to understand the binding of all NMDA receptor antagonists, i.e. the
phosphonate moieties of both AP5 and AP7 analogues are superimposable.
Ostensibly, this differs from the model of Hutchison *et al.* (1989) in which
the phosphonate groups of AP5 and AP7 analogues could not be superimposed, but as long as the phosphonate group can interact with the same
site on the receptor it is not essential for the phosphorus atoms of AP5 and
AP7 analogues to occupy exactly the same positions in space.

The potent antagonist CGP 40116 (Table 2.5, compound 151) was fitted
to the model and was taken to define the pharmacophore (see Fig. 2.9) for
all flexible fitting routines. The angle of the vector formed between the
phosphorus atom, the adjacent carbon atom, and the plane of the triangle
formed by joining the carboxylate carbon atom, the amine nitrogen atom,
and the carbon α to the phosphonate group (Fig. 2.9) was reported as
critical in order to define the pharmacophore.

A low-energy conformation for CGS-2-ene (Table 2.5, compound 159)
was found which was easily accommodated by the proposed pharmacophore, lending support to the theory that molecules with AP5 and AP7
chain length can be superimposed. However, AP6 could not be fitted to the
pharmacophore. Whitten *et al.* (1992) found that the piperidine ring of *cis*-
CGS-1-ene and *cis*-CGS-2-ene adopted a twist-boat conformation instead
of the usual chair conformation when fitted to the pharmacophore with
only a few kcal/mol expenditure of energy. The *trans* isomer of CGS-1-ene
(Table 2.5, compound 158) also fits the pharmacophore but in the chair
conformation.

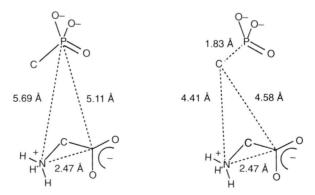

Fig. 2.9 Proposed pharmacophore for the phosphono amino acid NMDA receptor
antagonists. Reproduced with permission from Whitten *et al.* (1992).

By performing MAXIMIN2 calculations either using no electrostatic term or using a Coulomb's law term employing dielectric constants of 3.5 or 80 (to approximate any receptor environment from a lipophilic one to one which is hydrated) it was found that the omission of the electrostatic term had no significant effect and therefore could be safely omitted from the calculations. This approach for taking account of solvent effects in molecular mechanics calculations has been criticized (Gilson *et al.* 1985; Warwicker *et al.* 1985). Adjusting the dielectric constant in order to take account of solvent effects does not correct for the structural contribution of solvent introduced through hydrogen bonds. Additionally, applying a macroscopic dielectric function to individual molecules may be inappropriate. Even different parts of the same molecule may have completely different dielectric properties. One approach to this problem is a numerical solution of the Poisson–Boltzmann equation (Gilson *et al.* 1985; Warwicker *et al.* 1985; Warwicker 1986).

Mapping of the common Van der Waals volume of potent antagonists was contrasted with the exclusion volume map obtained from areas occupied by less active or inactive analogues. From these studies it was found that steric bulk on the carbon adjacent to the phosphonate moiety and in the vicinity of the nitrogen atom is not well tolerated, in agreement with findings from studies by Hutchison *et al.* (1989). Also in accordance with Hutchison *et al.* (1989), a number of less restricted regions were found, in particular around the 5-position of the piperidine-2-carboxylic acid nucleus.

Dorville *et al.* (1992) have also proposed a pharmacophore for the NMDA receptor antagonist recognition site (see Fig. 2.10). These authors

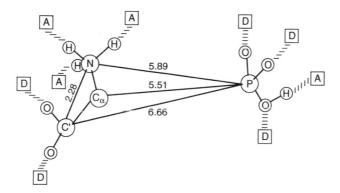

Fig. 2.10 Proposed configurations of the NMDA receptor–ligand complex in the antagonist preferring state including chemical and hydrogen bonds. Each of the interacting atoms may establish multiple interactions with the receptor atoms. In this model, permutation of the terminal groups bound to the phosphorus atom is allowed: D, proton, positive charge, proton donor, or water molecule; A, oxygen atom, negative charge, proton acceptor, or water molecule. Reproduced with permission from Dorville *et al.* (1992).

assumed that there will be multiple interactions between the oxygen, nitrogen, and hydrogen atoms of the ionized phosphonate, carboxylate, and amino functional groups with the contact points of the NMDA receptor locking the corresponding functional groups into a set conformation through hydrogen bonded interactions. In this study two receptor guide points were used for carboxylate oxygens (see Fig. 2.10) in analogy to the 'receptor fit point' method of Hughes and Andrews (1987). The MULTI-FIT option of SYBYL was used to superimpose the central atoms of the three functional groups (i.e. P, Nα, and C' (carbon atom of the CO_2H group)) of several potent NMDA receptor antagonists (see Table 2.8). The quality of superimposition of the P, Nα, and C' atoms was evaluated using the RMS deviation between atoms constituting the pharmacophore in the reference molecule, CGS 19755 (Table 2.5, compound 46) and the corresponding atoms in the molecules studied. As a result of these studies the bioactive structure of CGS 19755 was found to have a 4,7-*trans* conformation for torsion t_2 (see Fig. 2.11). In order to fit this model, CGS 19755 and (2R)-CGP 40116 (Table 2.5, compound 151) required an extended conformation, whereas CPP (Table 2.5, compound 59), CPPP (Table 2.5, compound 54), and CPP-ene (Table 2.5, compound 161) needed a folded conformation.

Dorville *et al.* (1992) were able easily to superimpose the three central atoms, Nα, C', and P, of *cis*-CPPP and CGS 19755. Thus only one location was found for the phosphorus atom for antagonists of both AP5 and AP7 chain length and not two as in the study by Hutchison *et al.* (1989). As described above, Hutchison *et al.* (1989) have favoured the (−)-*gauche* conformation for torsion t_2 of CGS 19755 (Fig. 2.11) and torsion t_4 of CPPP (Fig. 2.11). However, Dorville *et al.* (1992), as a result of their more extensive molecular modelling studies (which included the compounds studied by Hutchison *et al.* 1989), favour the *trans* or *anti* conformation for torsion t_2 of CGS 19755. Also, the use of twist-boat conformations for the *trans* C2/C4 isomers of CGS-1-ene (Table 2.5, compound 158), CGS-2-ene (Table 2.5, compound 160), CPPP, and CGS 19755 was not necessary since the pharmacophore proposed by Dorville *et al.* (1992) incorporates these molecules in their chair conformations.

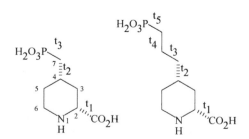

Fig. 2.11 Structures of CGS 19755 and CPPP and a definition of the torsions t_1 to t_5.

Volume mapping studies were undertaken with the initial compounds studied, the phenylalanine derivatives synthesized by Dorville *et al.* (1992) and also a set of active and inactive analogues from the work of Bigge *et al.* (1989*b*) and Hutchison *et al.* (1989). Through these studies, regions of forbidden volume were found around the amino group and extending from the carboxylate to the phosphonate groups. Also several sites were identified where bulk is tolerated to retain potent binding (e.g. around the 5-position of the piperidine-2-carboxylic acid ring, as found in other studies).

Ornstein and Klimkowski (1992) have briefly described their molecular modelling studies. The (−)-*gauche* conformation of (2R,4S)-CGS 19755 (Table 2.5, compound 46) was used as a starting template (in accordance with the suggestion of Hutchison *et al.* (1989) that this is the bioactive conformation) in order to derive low energy structures for the NMDA receptor antagonists studied. By superimposing the corresponding amino acid backbone atoms of the template and the molecules studied close structural similarities were revealed. Thus the phosphonate groups of (2R,4S)-CGS 19755 (AP5 chain length) and (2R)-AP5 (Table 2.5, compound 11) closely occupy the same region of space. Also the phosphonate groups of the AP7 analogues (3S,4aR,6S,8aR)-LY 235959 (an enantiomer of compound 82, Table 2.5) and (3R,4aS,6S,8aS)-LY 288534 (an enantiomer of compound 85, Table 2.5) overlap almost completely. At this stage the phosphonate centres of the AP5 and AP7 chain length analogues were 2.2 Å apart. This distance could be reduced to 1 Å if the phosphonomethyl group for each was rotated by 25° towards each other (resulting in an energy cost of less than 3 kcal/mol). Such a modification allows the phosphonate group of (2R)-CGP 40116 (Table 2.5, compound 151) to reside in the same region of space as that occupied by the phosphonate groups of the other four analogues (i.e. the oxygen atoms can overlap even where the phosphorus atoms of the group cannot). If the restriction that all backbone atoms of the amino acid must overlap exactly is relaxed, the phosphonate moieties of the analogues can overlap with even less energy cost and therefore AP7 and AP5 analogues were assumed to bind to a common receptor site. Another interesting fact to emerge is that the activity of (3S,4aR,6S,8aR)-LY235959, the potent antagonist with the unusual (S) configuration at the amino/carboxylate terminus, was accounted for using this model.

By far the most comprehensive molecular modelling study has been carried out by Ortwine *et al.* (1992). The hypothesis that competitive antagonists share a common binding mode with agonists was tested initially by modelling potent, rigid, NMDA receptor antagonists. It was assumed that the amino and the α-carboxylic acid groups in potent antagonists were binding to a common receptor site and therefore could be overlaid. A receptor site point was sought to account for the binding of the distal acidic

Table 2.8 Compounds and methods used in the antagonist modelling studies

Authors	Compounds used in modelling studies[1]	Software	State of ionization of compounds studied	Strategy
Hutchison et al. (1989)	AP5 (11); CGS 19755 (46); 3-Me-CGS 19755 (49); 5-Me-CGS 19755 (50); CPP (59); cis-CPPP (54); CGS-2-ene (159); CGS-1-ene (157)	AMBER force field (modified to take phosphonate groups into account MULTIC (onformer) submode of MacroModel program	not reported	Torsional grid method used to generate trial conformations which were then energy minimized (see Lipton and Still 1988)
Whitten et al. (1992)	AP5 (11); AP7 (15); CGS 19755 (46); CGS-1-ene (157); AP6 (13); CGP 40116 (151); CGS-2-ene (159)	SYBYL 5.3 (including SEARCH, a conformational analysis routine; MULTIFIT, which allows flexible fitting of molecules with energy minimization using the SYBYL force field and MAXIMIN2) AMPAC (AM1 Hamiltonian used to calculate charges)	NH_n^+ (n = 2 or 3); CO_2^-; PO_3^{2-}	vector maps used in order to find common conformations of compounds studied
Dorville et al. (1992)	CGS 19755 (46); cis-CPPP (54); (R)-CPP-ene (161); CPP (59); (2R)-CGP 40116 (151); CGS-1-ene (157); CGS-2-ene (159)	SYBYL 5.3 (including MULTIFIT and MAXIMIN2) AMPAC (PM3 Hamiltonian)[4]	NH_n^+ (n = 2, 3); CO_2^-; PO_3H^- (see Björkroth et al. 1991; Lehmann et al. 1988)	distance maps used in order to record allowed receptor atom locations (see Mayer et al. 1987)

Reference	Compounds	Software	Groups	Notes
Ornstein and Klimkowski (1992)	CGS 19755 (46); (2R)-CGP 40116 (151); (2R)-AP5 (11); (3S,4aR,6S,8aR)-LY 235959 (enantiomer of compound 82); (3R,4aS,6S,8aS)-LY 288534 (enantiomer of compound 85)	QUANTA/CHARMm 3.0 (Polygen Corporation, Waltham, MA)	not reported	(–)-gauche conformation of (2R,4S)-CGS 1975₅ used as a template on which all compounds studied were superimposed
Ortwine et al. (1992)	CGS 19755 (46); CPP (59); PD129635 (112); thiophene (131); quinoline (99); N-substituted glycine derivative (134); isoquinoline (81); p-PMPA (129); p-PPA (128); AP6 (13); CPEPz (57)[2]	SYBYL 5.3 (including MAXIMIN2, POTENTIAL (used to calculate electrostatic potentials), SEARCH, and MULTIFIT) CNDO/2 used to calculate charges (Pople and Beveridge 1970; Pearlstein; Childress 1985) as for agonist model (Table 2.7); also MOPAC (PM3 Hamiltonian in PRECISE mode (PM3 is better for heavier atoms such as phosphorus)[4]	NH_2; CO_2H; PO_3H_2	distance map method used
O'Callaghan (1993) and O'Callaghan et al. (1993)	to define primary pharmacophore used (2R,4S)-CGS 19755 (46); (R)-CGP 37849 (151); (R)-CGP-39653 (153); SC 48981 (75); LY 235959 (enantiomer of compound (82))[3]		partial charges assigned to the un-ionized forms of the molecules	SEARCH used to generate trial conformations; geometry optimized using MAXIMIN2; local minima optimized using PM3 Hamiltonian; INTERVOL analysis used to determine location of interaction points for NH_2, CO_2H, and PO_3H_2 groups on the receptor

[1] Figures in parenthesis refer to compound numbers in Table 2.5 except where stated.
[2] Approximately one hundred compounds were added to define the pharmacophore more accurately.
[3] More compounds were added in order to define the pharmacophore more accurately.
[4] Stewart (1990).

groups (carboxyl or phosphonate). This point of interaction was not assumed to have anything in common with the agonist distal acidic group interaction point.

Data from both the Cambridge Structural (Allen *et al.* 1979, 1983) and the Brookhaven Protein (Bernstein *et al.* 1977) databases were used to create the phosphonate-receptor site point geometry. An sp^3 nitrogen atom was added to one of the PO$_3$H$_2$ hydroxyl oxygens in the geometry obtained from database searches, replacing that hydroxyl's hydrogen in order to act as a hypothetical receptor atom. After superimposing the basic amine, its lone pair and the α-carboxyl of potent antagonists (see Table 2.8) conformational searches were run on phosphonate side chains using the SYBYL SEARCH module. The energetically allowed positions in space of the receptor atom relative to the amine and α-carboxyl were recorded as conformational searches of the flexible phosphonate side chains of potent antagonists proceeded.

The distance map method (for full details see Ortwine *et al.* 1992) proved successful in locating a unique area of space for the hypothetical receptor atom. A representative set of distances from this area was chosen as the location of a primary receptor interaction point. The potent antagonists, CPP (Table 2.5, compound 59), CGS 19755 (Table 2.5, compound 46), PD129635 (Table 2.5, compound 112), thiophene analogue (Table 2.5, compound 131), quinoline analogue (Table 2.5, compound 99), *N*-substituted glycine derivative (Table 2.5, compound 134), and isoquinoline analogue (Table 2.5, compound 81) were added to the model, leading to the discovery of a secondary receptor interaction point which could hydrogen bond to the other hydroxy group of the phosphonate moiety, or to a lone pair attached to the ketonic oxygen atom of antagonists bearing a distal carboxylic acid moiety.

Computation of electrostatic potentials revealed that the presence and direction of projection of the potential associated with the third 'ketonic' (P=O) oxygen of the phosphonate group appeared to be related to antagonist potency. Evidence for this proposal arose from the fact that antagonists possessing distal carboxylates (which lack this potential) are approximately 10 times less potent than those with phosphonates. Also the phosphinic acid analogue of CGS 19755, which has a methyl group in the same position as the third, 'ketonic' (P=O), phosphonate oxygen atom, is also 10 times less potent. When AP6 (Table 2.5, compound 13) and CPEPz (Table 2.5, compound 57) were fitted to the model, the 'ketonic' oxygen atom of the phosphonate moiety projected a negative potential towards the basic amine. This negative potential was assumed to inhibit the approach of a negatively charged receptor atom that must interact with the amine for strong binding. The periodicity in binding affinity observed as the phosphonate side chains are lengthened (from AP4 to AP7) can be rationalized on the basis of these observations.

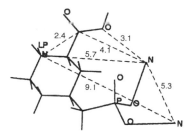

Fig. 2.12 Distances between pharmacophoric groups in the antagonist model illustrated using CGS 19755 in its fit conformation (distances are in Å). The nitrogen atoms attached to the PO_3 group represent receptor interaction points. Reproduced with permission from Ortwine *et al.* (1992).

The proposed competitive antagonist pharmacophore model (Fig. 2.12) consists of a folded conformation and contains two specific receptor interaction points off the distal phosphonic acid moiety. Both points are roughly in the plane of the piperazine ring of CPP, and one is positioned such that a receptor moiety could simultaneously hydrogen bond to oxygens on both the phosphonate and α-carboxyl groups. This point is also proximal to the distal acidic hydroxyl of the agonist model described by Ortwine *et al.* (1992). Indeed, these authors have proposed that both agonists and antagonists interact with the same receptor moieties at the same receptor site off one face (west and north-west) but the antagonists bind also to additional sites to the north, thus preventing the conformational change responsible for agonist activity.

Approximately one hundred structures were added to the model in order to allow the computation of the receptor tolerated and exclusion volumes. As in other models strict volume requirements are found near the basic amine, around the carbon α to the phosphonate moiety, and surrounding the receptor interaction sites. Volume tolerances were noted off positions 4–6 of the piperidine ring of cyclic antagonists such as CGS 19755. On adding (S)-SDZ EAB 515 (Table 2.5, compound 117) to the antagonist model it was found that the biphenyl moiety of (S)-SDZ EAB 515 did not conflict with any known excluded volume (whereas (R)-SDZ EAB 515 (Table 2.5, compound 118) could not be fitted to the model without encountering excluded volume) (Bigge 1993). This observation is in agreement with the finding that the potent antagonist activity resides in the (S) enantiomer of SDZ EAB 515. The fact that SDZ EAB 515 is more than 10 times more potent than the parent compound ((S)-*m*-PMPA, Table 2.5, compound 126) led Bigge (1993) to conclude that the biphenyl ring system must provide additional hydrophobic sites of interaction with the receptor, thus enhancing binding. On the basis of the modelling studies of Ortwine *et al.* (1992) a phosphono isoquinoline (Table 2.5, compound 77) (which has an IC_{50} of 0.27 μM versus [³H]CPP binding) was synthesized in order to obtain a more potent lipophilic antagonist. Relative to the compound with which they began their modelling efforts (NPC451 (Table 2.5, compound 114), IC_{50} of 61 μM versus [³H]CPP binding) they thus produced a compound with markedly enhanced potency.

Recently, O'Callaghan *et al.* (1993) (see also O'Callaghan 1993) have extended their modelling studies to include a receptor model of the antagonist site as well as the agonist site discussed earlier. In agreement with the studies of Ortwine *et al.* (1992), O'Callaghan and colleagues (1993) have proposed the existence of a primary interaction point, which is essential for binding both AP5 and AP7 analogues, as well as a secondary interaction point which is accessed by potent AP5 and AP7 analogues. The phosphonate groups of AP5 and AP7 analogues were found to lie in different regions of space but common receptor interaction points were proposed to lie between these regions.

Conformational analysis of the decahydroisoquinoline LY 235959 (the (3S) enantiomer of compound 82, Table 2.5) indicated that it adopts a double chair conformation (shaped rather like a hammock) in order to relieve ring strain. Inclusion of this compound in the receptor model provided evidence for the curvature of the binding site. Thus it was concluded that longer chain antagonists need to curve in the right direction in order to access the antagonist interaction sites (inclusion of *p*-PPG (Table 2.5, compound 111), a weak antagonist which is almost linear between the α-C and P atoms, supported this conclusion). The authors had no difficulty in superimposing (2R)-CPP-ene (Table 2.5, compound 161) on to LY 235959, despite the (S) stereochemistry at the amino carboxylate terminus of the latter compounds. Conformational analysis revealed the existence of two low energy conformations of CPP-ene; *cis*-(2R; 2 equatorial, 4 equatorial) and *trans*-(2S; 2 equatorial, 4 axial). The former conformation was assumed to be the bioactive one since it aligned extremely well with LY 235959 whereas the latter would not. Additionally (2S)-CPP-ene was proposed to be less potent on the grounds that it adopted the less energetically favourable *trans*-(2S; 2 equatorial, 4 axial) conformation.

Incorporation of the recently reported (Müller *et al.* 1992) phenylalanine, SDZ EAB 515 (Table 2.5, compound 117), and its analogues into the model led to the discovery of a deep cleft in the receptor cavity defined by the biphenyl side chain of these compounds. Since the triphenyl analogue (Table 2.5, compound 124) is seven times more potent than SDZ EAB 515, the channel was deduced to be very long and straight (at least as long as a biphenyl group i.e. about 9 Å). The *t*-butyl group was reported to be an acceptable replacement for the third phenyl ring of the triphenyl analogue and therefore lipophilic interactions were assumed to be important for enhanced binding potency. Derivatives of stizolobic acid (Table 2.6, compounds 27–29) were cited as further evidence for the existence of a region in the NMDA receptor which binds lipophilic side chains with large regions of π-electron density.

Summary of NMDA antagonist modelling studies

Hutchison *et al.* (1989) proposed that the 4,5-(−)-*gauche* conformation of AP5 analogues is the bioactive one and this has been supported by the findings of Ornstein and Klimkowski (1992). However, Dorville *et al.* (1992) prefer the 4,5-*anti* conformation for AP5 analogues. In addition, Hutchison *et al.* (1989) favour the (−)-*gauche* for the C(4)–C(5) bond but the *anti* conformation for the C(5)–C(6) and C(6)–C(7) bonds as depicting the bioactive form of AP7 analogues.

Hutchison *et al.* (1989) concluded that the *cis* forms of the 2,4-substituted piperidine antagonists (CGS 19755, CPPP, CGS-1-ene, and CGS-2-ene) were locked in a chair conformation whereas the *trans* forms adopted a twist-boat conformation. This differs from the conclusions of Whitten *et al.* (1992) that the *cis* isomers adopted a twist-boat conformation whereas the *trans* isomer of CGS-1-ene adopted a chair conformation. Dorville *et al.* (1992) found that both *cis* and *trans* 2,4-substituted piperidines could be fitted to their pharmacophore model in the chair conformation.

Both Whitten *et al.* (1992) and Dorville *et al.* (1992) were able to superimpose the basic nitrogen atom, the carboxyl carbon atom, and the phosphorus atom of the phosphonate group for all compounds studied (i.e. both AP5 and AP7 chain length compounds). This apparently contrasts with the findings of Hutchison *et al.* (1989) and Ornstein and Klimkowski (1992) who could not superimpose these atoms completely but nevertheless concluded that the phosphonate groups were close enough to each other in space to interact with the same receptor site.

The different results obtained in these modelling studies, as outlined above, could be due to differences in the methods used in generating the pharmacophores. Hutchison *et al.* (1989) used the torsional grid search method, whereas Dorville *et al.* (1992), Whitten *et al.* (1992), and Ortwine *et al.* (1992) employed conformational searching, multifitting, and energy minimization techniques. Ornstein and Klimkowski (1992) used the 4,5-(−)-*gauche* conformer of (2R,4S)-CGS 19755 as a starting template upon which all other compounds studied were superimposed in order to derive their pharmacophore. Alternatively, the reasons for these differences may lie in the different states of ionization of the molecules used in the molecular mechanics calculations (see Table 2.8 for details).

Ortwine *et al.* (1992), as a result of their extensive molecular modelling study, proposed that antagonists bind in a folded conformation in their pharmacophore model. The primary interaction site of the phosphonate group was proposed to be proximal to the distal NMDA receptor agonist binding site, and to be positioned so that a receptor moiety could simultaneously hydrogen bond to oxygens on both the phosphonate and α-carboxyl groups. A secondary interaction site was also defined which was thought to be responsible for preventing a conformational change necessary for NMDA receptor activation. The results of electrostatic potential calculations were used by Ortwine *et al.* (1992) in order to explain the periodicity in affinity found when phosphonate side chains are lengthened in the AP4–AP7 series.

All the authors (except Ornstein and Klimkowski (1992), who did not map receptor exclusion or tolerated volumes) who have undertaken modelling studies have reported receptor tolerated volume around position 5 of the 2,4-substituted piperidine antagonists. Ortwine *et al.* (1992), presumably as a result of the inclusion of many more compounds in their study, have also reported receptor tolerated volume around positions 4 and 6 of the piperidine ring. Receptor exclusion volumes were reported around the carbon atom α to the phosphonate group and in the vicinity of the basic nitrogen atom in most of the models. Additionally, Hutchison *et al.* (1989) and Whitten *et al.* (1992) have reported receptor exclusion volume around position 6 of the piperidine ring (the difference between these findings may be due to the much larger data set used by Ortwine *et al.* (1992) which would be expected to give a more accurate picture of the receptor site). Both Bigge (1993) and O'Callaghan and colleagues (1993) have reported the existence of a deep hydrophobic pocket in the receptor as a result of including SDZ EAB 515 and its analogues in their models.

As has been mentioned above and reviewed in Chapter 6, there is mounting evidence for the existence of subtypes of the NMDA receptor. Molecular modelling work will need to be repeated with subtype-specific agonists and antagonists in order to gain an accurate picture of the antagonist binding sites of these subtypes. This will probably require the development of a new generation of compounds which, along with existing compounds, will need to be tested on pure populations of NMDA receptor subtypes and NMDA receptors in discrete brain areas and neuronal pathways.

In most of the models described above attention has been given to the problems of modelling highly charged compounds. Neither Ortwine *et al.* (1992) nor O'Callaghan and colleagues (1993) employed ionized species in their calculations due to the problems associated with parameterization of charged species within the force fields and deciding how to include solvent or counter-ions such as salts in the calculations. In the absence of any information on the situation at the active site of the NMDA receptor this seems like the best option. Advances in molecular biology may' help to provide an understanding of the three-dimensional structure and environment of the active site of the NMDA receptor complex as well as information on the composition of receptor subtypes. This may in turn lead to the discovery of therapeutically useful potent and subtype-specific NMDA receptor antagonists.

Acknowledgements

We thank Miss Audrey Kerr and Mrs Joan Keeling for typographical assistance. Our own experimental work described in this review was generously supported by the Medical Research Council and the Scottish Hospital Endowments Research Trust.

References

Aebischer, B., Frey, P., Haerter, H. P., Herrling, P. L., Mueller, W. A., Olverman, H. J., and Watkins, J. C. (1989). Synthesis and NMDA antagonist properties of the enantiomers of 4-(3-phosphonopropyl)-piperazine-2-carboxylic acid (CPP) and of the unsaturated analogue (E)-4-(3-phosphonoprop-2-enyl)piperazine-2-carboxylic acid (CPP-ene). *Helvetica Chimica Acta*, **72**, 1043–51.

Allan, R. D., Bornstein, J. C., Curtis, D. R., Johnston, G. A. R., and Lodge, D. (1980). Selective antagonist activity of 5-aminohex-2-enedioic acid on amino acid excitation of cat spinal neurones. *Neuroscience Letters*, **16**, 17–20.

Allen, F. H., Bellard, S., Brice, M. D., Cartwright, B. A., Doubleday, A., Higgs, H., Hummelink, T., Hummelink-Peters, B. G., Kennard, O., Motherwell, W. D. S., Rodgers, J. R., and Watson, D. G. (1979). The Cambridge crystallographic data centre: computer-based search, retrieval, analysis, and display of information. *Acta Crystallographica*, **B35**, 2231–9.

Allen, F. H., Kennard, O., and Taylor, R. (1983). Systematic analysis of structural data as a research technique in organic chemistry. *Accounts of Chemical Research*, **16**, 146–53.

Baudy, R. B., Greenblatt, L. P., Jirkovsky, I. L., Conklin, M., Russo, R. J., Bramlett, D. R., Emrey, T. A., Simmonds, J. T., Kowal, D. M., Stein, R. P., and Tasse, R. P. (1993). Potent quinoxaline-spaced phosphono α-amino acids of the AP6 type as competitive NMDA antagonists: synthesis and biological evaluation. *Journal of Medicinal Chemistry*, **36**, 331–42.

Bernstein, F. C., Koetzle, T. F., Williams, G. J. B., Meyer, E. F., Jr, Brice, M. D., Rodgers, J. R., Kennard, O., Shimanouchi, T., and Tasumi, M. (1977). The protein data bank: a computer-based archival file for macromolecular structures. *Journal of Molecular Biology*, **112**, 535–42.

Bigge, C. F. (1993). Structural requirements for the development of potent N-methyl-D-aspartic acid (NMDA) receptor antagonists. *Biochemical Pharmacology*, **45**, 1547–61.

Bigge, C. F., Drummond, J. T., and Johnson, G. (1989a). Synthesis and NMDA receptor binding of 2-amino-7,7-difluoro-7-phosphonoheptanoic acid. *Tetrahedron Letters*, **30**, 7013–16.

Bigge, C. F., Drummond, J. T., Johnson, G., Malone, T., Probert, A. W., Jr, Marcoux, F. W., Coughenour, L. L., and Brahce, L. J. (1989b). Exploration of phenyl-spaced 2-amino-(5-9)-phosphonoalkanoic acids as competitive N-methyl-D-aspartic acid antagonists. *Journal of Medicinal Chemistry*, **32**, 1580–90.

Bigge, C. F., Wu, J.-P., Drummond, J. T., Coughenour, L. L., and Hanchin,

C. M. (1992*a*). Excitatory amino acids: 6-phosphonomethyltetrahydro-4-pyrimidinecarboxylic acids and their acyclic analogues are competitive *N*-methyl-D-aspartic acid receptor antagonists. *Bioorganic and Medicinal Chemistry Letters*, **2**, 207–21.

Bigge, C. F., Johnson, G., Ortwine, D. F., Drummond, J. T., Retz, D. M., Brahce, L. J., Coughenour, L. L., Marcoux, F. W., and Probert, A. W. (1992*b*). Exploration of *N*-phosphonoalkyl-, *N*-phosphonoalkenyl-, and *N*-(phosphono-alkyl)phenyl-spaced α-amino acids as competitive *N*-methyl-D-aspartic acid antagonists. *Journal of Medicinal Chemistry*, **35**, 1371–84.

Bigge, C. F., Wu, J.-P., Malone, T. C., Taylor, C. P., and Vartanian, M. G. (1993). Synthesis and anticonvulsant activity of the (+)- and (−)-enantiomers of 1,2,3,4-tetrahydro-5-(2-phosphonoethyl)-3-isoquinolinecarboxylic acid, a competitive NMDA antagonist. *Bioorganic and Medicinal Chemistry Letters*, **3**, 39–42.

Björkroth, J.-P., Pakkanen, T. A., and Lindroos, J. (1991). Comparative molecular field analysis of some clodronic acid esters. *Journal of Medicinal Chemistry*, **34**, 2338–43.

Burton, N. R., Smith, D. A. S., and Stone, T. W. (1988). A quantitative pharmacological analysis of some excitatory amino acid receptors in the mouse neocortex *in vitro*. *British Journal of Pharmacology*, **93**, 381–91.

Chenard, B. L., Lipinski, C. A., Dominy, E. W., Mena, E. E., Ronau, R. T., Butterfield, G. C., Marinovic, L. C., Pagnozzi, M., Butler, T. W., and Tsang, T. (1990). A unified approach to systematic isosteric substitution for acidic groups and application to NMDA antagonists related to 2-amino-7-phosphonoheptanoate. *Journal of Medicinal Chemistry*, **33**, 1077–83.

Childress, R. (ed.) (1985). Revised MDL Edition, March 1985; Molecular Design Ltd, San Leandro, CA.

Claesson, A., Swahn, B.-M., Edvinsson, K. M., Molin, H., and Sandberg, M. (1992). Competitive NMDA antagonists that base their activity on a unique conformation effect. *Bioorganic and Medicinal Chemistry Letters*, **2**, 1247–50.

Clark, M., Cramer, R. D., and Van Opdenbosch, N. (1989). Validation of the Tripos 5.2. force field. *Journal of Computational Chemistry*, **10**, 982–1012.

Collingridge, G. L., Kehl, S. J., and McLennan, H. (1983). Excitatory amino acids in synaptic transmission in the Schaffer collateral-commissural pathway of the rat hippocampus. *Journal of Physiology* (Lond.), **334**, 33–46.

Collingridge, G. L. and Lester, R. A. J. (1989). Excitatory amino acid receptors in the vertebrate central nervous system. *Pharmacological Reviews*, **40**, 143–210.

Croucher, M. J., Collins, J. F., and Meldrum, B. S. (1982). Anticonvulsant action of excitatory amino acid antagonists. *Science*, **216**, 899–901.

Curry, K., Peet, M. J., Magnuson, D. S. K., and McLennan, H. (1988). Synthesis, resolution and absolute configuration of the isomers of the neuronal excitant 1-amino-1,3-cyclopentanedicarboxylic acid. *Journal of Medicinal Chemistry*, **31**, 864–7.

Curtis, D. R. and Watkins, J. C. (1960). The excitation and depression of spinal neurones by structurally related amino acids. *Journal of Neurochemistry*, **6**, 117–41.

Dappen, M. S., Pellicciari, R., Natalini, B., Monahan, J. B., Chiorri, C., and Cordi, A. A. (1991). Synthesis and biological evaluation of cyclopropyl analogues of 2-amino-5-phosphonopentanoic acid. *Journal of Medicinal Chemistry*, **34**, 161–8.

Davies, J. and Watkins, J. C. (1982). Actions of D and L forms of 2-amino-5-phosphonovalerate and 2-amino-4-phosphonobutyrate in the cat spinal cord. *Brain Research*, **235**, 378–86.

Davies, J., Francis, A. A., Jones, A. W., and Watkins, J. C. (1981). 2-Amino-5-phosphonovalerate (2APV), a potent and selective antagonist of amino acid-induced and synaptic excitation. *Neuroscience Letters*, **21**, 77–81.

Davies, J., Evans, R. H., Francis, A. A., Jones, A. W., Smith, D. A. S., and Watkins, J. C. (1982). Conformational aspects of the actions of some piperidine dicarboxylic acids at excitatory amino acid receptors in the mammalian and amphibian spinal cord. *Neurochemical Research*, **7**, 1119–33.

Davies, J., Evans, R. H., Herrling, P. L., Jones, A. W., Olverman, H. J., Pook, P., and Watkins, J. C. (1986). CPP, a new and selective NMDA antagonist. Depression of central neuron responses, affinity for [^{3}H]D-AP5 binding sites on brain membranes and anticonvulsant activity. *Brain Research*, **382**, 169–73.

Dewar, M. J. S., Zoebisch, E. G., Healy, E. F., and Stewart, J. J. P. (1985). AM1: a new general purpose quantum mechanical molecular model. *Journal of the American Chemical Society*, **107**, 3902–9.

Dorville, A., McCort-Tranchepain, I., Vichard, D., Sather, W., Maroun, R., Ascher, P., and Roques, B. P. (1992). Preferred antagonist binding state of the NMDA receptor: synthesis, pharmacology, and computer modelling of (phosphonomethyl)phenylalanine derivatives. *Journal of Medicinal Chemistry*, **35**, 2551–62.

Evans, R. H. and Watkins, J. C. (1981). Pharmacological antgonists of excitant amino acids. *Life Sciences*, **28**, 1303–8.

Evans, R. H., Francis, A. A., Hunt, K., Oakes, D. J., and Watkins, J. C. (1979). Antagonism of excitatory amino acid-induced responses and of synaptic excitation in the isolated spinal cord of the frog. *British Journal of Pharmacology*, **67**, 591–603.

Evans, R. H., Francis, A. A., Jones, A. W., Smith, D. A. S., and Watkins, J. C. (1982a). The effects of a series of ω-phosphonic α-carboxylic amino acids on electrically evoked and amino acid induced responses in isolated spinal cord preparations. *British Journal of Pharmacology*, **75**, 65–75.

Evans, R. H., Nunn, P. B., and Pearson, S. (1982b). γ-N-Oxalyl-L-α, γ-diaminobutyrate (γ-L-ODAB) a naturally occurring N-methyl-D-aspartate antagonist. *Journal of Physiology* (Lond.), **327**, 81P.

Fagg, G. E. and Baud, J. (1988). Characterization of NMDA receptor–ionophore complexes in the brain. In *Excitatory amino acids in health and disease*, (ed. D. Lodge), pp. 63–90. John Wiley, Chichester, UK.

Fagg, G. E. and Matus, A. (1984). Selective association of N-methyl-D-aspartate and quisqualate types of L-glutamate receptor with brain postsynaptic densities. *Proceedings of the National Academy of Science, USA*, **21**, 6876–80.

Fagg, G. E., Olpe, H.-R., Pozza, M. F., Baud, J., Steinmann, M., Schmutz, M., Portet, C., Baumann, P., Thedinga, K., Bittiger, H., Allgeier, H., Heckendorn, R., Angst, C., Brundish, D., and Dingwall, J. G. (1990). CGP 37849 and CGP 39551: novel and competitive N-methyl-D-aspartate receptor antagonists with oral activity. *British Journal of Pharmacology*, **99**, 791–7.

Ferkany, J. W., Kyle, D. J., Willets, J., Rzeszotarski, W. J., Guzewska, M. E., Ellenberger, S. R., Jones, S. M., Sacaan, A. I., Snell, L. D., Borosky, S., Jones, B. E., Johnson, K. M., Balster, R. L., Burchett, K., Kawasaki, K., Hoch, D. B., and Dingledine, R. (1989). Pharmacological profile of NPC 12626, a novel, competitive *N*-methyl-D-aspartate receptor antagonist. *Journal of Pharmacology and Experimental Therapeutics*, **250**, 100–9.

Ferkany, J. W., Hamilton, G. S., Patch, R. J., Huang, Z., Borosky, S. A., Bednar, D. L., Jones, B. E., Zubrowski, R., Willets, J., and Karbon, E. W. (1993*a*). Pharmacological profile of NPC 17742 [2R, 4R, 5S-(2-amino-4,5-(1,2-cyclohexyl)-7-phosphonoheptanoic acid)], a potent, selective and competitive *N*-methyl-D-aspartate receptor antagonist. *Journal of Pharmacology and Experimental Therapeutics*, **264**, 256–64.

Ferkany, J. W., Willetts, J., Borosky, S. A., Clissold, D. B., Karbon, E. W., and Hamilton, G. S. (1993*b*). Pharmacology of (2R, 4R, 5S)-2-amino-4,5-(1,2-cyclohexyl)-7-phosphonoheptanoic acid (NPC 17742); A selective, systemically active, competitive NMDA antagonist. *Bioorganic and Medicinal Chemistry Letters*, **3**, 33–8.

Foster, A. C. and Fagg, G. E. (1987). Comparison of L-[³H]glutamate, D-[³H]aspartate, DL-[³H]AP5 and [³H]NMDA as ligands for NMDA receptors in crude postsynaptic densities from rat brain. *European Journal of Pharmacology*, **133**, 291–300.

Gilson, M. K., Rashin, A., Fine, R., and Honig, B. (1985). On calculation of electrostatic interactions in proteins. *Journal of Molecular Biology*, **184**, 503–16.

Grimwood, S., Foster, A. C., and Kemp, J. A. (1991). The pharmacological specificity of *N*-methyl-D-aspartate receptors in rat cerebral cortex: correspondence between radioligand binding and electrophysiological measurements. *British Journal of Pharmacology*, **103**, 1385–92.

Hamilton, G. S., Huang, Z., Patch, R. J., Narayanan, B. A., and Ferkany, J. W. (1993). Enzymatic asymmetric synthesis of (2R, 4R, 5S)-2-amino-4,5-(1,2-cyclohexyl)-7-phosphonoheptanoic acid. A potent, selective and competitive NMDA antagonist. *Bioorganic and Medicinal Chemistry Letters*, **3**, 27–32.

Harris, E. W., Ganong, A. H., and Cotman, C. W. (1984). Long-term potentiation in the hippocampus involves activation of *N*-methyl-D-aspartate receptors. *Brain Research*, **323**, 132–7.

Harris, E. W., Ganong, A. H., Monaghan, D. T., Watkins, J. C., and Cotman, C. W. (1986). Action of 3-([±]-2-carboxypiperazin-4-yl)-propyl-1-phosphonic acid (CPP): a new and highly potent antagonist of *N*-methyl-D-aspartate receptors in the hippocampus. *Brain Research*, **382**, 174–7.

Harrison, N. L. and Simmonds, M. A. (1985). Quantitative studies on some antagonists of NMDA in slices of rat cerebral cortex. *British Journal of Pharmacology*, **84**, 381–93.

Hays, S. J., Bigge, C. F., Novak, P. M., Drummond, J. T., Bobovski, T. P., Rice, M. J., Johnson, G., Brahce, L. J., and Coughenour, L. L. (1990*a*). New and versatile approaches to the synthesis of CPP-related competitive NMDA antagonists. Preliminary structure–activity relationships and pharmacological evaluation. *Journal of Medicinal Chemistry*, **33**, 2916–24.

Hays, S. J., Bigge, C. F., Drummond, J. T., Johnson, G., Brahce, L. J., Coughenour, L. L., and Robichaud, L. J. (1990*b*). Novel heteroaryl-spaced APV and APH analogues as ligands for the NMDA receptor. *Neurochemistry International*, **16**, 43.

Herrling, P. L. and Müller, W. (1988). UK patent GB(A) 2 198 134.

Hughes, R. A. and Andrews, P. R. (1987). Structural and conformational analogy between cholecystokinin and ergopeptines. *Journal of Pharmacy and Pharmacology*, **39**, 339–43.

Hutchison, A. J., Shaw, K. R., and Schneider, J. A. (1986). European patent 0 203 891 A2.

Hutchison, A. J., Williams, M., Angst, C., de Jesus, R., Blanchard, L., Jackson, R. H., Wilusz, E. J., Murphy, D. E., Bernard, P. S., Schneider, J., Campbell, T., Guida, W., and Sills, M. A. (1989). 4-(Phosphonoalkyl)- and 4-(phosphono-alkenyl)-2-piperidinecarboxylic acids: synthesis, activity at *N*-methyl-D-aspartic acid receptors, and anticonvulsant activity. *Journal of Medicinal Chemistry*, **32**, 2171–8.

Irving, A. J., Schofield, J. G., Watkins, J. C., Sunter, D. C., and Collingridge, G. L. (1990). 1S, 3R-ACPD stimulates and L-AP3 blocks Ca^{2+} mobilisation in rat cerebellar neurons. *European Journal of Pharmacology*, **186**, 363–5.

Iwama, T., Nagai, Y., Tamura, N., Harada, S., and Nagaoke, A. (1991). A novel glutamate agonist, TAN-950A, isolated from streptomycetes. *European Journal of Pharmacology*, **197**, 187–92.

Jaarsma, D., Sebens, J. B., and Korf, J. (1993). Glutamate dehydrogenase improves binding of [^{3}H]CGP 39653 to NMDA receptors in the autoradiographic assay. *Journal of Neuroscience Methods*, **46**, 133–40.

Jones, A. W., Smith, D. A. S., and Watkins, J. C. (1984). Structure–activity relations of dipeptide antagonists of excitatory amino acids. *Neuroscience*, **13**, 573–81.

Jones, P. L. St J., Birse, E. F., Jane, D. E., Jones, A. W., Mewett, K. N., Pook, P. C.-K., Sunter, D. C., Udvarhelyi, P. M., Wharton, B., and Watkins, J. C. (1993). Agonist and antagonist actions of phenylglycine derivatives at depolarizing mediating (1S,3R)-ACPD receptors in neonatal rat motoneurones. *British Journal of Pharmacology* (*Proceedings Supplement*), **108**, 86P.

Kawai, M., Horikawa, Y., Ishihara, T., Shimamoto, K., and Ohfune, Y. (1992). 2-(Carboxycyclopropyl)glycines: binding, neurotoxicity and induction of intracellular free Ca^{2+} increase. *European Journal of Pharmacology*, **211**, 195–202.

Kinney, W. A., Lee, N. E., Garrison, D. T., Podlesney, F. J., Jr, Simmonds, J. T., Bramlett, D., Notvest, R. R., Kowal, D. M., and Tasse, R. P. (1992). Bioisosteric replacement of the α-amino carboxylic acid functionality in 2-amino-5-phosphonopentanoic acid yields unique 3,4-diamino-3-cyclobutene-1,2-dione containing NMDA antagonists. *Journal of Medicinal Chemistry*, **35**, 4720–6.

Koerner, J. F. and Cotman, C. W. (1982). Response of Schaffer collateral-CA1 pyramidal cell synapses of the hippocampus to analogues of acidic amino acids. *Brain Research*, **251**, 105–15.

Krogsgaard-Larsen, P., Madsen, U., Ebert, B., and Hansen, J. J. (1992). Excitatory amino acid receptors: multiplicity and ligand selectivity of receptor subtypes. In *Excitatory amino acid receptors. Design of agonists and antagonists*, (ed. P. Krogsgaard-Larsen and J. J. Hansen), pp. 34–55. Ellis Horwood Ltd, Chichester, UK.

Kyle, D. J., Patch, R. J., Karbon, E. W., and Ferkany, J. W. (1992). NMDA receptors: heterogeneity and agonism. In *Excitatory amino acid receptors. Design of agonists and antagonists*, (ed. P. Krogsgaard-Larsen and J. J. Hansen), pp. 121–62. Ellis Horwood Ltd, Chichester, UK.

Leach, M. J., Marsen, C. M., and Canning, H. M. (1986). (±)*cis*-2,3-Piperidine dicarboxylic acid is a partial NMDA agonist in the *in vitro* rat cerebellar cGMP model. *European Journal of Pharmacology*, **121**, 173–9.

Lehmann, J., Schneider, J., McPherson, S., Murphy, D. E., Bernard, P., Tsai, C., Bennett, D. A., Pastor, G., Steel, D. J., Boehm, C., Cheney, D. L., Liebman, J. M., Williams, M., and Wood, P. L. (1987). CPP, A selective *N*-methyl-D-aspartate (NMDA)-type receptor antagonist. Characterization *in vitro* and *in vivo. Journal of Pharmacology and Experimental Therapeutics*, **240**, 737–46.

Lehmann, J., Hutchison, A. J., McPherson, S. E., Mondadori, C., Schmutz, M., Sinton, C. M., Tsai, C., Murphy, D. E., Steel, D. J., Williams, M., Cheney, D. L., and Wood, P. L. (1988). CGS 19755, a selective and competitive N-methyl-D-aspartate-type excitatory amino acid receptor antagonist. *Journal of Pharmacology and Experimental Therapeutics*, **246**, 65–75.

Lipton, M. and Still, W. C. (1988). The multiple minimum problem in molecular modelling. Tree searching internal coordinate conformational space. *Journal of Computational Chemistry*, **9**, 343–55.

Lodge, D., Davies, S. N., Jones, M. G., Millar, J., Manallack, D. T., Ornstein, P. L., Verberne, A. J. M., Young, N., and Beart, P. M. (1988). A comparison between the *in vivo* and *in vitro* activity of five potent and competitive NMDA antagonists. *British Journal of Pharmacology*, **95**, 957–65.

Lunn, W. H. W., Schoepp, D. D., Calligaro, D. O., Vasileff, R. T., Heinz, L. J., Salhoff, C. R., and O'Malley, P. J. (1992). D,L-Tetrazol-5-ylglycine, a highly potent NMDA agonist: its synthesis and NMDA receptor efficacy. *Journal of Medicinal Chemistry*, **35**, 4608–12.

Madsen, U., Ferkany, J. W., Jones, B. E., Ebert, B., Johansen, T. N., Holm, T., and Krogsgaard-Larsen, P. (1990). NMDA receptor agonists derived from ibotenic acid: preparation, neuroexcitation and neurotoxicity. *European Journal of Pharmacology*, **189**, 381–91.

Magnusson, D. S. K., Curry, K., Peet, M. J., and McLennan, H. (1988). Structural requirements for the activation of excitatory amino acid receptors in the rat spinal cord *in vitro. Experimental Brain Research*, **73**, 541–5.

Mayer, D., Naylor, C., Motoc, I., and Marshall, G. R. (1987). A unique geometry of the active site of angiotensin-converting enzyme consistent with structure–activity studies. *Journal of Computer-Aided Molecular Design*, **1**, 3–16.

Mayer, M. L. and Westbrook, G. L. (1987). The physiology of excitatory amino acids in the vertebrate CNS. *Progress in Neurobiology*, **28**, 197–296.

Meldrum, B. S. (1985). Possible therapeutic applications of antagonists of excitatory amino acid neurotransmitters. *Clinical Science*, **68**, 113–22.

Monaghan, D. T. and Cotman, C. W. (1986). Identification and properties of NMDA receptors in rat brain synaptic plasma membranes. *Proceedings of the National Academy of Science, USA*, **83**, 7532–6.

Monaghan, D. T., Olverman, H. J., Nguyen, L., Watkins, J. C., and Cotman, C. W. (1988). Two classes of NMDA recognition sites: differential distribution and differential regulation by glycine. *Proceedings of the National Academy of Science, USA*, **85**, 9836–40.

Monaghan, D. T., Bridges, R. J., and Cotman, C. W. (1989). The excitatory amino acid receptors: their classes, pharmacology, and distinct properties in the function of the central nervous system. *Annual Review of Pharmacology and Toxicology*, **29**, 365–402.

Monahan, J. B. and Michel, J. (1987). Identification and characterisation of an N-methyl-D-aspartate specific L-[^{3}H]glutamate recognition site in synaptic plasma membranes. *Journal of Neurochemistry*, **48**, 1699–708.

Monahan, J. B., Hood, W. F., Compton, R. P., Cordi, A. A., Snyder, J. P., Pellicciari, R., and Natalina, B. (1990). Characterisation of D-3,4-cyclopropylglutamates as N-methyl-D-aspartate receptor agonists. *Neuroscience Letters*, **112**, 328–32.

Morris, R. G. M., Anderson, E., Lynch, G. S., and Baudry, M. (1986). Selective impairment of learning and blockade of long-term potentiation by an NMDA receptor antagonist AP5. *Nature* (Lond.), **319**, 774.

Müller, W. and Herrling, P. L. (1985). UK patent GB (A) 2 156 818.

Müller, W., Lowe, D. A., Neijt, H., Urwyler, S., Herrling, P. L., Blaser, D., and Seebach, D. (1992). Synthesis and *N*-methyl-D-aspartate (NMDA) antagonist properties of the enantiomers of α-amino-5-(phosphonomethyl)[1,1'-biphenyl]-3-propanoic acid. Use of a new chiral glycine derivative. *Helvetica Chimica Acta*, **75**, 855–64.

Murphy, D. E., Schneider, J., Boehm, C., Lehmann, J., and Williams, M. (1987). Binding of [³H]-3-(2-carboxypiperazin-4-yl)propyl-1-phosphonic acid to rat brain membranes: a selective high affinity ligand for *N*-methyl-D-aspartate receptors. *Journal of Pharmacology and Experimental Therapeutics*, **240**, 778–84.

Murphy, D. E., Hutchison, A. J., Hurt, S. D., Williams, M., and Sills, M. A. (1988). Characterization of the binding of [³H]-CGS 19755: a novel *N*-methyl-D-aspartate antagonist with nanomolar affinity in rat brain. *British Journal of Pharmacology*, **95**, 932–8.

Nakanishi, S. (1992). Molecular diversity of glutamate receptors and implications of brain function. *Science*, **258**, 597–603.

O'Callaghan, D. (1993). The neuropharmacology and computer-aided structural analysis of *N*-methyl-D-aspartate receptor ligands. Unpublished D.Phil. thesis, University of Sydney, Australia.

O'Callaghan, D., Wong, M. G., and Beart, P. M. (1992). Molecular modelling of *N*-methyl-D-aspartate receptor agonists. *Molecular Neuropharmacology*, **2**, 89–92.

O'Callaghan, D., Wong, M. G., and Beart, P. M. (1993). Unpublished observations.

Olverman, H. J. and Watkins, J. C. (1989). NMDA agonists and competitive antagonists. In *The NMDA receptor*, (ed. J. C. Watkins and G. L. Collingridge), pp. 19–36. IRL Press at Oxford University Press, Oxford, UK.

Olverman, H. J., Jones, A. W., and Watkins, J. C. (1984). L-Glutamate has higher affinity than other amino acids for [³II]-D-AP5 binding sites in rat brain membranes. *Nature* (Lond.), **307**, 460–2.

Olverman, H. J., Monaghan, D. T., Cotman, C. W., and Watkins, J. C. (1986). [³H]-CPP, a new competitive ligand for NMDA receptors. *European Journal of Pharmacology*, **131**, 161–2.

Olverman, H. J., Jones, A. W., Mewett, K. N., and Watkins, J. C. (1988a). Structure/activity relations of NMDA receptor ligands as studied by their inhibition of ³H-D-AP5 binding in rat brain membranes. *Neuroscience*, **26**, 17–31.

Olverman, H. J., Jones, A. W., and Watkins, J. C. (1988b). [³H]D-2-Amino-5-phosphonopentanoate as a ligand for *N*-methyl-D-aspartate receptors in the mammalian central nervous system. *Neuroscience*, **26**, 1–15.

Ornstein, P. L. and Klimkowski, V. J. (1992). Competitive NMDA receptor antagonists. In *Excitatory amino acid receptors. Design of agonists and antagonists*, (ed. P. Krogsgaard-Larsen and J. J. Hansen), pp. 183–201. Ellis Horwood Ltd, Chichester, UK.

Ornstein, P. L., Schaus, J. M., Chambers, J. W., Huser, D. L., Leander, J. D., Wong, D. T., Paschal, J. W., Jones, N. D., and Deeter, J. B. (1989). Synthesis and pharmacology of a series of 1-and 4-(phosphonoalkyl)pyridine- and-piperidine-2-carboxylic acids. Potent *N*-methyl-D-aspartate receptor antagonists. *Journal of Medicinal Chemistry*, **32**, 827–33.

Ornstein, P. L., Schoepp, D. D., Leander, J. D., and Lodge, D. (1990). Development of novel competitive NMDA antagonists as useful therapeutic agents. Discovery of LY 274614 and LY 233536. *Neuroscience International*, **16**, Suppl. 1, 8.

Ornstein, P. L., Schoepp, D. D., Arnold, M. B., Leander, J. D., Lodge, D., Paschal, J. W., and Elzey, T. (1991). 4-(Tetrazolylalkyl)piperidine-2-carboxylic acids. Potent and selective N-methyl-D-aspartic acid receptor antagonists with a short duration of action. *Journal of Medicinal Chemistry*, **34**, 90–7.

Ornstein, P. L., Schoepp, D. D., Arnold, M. B., Augenstein, N. K., Lodge, D., Millar, J. D., Chambers, J., Campbell, J., Paschal, J. W., Zimmerman, D. M., and Leander, J. D. (1992a). 6-Substituted decahydroisoquinoline-3-carboxylic acids as potent and selective conformationally constrained NMDA receptor antagonists. *Journal of Medicinal Chemistry*, **35**, 3547–60.

Ornstein, P. L., Schoepp, D. D., Arnold, M. B., Jones, N. D., Deeter, J. B., Lodge, D., and Leander, J. D. (1992b). NMDA antagonist activity of (±)-(2SR, 4RS)-4-(1H-tetrazol-5-ylmethyl)piperidine-2-carboxylic acid resides with the (−)-2R, 4S-isomer. *Journal of Medicinal Chemistry*, **35**, 3111–15.

Ornstein, P. L., Arnold, M. B., Evrard, D., Leander, J. D., Lodge, D., and Schoepp, D. D. (1993). Tetrazole amino acids as competitive NMDA antagonists. *Bioorganic and Medicinal Chemistry Letters*, **3**, 43–8.

Ortwine, D. F., Malone, T. C., Bigge, C. F., Drummond, J. T., Humblet, C., Johnson, G., and Pinter, G. W. (1992). Generation of N-methyl-D-aspartate agonist and competitive antagonist pharmacophore models. Design and synthesis of phosphonoalkyl-substituted tetrahydroisoquinolines as novel antagonists. *Journal of Medicinal Chemistry*, **35**, 1345–70.

Palmer, E., Monaghan, D. T., and Cotman, C. W. (1989). Trans-ACPD, a selective agonist of the phosphoinositide-coupled excitatory amino acid receptor. *European Journal of Pharmacology*, **166**, 585–7.

Pearlstein, R. A. CHEMLAB-II Reference Manual. Chemlab Inc. (Software available from Molecular Design Ltd, San Leandro, California).

Perkins, M. N., Collins, J. F., and Stone, T. W. (1982). Isomers of 2-amino-7-phosphonoheptanoic acid as antagonists of neuronal excitants. *Neuroscience Letters*, **32**, 65–8.

Pople, J. A. and Beveridge, D. L. (1970). *Approximate molecular orbital theory*. McGraw Hill, New York.

Sakurai, S. Y. and Young, A. B. (1992). Receptor autoradiography of excitatory amino acid receptors: basic and clinical aspects. In *Excitatory amino acid receptors. Design of agonists and antagonists*, (ed. P. Krogsgaard-Larsen and J. J. Hansen), pp. 101–20. Ellis Horwood Ltd, Chichester, U.K.

Schoepp, D. D. and Conn, P. J. (1993). Metabotropic glutamate receptors in brain function and pathology. *Trends in Pharmacological Sciences*, **14**, 13–20.

Schoepp, D. D., Smith, C. L., Lodge, D., Millar, J. D., Leander, J. D., Sacaan, A. I., and Lunn, W. H. W. (1991a). D,L-(Tetrazol-5-yl)glycine: a novel and highly potent NMDA receptor agonist. *European Journal of Pharmacology*, **203**, 237–43.

Schoepp, D. D., Bockaert, J., and Sladeczek, F. (1991b). Pharmacological and functional characteristics of metabotropic excitatory amino acid receptors. In *Trends in Pharmacological Sciences: A special report*, (ed. D. Lodge and G. L. Collingridge), pp. 74–81.

Shinozaki, H. (1992a). Kainic acid receptor agonists. In *Excitatory amino acid receptors. Design of agonists and antagonists*, (ed. P. Krogsgaard-Larsen and J. J. Hansen), pp. 34–55. Ellis Horwood Ltd, Chichester, UK.

Shinozaki, H. (1992*b*) Structure–activity studies of glutamate agonists and antagonists. In *Excitatory amino acids*, Fidia Research Foundation Symposium Series 9 (ed. R. P. Simon), pp. 63–71. Thieme Medical Publishers, Inc., New York.

Sills, M. A., Fagg, G., Pozza, M., Angst, C., Brundish, D. E., Hurt, S. D., Wilusz, E. J., and Williams, M. (1991). [^{3}H]CGP 39653: a new *N*-methyl-D-aspartate antagonist radioligand with low nanomolar affinity in rat brain. *European Journal of Pharmacology*, **192**, 19–24.

Simon, R. P., Swan, J. H., Griffiths, T., and Meldrum, B. S. (1984). Blockade of *N*-methyl-D-aspartate receptors may protect against ischaemic damage in the brain. *Science*, **226**, 850–2.

Stewart, J. J. P. (1990). Semiempirical molecular orbital methods. In *Reviews in Computational Chemistry*, (ed. K. B. Lipkowitz and D. B. Boyd), pp. 45–82. VCH, New York.

Stone, T. W. and Burton, N. R. (1988). NMDA receptors and ligands in the vertebrate CNS. *Progress in Neurobiology*, **30**, 333–68.

Sunter, D. C., Edgar, G. E., Pook, P. C.-K., Howard, J. A. K., Udvarhelyi, P. M., and Watkins, J. C. (1991). Actions of the four isomers of 1-aminocyclopentane-1,3-dicarboxylate (ACPD) in the hemisected spinal cord of the neonatal rat. *British Journal of Pharmacology* (Proceedings supplement), **104**, 377P.

Taylor, R., Kennard, O., and Verschel, W. (1984). The geometry of the N–H...O=C hydrogen bond. 3: hydrogen-bond distances and angles. *Acta Crystallographica*, **B40**, 280–8.

Tsai, C., Schneider, J. A., and Lehmann, J. (1988). *Trans*-2-carboxy-3-pyrrolidineacetic acid (CPAA), a novel agonist at NMDA-type receptors. *Neuroscience Letters*, **92**, 298–302.

Warwicker, J. (1986). Continuum dielectric modelling of the protein-solvent system, and calculation of the long-range electrostatic field of the enzyme phosphoglycerate mutase. *Journal of Theoretical Biology*, **121**, 199 210.

Warwicker, J., Ollis, D., and Richards, H. (1985). Electrostatic field of the large fragment of *Escherichia coli* DNA polymerase I. *Journal of Molecular Biology*, **186**, 645–9.

Watkins, J. C. (1962). The synthesis of some acidic amino acids possessing neuropharmacological activity. *Journal of Medicinal and Pharmaceutical Chemistry*, **5**, 1187–99.

Watkins, J. C. (1981). Pharmacology of excitatory amino acid receptors. In *Glutamate: transmitter in the central nervous system*, (ed. P. J. Roberts, J. Storm-Mathisen, and G. A. R. Johnston), pp. 1–24. Wiley, Chichester, UK.

Watkins, J. C. (1990). Chemical highlights in the development of excitatory amino acid pharmacology. *Canadian Journal of Physiology and Pharmacology*, **69**, 1064–75.

Watkins, J. C. (1991). Structure/activity relations of competitive NMDA receptor antagonists. In *Excitatory amino acid antagonists*, (ed. B. Meldrum), pp. 84–100. Blackwell Scientific Publications, Oxford.

Watkins, J. C. and Evans, R. H. (1981). Excitatory amino acid transmitters. *Annual Review of Pharmacology and Toxicology*, **21**, 165–204.

Watkins, J. C. and Olverman, H. J. (1987). Agonists and antagonists for excitatory amino acid receptors. *Trends in Neurosciences*, **10**, 265–72.

Watkins, J. C. and Olverman, H. J. (1988). Structural requirements for activation and blockade of EAA receptors, In *Excitatory amino acids in health and disease*, (ed. D. Lodge), pp. 13–45. John Wiley, Chichester, UK.

Watkins, J. C., Krogsgaard-Larsen, P. and Honoré, T. (1991). Structure–activity relationships in the development of excitatory amino acid receptor agonists and competitive antagonists. In *The pharmacology of excitatory amino acids*, (ed. D. Lodge and G. L. Collingridge), special issue of *Trends in Pharmacological Sciences*, pp. 4–12.

Wedler, F. C., Farrington, G. K., Kumar, A., Bigge, C. F., Ortwine, D. F., and Johnson, G. (1992). 3-[(Phosphonomethyl)sulfinyl]-D,L-alanine, a potent *N*-methyl-D-aspartate receptor antagonist. *Life Sciences Advances in Neurochemistry*. (In press.)

Wheatley, P. L. and Collins, K. J. (1986). Quantitative studies of NMDA, 2-amino-5-phosphonovalerate and *cis*-2,3-piperidine dicarboxylate interactions on the neonatal rat spinal cord *in vitro*. *European Journal of Pharmacology*, **121**, 257–63.

Whitten, J. P., Baron, B. M., Miller, D. M. F., White, H. S., and McDonald, I. A. (1990). (R)-4-Oxo-5-phosphononorvaline: A new competitive glutamate antagonist at the NMDA receptor complex. *Journal of Medicinal Chemistry*, **33**, 2961–3.

Whitten, J. P., Muench, D., Cube, R. V., Nyce, P. L., Baron, B. M., and McDonald, I. A. (1991). Synthesis of 3(S)-phosphonoacetyl-2(R)-piperidine-carboxylic acid, a conformationally-restricted glutamate antagonist. *Bioorganic and Medicinal Chemistry Letters*, **1**, 441–4.

Whitten, J. P., Harrison, B. L., Weintraub, H. J. R., and McDonald, I. A. (1992). Modelling of competitive phosphono amino acid NMDA receptor antagonists. *Journal of Medicinal Chemistry*, **35**, 1509–14.

Whitten, J. P., Baron, B. M., and McDonald, I. A. (1993*a*). Competitive NMDA receptor antagonists: (R)-4-oxo-5-phosphononorvaline structure–activity relationships. *Bioorganic and Medicinal Chemistry Letters*, **3**, 23–6.

Whitten, J. P., Cube, R. V., Baron, B. M., and McDonald, I. A. (1993*b*). Competitive NMDA receptor antagonists: synthesis of β-ketophosphonate-substituted piperidine carboxylic acid derivatives. *Bioorganic and Medicinal Chemistry Letters*, **3**, 19–22.

Wieloch, T. (1985). Hypoglycemia-induced neuronal damage prevented by an NMDA antagonist. *Science*, **230**, 681–3.

Young, A. B. and Fagg, G. E. (1991). Excitatory amino acid receptors in the brain: membrane binding and receptor autoradiographic approaches. In *The pharmacology of excitatory amino acids*, (ed. D. Lodge and G. L. Collingridge), special issue of *Trends in Pharmacological Sciences*, pp. 18–24.

3 Non-competitive antagonists of N-methyl-D-aspartate

DAVID LODGE, MARTYN JONES AND
ELIZABETH FLETCHER

Introduction

Identifying the chemicals that act as the main excitatory transmitters in the central nervous system (CNS) has been a scientific goal since synaptic transmission between most nerve cells was accepted as being chemical rather than electrical (Eccles 1963). Acetylcholine and monoamines such as noradrenaline, which are transmitters at synapses in the peripheral nervous system, also act in the CNS but only at a small proportion of the total number of synapses.

Interest in the acidic amino acids, glutamate and aspartate, arose from the pioneering observations that they caused muscle contractions when applied to the surface of the cerebral cortex (Hayashi 1952) and excitation when administered to single spinal neurones using the technique of microelectrophoresis (Curtis and Watkins 1960; see also Chapter 1). A full structure–activity study showed that some analogues of aspartate and glutamate, e.g. N-methyl-D-aspartate (NMDA) and other D isomers were more potent than L-aspartate and L-glutamate. These observations (Curtis and Watkins 1960), together with the fact that such compounds excited all neurones tested and that they were neurotoxic following systemic administration to neonatal rats (Olney 1969), appeared to reduce their candidature for a synaptic role. Considerable neurochemical and neuroanatomical evidence, however, now suggests that excitatory amino acids do have a transmitter role (Fonnum 1984), but the most compelling evidence comes from the development of pharmacological probes for glutamate receptors.

The acceptance of different receptor subtypes followed reports of regional differences in potency between the glutamate analogues, NMDA and kainate, and substances that could selectively antagonize excitation by particular amino acids (Curtis and Johnson 1964; Evans et al. 1978; Davies and Watkins 1979; McLennan and Lodge 1979; Watkins and Evans 1981; McLennan 1983; see also Chapter 1). Some of these substances, glutamic acid diethyl ester (GDEE), D-α-aminoadipate (DAA), 1-hydroxy-3-amino-pyrrolidone-2 (HA-966), and magnesium ions were used to develop the present, almost certainly oversimplified view that there are three major receptor subtypes, which mediate the post-synaptic depolarizing actions of glutamate and aspartate (McLennan and Lodge 1979; Watkins and Evans 1981). They were named the NMDA, quisqualate, and kainate receptors since these three glutamate analogues were potent agonists displaying a differential sensitivity to a variety of antagonists. For example, the excitatory action of NMDA was reduced by DAA, HA-966, and Mg^{2+}, and that of quisqualate by GDEE, whereas excitation by kainate was relatively resistant to all these antagonists. Although this general scheme has many flaws, the idea of a separate NMDA receptor subtype is almost universally accepted.

In general the ability of DAA and a range of related substances to act as amino acid antagonists has been found to parallel the ability of these substances to displace binding of tritiated ligands from the recognition site of the NMDA receptor (Watkins and Olverman 1988; see also Chapter 2). Important exceptions include Mg^{2+} and HA-966, which do not displace [^{3}H]D-2-amino-5-phosphonovalerate (D-AP5), a competitive-type NMDA receptor antagonist, from rat brain binding sites. Several other groups of compounds have joined this 'non-competitive' list in the 1980s and 1990s. In the remainder of this chapter we will concentrate on chemicals acting at sites other than that for NMDA recognition but which nevertheless influence the functions of the NMDA receptor channel complex.

The actions of magnesium

The observation that magnesium is a selective but non-competitive antagonist of NMDA was first made by Evans *et al.* (1978) on isolated frog and rat spinal cords. They showed that magnesium, 10^{-4}–10^{-3} M, decreased NMDA-induced depolarizations recorded from ventral roots to a far greater extent than those induced by kainate and quisqualate (which were hardly affected) with intermediate effects on responses to L-glutamate and L-aspartate. The mechanism of this action was not understood but the possibility that magnesium was acting as a channel blocker and/or calcium antagonist were considered.

When electrophysiologists began studying the intracellular potential changes following administration of NMDA receptor agonists, it was clear that the ensuing depolarizations were not simply due to an ohmic conductance increase to sodium and potassium. J-shaped current–voltage curves were obtained. There were suggestions about reduced potassium conductances and active calcium currents to try to explain some of the unusual features. It was not until studies of Nowak *et al.* (1984) using patch-clamp technology and those of Mayer *et al.* (1984) using voltage clamp that the essential role of magnesium was elucidated (Chapter 7).

In the presence of extracellular magnesium, the patch-clamp studies showed large, 50 pS, channels opened by NMDA and by L-glutamate, the events occurring in bursts of rapid openings and closings. In the absence of added magnesium, each burst became a single, long-lasting opening. Thus the rapid closures during bursts were induced by magnesium ions. This leads to a 'flickery' appearance of channel opening as magnesium presumably blocks the channel intermittently. This may represent magnesium ions oscillating in and out of the channel mouth or, as seems more likely, temporarily blocking the channel whilst they proceed through to the inner surface.

This latter suggestion seems particularly likely since the magnesium block is highly voltage-dependent with maximum block occurring at around -80 mV. This voltage-dependent block of the NMDA channel by normal extracellular fluid concentrations of magnesium is important for the physiological role of such synapses. A hyperpolarized neurone will only be slightly depolarized on activation of post-synaptic receptors of the NMDA subtype whereas on a partly depolarized neurone similar activation will have a much greater effect. Thus repetitive activation of an NMDA receptor-mediated synapse will produce a non-linear summating effect, a type of positive feedback or regenerative depolarization.

Other divalent cations such as nickel, cobalt, zinc, and manganese also block NMDA-induced depolarizations. Part of their actions may be via other sites on the membrane (see below) or via block of voltage-activated calcium channels but the actions of manganese and nickel are probably akin to those described for magnesium.

On cortical wedges (Harrison and Simmonds 1985), nickel, magnesium, and manganese gave selective and reversible reductions of responses to 40 µM NMDA with IC_{50}s of about 200, 600, and 700 µM respectively. Cobalt, cadmium, and zinc, although on some slices showing selectivity towards NMDA, were mostly non-selective and appeared to be toxic since responses to NMDA and to quisqualate continued to decline after removing these cations from the superfusate (D. Lodge and J. Millar, unpublished observations).

The NMDA channel is, however, permeable to the divalent cation, calcium (see Chapters 7 and 13 in this book). The resultant increase in cytoplasmic calcium on NMDA receptor activation has several important consequences, one of which is to limit conductance of the NMDA-coupled channel. Activation of calcium-dependent potassium channels will result in hyperpolarization which in turn will increase magnesium block of the channel.

Thus magnesium-dependent regenerative depolarization of the NMDA receptor–channel complex coupled with the consequent calcium-dependent potassium conductances leads to depolarization–hyperpolarization sequences which underpin neural rhythmicity, such as pattern generation for locomotion (Sigvart *et al.* 1985; see also Chapter 12) and abnormal burst discharges of epilepsy (Patel *et al.* 1988; Aram *et al.* 1989 and Chapter 17).

The action of phencyclidine

As was known previously, we reported that dissociative anaesthetics reduced polysynaptic reflexes and excitations of spinal neurones (Lodge and Anis 1984) and we further showed that ketamine and phencyclidine (PCP) selectively reduced the excitatory action of NMDA (Lodge and Anis 1982; Anis *et al.* 1983) which would explain the reduction of polysynaptic excitations. Reduction of reflex activity by low (NMDA-selective) systemic doses of ketamine has now been demonstrated more elegantly on responses in single ventral root afferents to natural stimulation of the peripheral receptive fields (Headley *et al.* 1987).

The NMDA blocking action of the dissociative anaesthetics was stereoselective in that the (+) isomers of ketamine and methyl-phencyclidine were more potent than the equivalent (−) isomer (Berry *et al.* 1983; Berry and Lodge 1985). Other dissociative anaesthetics, tiletamine (see Fig. 3.1), etoxadrol, and dexoxadrol, were similarly selective as NMDA antagonists as were sigma opiates such as cyclazocine and SKF 10,047 (Berry *et al.* 1984*a,b*). Even pentazocine shows weak NMDA antagonist activity. This action of the sigma opiates is not blocked by naloxone and, unlike effects at classical opiate receptors, does not reside exclusively in the (−) isomer (Berry *et al.* 1984*b*). Morphinans, such as dextrorphan and dextromethorphan, also display clear NMDA antagonism although levorphanol is weak

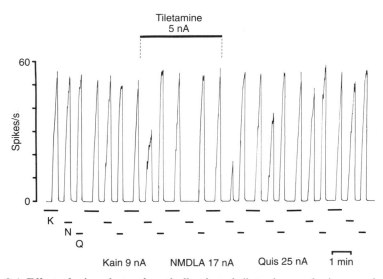

Fig. 3.1 Effect of microelectrophoretically ejected tiletamine on the increase in firing rate of a rat spinal neurone in response to the ejection of kainate, NMDLA, and quisqualate at the times and with the currents indicated. Tiletamine produces a selective and reversible abolition of the NMDLA response.

in this respect (Church *et al.* 1985). Benz(f)isoquinolines (Berry and Lodge 1984) and methyldiphenylpropanolamines (Blake *et al.* 1986) also are selective and potent NMDA antagonists. Memantine, an adamantane derivative used in the treatment of Parkinson's disease, is also a PCP-like NMDA antagonist (Chen *et al.* 1992) with a potency not dissimilar to that of ketamine. The most potent of this series of PCP-like compounds is the dibenzocyloalkenimine, (+)-MK-801 (Wong *et al.* 1986; Davies *et al.* 1988). The structure of several of these PCP-like non-competitive NMDA antagonists is shown in Fig. 3.2.

More or less coincident with the above studies, the specific binding of

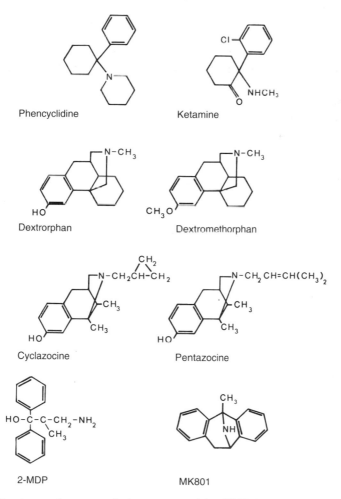

Phencyclidine

Ketamine

Dextrorphan

Dextromethorphan

Cyclazocine

Pentazocine

2-MDP

MK801

Fig. 3.2 Structures of some typical non-competitive NMDA antagonists which are known to act at the PCP site.

[^{3}H]PCP to rat brain membranes was being described (Vincent *et al.* 1979; Zukin and Zukin 1979). It was thus of considerable interest to us that of all the drugs tested only dissociative anaesthetics and sigma opiates displaced PCP binding and that glutamate did not displace PCP binding. Since then extensive structure–activity studies have been performed and we have compared the potencies of these drugs as NMDA antagonists with their potencies in binding studies. Relative potencies from the above experiments on spinal neurones *in vivo* (Berry and Lodge 1985; Lodge *et al.* 1988*a*) and on cortical wedges (Snell and Johnson 1985; Lodge *et al.* 1987; Martin and Lodge 1988; Aram *et al.* 1989) correlate well with that in binding studies (see Table 3.1), although the absolute values are larger in the electropharmacological experiments on more intact tissues. There appears, however, to be no correlation with other known binding sites, including that at opiate, sigma, or other recognized neurotransmitter receptors (Berry and Lodge 1984; Snell and Johnson 1985; Lodge *et al.* 1987; Martin and Lodge 1988). The density of NMDA and PCP binding sites in different brain areas is similar (Greemayre *et al.* 1983; Cotman *et al.* 1987). Thus the binding for both types of ligands is high, for example, in the CA1 region of the hippocampus and in superficial layers of the cerebral cortex, and is low in striatum and cerebellum.

With relevance to functional aspects of NMDA and PCP receptors, a good correlation exists between NMDA antagonism and various behavioural effects of PCP-like compounds (see Table 3.1). Animals trained to discriminate between PCP and saline produce PCP-appropriate responses

Table 3.1 Relative potencies of phencyclidine-like compounds in electrophysiological biochemical and behavioural tests

	As NMDA antagonists			PCP		
	Cortex *in vitro*	Cord *in vitro*	Cord *in vivo*	PCP binding	Discrimination	PCP catalepsy
MK-801	8.5	1.5	3.5	30	3–10	3.2
TCP	1.88	NT	1.7	1.57	1.46	NT
(−)CYC	1.54	0.95	0.8	0.36	1.09	2.0
PCP	1.0	1.0	1.0	1.0	1.0	1.0
(+)PCMP	0.69	2.6	1.2	NT	1.0	NT
(+)SKF	0.43	0.58	0.3	0.2	0.45	0.25
(+)CYC	0.36	0.65	0.4	0.1	0.13	0.5
(±)KET	0.15	0.6	0.1	0.15	0.10	0.25
(−)SKF	0.08	0.18	0.2	0.18	0.18	0.25
(−)PCMP	0.06	0.16	0.1	NT	0.3	NT

Reproduced from Martin and Lodge (1988) where details can be found.
NT = not tested; TCP = thienylcyclohexylpiperidine.

when tested with other members of the series (Brady *et al.* 1982; Herling and Woods 1982; Holzman 1982; Leander 1982; Shannon 1983). The potency of drugs in these behavioural studies parallels the intravenous doses required to antagonize NMDA on central neurones (Lodge *et al.* 1988*a*). Such results suggest that reduced efficiency at synapses operated via NMDA receptors explains some of the behavioural effects of PCP-like compounds. This idea is given further support by the finding that competitive NMDA antagonists are also able to mimic some of the behavioural effects of PCP (Woods *et al.* 1986; Tricklebank *et al.* 1987).

When tested *in vitro*, the action of PCP-like compounds appeared not to be competitive, since dose–response curves were not shifted in a parallel manner (Lodge and Johnston 1985, 1990; Snell and Johnson 1985). The non-additive nature of combinations of ketamine both with competitive antagonists and with magnesium suggests that ketamine acts at a site distinct from the NMDA recognition site and from the magnesium site (Harrison and Simmonds 1985; Martin and Lodge 1985; but see Mori *et al.* 1992). The block of NMDA by ketamine was dependent on the membrane potential although with a flatter current–voltage relationship than that for magnesium (MacDonald *et al.* 1987; MacDonald and Nowak 1990). It has also been shown that the development and recovery from the block was dependent on the presence of an NMDA receptor agonist (Huettner and Bean 1988). This agonist- or use-dependency of the block was also demonstrated on cortical slices with other PCP-like compounds (Wong *et al.* 1986; Davies *et al.* 1988). That use-dependency is difficult to demonstrate *in vivo* (Davies *et al.* 1988) is probably due to the faster rate of reactions at the higher temperature in these experiments. In neurochemical studies, the binding of these compounds was shown to be similarly dependent on presence of endogenous glutamate or addition of other NMDA agonists (Loo *et al.* 1986; Kloog *et al.* 1988). Such results support the concept that PCP-like compounds antagonize NMDA by entering and blocking the open channel, and that they may then be trapped within the channel until it is activated again. In passing, the fact that PCP blocks the NMDA-associated channel and does not affect the responses of neurones to quisqualate and kainate suggests to us that no appreciable part of the inward currents evoked by these latter two agonists is via the NMDA receptor coupled channel.

As with other receptors there has been an intensive and systematic search for antagonists and for endogenous ligands.

Beside some interest in an alkylating agent called metaphit, which proved to be a PCP-like NMDA antagonist (Davies *et al.* 1986) with effects on other channels, there have been no reports of drugs which block the actions of PCP. This is perhaps not surprising, if the site for PCP is deep in the channel coupled to the NMDA receptor. All compounds binding at such a site are likely to have similar effects on the channel conductance.

With respect to endogenous ligands, there have been several reports of compounds isolated from the brain that are able to displace PCP binding (DiMaggio *et al*. 1986; Zukin *et al*. 1987). These appear to be high molecular weight peptides. Little progress appears to have been made in this direction in the past 5 years. With the discovery of several sites that are able to influence binding at the PCP receptor (see below), such compounds will have to be rigorously tested before they can be said to be truly endogenous PCP receptor ligands. Further study of these interesting peptides is required.

Whilst discussing channel blockers, it should be mentioned that the spider toxin, argiotoxin 636 (Priestley *et al*. 1989), and agatoxin 489 (Kiskin *et al*. 1992) have been shown to produce a use- and voltage-dependent block of channels coupled to the NMDA receptor on neurones in culture. In experiments on brainstem neurones *in vivo*, we found that argiotoxin 636, like philanthotoxin (Jones and Lodge 1991), from the venom of the digger wasp, reduced responses to quisqualate and kainate more than those to NMDA. The latter results concur with previous studies of such toxins on invertebrate and vertebrate tissues. For a recent review of this area, see Scott *et al*. (1993).

The action of HA-966

HA-966 is a pyrrolidone compound first described by Bonta *et al*. (1971) as producing increased locomotor activity and some central sympathomimetic effects. This compound was later shown to have glutamate antagonist properties, preferentially reducing the actions of NMDA (Curtis and Johnson 1974; Evans *et al*. 1978; Watkins and Evans 1981). Subsequently, however, as judged by displacement of binding of the selective NMDA antagonist, [^{3}H]D-AP5, HA-966 was shown not to act at the NMDA recognition site (Watkins and Olverman 1988). HA-966 was thus an NMDA antagonist without a known site of action.

The discovery in 1987 that glycine in submicromolar concentrations facilitated NMDA-evoked currents in cultured neurones (Johnson and Ascher 1987) has eventually led to an explanation of the action of HA-966 and some other atypical NMDA antagonists.

The increase in NMDA-activated channel opening by glycine was also seen with D-serine, but not with GABA, and was not antagonized by strychnine. This action is therefore distinct from that at the classical strychnine-sensitive receptors that mediate inhibitory synaptic transmission (Curtis and Johnson 1974).

These observations have been confirmed by other electrophysiologists working with isolated systems (Mayer *et al*. 1984; Kleckner and Dingledine 1988; Kushner *et al*. 1988) but not by those working with more intact preparations (Birch *et al*. 1988; Fletcher and Lodge 1988; Watson *et al*.

1988; for reviews see Foster and Kemp 1989; Kemp and Leeson 1993; Wong and Kemp 1991). Parallel results show that glycine facilitates binding of PCP-like ligands to well washed brain membranes (Loo *et al.* 1986; Snell *et al.* 1987; Ranson and Stec 1988; Reynolds *et al.* 1988; Foster and Kemp 1989). These data indicate, as suggested by Johnson and Ascher (1987) and by neurochemical estimates, that extracellular levels of glycine are normally sufficient to occupy all the glycine receptors.

We hypothesized that, if this were the case, some non-competitive NMDA antagonists with unknown sites of action could act by displacing endogenous glycine. We decided initially to examine HA-966 since this fitted some of the above criteria and could be regarded as a glycine analogue.

Both on cortical wedges and with iontophoresis *in vivo*, the NMDA antagonism induced by HA-966 could be reversed by the co-administration of glycine (Fletcher and Lodge 1988; Fletcher *et al.* 1989), whereas similar antagonism by ketamine, magnesium, or D-AP5 was not affected. D-serine mimicked this action and these effects were not reversed by strychnine. In fact on most spinal and brain stem neurones *in vivo*, it was necessary to perform the experiment in the presence of strychnine to prevent the inhibitory effect of glycine. HA-966 has now been shown to displace [^{3}H]glycine binding (Foster and Kemp 1989).

Several other substances are now known to act as NMDA antagonists at least in part by an interaction at the glycine site. Kynurenic acid is an NMDA antagonist (Birch *et al.* 1988; Stone and Burton 1988) which displaces glycine binding (Kessler *et al.* 1987; Marvizon and Skolnick 1988) *but* also acts competitively at the NMDA receptor (Ascher *et al.* 1988; Stone and Burton 1988; Watkins and Olverman 1988). The 7-chloro derivative of kynurenate is more selective and potent at the glycine site than is the parent compound (Kemp *et al.* 1988; Elizabeth Fletcher, unpublished observations). 6-Cyano-7-nitro-quinoxalinedione (CNQX), a potent antagonist at non-NMDA receptors (Fletcher *et al.* 1988; Honoré *et al.* 1988), has little action on binding at the NMDA recognition site (Honoré *et al.* 1988) but has weak NMDA antagonist properties (Birch *et al.* 1988; Fletcher *et al.* 1988). As with HA-966, the NMDA antagonist actions of the above drugs can be reversed by glycine and D-serine *in vitro* (Ascher *et al.* 1988; Birch *et al.* 1988; Fletcher and Lodge 1988; Kemp *et al.* 1988; Fletcher *et al.* 1989; Foster and Kemp 1989) and *in vivo* (Martyn Jones, unpublished observations). An example from an *in vivo* experiment of the reversal by glycine of kynurenate's antagonism of NMDA but not of quisqualate is shown in Fig. 3.3. Most of these compounds also reduce responses to quisqualate and/or kainate but this part of their action is not reversed by glycine.

Structure–activity relationships at the glycine receptor are now well established (Wong and Kemp 1991; Kemp and Leeson 1993; Yoneda *et al.*

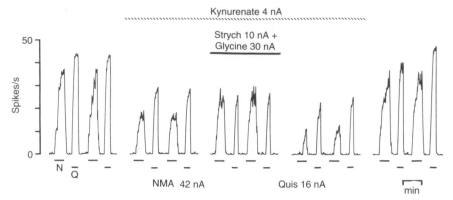

Fig. 3.3 Effect of kynurenate and glycine on responses of a rat trigeminal neurone to the electrophoretic administration of NMDA and quisqualate ejected for the times and with the currents indicated. Kynurenate non-selectively reduces responses to both agonists. Glycine, co-ejected with strychnine (Strych.) to prevent its classical inhibitory actions, increases only the action of NMDA. Recovery from this effect of glycine and of kynurenate's action are also shown.

1993; see also Table 3.2). The D isomers of serine and alanine are nearly as potent as glycine and considerably more than the L isomers; larger amino acids are less effective (Johnson and Ascher 1987; Snell *et al.* 1987; Fletcher *et al.* 1989; Foster and Kemp 1989). Cyclopropane-aminocarboxylate is another potent agonist (Nadler *et al.* 1988) whereas cycloleucine, which has a larger cyclic substituent for the α carbon of glycine, shows some antagonistic activity at this site. Cycloserine, which is structurally similar to HA-966, shows up as a relatively potent glycine agonist. These structure–activity studies and the interaction between the glycine, NMDA, and PCP binding sites have recently been well reviewed (Snell *et al.* 1987; Kemp and Leeson 1993). Tetrahydroquinoline derivatives from kynurenic acid are thus pure antagonists with nanomolar affinity for the glycine site but do not cross the blood–brain barrier, whereas the (+)-4-methyl-HA-966, although a partial agonist with micromolar affinity, acts as a systemically active glycine site antagonist (Kemp and Leeson 1993). Figure 3.4 shows the structures of these and other new antagonists acting at the glycine site.

The debate as to whether occupation of the glycine site is an essential requirement for activation of the NMDA receptor channel complex or whether it prevents desensitization is still active (Kleckner and Dingledine 1988; Kushner *et al.* 1988; Wong and Kemp 1991; Kemp and Leeson 1993). Glycine has been observed to decrease the desensitization of NMDA receptors in some (Mayer *et al.* 1989*a*) but not all (Sather *et al.* 1992) neuronal cultures (Kemp and Leeson 1993). This anomaly may in part be explained by the presence of both fast, glycine-sensitive and slow, glycine-insensitive phases of desensitization observed in outside-out patches of

Table 3.2 Comparison of potencies of numerous Gly ligands to displace binding of [³H]Gly and [³H]DCKA

Drug	[³H]Gly binding		[³H]DCKA binding	
	K_i (μM)	Hill	K_i (μM)	Hill
Agonists				
Gly	0.15 ± 0.003	0.98 ± 0.04	0.17 ± 0.03	0.83 ± 0.01
D-Ser	0.30 ± 0.16	0.88 ± 0.08	0.16 ± 0.06	0.83 ± 0.06
D-Ala	0.42 ± 0.20	0.97 ± 0.22	0.96 ± 0.34	0.90 ± 0.16
L-Ser	12.6 ± 2.3	1.04 ± 0.10	19.2 ± 3.4	0.89 ± 0.04
L-Ala	38.8 ± 9.2	0.92 ± 0.05	41.8 ± 8.4	1.39 ± 0.27
β-Ala	>100	—	>100	—
ACPC	0.21 ± 0.04	0.93 ± 0.07	0.23 ± 0.05	1.07 ± 0.08
GME	0.80 ± 0.14	0.97 ± 0.06	0.50 ± 0.05	1.04 ± 0.07
γ-LGG	51.6 ± 7.1	1.10 ± 0.15	24.8 ± 8.4	0.64 ± 0.15
NMG	59.8 ± 9.4	1.12 ± 0.09	37.6 ± 5.4	0.84 ± 0.08
γ-DGG	78.2 ± 3.3	0.95 ± 0.22	36.2 ± 5.2	0.67 ± 0.06[a]
Antagonists				
L-689,560	0.0028 ± 0.0004	0.93 ± 0.16	0.0020 ± 0.0003	1.12 ± 0.14
DCKA	0.06 ± 0.01	0.65 ± 0.16	0.04 ± 0.01	0.98 ± 0.22
7-ClKYNA	0.34 ± 0.06	0.68 ± 0.13	0.11 ± 0.03	0.74 ± 0.16
KYNA	13.1 ± 1.1	0.99 ± 0.06	4.42 ± 0.50	1.08 ± 0.10
MNQX	0.32 ± 0.08	0.66 ± 0.07[a]	0.03 ± 0.01	0.58 ± 0.04[b]
DHQXC	0.47 ± 0.07	0.69 ± 0.11	0.11 ± 0.01	0.81 ± 0.05
DCQX	0.59 ± 0.10	1.05 ± 0.21	0.16 ± 0.04	0.82 ± 0.07
DNQX	1.35 ± 0.26	0.89 ± 0.13	0.12 ± 0.01	0.89 ± 0.08
CNQX	5.06 ± 0.97	0.96 ± 0.24	2.88 ± 1.28	0.92 ± 0.09
CQX	5.84 ± 0.85	1.18 ± 0.21	0.50 ± 0.09	0.70 ± 0.06[a]
QX	42.0 ± 3.1	0.98 ± 0.09	4.66 ± 0.45	0.68 ± 0.09[a]
NBQX	100	—	29.7 ± 2.6	0.88 ± 0.06
HA-966	7.86 ± 2.05	1.06 ± 0.07	13.2 ± 1.1	0.88 ± 0.02

K_i values were obtained according to the equation $K_i = IC_{50}/(1 + [L]/K_D)$, where [L] is the concentration of the ligand used.
[a] $P < 0.05$; [b] $P < 0.01$, significantly different from unity.
(Table taken from Yoneda *et al.* (1993) with permission.)

hippocampal neurones (Lester *et al.* 1993). The glycine-sensitive desensitization appears at first to be at odds with the binding experiments which show mutual facilitation at the NMDA and glycine recognition sites (Kemp and Leeson 1993), but one might expect the desensitized state of the NMDA receptor to show a higher affinity for the agonist. How this all relates to the situation in more intact adult preparations is still not known; within the limitations of the time resolution of our techniques *in vivo* and in slices, desensitization is not a recognizable feature of the response to NMDA. On

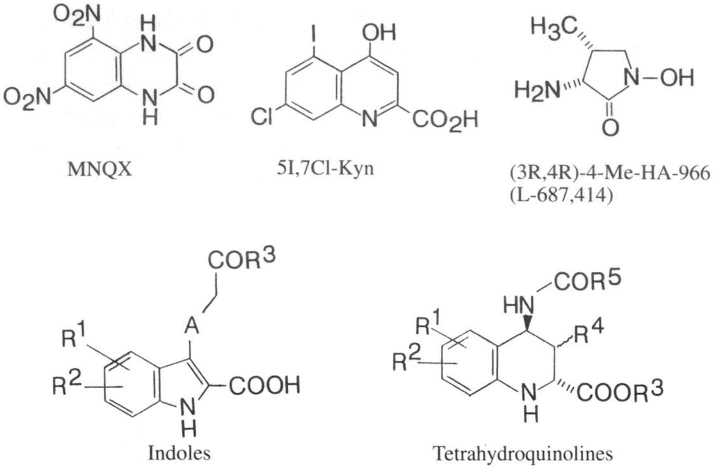

MNQX   5I,7Cl-Kyn   (3R,4R)-4-Me-HA-966
                                                (L-687,414)

Indoles   Tetrahydroquinolines

Fig. 3.4 Antagonists acting at the glycine site of the NMDA receptor. MNQX, 6,8-dinitroquinoxaline-2,3-dione; 5I,7Cl-Kyn, 5-iodo-7-chlorokynurenic acid; L-687,414, (3R,4R)-3-amino-1-hydroxy-4-methylpyrrolid-2-one. A = CH_2, NH or S; R^1–R^5, various. (From Sheardown *et al.* 1989; Salituro *et al.* 1990, 1991; Singh *et al.* 1990; Leeson *et al.* 1991, 1992; Foster *et al.* 1992.)

cortical wedges, HA-966 does not completely block NMDA-evoked depolarizations even at high concentrations (Fletcher and Lodge 1988; Foster and Kemp 1989) suggesting that either activation of glycine receptors is not essential for the expression of NMDA actions or that HA-966 acts as a partial agonist at the glycine receptor. This latter interpretation receives some support from preliminary binding experiments with [³H]MK-801 (Fletcher *et al.*, unpublished observation, and see Kemp and Leeson 1993). Further experiments are required to resolve many of the above issues.

The zinc binding site

Zinc and other Group IIb cations produce selective and non-competitive antagonism of NMDA in cultured neurones (Peters *et al.* 1987; Westbrook and Mayer 1987; Mayer *et al.* 1989*b*), in TCP binding studies (Reynolds and Miller 1989) and in neurotoxicity studies (Peters *et al.* 1987). Its action is distinct from that of magnesium in that the reduction of NMDA currents is not voltage-dependent but is due to reduced channel open time (Mayer *et al.* 1988). Thus it appears that zinc acts at a site separate from that of any of the antagonists described above. Interestingly there are areas in the CNS where zinc is present in relatively high amounts, e.g. the hippocampus, and it may be that in such areas zinc modulates the function of NMDA receptor channel complexes.

Recent kinetic studies on the binding of MK-801 (see above) suggest that some tricyclic antidepressants (TCA), eg. desmethylimipramine, have similar properties to zinc and hence may bind at the same site (Reynolds and Miller 1989), although the voltage-dependency of NMDA block by tricyclics (Sernagor *et al.* 1989) suggests otherwise.

Selective effects of TCAs as NMDA antagonists have yet to be demonstrated electrophysiologically *in vivo* or in more intact preparations *in vitro* (Martyn Jones, unpublished observations). Presumably the non-specific actions of zinc and TCAs prevent demonstration of the phenomena described in more isolated preparations. Alternatively, the neonatal cultures and membrane fragments used for binding experiments may lack endogenous substances which interact with the zinc/TCA site in more intact preparations. Recently, however, TCAs have been shown to block the lethal convulsant effects of NMDA (Leander 1989). The concentrations of TCAs likely to be required for such actions *in vivo* are, however, well above those that affect monoamine systems and are thus unlikely to contribute anything to the pharmacological profile of these drugs in normal clinical use as antidepressants. Development of more specific and potent tricyclic drugs with actions similar to those of zinc is awaited with interest. Desmethylimipramine may act as a lead compound in developments of such drugs with which to probe the physiological function of this site.

Intracellular manipulation of NMDA-mediated actions

NMDA receptor activation, presumably as a result of calcium entry, triggers several second messenger systems, including protein kinase C, phospholipase C, ornithine decarboxylase (ODC), cyclases, and arachidonic acid cascades, with resulting increases in phosphoinositides, cyclic nucleotides, polyamines, and endothelium-derived relaxing factor (see Sladeczek *et al.* 1985; Garthwaite *et al.* 1988; MacDonald *et al.* 1989). Such second messengers, which may also act as mediators for other receptors (Chen and Huang 1991; Rusin and Randic 1991; Schoepp and Conn 1993), may lead to further changes in the properties of NMDA receptor channel complexes. For example, stimulation of the NMDA receptors may, by activating protein kinase C (Chen and Huang 1992) and arachidonate synthesis (Miller *et al.* 1992), lead to further facilitation of the NMDA receptor-induced calcium flux. Fortunately, increases in intracellular calcium directly inactivate NMDA receptors (see Legendre *et al.* 1993) and hence limit intracellular accumulation of this potentially toxic action. Excessive or prolonged NMDA receptor stimulation may also stimulate other enzyme systems, e.g. proteases, which result in cell necrosis (Schwarcz and Meldrum 1985; Rothman and Olney 1987). Functional antagonists of these NMDA receptor-coupled processes are coming to light. Actions of protein kinase C and phospholipases and their inhibitors, for example in NMDA receptor-mediated long-term potentiation, are discussed elsewhere in this book (Chapter 13).

Polyamines, presumably via an intracellular site, affect the NMDA receptor–channel complex. Spermidine potentiates MK-801/PCP binding, an effect which is potentiated by glycine and glutamate (Ransom and Stec 1988). This may be part of a positive feedback system since NMDA also stimulates the activity of ODC, the enzyme responsible for the synthesis of such polyamines. Similarly, inhibition of ODC reduces NMDA-induced calcium fluxes (Siddiqui *et al*. 1988), whereas other polyamines appear to antagonize the neurotoxic effects of glutamate (Markwell *et al*. 1990). The precise mechanisms and physiological significance of these effects of polyamines remains to be determined (for review see Scott *et al*. 1993). A similar situation exists with respect to the gangliosides.

Changes in metabolic status also affect NMDA receptor channel function. For instance it has been recognized for many years that alkalosis increases seizure susceptibility which from work on cortical slices could in part be explained by facilitation of responses to NMDA (Aram and Lodge 1987). The partial block of the NMDA receptor channel by protons at physiological pH has now been established (Traynelis and Cull-Candy 1990). Furthermore, the redox state of the receptor is also critical for normal functioning. Reducing and oxidizing agents, such as dithiothreitol and ascorbic acid, potentiate and inhibit the NMDA complex respectively (Aizenman *et al*. 1989; Majewska *et al*. 1990).

Actions of non-competitive NMDA antagonists on physiological processes

One sometimes hears advanced the view that NMDA receptors do not play an important role in normal synaptic transmission (but see Chapters 8 and 10–13) and hence it might be predicted that NMDA antagonists would have little effect except in abnormal situations. It is argued that, because of the voltage-dependency of the associated ionophore, in order for NMDA receptor activation to have any substantial effects the neuronal membrane needs to be markedly depolarized by other mechanisms. These may be:

(1) prolonged or intense depolarization via other post-synaptic receptors;

(2) reduced synaptic inhibition or membrane rectification;

(3) reduced activity of ion pumps that maintain membrane polarization;

(4) increased extracellular levels of depolarizing agents such as potassium or glutamate.

Two reasonable arguments may be cited against such assertions. Firstly, NMDA excites neurones as shown by the rapid increase in spike firing rate of otherwise quiescent spinal (Curtis and Watkins 1960; Davies and Watkins 1979; McLennan and Lodge 1979), thalamic (Kemp and Leeson 1993), and cortical (Stone and Burton 1988) neurones in anaesthetized rats and cats. This action is blocked by selective NMDA antagonists and not affected by non-NMDA antagonists.

Secondly, it is clear from current–voltage plots for NMDA-induced conductances that even at −90 mV, although the current becomes very small, it is never completely blocked by magnesium (Mayer *et al.* 1984; Nowak *et al.* 1984; MacDonald *et al.* 1987). Since neurones are often spontaneously active *in vivo*, their membrane potentials may be assumed to be in the −60 to −70 mV range. Thus for many central neurones, synaptic activation of NMDA receptors will result in finite current flow, the large 50 pS channels producing substantial depolarizations. Since many neurones are near threshold or indeed spontaneously active, any such current flow is bound to increase their probability of firing.

Other observations support these arguments. Thus, selective doses of NMDA antagonists such as D-AP5 and ketamine reduce the firing rate of spinal motoneurones in response to gentle and natural stimulation of skin (Headley *et al.* 1987). There are many other previous *in vivo* and *in vitro* observations of NMDA receptor-mediated synaptic events following electrical stimulation of afferent pathways (Watkins and Evans 1981); an early example is the reduction of the dorsal root stimulation of Renshaw cells and other spinal interneurones (Watkins and Evans 1981). (For further discussion of the role of NMDA receptors in normal synaptic transmission see Chapters 8 and 10–13.)

This is not to say that the voltage-dependency of these channels does not introduce important and interesting properties to NMDA receptor mediated events. It undoubtedly does, but it does not stop neurones responding to NMDA receptor activation *in vivo*.

It is therefore not surprising that competitive and non-competitive NMDA antagonists have noticeable effects on animal (see above) and human (Domino and Luby 1981 and see Chapter 16) behaviour, on blood pressure regulation (see Lodge *et al.* 1988*b*), on locomotion (Sigvart *et al.* 1985), on long-term potentiation (Collingridge and Bliss 1987; Chapter 13), and on learning and memory (Morris *et al.* 1986; Kleinschmidt *et al.* 1987; Rauschecker and Hahn 1987; Chapter 15). Even the organization of normal neuronal circuitry may depend on the presence of NMDA receptors in the target areas during synaptogenesis (Constantine-Paton *et al.* 1990 and see Chapter 14).

Such effects may limit the therapeutic usefulness of all NMDA antagonists but providing clinicians are aware of them, they may be controlled (White *et al.* 1982).

Potential of non-competitive NMDA antagonists in neurological conditions

Whether abnormal functioning of NMDA receptors contributes to human neurological conditions is highly speculative. There is, however, a lot of experimental animal evidence that points to such a contribution, some of which has been indicated above.

There is, for example, evidence to suggest that NMDA antagonists might help relieve the signs of epilepsy and other types of convulsions (Croucher *et al.* 1982; Hayes and Balster 1985; Aram and Lodge 1988; Leander *et al.* 1988; Patel *et al.* 1988; Aram *et al.* 1989) and reduce the neuronal damage that follows hyperactivity (Sloviter 1983; Schwarcz and Meldrum 1985; Rothman and Olney 1987) and the intracellular calcium accumulation (Schwarcz and Meldrum 1985; Rothman and Olney 1987; Choi 1988) that results in neuronal death following a variety of hypoxic, ischaemic, and hypoglycaemic insults (Schwarcz and Meldrum 1985; Rothman and Olney 1987; Choi 1988; Church *et al.* 1989). Huntington's chorea, Alzheimer's disease, motor neurone disease, olivo-cerebellar-pontine atrophy, and other degenerative diseases may have an NMDA receptor involvement (Schwarcz and Meldrum 1985; Bridges *et al.* 1988; Ross and Spencer 1988). Much of this will be reviewed in detail in other sections of this book. It is, however, pertinent to ask here which NMDA antagonists are likely to have the most therapeutic potential in relation to side effects, modes of action, and pharmacodynamics.

Although superficially it might be thought that reducing NMDA receptor efficiency by whatever means will produce the same final effects, evidence from other transmitter systems suggest that this may not be so. For example, drugs which facilitate $GABA_A$ receptor function, such as benzodiazepines, barbiturates, and steroids, have quite different therapeutic uses.

Because PCP is a potent NMDA antagonist and produces psychotic reactions in man (Domino and Luby 1981), a cause and effect relationship would imply that all NMDA antagonists will induce psychotomimetic effects. This possibility needs exploration. Many other PCP receptor ligands, including cyclazocine, pentazocine, ketamine, dexoxadrol, dextrorphan, and dextromethorphan also induce similar perceptual abnormalities in man. Interactions with other neuronal processes, for example with acetylcholine, monoamine, mu, sigma, and kappa receptors, with monoamine transport processes and with voltage-dependent potassium channels cannot be excluded in the genesis of psychomimetic activity. Scientifically it would be valuable to compare the ability of drugs from different classes of NMDA antagonist to induce psychotomimetic activity in man with their ability to reduce the depolarizing actions of NMDA. This is of course ethically unacceptable (but see Chapter 16). So scientists have used animals for evaluating the subjective effects of such drugs. They are easily trained to discriminate PCP from saline or from other neuroactive drugs. As outlined above, the ability of the above drugs to mimic PCP in such PCP-trained animals compares favourably with their potency in PCP binding studies and as NMDA antagonists. These animals do not respond to drugs such as morphine, cocaine, LSD, etc., which do not displace PCP binding, which produce different subjective effects in man, and which do not antagonize NMDA. Furthermore, competitive NMDA antagonists, at least in part, also produce PCP-appropriate responses (see Willetts and Balster 1988). These results are highly suggestive that the discrimination cues arise from changes in synaptic function mediated by NMDA receptors. Other overt behavioural effects of PCP-like drugs are also shared by competitive NMDA antagonists (Woods *et al.* 1986; Tricklebank *et al.* 1987) and possibly by HA-966 (Bonta *et al.* 1971).

Is this relevant to man? Only in so far as animal models are predictive. But, since NMDA receptors mediate some synaptic function in the cerebral cortex, it is likely that all NMDA antagonists, not just PCP, will induce perceptual abnormalities in man. In the therapeutic setting, at least in hospitalized patients, such symptoms should be controllable by keeping patients in a quiet environment and by the use of other drugs, regimens which have been successful in anaesthetic recovery rooms in the past (White *et al.* 1982).

Related to the above is the question of NMDA receptors and schizophrenia. Because PCP produces schizophrenia-like symptoms (Domino and Luby 1981), derangements of glutamate neurotransmitter systems may contribute to psychoses in man (Lodge and Berry 1984). Levels of glutamate in cerebrospinal fluid are said to be low in some schizophrenic patients (Kim *et al.* 1989); this needs confirmation. Nevertheless, it remains an intriguing possibility that potentiation of glutamatergic neurotransmission, particularly that mediated by NMDA receptors, with uptake inhibitors or agonists may help alleviate some types of psychosis (Lodge and Berry 1984).

So will non-competitive antagonists have a place in therapy? They offer some advantages over competitive ones.

Firstly, in general, PCP-like drugs appear to cross the blood–brain barrier more easily. The time course of onset of NMDA antagonism in the spinal cord following intravenous systemic administration of MK-801 is, however, not that different from that of the more potent and systemically active competitive NMDA antagonists (Davies *et al.* 1988; Lodge *et al.* 1988*b*).

Secondly, there is a lot of variety in the time course of action within the non-competitive drugs (Berry *et al.* 1984*a*; Lodge and Anis 1984; Lodge *et al.* 1987; Davies *et al.* 1988) whereas most competitive NMDA antagonists have long-lasting effects if they cross the blood–brain barrier (Lodge *et al.* 1988*b*). A short half-life is regarded as valuable for clinicians in intensive care wards who might wish to titrate dose against effect on an hourly basis.

Thirdly, the effects of non-competitive antagonists, particularly of the channel blocking type, are not likely to be overcome by high levels of extracellular glutamate which would displace competitive antagonists. It should therefore be easier to predict a useful therapeutic dose of non-competitive antagonists.

Fourthly, the ability of some antagonists to act downstream from the receptor site may allow for normal physiological functioning of NMDA receptors while preventing the effects of their excessive stimulation in other areas. Ornithine decarboxylase inhibition and administration of gangliosides will undoubtedly receive attention in the near future.

Finally, since as well as being NMDA antagonists many of the non-competitive antagonists interact with other neuronal processes, these other properties may be employed usefully in the clinical setting.

If psychotomimetic and other known behavioural effects of PCP-like drugs are not produced by competitive NMDA antagonists, these latter drugs and others such as glycine antagonists that act on the NMDA receptor complex will have greater therapeutic potential.

With the cloning of several subtypes of NMDA receptor (see other chapters), it will be interesting to see whether all express the same modulatory sites. This is surely an unlikely outcome and hence the possibilities for drugs selective between NMDA subtypes (Monyer *et al.* 1992). Molecular biology techniques will help determine which amino acids are responsible for binding the various modulatory agents (Durand *et al.* 1992; Mori *et al.* 1992).

Acknowledgements

We wish to thank our previous collaborators and assistants who are cited in the references, our sources of financial support including MRC, Wellcome Trust, Eli Lilly Co., and Merck Sharp and Dohme and the many people who have given us generous supplies of compounds and advice during this study.

References

Aizenman, E., Lipton, S. A., and Loring, R. E. (1989). Selective modulation of NMDA responses by reduction and oxidation. *Neuron*, **2**, 1257–63.

Anis, N. A., Berry, S. C., Burton, N. R., and Lodge, D. (1983). The dissociative anaesthetics, ketamine and phencyclidine, selectively reduce excitation of central mammalian neurones by *N*-methyl-aspartate. *British Journal of Pharmacology*, **79**, 565–75.

Aram, J. A. and Lodge, D. (1987). Epileptiform activity induced by alkalosis in rat neocortical slices: block by antagonists of *N*-methyl-D-aspartate. *Neuroscience Letters*, **83**, 345–50.

Aram, J. A. and Lodge, D. (1988). Validation of neocortical slice preparation for the study of epileptiform activity. *Journal of Neuroscience Methods*, **23**, 211–24.

Aram, J. A., Martin, D., Tomczyk, M., Zeman, S., Millar, J., Pohler, G., and Lodge, D. (1989). Neocortical epileptogenesis *in vitro*: Studies with NMDA,

PCP, sigma and dextromethorphan receptor ligands. *Journal of Pharmacology and Experimental Therapeutics*, **248**, 320–8.

Ascher, P., Henderson, G., and Johnson, J. W. (1988). Dual inhibitory actions of kynurenate on the *N*-methyl-D-aspartate (NMDA)-activated response of cultured mouse cortical neurones. *Journal of Physiology*, **406**, 141P.

Berry, S. C. and Lodge, D. (1984). Benz(f)isoquinolines as excitatory amino acid antagonists: an indication of their mode of action? *Biochemical Pharmacology*, **33**, 3829–32.

Berry, S. C. and Lodge, D. (1985). Correlating some biochemical, pharmacological and behavioural properties of dissociative anaesthetics and sigma opiates in the rat and cat. *Journal of Physiology*, **364**, 36P.

Berry, S. C., Burton, N. R., Anis, N. A., and Lodge, D. (1983). Stereoselective effects of two phencyclidine derivatives on *N*-methylaspartate excitation of spinal neurones in the cat and rat. *European Journal of Pharmacology*, **96**, 261–7.

Berry, S. C., Anis, N. A., and Lodge, D. (1984*a*). The effect of the dioxolanes on amino acid induced excitation in the mammalian spinal cord. *Brain Research*, **307**, 85–90.

Berry, S. C., Dawkins, S. L., and Lodge, D. (1984*b*). Comparison of sigma and kappa opioids as excitatory amino acid antagonists. *British Journal of Pharmacology*, **83**, 179–85.

Birch, P. J., Grossman, C. J., and Hayes, A. G. (1988). Kynurenate and FG9041 have both competitive and non-competitive actions at excitatory amino acid receptors. *European Journal of Pharmacology*, **151**, 313–15.

Blake, J. C., Davies, S. N., Church, J., Martin, D., and Lodge, D. (1986). 2-methyl-3, 3-diphenyl-3-propanolamine (2-MDP) selectively antagonises *N*-methyl-aspartate (NMA). *Pharmacology, Biochemistry and Behaviour*, **24**, 23–5.

Bonta, I. L., De Vos, C. J., Grijsen, H., Hillen, E. L., Noach, E. L., and Sim, A. W. (1971). 1-Hydroxy-3-amino-pyrollidone (HA-966). A new GABA-like compound, with potential use in extrapyramidal diseases. *British Journal of Pharmacology*, **43**, 514–35.

Brady, K. T., Balster, R. L., and May, E. L. (1982). Discriminative stimulus properties of stereoisomers of *N*-allylnormetazocine in phencyclidine-trained squirrel monkeys and rats. *Science*, **215**, 178–80.

Bridges, R. J., Geddes, J. W., Monaghan, D. T., and Cotman, C. W. (1988). Excitatory amino acid receptors in Alzheimer's disease. In *Excitatory amino acids in health and disease*, (ed. D. Lodge), pp. 321–35. John Wiley, London.

Chen, H.-S. V., Pellegrini, J. W., Aggarwal, S. K., Lei, S. Z., Warach, S., Jensen, F. E., and Lipton, S. A. (1992). Open channel block of *N*-methyl-D-aspartate (NMDA) responses by memantine: therapeutic advantage against NMDA receptor-mediated neurotoxicity. *Journal of Neuroscience*, **12**, 4427–36.

Chen, L. and Huang, L.-Y. M. (1991). Sustained potentiation of NMDA receptor-mediated glutamate responses through activation of protein kinase C by a μ opioid. *Neuron*, **7**, 319–26.

Chen, L. and Huang, L.-Y. M. (1992). Protein kinase C reduces Mg^{2+} block of NMDA receptor channels as a mechanism of modulation. *Nature*, **356**, 521–3.

Choi, D. W. (1988). Calcium-mediated neurotoxicity: Relationship to specific channel types and role in ischaemic damage. *Trends in Neuroscience*, **11**, 465–9.

Church, J., Lodge, D., and Berry, S. C. (1985). Differential effects of dextrorphan and levorphanol on the excitation of rat spinal neurones by amino acids. *European Journal of Pharmacology*, **111**, 185–90.

Church, J., Zeman, S., and Lodge, D. (1989). Comparison of the neuroprotective action of ketamine and MK-801 following transient cerebral ischemia in rats. *Anesthesiology*, **69**, 702–9.

Collingridge, G. L. and Bliss, T. V. P. (1987). NMDA receptors—their role in long-term potentiation. *Trends in Neuroscience*, **10**, 288–93.

Constantine-Paton, M., Cline, H. T., and Debski, E. A. (1990). Patterned activity, synaptic convergence, and the NMDA receptor in developing visual pathways. *Annual Review of Neuroscience*, **13**, 129–54.

Cotman, C. W., Monaghan, D. T., Ottersen, O. P., and Storm-Mathisen, J. (1987). Anatomical organization of excitatory amino acid receptors and their pathways. *Trends in Neuroscience*, **10**, 273–80.

Croucher, M. J., Collins, J. F., and Meldrum, B. S. (1982). Anticonvulsant action of excitatory amino acid antagonists. *Science*, **216**, 899–901.

Curtis, D. R. and Johnston, G. A. R. (1974). Amino acid transmitters in the mammalian central nervous system. *Ergebnisse der Physiologie*, **69**, 97–188.

Curtis, D. R. and Watkins, J. C. (1960). The chemical excitation of spinal neurones by certain acidic amino acids. *Journal of Physiology*, **150**, 656–82.

Davies, J. and Watkins, J. C. (1979). Selective antagonism of amino acid-induced and synaptic excitation in the cat spinal cord. *Journal of Physiology*, **297**, 621–36.

Davies, S. N., Church, J., Blake, J., Lodge, D., Lessor, R. A., Rice, K. C., and Jacobson, A. E. (1986). Is metaphit a phencyclidine antagonist? Studies with ketamine and *N*-methylaspartate. *Life Sciences*, **38**, 2441–5.

Davies, S. N., Martin, D., Millar, J. D., Aram, J. A., and Lodge, D. (1988). Differences in results from *in vivo* and *in vitro* studies on the use-dependency of *N*-methylaspartate antagonism by MK-801 and other phencyclidine receptor ligands. *European Journal of Pharmacology*, **145**, 141–51.

DiMaggio, D. A., Contreras, P. C., Quirion, R., and O'Donohue, T. L. (1986). Isolation and identification of an endogenous ligand for the phencyclidine receptor. *NIDA Research Monograph*, **64**, 24–35.

Domino, E. F. and Luby, E. D. (1981). Abnormal mental states induced by phencyclidine as a model of schizophrenia. In *PCP (Phencyclidine): historical and current perspectives*, (ed. E. F. Domino), pp. 401–13. NPP Books, Ann Arbor, MI.

Durand, G. M., Gregor, P., Zheng, X., Bennett, M. V. L., Uhl, G. R., and Zukin, R. S. (1992). Cloning of an apparent splice variant of the rat *N*-methyl-D-aspartate receptor NMDAR1 with altered sensitivity to polyamines and activators of protein kinase C. *Proceedings of the National Academy of Sciences, USA*, **89**, 9359–63.

Eccles, J. C. (1963). *The physiology of synapses*. Springer, Berlin.

Evans, R. H., Francis, A. A., and Watkins, J. C. (1978). Mg^{2+}-like antagonism of excitatory amino acid-induced responses by diaminopimelic acid, D-aminoadipate and HA-966 in isolated spinal cord of frog and immature rat. *Brain Research*, **148**, 536–42.

Fletcher, E. J. and Lodge, D. (1988). Glycine reverses antagonism of *N*-methyl-D-aspartate (NMDA) by 1-hydroxy-3-aminopyrrolidone-2 (HA-966) but not by D-2-amino-5-phophonovalerate (D-AP5) on rat cortical slices. *European Journal of Pharmacology*, **151**, 161–2.

Fletcher, E. J., Martin, D., Aram, J. A., Lodge, D., and Honore, T. (1988). Quinoxalinediones selectively block quisqualate and kainate receptors and synaptic events in rat neocortex and hippocampus and frog spinal cord *in vitro*. *British Journal of Pharmacology*, **95**, 585–97.

Fletcher, E. J., Millar, J. D., Zeman, S., and Lodge, D. (1989). Non-competitive antagonism of N-methyl-D-aspartate by displacement of an endogenous glycine-like substance. *European Journal of Neuroscience*, **1**, 196–203.

Fonnum, F. (1984). Glutamate: a neurotransmitter in mammalian brain. *Journal of Neurochemistry*, **42**, 1–11.

Foster, A. C. and Kemp, J. A. (1989). HA-966 antagonizes N-methyl-D-aspartate receptors through a selective interaction with the glycine modulatory site. *Journal of Neuroscience*, **9**, 2191–6.

Foster, A. C., Kemp, J. A., Leeson, P. D., Grimwood, S., Donald, A. E., Marshall, G. R., Priestley, T., Smith, J. D., and Carling, R. W. (1992). Kynurenic acid analogues with improved affinity and selectivity for the glycine site on the N-methyl-D-aspartate receptor from rat brain. *Molecular Pharmacology*, **41**, 914–22.

Garthwaite, J., Charles, S. L., and Chess-Williams, R. (1988). Endothelium-derived relaxing factor release on activation of NMDA receptors suggests role as intercellular messenger in the brain. *Nature*, **336**, 385–8.

Greenmayre, J. T., Young, A. B., and Penney, J. B. (1983). Quantitative auto-radiography of L-[^{3}H]-glutamate binding to rat brain. *Neuroscience Letters*, **37**, 155–60.

Harrison, N. L. and Simmonds, M. A. (1985). Quantitative studies on some antagonists of N-methyl-D-aspartate in slices of rat cerebral cortex. *British Journal of Pharmacology*, **323**, 132–7.

Hayashi, T. (1952). A physiological study of epileptic seizures following cortical stimulation in animals and its application to human clinics. *Japanese Journal of Physiology*, **3**, 46–64.

Hayes, B. A. and Balster, R. L. (1985). Anticonvulsant properties of phencyclidine-like drugs in mice. *European Journal of Pharmacology*, **117**, 121–5.

Headley, P. M., Parsons, C. G., and West, D. C. (1987). The role of N-methyl-aspartate receptors in mediating responses of rat and cat spinal neurones to defined sensory stimuli. *Journal of Physiology*, **385**, 169–88.

Herling, S. and Woods, J. H. (1982). Discriminative effects of narcotics: evidence for multiple receptor-mediated actions. *Life Sciences*, **28**, 1571–87.

Holzman, S. G. (1982). Phencyclidine-like discriminative stimulus properties of opioids in the squirrel monkey. *Psychopharmacology*, **77**, 295–300.

Honoré, T., Davies, S. N., Drejer, J., Fletcher, E. J., Jacobsen, P., Lodge, D., and Nielsen, F. E. (1988). Quinoxalinediones: Potent competitive non-N-methyl-D-aspartate glutamate receptor antagonists. *Science*, **241**, 701–3.

Huettner, J. E. and Bean, B. P. (1988). Block of N-methyl-D-aspartate-activated current by the anticonvulsant MK-801: Selective binding to open channels. *Proceedings of the National Academy of Sciences, USA*, **85**, 1307–11.

Johnson, J. W. and Ascher, P. (1987). Glycine potentiates the NMDA response in cultured mouse brain neurones. *Nature*, **325**, 529–31.

Jones, M. G. and Lodge, D. (1991). Comparison of some arthropod toxins and toxin fragments as antagonists of excitatory amino acid-induced excitation of rat spinal neurones. *European Journal of Pharmacology*, **204**, 203–9.

Kemp, J. A. and Leeson, J. D. (1993). The glycine site of the NMDA receptor—five years on. *Trends in Pharmacological Science*, **14**, 20–5.

Kemp, J. A., Foster, A. C., Leeson, P. D., Priestley, T., Tridgett, R., and Iversen, L. L. (1988). 7-Chlorokynurenic acid is a selective antagonist at the glycine modulatory site of the *N*-methyl-D-aspartate receptor complex. *Proceedings of the National Academy of Sciences, USA*, **85**, 6547–50.

Kessler, M., Baudry, M., Terramani, T., and Lynch, G. (1987). A glycine site associated with *N*-methyl-D-aspartic acid receptors: Characterisation and identification of a new class of antagonists. *Journal of Neurochemistry*, **52**, 1319–29.

Kim, J. S., Kornhuber, H. H., Schmid-Berger, W. and Holzmuller, B. (1989). Low cerebrospinal fluid glutamate in schizophrenic patients and a new hypothesis of schizophrenia. *Neuroscience Letters*, **20**, 379–82.

Kiskin, N. I., Chizhmakov, I. V., Tysndrenko, A. Ya, Mueller, A. L., Jackson, H., and Krishtal, O. A. (1992). A highly potent and selective *N*-methyl-D-aspartate receptor antagonist from the venom of the *Agelenopsis aperta* spider. *Neuroscience*, **51**, 11–18.

Kleckner, N. W. and Dingledine, R. (1988). Requirement for glycine in activation of NMDA-receptors expressed in Xenopus oocytes. *Science*, **241**, 835–7.

Kleinschmidt, A., Bear, M. F., and Singer, W. (1987). Blockade of "NMDA" receptors disrupts experience-dependent plasticity of kitten striate cortex. *Science*, **238**, 355–8.

Kloog, Y., Haring, R., and Sokolovsky, M. (1988). Kinetic characterization of the phencyclidine–NMDA receptor interaction: Evidence for a steric blockade of the channel. *Biochemistry*, **27**, 843–8.

Kushner, L., Lerma, J., Zukin, R. S., and Bennett, M. V. L. (1988). Coexpression of *N*-methyl-D-aspartate and phencyclidine receptors in Xenopus oocytes injected with rat brain mRNA. *Proceedings of the National Academy of Sciences, USA*, **85**, 3250–4.

Leander, J. D. (1982). Comparison of phencyclidine, etoxadrol and dexoxadrol in the pigeon. *Substance, Alcohol Actions and Misuse*, **2**, 197–203.

Leander, J. D. (1989). Tricyclic antidepressants block *N*-methyl-D-aspartic acid-induced lethality in mice. *British Journal of Pharmacology*, **96**, 256–8.

Leander, J. D., Rathbun, R. C., and Zimmerman, D. M. (1988). Anticonvulsant effects of phencyclidine-like drugs: Relation to *N*-methyl-D-aspartic acid antagonism. *Brain Research*, **454**, 368–72.

Leeson, P. D., Baker, R., Carling, R. W., Curtis, N. R., Moore, K. W., Williams, B. J., Foster, A. C., Donald, A. E., Kemp, J. A., and Marshall, G. R. (1991). Kynurenic acid derivatives. Structure–activity relationships for excitatory amino acid antagonism and identification of potent and selective antagonists at the glycine site on the *N*-methyl-D-aspartate receptor. *Journal of Medicinal Chemistry*, **34**, 1243–52.

Leeson, P. D., Carling, R. W., Moore, K. W., Moseley, A. M., Smith, J. D., Stevenson, G., Chan, T., Baker, R., Foster, A. C., Grimwood, S., Kemp, J. A., Marshall, G. R., and Hoogsteen, K. (1992). 4-Amido-2-carboxytetrahydroquinolines. Structure–activity relationships for antagonism at the glycine site of the NMDA receptor. *Journal of Medicinal Chemistry*, **35**, 1954–68.

Legendre, P., Rosenmund, C., and Westbrook, G. L. (1993). Inactivation of NMDA channels in cultured hippocampal neurons by intracellular calcium. *Journal of Neuroscience*, **13**, 674–84.

Lester, R. A. J., Tong, G., and Jahr, C. E. (1993). Interaction between the glycine and glutamate binding sites of the NMDA receptors. *Journal of Neuroscience*, **13**, 1088–96.

Lodge, D. and Anis, N. A. (1982). Effects of phencyclidine on excitatory amino acid activation of spinal interneurones in the cat. *European Journal of Pharmacology*, **77**, 203–4.

Lodge, D. and Anis, N. A. (1984). Effects of ketamine and three other short acting anaesthetics on spinal reflexes and inhibitions in the cat. *British Journal of Anaesthesia*, **56**, 1143–51.

Lodge, D. and Berry, S. C. (1984). Psychotomimetic effects of sigma opiates may be mediated by block of central excitatory synapses utilising receptors for aspartate-like amino acids. In *Modulation of sensory motor activity during altered behavioural states*, (ed. R. Bandler), pp. 503–18. Alan R. Liss Inc., New York.

Lodge, D. and Johnson, K. M. (1990). Noncompetitive excitatory amino acid antagonists. *Trends in Pharmacological Science*, **11**, 81–6.

Lodge, D. and Johnston, G. A. R. (1985). Effect of ketamine on amino acid evoked release of acetylcholine from rat cerebral cortex *in vitro*. *Neuroscience Letters*, **56**, 371–5.

Lodge, D., Davies, S. N., Aram, J. A., Church, J., and Martin, D. (1987). Sigma opiates and excitatory amino acids. In *Excitatory amino acids in health and disease*, (ed. D. Lodge), pp. 237–59. John Wiley, London.

Lodge, D., Aram, J. A., Church, J., Davies, S. N., Fletcher, E., and Martin, D. (1988*a*). Electrophysiological studies of the interaction between phencyclidine/sigma receptor agonists and excitatory amino acid neurotransmission on central mammalian neurones. In *Sigma and phencyclidine-like compounds as molecular probes in biology*, (ed. E. F. Domino and J.-M. Kamenka), pp. 239–50. NPP Books, Ann Arbor, MI.

Lodge, D., Davies, S. N., Jones, M. G., Millar, J., Manallack, D. T., Ornstein, P. L., Verberne, A. J. M., Young, N., and Beart, P. M. (1988*b*). A comparison between the *in vivo* and *in vitro* activity of five potent and competitive NMDA antagonists. *British Journal of Pharmacology*, **95**, 957–65.

Loo, P., Braunwalder, A., Lehmann, J., and Williams, M. (1986). Radioligand binding to central phencyclidine recognition sites is dependent on excitatory amino acid receptor agonists. *European Journal of Pharmacology*, **123**, 467–8.

MacDonald, J. F. and Nowak, L. M. (1990). Mechanisms of blockade of excitatory amino acid receptor channels. *Trends in Pharmacological Science*, **11**, 167–72.

MacDonald, J. F., Miljkovic, Z., and Pennefather, P. (1987). Use-dependent block of excitatory amino acid currents in cultured spinal cord neurones. *Journal of Neurophysiology*, **58**, 251–66.

MacDonald, J. F., Mody, I., and Salter, M. W. (1989). Regulation of N-methyl-D-aspartate receptors revealed by intracellular dialysis of murine neurones in culture. *Journal of Physiology*, **414**, 17–34.

McLennan, H. (1983). Receptors for excitatory amino acids in the mammalian central nervous system. *Progress in Neurobiology*, **20**, 251–71.

McLennan, H. and Lodge, D. (1979). The antagonism of amino acid-induced excitation of spinal neurones in the cat. *Brain Research*, **169**, 83–90.

Majewska, M. D., Bell, J. A., and London, E. D. (1990). Regulation of NMDA receptor by redox phenomena: inhibitory role of ascorbate. *Brain Research*, **537**, 328–32.

Markwell, M. A. K., Berger, S. P., and Paul, S. M. (1990). The polyamine synthesis inhibition of d-difluoromethylornithine blocks NMDA-induced neurotoxicity. *European Journal of Pharmacology*, **182**, 607–9.

Martin, D. and Lodge, D. (1985). Ketamine acts as a non-competitive N-methyl-D-aspartate antagonist on frog spinal cord *in vitro. Neuropharmacology*, **24**, 999–1003.

Martin, D. and Lodge, D. (1988). Phencyclidine receptors and N-methyl-D-aspartate antagonism: Electrophysiologic data correlates with known behaviours. *Pharmacology, Biochemistry and Behaviour*, **31**, 279–86.

Marvizon, J. C. G. and Skolnick, P. (1988). [³H]-Glycine binding is modulated by Mg2+ and other ligands of the NMDA receptor–cation complex. *European Journal of Pharmacology*, **151**, 157–8.

Mayer, M. L., Westbrook, G. L., and Guthrie, P. B. (1984). Voltage-dependent block by Mg^{2+} of NMDA responses in spinal cord neurones. *Nature*, **309**, 261–3.

Mayer, M. L., Westbrook, G. L., and Vycklicky, L., Jr (1988). Sites of action on N-methyl-D-aspartic acid receptors studied using fluctuation analysis and a rapid perfusion technique. *Journal of Neurophysiology*, **60**, 645–53.

Mayer, M. L., Vyclicky, L., Jr, and Clements, J. (1989*a*). Regulation of NMDA receptor desensitization in mouse hippocampal neurons by glycine. *Nature*, **338**, 425–7.

Mayer, M. L., Vyklicky, L., Jr, and Westbrook, G. L. (1989*b*). Modulation of excitatory amino acid receptors by group IIB metal cations in cultured mouse hippocampal neurones. *Journal of Physiology*, **415**, 329–50.

Miller, B., Sarantis, M., Traynelis, S. F., and Attwell, D. (1992). Potentiation of NMDA receptor currents by arachidonic acid. *Nature*, **355**, 722–5.

Monyer, H., Sprengel, R., Shoepfer, R., Herb, A., Higuchi, M., Lomeli, H., Burnashev, N., Sakmann, B., and Seeburg, P. H. (1992). Heteromeric NMDA receptors: molecular and functional distinction of subtypes. *Science*, **256**, 36–41.

Mori, H., Masaki, H., Yamakura, T., and Mishina, M. (1992). Identification by mutagenesis of a Mg^{2+}-block site of the NMDA receptor channel. *Nature*, **358**, 673–5.

Morris, R. G. M., Anderson, E., Lynch, G. S., and Baudry, M. (1986). Selective impairment of learning and blockade of long term potentiation by an N-methyl-D-aspartate receptor antagonist. *Nature*, **319**, 774–6.

Nadler, V., Kloog, Y., and Sokolovsky, M. (1988). 1-Aminocyclopropane-1-carboxylic acid (ACC) mimics the effects of glycine on the NMDA receptor ion channel. *European Journal of Pharmacology*, **157**, 115–16.

Nowak, L., Bregestovski, P., Ascher, P., Herbet, A., and Prochiantz, A. (1984). Magnesium gates glutamate-activated channels in mouse central neurones. *Nature*, **307**, 462–5.

Olney, J. W. (1969). Brain lesions, obesity and other disturbances in mice treated with monosodium glutamate. *Science*, **164**, 719–21.

Patel, S., Chapman, A. G., Millan, M. H., and Meldrum, B. S. (1988). Epilepsy and excitatory amino acid antagonists. In *Excitatory amino acids in health and disease*, (ed. D. Lodge), pp. 353–78. Wiley, London.

Peters, S., Koh, J., and Choi, D. W. (1987). Zinc selectively blocks the action of N-methyl-D-aspartate on cortical neurones. *Science*, **236**, 589–93.

Priestley, T., Woodruff, G. N., and Kemp, J. A. (1989). Antagonism of responses to excitatory amino acids on rat cortical neurones by the spider toxin, argiotoxin-636. *British Journal of Pharmacology*, **97**, 1315–23.

Ransom, R. W. and Stec, N. L. (1988). Cooperative modulation of [³H]MK-801 binding to the N-methyl-D-aspartate receptor-ion complex by L-glutamate, glycine and polyamines. *Journal of Neurochemistry*, **51**, 830–6.

Rauschecker, J. P. and Hahn, S. (1987). Ketamine-xylazine anaesthesia blocks consolidation of ocular dominance changes in kitten visual cortex. *Nature*, **326**, 183–5.

Reynolds, I. J. and Miller, R. J. (1989). Multiple sites for the regulation of the *N*-methyl-D-aspartate receptor. *Molecular Pharmacology*, **33**, 581–4.

Reynolds, I. J., Murphy, S. N., and Miller, R. J. (1988) ^{3}H-labelled MK-801 binding to the excitatory amino acid complex from rat brain is enhanced by glycine. *Proceedings of the National Academy of Sciences, USA*, **84**, 7744–8.

Ross, S. M. and Spencer, P. S. (1988). Excitotoxic principles of plants linked to neuronal diseases involving motor and other systems. *Neurology and Neurobiology*, **46**, 514–24.

Rothman, S. M. and Olney, J. W. (1987). Excitotoxicity and the NMDA receptor. *Trends in Neuroscience*, **10**, 299–302.

Rusin, K. I. and Randic, M. (1991). Modulation of NMDA-induced currents by μ-opioid receptor agonist DAGO in acutely isolated rat spinal dorsal horn neurons. *Neuroscience Letters*, **124**, 208–12.

Salituro, F. G., Harrison, B. L., Baron, B. M., Nyce, P. L., Stewart, K. T., and McDonald, I. A. (1990). 3-(2-Carboxyindol-3-yl) propionic acid derivatives: antagonists of the strychnine-insensitive glycine receptor associated with the *N*-methyl-D-aspartate receptor complex. *Journal of Medicinal Chemistry*, **33**, 2944–6.

Salituro, F. G., Tomlinson, R. C., Baron, B. M., Demeter, D. A., Weintraub, H. J. R., and McDonald, I. A. (1991). Design, synthesis and molecular modeling of 3-acylamino-2-carboxyindole NMDA receptor glycine-site antagonists. *Bioorganic and Medicinal Chemistry Letters*, **1**, 455–60.

Sather, W., Dieudonné, S., MacDonald, J. F., and Ascher, P. (1992). Activation and desensitization of *N*-methyl-D-aspartate receptors in nucleated outside-out patches of mouse neurones. *Journal of Physiology*, **450**, 643–72.

Schoepp, D. D. and Conn, J. (1993). Metabotropic glutamate receptors in brain function and pathology. *Trends in Pharmacological Science*, **14**, 13–19.

Schwarcz, R. and Meldrum, B. S. (1985). Excitatory amino acid antagonists provide a therapeutic approach to neurological disorders. *Lancet*, **ii**, 140–3.

Scott, R. H., Sutton, K. G., and Dolphin, A. C. (1993). Interactions of polyamines with neuronal ion channels. *Trends in Neuroscience*, **16**, 153–60.

Sernagor, E., Kuhn, D., Vyklicky, L., Jr, and Mayer, M. L. (1989). Open channel block of NMDA receptor responses evoked by tricyclic antidepressants. *Neuron*, **2**, 1221–7.

Shannon, H. E. (1983). Pharmacological evaluation of *N*-allylnor-metazocine (SKF 10,047) on the basis of its discriminative properties. *Journal of Pharmacology and Experimental Therapeutics*, **255**, 144–52.

Sheardown, M. J., Drejer, J., Jensen, L. H., Stidsen, C. E., and Honoré, T. (1989). A potent antagonist of the strychnine insensitive glycine receptor has anticonvulsant properties. *European Journal of Pharmacology*, **174**, 197–204.

Siddiqui, F., Iqbal, Z., and Koenig, H. (1988). Polyamine dependence of NMDA receptor-mediated Ca^{2+} fluxes and transmitter release from rat hippocampus. *Society of Neuroscience Abstracts*, **14**, 1048.

Sigvart, K. G., Grillner, S., Wallen, P., and Vandongen, P. A. M. (1985). Activation of NMDA receptors elicits fictive locomotion and bistable membrane properties in the lamprey spinal cord. *Brain Research*, **336**, 390–5.

Singh, L., Donald, A. E., Foster, A. C., Huston, P. H., Iversen, L. L., Iversen, S. D., Kemp, J. A., Leeson, P. D., Marshall, G. R., Oles, R. J., Priestley, T., Thorn, L., Tricklebank, M. D., Vass, C. A. and Williams, B. J. (1990).

Enantiomers of HA-966 (3-amino-1-hydroxyoyrrolid-2-one) exhibit distinct central nervous system effects: (+)-HA-966 is a selective glycine/N-methyl-D-aspartate receptor antagonist, but (−)-HA-966 is a potent γ-butyrolactone-like sedative. *Proceedings of the National Academy of Science, USA*, **87**, 347–51.

Sladeczek, F., Pink, J. P., Recasens, M., Bockaert, J., and Weiss, S. (1985). A new mechanism for glutamate receptor action: Phosphoinositide hydrolysis. *Trends in Neuroscience*, **11**, 545–9.

Sloviter, R. S. (1983). "Epileptic" brain damage in rats induced by sustained electrical stimulation of the perforant pathway. 1. Acute electrophysiological and light microscopy studies. *Brain Research Bulletin*, **10**, 675–97.

Snell, L. D. and Johnson, K. M. (1985). Antagonism of N-methyl-D-aspartate induced transmitter release in the rat striatum and its relationship to turning behavior. *Journal of Pharmacology and Experimental Therapeutics*, **235**, 50–7.

Snell, L. D., Morter, R. S., and Johnson, K. M. (1987). Glycine potentiates N-methyl-D-aspartate-induced [^{3}H]-TCP binding to rat cortical membranes. *Neuroscience Letters*, **83**, 313–17.

Stone, T. W. and Burton, N. R. (1988). NMDA receptors and ligands in the vertebrate CNS. *Progress in Neurobiology*, **30**, 333–68.

Thomson, A. M. (1990). Glycine is a coagonist at the NMDA receptor/channel complex. *Progress in Neurobiology*, **35**, 53–76.

Traynelis, S. F. and Cull-Candy, S. G. (1990). Proton inhibition of N-methyl-D-aspartate receptors in cerebral neurones. *Nature*, **345**, 347–50.

Tricklebank, M. D., Singh, L., Oles, R. J., Wong, E. H. F., and Iversen, L. L. (1987). A role for receptors of N-methyl-D-aspartic acid in the discriminative stimulus of phencyclidine. *European Journal of Pharmacology*, **141**, 497–501.

Vincent, J. P., Kartalovski, B., Geneste, P., Kamenka, J.-M., and Lazdunski, M. (1979). Interaction of phencyclidine ('angel dust') with a specific receptor in rat brain membranes. *Proceedings of the National Academy of Sciences, USA*, **76**, 4678–82.

Watkins, J. C. and Evans, R. H. (1981). Excitatory amino acid transmitters. *Annual Review of Pharmacology and Toxicology*, **21**, 165–204.

Watkins, J. C. and Olverman, H. (1988). Structural requirements for activation and blockade of EAA receptors. In *Excitatory amino acids in health and disease*, (ed. D. Lodge), pp. 13–45. Wiley, London.

Watson, G. B., Hood, W. F., Monahan, J. B., and Lanthorn, T. H. (1988). Kynurenate antagonizes N-methyl-D-aspartate through a glycine-sensitive receptor. *Neuroscience Research Communications*, **2**, 169–74.

Westbrook, G. L. and Mayer, M. L. (1987). Micromolar concentrations of Zn^{2+} antagonize NMDA and GABA responses of hippocampal neurones. *Nature*, **328**, 640–3.

White, P. F., Way, W. L., and Trevor, A. J. (1982). Ketamine: Its pharmacology and therapeutic uses. *Anesthesiology*, **56**, 119–36.

Willetts, J. and Balster, R. L. (1988). Role of NMDA receptor stimulation and antagonism in phencyclidine discrimination in rats. In *Sigma and phencyclidine-like compounds as molecular probes in biology*, (ed. E. F. Domino and J.-M. Kamenka), pp. 397–406. NPP Books, Ann Arbor, MI.

Wong, E. H. F. and Kemp, J. A. (1991). Sites for antagonism of the N-methyl-D-aspartate receptor channel complex. *Annual Review of Pharmacology and Toxicology*, **31**, 401–25.

Wong, E. H. F., Kemp, J. A., Priestley, T., Knight, A. R., Woodruff, G. N., and

Iverson, L. L. (1986). The anticonvulsant MK-801 is a potent *N*-methyl-D-aspartate antagonist. *Proceedings of the National Academy of Sciences, USA*, **83**, 7104–8.

Woods, J. H., France, C. P., Hartman, J., Baron, S., and Cook, J. (1986). Similarity of the discriminative stimulus effects of *N*-methyl-D-aspartate and beta-carboline ethyl ester in pigeons. *Journal of Neurology and Neurobiology*, **46**, 317–23.

Yoneda, Y., Suzuki, T., Ogita, K., and Han, D. (1993). Support for radiolabelling of a glycine recognition domain on the *N*-methyl-D-aspartate receptor ionophore complex by 5,7-[^{3}H]dichloro-kynurenate in rat brain. *Journal of Neurochemistry*, **60**, 634–45.

Zukin, R. S. and Zukin, R. S. (1979). Specific [^{3}H]-phencyclidine binding in rat central nervous system. *Proceedings of the National Academy of Sciences, USA*, **76**, 5372–6.

Zukin, S. R., Zukin, R. S., Vale, W., Rivier, J., Nichtenhauser, R., Snell, L. D., and Johnson, K. M. (1987). An endogenous ligand for the brain sigma/PCP receptor antagonizes NMDA-induced transmitter release. *Brain Research*, **41**, 84–9.

4 NMDA receptor agonists and competitive antagonists

MARK L. MAYER, MORRIS BENVENISTE,
AND DORIS K. PATNEAU

Introduction

NMDA receptors have a rich and diverse pharmacology reflecting the presence of multiple ligand binding sites at which agonists, antagonists, and modulators interact in an allosteric manner. In addition to opening many approaches for the therapeutic manipulation of NMDA receptor activity, studies on drug action at NMDA receptors lay the groundwork for analysis of NMDA receptor function during synaptic transmission. This chapter will describe concentration jump experiments used to characterize the activation of NMDA receptors by agonists and the block of NMDA receptor activity by competitive antagonists. These results were obtained before cDNAs for multiple families of NMDA receptor subunits were identified, and although our experiments illustrate important principles which would be expected to apply to all subtypes of NMDA receptor, a challenging task for the future will be to characterize in detail the ligand binding characteristics of native NMDA receptor subtypes in different areas of the brain.

Selective activation of NMDA receptors at low concentrations of glutamate

L-glutamate has been known for many years to act as a non-selective (mixed) agonist with activity at both NMDA- and AMPA-preferring subtypes of glutamate receptors (Watkins *et al*. 1981; Mayer and Westbrook 1984; Patneau and Mayer 1990). To determine experimental conditions which allow the analysis of agonist responses at individual subtypes of glutamate receptor we initially studied responses to the selective agonists kainate, NMDA, and quisqualate (similar results were obtained with AMPA). Figure 4.1(A) shows responses to these agonists under conditions which permit activation of both NMDA and AMPA receptors (3 μM glycine present continuously, no added Mg, and, to prevent Ca-mediated inactivation of NMDA receptor activity, only 0.2 mM Ca). Figure 4.1(B) shows responses under conditions where responses at NMDA receptors are blocked, while responses at AMPA receptors are unaffected (no added

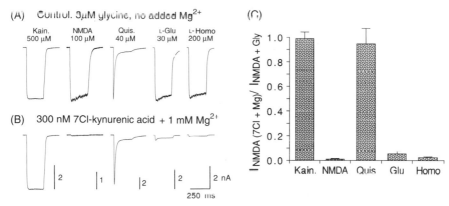

Fig. 4.1 Selective activation of NMDA receptors at low concentrations of glutamate. (A) Responses under conditions which permit activation of both NMDA and AMPA receptors. In (B) responses at NMDA receptors were suppressed; note that responses to 30 μM L-glutamate (L-Glu) and 200 μM L-homocysteate (L-Homo) are nearly abolished. (C) Mean ± SD from experiments on six cells. Adapted from Patneau and Mayer (1990).

glycine, 300 nM 7-Cl-kynurenic acid, and 1 mM Mg). Using these conditions we then recorded responses to L-glutamate and L-homocysteate, applied at doses producing close to maximal activation of NMDA receptors; these experiments showed that less than 10 per cent of the total response to L-glutamate and L-homocysteate occurs at AMPA receptors. Thus, much higher concentrations of L-glutamate and L-homocysteate are required for efficient activation of AMPA versus NMDA receptors.

Similar experiments were performed for a series of 15 excitatory amino acid agonists, of which seven produced marked activation of both NMDA and AMPA receptors. For each of these mixed agonists (L-glutamate, *S*-sulfo-L-cysteine, L-homocysteate, L-homocysteine sulphinate, L-cysteine sulphinate, L-serine-*O*-sulphate and L-cysteate) there was selective activation of NMDA receptors at low concentrations of agonist (Patneau and Mayer 1990), with substantial mixed agonist action developing only at agonist concentrations above saturation for activation of NMDA receptors. It is of interest that L-aspartate is inactive at AMPA receptors in hippocampal neurones, while at high concentrations the 'selective' agonist quisqualic acid can produce weak activation of NMDA receptors (Grudt and Jahr 1990).

Glutamate is a potent agonist at NMDA receptors

Dose response analysis was performed for a series of 11 agonists producing strong activation of NMDA receptors, and revealed a 1000-fold range of potency, with L-glutamate (EC$_{50}$ 2.3 μM) the most potent and quinolinic acid (EC_{50} 2.3 mM) the least potent; L-aspartate (EC_{50} 16.9 μM) and L-cysteate (EC_{50} 302 μM) were of intermediate potency. Dose–response curves for these agonists were initially analysed using the logistic equation

$$I = I_{max} \times \frac{1}{1 + \left\{ \dfrac{EC_{50}}{[\text{dose}]} \right\}^n}$$

where I is the amplitude of the current response at a given dose of agonist, I_{max} the response to a saturating dose of agonist, EC_{50} the concentration of agonist which produces 50 per cent of the maximum response, and n the Hill coefficient. In every case Hill coefficients were greater than one, indicating that two or more molecules of agonist must bind to the NMDA receptor to permit activation of ion channel gating; consistent with this, measurement of the limiting slope of the dose response curve for NMDA gave an estimate of two molecules required for activation (Patneau and Mayer 1990). Kinetic analysis of responses to L-glutamate revealed a sigmoidal activation time course, which also was well fitted by a model requiring two molecules of agonist for activation of NMDA receptors (Clements and Westbrook 1991). Similar experiments for the coagonist glycine also revealed a stoichiometry of two for NMDA receptors expressed in hippocampal neurones (Benveniste *et al.* 1990; Benveniste and Mayer 1991; Clements and Westbrook 1991).

Dose–response curves for all 11 NMDA receptor agonists examined in our experiments were fitted well by a two binding site model:

$$A + R \underset{k_{off}}{\overset{2k_{on}}{\rightleftharpoons}} AR + A \underset{2k_{off}}{\overset{k_{on}}{\rightleftharpoons}} A_2R^* \quad \text{for which} \quad I = I_{max} \times \frac{C^2}{1 + 2C + C^2}$$

where C is the agonist concentration divided by the microscopic equilibrium dissociation constant for an individual agonist binding site ($K_d = k_{off}/k_{on}$, where k_{off} and k_{on} are the apparent dissociation and association rate constants respectively). Figure 4.2 shows that the microscopic K_ds for L-glutamate (1.1 μM), L-aspartate (7.5 μM), L-cysteate (138 μM), and the other agonists examined were, with the exception of quinolinate, in excellent agreement with equilibrium dissociation constants determined from displacement of the binding of radiolabelled [³H]D-AP5 from NMDA receptors in adult rat brain membrane preparations (Olverman *et al.* 1988). Given that it is likely that several subtypes of NMDA receptor are present in the membrane preparations used for binding assays, this result suggests either that the agonists examined discriminate little between NMDA receptor subtypes, or that a single receptor species predominates in adult rat brain and that hippocampal neurones in culture provide a good assay system for its study by patch-clamp techniques.

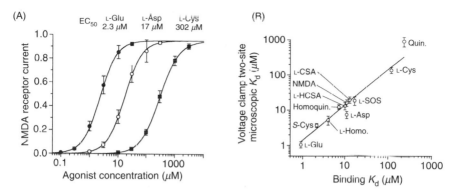

Fig. 4.2 Dose–response curves for NMDA receptor agonists. (A) Mean ± SD from experiments on six to 11 cells. (B) Microscopic K_ds from dose–response curves like those in (A), fitted with a two-site model for activation of NMDA receptors and plotted versus K_ds obtained from ligand binding experiments. Abbreviations for this and subsequent figures: L-glutamate, L-Glu; L-aspartate, L-Asp; L-homocysteic acid, L-Homo; L-homocysteine sulphinic acid, L-HCSA; L-cysteic acid, L-cys; L-cysteine sulphinic acid, L-CSA; L-serine-*O*-sulphate, L-SOS; *N*-methyl-D-aspartic acid, NMDA; *S*-sulpho-L-cysteine, *S*-Cys; quinolinic acid, Quin; and homoquinolinic acid, Homoquin. Adapted from Patneau and Mayer (1990).

Agonist selectivity for activation of NMDA versus AMPA receptors

At excitatory synapses in the cerebellum (Silver *et al.* 1992), cerebral cortex (Sah and Nicoll 1991), and hippocampus (Hestrin *et al.* 1990), there is substantial evidence for simultaneous activation of both NMDA- and AMPA-preferring subtypes of glutamate receptor. The simplest explanation for this would be that both receptor species are colocalized at individual synaptic boutons (Bekkers and Stevens 1989), and that the excitatory neurotransmitter in synaptic vesicles is a mixed agonist. L-glutamate is the transmitter candidate which best fulfils this role. Surprisingly, two sets of experimental results suggest that L-aspartate is unlikely to function as an excitatory synaptic transmitter, at least in the hippocampus. First, L-aspartate is a highly selective NMDA receptor agonist, producing responses comparable to that of NMDA itself, with essentially no activity at AMPA receptors (Patneau and Mayer 1990). Second, the amino acid transporter in synaptic vesicles is highly selective, and does not bind L-aspartate (Naito and Ueda 1985).

Like L-glutamate, several other amino acids, notably the sulphinate and sulphonate analogues of glutamate and aspartate, activate both NMDA and non-NMDA receptors, and are potential transmitter candidates (Mayer and Westbrook 1984; Patneau and Mayer 1990). For responses measured at equilibrium the structure–activity relationship for agonist activity at NMDA receptors is comparable to that for AMPA receptors, with L-glutamate being the most, and L-cysteate the least potent agonist (Fig. 4.3). Equilibrium responses at AMPA receptors occur with EC_{50} values approximately 8-fold higher than for responses at NMDA receptors (Fig. 4.3), although L-homocysteate (EC_{50} ratio of 37), and L-cysteine sulphinate (EC_{50} ratio of 93) show stronger selectivity for agonist action at NMDA receptors. Because NMDA receptors bind sulphur amino acids with relatively high affinity, it is plausible that any of these compounds could be released at sufficiently high concentrations to allow efficient activation of NMDA receptors during synaptic transmission, with the exception perhaps of L-cysteate ($EC_{50} = 300 \, \mu M$). However, although such equilibrium measurements provide little evidence on which to discriminate between transmitter candidates, kinetic measurements (Lester *et al.* 1990; Lester and Jahr 1992) strongly suggest that in the hippocampus only L-glutamate can produce synaptic responses with an appropriately long time course. Given that L-glutamate is the most potent agonist at NMDA receptors, one functional advantage which would arise if more than one amino acid were released during synaptic transmission would be NMDA receptor synaptic responses of shorter duration. Since L-glutamate already has a low potency for activation of AMPA receptors, should other amino acids be used as synaptic transmitters it is likely that they would be extremely inefficient at activating AMPA receptors, and thus would greatly alter the ratio of NMDA to AMPA receptor current; with L-aspartate there would be selective activation of NMDA but not AMPA receptors. No evidence is available concerning these points at present, and L-glutamate remains the most likely transmitter candidate at the majority of excitatory synapses.

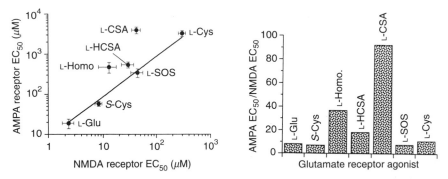

Fig. 4.3 Potency ratios for activation of NMDA versus AMPA receptors. Equilibrium EC_{50} values for agonist responses at NMDA receptors versus those for responses at AMPA receptors; data points show mean ± SD. The ratio EC_{50} AMPA/EC_{50} NMDA was approximately 8 for L-Glu, *S*-Cys, L-SOS, and L-Cys, but nearly 40 and 100 for L-Homo and L-CSA respectively. Adapted from Patneau and Mayer (1990).

The kinetics of action of competitive antagonists

Because agonists and competitive antagonists are thought to interact with common sites on a receptor surface, their binding is mutually exclusive. This has the consequence that when a competitive antagonist is applied rapidly to a receptor which has bound agonist, the antagonist will be unable to bind until after the agonist has dissociated from the receptor. During our studies on NMDA receptors we realized that knowledge of the kinetics of the binding of agonists and antagonists was essential if we were to be able to understand the action of drugs applied with rapid perfusion techniques. Both glutamate and glycine bind with high affinity to NMDA receptors (Johnson and Ascher 1992; McBain *et al.* 1989; Benveniste *et al.* 1990*a*), and thus would be expected to have relatively slow dissociation rate constants, as has been confirmed experimentally (Benveniste *et al.* 1990*a,b*; Lester *et al.* 1990; Johnson and Ascher 1992; Lester and Jahr 1992). This has the consequence that although glutamate and glycine are the natural agonists at NMDA receptors, their slow kinetics of binding can seriously interfere with attempts to study the kinetics of action of antagonists. An example of this is shown in Fig. 4.4 which illustrates responses to concentration jump application of the glycine antagonist 7-Cl-kynurenic acid, with NMDA applied continuously and either glycine, or the lower affinity, more rapidly dissociating agonist L-alanine used to activate ion channel gating. In the presence of glycine, block by 7-Cl-kynurenic acid develops slowly, and the kinetics of onset of block do not increase with concentration of antagonist (Benveniste *et al.* 1990*b*), as required by the law of mass action. However, when L-alanine is used as an agonist, 7-Cl-

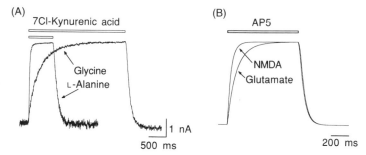

Fig. 4.4 Antagonist binding at NMDA receptors limited by dissociation of agonist. (A) Responses to 30 µM 7-Cl-kynurenic acid applied by concentration jump, in the presence of 100 µM NMDA and either 3 µM glycine or 100 µM L-alanine. (B) Simulation of responses to 30 µM ⁻AP5 applied in the presence of either 35 µM L-glutamate, or 400 µM NMDA, using the model illustrated in Fig. 4.5, and rate constants for k_{on} (in µM⁻¹ s⁻¹) being 5 for L-Glu, 2 for NMDA, and 22 for AP5; and for k_{off} (in s⁻¹) being 5 for L-Glu, 23 for NMDA, and 19 for AP5. Adapted from Benveniste *et al.* (1990*b*).

kynurenic acid acts rapidly, and the rate of onset of block becomes faster with increase in concentration (Benveniste *et al.* 1990*b*). Similar effects occurred during analysis of the action of competitive antagonists acting at the glutamate binding site, and could be predicted by a model with two binding sites for glutamate at which the binding of agonist and antagonist is mutually exclusive (Benveniste and Mayer 1991*a*,*b*; Clements and West-brook 1991). Such experiments show that to study the kinetics of action of competitive antagonists, it is necessary to use agonists of low affinity, with rapid association and dissociation kinetics.

   Although these principles were well established during the classical era of receptor theory (Rang 1966), their consequences are not usually appar-ent in many experimental situations when agonists and antagonists are applied with slow perfusion systems, and thus are always at equilibrium. However, the kinetics of drug action have a large influence on the results of concentration jump experiments. Figure 4.5 shows responses obtained using two protocols for the application to NMDA receptors of equipotent doses of the NMDA antagonists AP7, and the CPP analogue LY 257883 (Ornstein *et al.* 1989). When an agonist and antagonist are applied simul-taneously, and the antagonist is present at a lower concentration than the agonist, initially more receptors bind agonist than occurs at equilibrium; as a result there is an initial overshoot in the response to NMDA. The effect is more marked for LY 257883 because this CPP analogue is a more potent antagonist than AP7, and thus could be applied at an 11-fold lower con-centration, lowering the effective rate at which LY 257883 binds to the

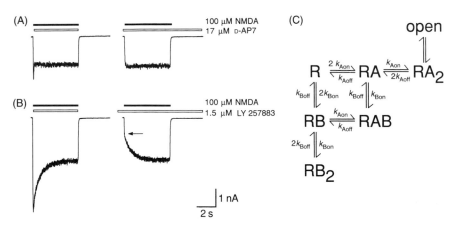

Fig. 4.5 The influence of antagonist binding kinetics on the activation of NMDA receptors. (A) and (B) show responses from the same neurone to NMDA and two competitive antagonists applied either simultaneously with agonist (left) or before and during the application of NMDA (right). (C) illustrates the state diagram for a two-site model for competitive antagonism, where A indicates agonist, and B antagonist. Adapted from Benveniste and Mayer (1991*b*).

population of NMDA receptors. However, at equilibrium, both drugs produce the same degree of block and hence the number of AP7 and LY 257883 molecules bound to the NMDA receptor population is equal. Conversely, when the antagonists are applied before NMDA, their kinetics of dissociation limit the rate at which agonist can bind to and activate the receptor. The concentrations of antagonist used for the experiments in Fig. 4.5 are non-saturating, and thus there exists two populations of NMDA receptors, with, and without antagonist bound. As a result, there is rapid activation by NMDA of those receptors which have not bound antagonist, followed by a slower increase in the response as the binding of agonist and antagonist approaches equilibrium. The dissociation rate constant for AP7 is approximately 16 times faster than that for LY 257883, and as a result it is difficult to distinguish the two phases for AP7 (Benveniste and Mayer 1991*b*).

Structure–activity analysis for competitive antagonists acting at the glutamate binding site

Using the two-site model of NMDA receptor activation shown in Fig. 4.5, we were able to analyse the kinetics of action of a series of 16 structurally related antagonists acting at the glutamate binding site on NMDA receptors (Benveniste and Mayer 1991*b*). The rate constants for the binding (k_{Bon}) and dissociation of antagonist (k_{Boff}) were obtained by analysis with a two-site model of responses to the removal and reapplication of antagonist; equilibrium dose inhibition curves fitted by a two-site model were used to confirm that the antagonist equilibrium dissociation constant was similar to the ratio k_{Boff}/k_{Bon}. Figure 4.6 shows kinetic analysis of responses to the D and L isomers of CPP applied at equieffective concentrations, and the equilibrium dose inhibition curves obtained over a wide range of block. The two-site model predicts that following the removal of antagonist, recovery from block will occur with sigmoidal kinetics, as can clearly be seen for concentration jump responses to D-CPP. Kinetic analysis revealed no difference between the association rate constant for D-CPP (3.6×10^6 M^{-1} s^{-1}) and that for L-CPP (3.8×10^6 M^{-1} s^{-1}), but a 10.3-fold difference in the dissociation rate constant for D-CPP (1.1 s^{-1}) and that for L-CPP (11.3 s^{-1}). The lower equilibrium potency of L-CPP thus results nearly exclusively from faster dissociation of this antagonist, suggesting that stereochemistry at the α-carbon atom plays a critical role in stabilizing the binding of NMDA receptor antagonists. Similar experiments were performed for a series of AP5 and AP7 derivatives, with ω-phosphonate, ω-carboxyl, and ω-tetrazole acidic groups, and revealed that although there was excellent correlation between the ratio k_{Boff}/k_{Bon} and equilibrium K_i values for individual antagonists, values for k_{Boff} and k_{Bon} were widely scattered, and showed little correlation with antagonist potency

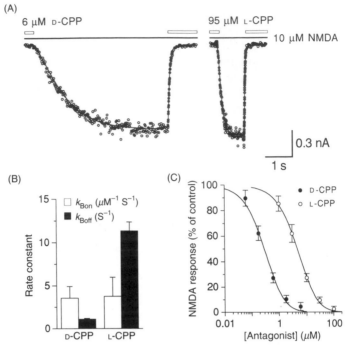

Fig. 4.6 Kinetic analysis of responses to NMDA receptor antagonists. (A) Responses to the D and L isomers of CPP applied at equipotent doses and fitted to a two-site model for competitive antagonism. Panel (B) summarizes results from experiments on four to seven cells. (C) Analysis of equilibrium dose–inhibition curves with a two-site model for competitive antagonism. Adapted from Benveniste and Mayer (1991*b*).

(Fig. 4.7). Two trends emerged from this structure–activity analysis for antagonist binding kinetics. First, both the association and dissociation rate constants for antagonists decrease with increasing conformational restriction, and hence have opposite effects on antagonist potency. Although highly constrained antagonists stay bound to NMDA receptors for long periods of time, the rate at which they are able to bind to NMDA receptors is slower than for more flexible molecules. Second, the association rate constants for antagonists with an ω-phosphonate group was on average two to three times slower than for antagonists of otherwise similar structure, but with an ω-carboxyl or ω-tetrazole acidic group. We considered several plausible explanations for this effect, and noted that at physiological pH the ω-phosphonate group in NMDA receptor antagonists was not fully ionized (Bigge *et al.* 1989; Chenard *et al.* 1990). This raised the possibility that there might be a difference between the potency of antagonist molecules in which the ω-phosphonate group has one negative charge and those with two negative charges.

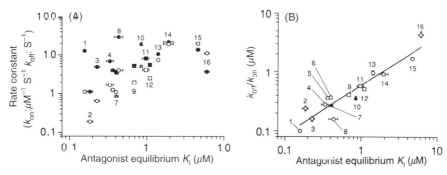

Fig. 4.7 Rate constants for the binding of NMDA receptor antagonists reflect conformational restriction. (A) Paired values for k_{on} (filled circles) and k_{off} (open circles) for 16 antagonists structurally related to AP5 and AP7. (B) plots the ratio k_{off}/k_{on} versus K_i values determined from analysis of equilibrium dose–inhibition curves. Key: 1, CGP 37849; 2, LY 235959; 3, D-CPP-ene; 4, CGS 19755; 5, LY 257883; 6, D-CPP; 7, LY 202157; 8, *trans*-APPA; 9, D-CPC; 10, LY 233053; 11, D-CPC-ene; 12, LY 221501; 13, D-CMP; 14, D-AP5; 15, D-AP7; 16, L-CPP. In A and B circles, squares and triangles represent values for antagonists with ω-phosphono, ω-carboxylate, and ω-tetrazolyly groups respectively. Adapted from Benveniste and Mayer (1991*b*).

ω-phosphonate antagonists are only partially active at physiological pH

Experiments with AP7, for which ionization of the second hydroxyl group occurs with a pK_a of 7.8 (Bigge *et al.* 1989; Chenard *et al.* 1990), showed that the antagonist potency increased 3.7-fold on raising the extracellular pH from 7.3 to 8.2 (Fig. 4.8). Control experiments revealed no change in the potency of NMDA over this range of pH, and much smaller changes in the potency of LY 221501, an antagonist containing an ω-carboxyl group (Ornstein *et al.* 1989). These results suggest that antagonist molecules in which the ω-phosphonate group is fully ionized bind to NMDA receptors with higher affinity than antagonist molecules in which the ω-phosphonate group has only a single negative charge. NMDA receptor block by the doubly but not singly charged phosphonate moiety seems to conflict with the observation that drugs with ω-carboxyl and ω-tetrazole acidic groups, which have only a single negative charge, are also potent NMDA receptor antagonists. Differences in the geometry between the planar, but charge-delocalized ω-carboxyl and ω-tetrazole groups on one hand and the tetrahedral ω-phosphonate moiety on the other could underlie differences in the charge dependence for binding these ω-acidic groups. Support for our proposal that the doubly charged ionic form of the phosphonate moiety is the active species at NMDA receptors comes from the work of Fagg and Baud (1988) who reported that the tetrahedral phosphinate moiety, which is similar in structure to the phosphonate group, but which has only a single

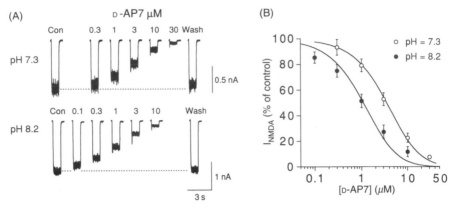

Fig. 4.8 Ionization of AP7 increases NMDA receptor antagonist potency. (A) Responses to 10 μM NMDA and block by various doses of AP7 at pH 7.3 and 8.2. (B) Analysis of dose–inhibition curves for AP7 fitted by a two-site model for competitive antagonism; the IC_{50} values at pH 8.2 and 7.3 were 1.1 and 3.4 μM respectively. Adapted from Benveniste and Mayer (1992).

negative charge when fully ionized, is inactive, or of very low potency when used as the ω-acidic group in NMDA receptor antagonists.

Our observation that at physiological pH NMDA receptor antagonists exist in two ionic forms, only one of which is active, provides an explanation for the unusually slow association rate constant of drugs with an ω-phosphonate versus ω-carboxyl or ω-tetrazole groups. Since association rates are concentration-dependent, attempts to determine the rate constant require accurate knowledge of the species of antagonist. Figure 4.9 shows structures for some antagonists of differing degrees of conformational restraint, with ω-phosphonate or ω-tetrazole groups, and the corresponding values for experimentally determined association rate constants measured at pH 7.3, and the association rate constants predicted for the fully ionized species of antagonist (Benveniste and Mayer 1992). For AP5, the corrected value for k_{on} (6.3×10^7 M^{-1} s^{-1}) is close to the diffusion limit, while for CGS 19755 and for LY 235959 the rate constants are slower, but similar to those measured for the corresponding ω-tetrazoles.

Conclusions

Measurements of the kinetics of action of NMDA receptor agonists and antagonists provides a necessary framework for the analysis of synaptic responses, but in addition reveals some unexpected results. The unusually high affinity of NMDA but not AMPA receptors for L-glutamate has the consequence that because there is likely to exist a low (micromolar) concentration of agonist in the extracellular space (Benveniste *et al.* 1984),

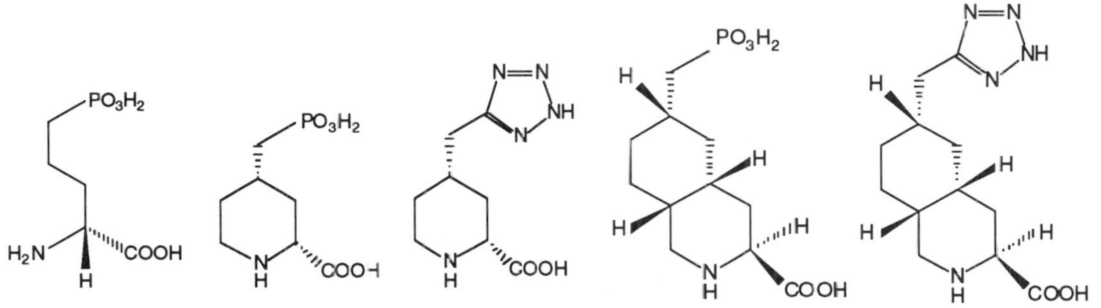

D-AP5　　CGS 19755*　　LY 233053*　　LY 235959　　LY 202157

	D-AP5	CGS 19755*	LY 233053*	LY 235959	LY 202157
k_{on} μM^{-1} s^{-1} (pH 7.3)	22.2 ± 6.5	7.0 ± 2.3	19.6 ± 11.4	1.1 ± 0.6	3.4 ± 1.0
k_{on} μM^{-1} s^{-1} (corrected)	63.4	20.0	19.6	3.1	3.4
k_{off} s^{-1}	19.4 ± 4.1	1.7 ± 0.2	5.2 ± 0.4	0.19 ± 0.03	0.87 ± 0.10

Fig. 4.9 The influence of conformational restriction and the ω-acidic group on the binding kinetics of NMDA receptor antagonists. Values for k_{on} (μM^{-1} s^{-1}) were determined at pH 7.3, and then corrected for incomplete ionization, assuming that ionization of the ω-phosphonate group occurs with a pK$_a$ value of 7.8. The association rate constant was highest for the least constrained antagonist (AP5), of intermediate kinetics for the piperidine derivatives CGS 19755 and LY 233053, and lowest for the bicyclic decahydroisoquinolines LY 235959 and LY 202157. Note that when corrected for incomplete ionization the association rate constants for the ω-phosphonates CGS 19755 and LY 235959 are similar to those for the corresponding tetrazoles LY 233053 and LY 202157. Adapted from data in Benveniste and Mayer (1991*b*, 1992).

there will be a selective, possibly substantial, tonic activation of NMDA receptors. Such responses will be counteracted to some extent by Mg block of the NMDA receptor ion channel, but would be expected to regulate the firing pattern and excitability of central neurones. That this occurs has been confirmed in several studies on brain slice preparations (Sah *et al.* 1989; Blanton *et al.* 1990; LoTurco *et al.* 1991). It would be expected that changes in NMDA receptor subunit expression during development could alter the extent to which such responses are functionally important. An attractive hypothesis is that early in development Ca influx through high affinity NMDA receptors plays an important role in the control of gene expression and neuronal development (Blanton *et al.* 1990; LoTurco *et al.* 1991), and that in adult life NMDA receptors switch to a low affinity form, which are no longer activated at the micromolar extracellular concentrations of L-glutamate which exist as a consequence of the stoichiometry of ion-coupled glutamate transport (Nicholls and Atwell 1991). Studies on antagonists suggest that drugs with an ω-phosphonate group are not ideal, because they suffer a considerable loss of potency at physiological pH, due to incomplete ionization. However, once bound to NMDA receptors, drugs with an ω-phosphonate group form a more stable complex than the corresponding ω-carboxyl and ω-tetrazole analogues. At present only preliminary data have been reported concerning the functional properties of NMDA receptors assembled from different receptor subunit combinations (Kutsuwada *et al.* 1992; Monyer *et al.* 1992), but it would be expected that further study will identify important functional variation. A major challenge for the future will be to identify which of the possible receptor subunit combinations actually exist in native NMDA receptors, and to develop drugs which can be used to therapeutic advantage at NMDA receptor subtypes.

References

Bekkers, J. M. and Stevens, C. F. (1989). NMDA and non-NMDA receptors are co-localized at individual excitatory synapses in cultured rat hippocampus. *Nature*, **341**, 230–3.

Benveniste, M. and Mayer, M. L. (1991*a*). Kinetic analysis of antagonist action at *N*-methyl-D-aspartic acid receptors. *Biophysical Journal*, **59**, 560–73.

Benveniste, M. and Mayer, M. L. (1991*b*). Structure–activity analysis of binding kinetics for NMDA receptor competitive antagonists: the influence of conformational restriction. *British Journal of Pharmacology*, **104**, 207–21.

Benveniste, M. and Mayer, M. L. (1992). Effect of extracellular pH on potency of *N*-methyl-D-aspartic acid receptor competitive antagonists. *Molecular Pharmacology*, **42**, 679–86.

Benveniste, H., Drejer, J., Schousboe, A., and Diemer, N. H. (1984). Elevation of the extracellular concentrations of glutamate and aspartate in rat hippocampus during transient cerebral ischemia monitored by intracerebral microdialysis. *Journal of Neurochemistry*, **43**, 1369–74.

Benveniste, M., Clements, J., Vyklicky, L., and Mayer, M. L. (1990*a*). A kinetic analysis of the modulation of *N*-methyl-D-aspartic acid receptors by glycine in mouse cultured hippocampal neurones. *Journal of Physiology*, **428**, 333–57.

Benveniste, M., Mienville, J. M., Sernagor, E., and Mayer, M. L. (1990*b*). Concentration-jump experiments with NMDA antagonists in mouse cultured hippocampal neurons. *Journal of Neurophysiology*, **63**, 1373–84.

Bigge, C. F., Drummond, J. T., and Johnson, G. (1989). Synthesis and NMDA-receptor binding of 2-amino-7,7-difluoro-7-phosphonoheptanoic acid. *Tetrahedron Letters*, **30**, 7013–16.

Blanton, M. G., LoTurco, J. J., and Kriegstein, A. R. (1990). Endogenous neurotransmitter activates *N*-methyl-D-aspartate receptors on differentiating neurons in embryonic cortex. *Proceedings of the National Academy of Science, USA*, **87**, 8027–30.

Chenard, B. L., Lipinski, C. A., Dominy, B. W., Mena, E. E., Ronau, R. T., Butterfield, G. C., Marinovic, L. C., Pagnozzi, M., Butler, T. W., and Tzang, T. (1990). A unified approach to systematic isosteric substitution for acidic groups and application to NMDA antagonists related to 2-amino-7-phosphonoheptanoate. *Journal of Medicinal Chemistry*, **33**, 1077–83.

Clements, J. D. and Westbrook, G. L. (1991). Activation kinetics reveal the number of glutamate and glycine binding sites on the *N*-methyl-D-aspartate receptor. *Neuron*, **7**, 605–13.

Fagg, G. E. and Baud, J. (1988). Characterization of NMDA receptor–ionophore complexes in the brain. In *Excitatory amino acids in health and disease*, (ed. D. Lodge), pp. 63–90. Wiley, London.

Grudt, T. J. and Jahr, C. E. (1990). Quisqualate activates *N*-methyl-D-aspartate receptor-channels in hippocampal neurons maintained in culture. *Molecular Pharmacology*, **37**, 477–81.

Hestrin, S., Nicoll, R. A., Perkel, D., and Sah, P. (1990). Analysis of synaptic action in pyramidal cells using whole-cell recording from rat hippocampal slices. *Journal of Physiology*, **422**, 203–25.

Johnson, J. W. and Ascher, P. (1987). Glycine potentiates the NMDA response of mouse central neurones. *Nature*, **325**, 529–31.

Johnson, J. W. and Ascher, P. (1992). Equilibrium and kinetic study of glycine action on the *N*-methyl-D-aspartate receptor in cultured mouse brain neurons. *Journal of Physiology*, **455**, 339–65.

Kutsuwada, T., Kashiwabuchi, N., Mori, H., Sakimura, K., Kushiya, E., Araki, K., Meguro, H., Masaki, H., Kumanishi, T., Arakawa, M., and Mishina, M. (1992). Molecular diversity of the NMDA receptor channel. *Nature*, **358**, 36–41.

Lester, R. A. and Jahr, C. E. (1992). NMDA channel behavior depends on agonist affinity. *Journal of Neuroscience*, **12**, 635–43.

Lester, R. A., Clements, J. D., Westbrook, G. L., and Jahr, C. E. (1990) Channel kinetics determine the time course of NMDA receptor-mediated synaptic currents. *Nature*, **346**, 565–7.

LoTurco, J. J., Blanton, M. G., and Kriegstein, A. R. (1991). Initial expression and endogenous activation of NMDA channels in early neocortical development. *Journal of Neuroscience*, **11**, 792–9.

McBain, C. J., Kleckner, N. W., Wyrick, S., and Dingledine, R. (1989). Structural requirements for activation of the glycine coagonist site of NMDA receptors expressed in *Xenopus* oocytes. *Molecular Pharmacology*, **36**, 556–65.

Mayer, M. L. and Westbrook, G. L. (1984). Mixed-agonist action of excitatory amino acids on mouse spinal cord neurones under voltage clamp. *Journal of Physiology*, **354**, 29–53.

Monyer, H., Sprengel, R., Schoepfer, R., Herb, A., Higuchi, M., Lomeli, H., Burnashev, N., Sakmann, B., and Seeburg, P. H. (1992). Heteromeric NMDA receptors: molecular and functional distinction of subtypes. *Science*, **256**, 1217–21.

Naito, S. and Ueda, T. (1985). Characterization of glutamate uptake into synaptic vesicles. *Journal of Neurochemistry*, **44**, 99–109.

Nicholls, D. and Attwell, D. (1990). The release and uptake of excitatory amino acids. *Trends in Pharmacological Science*, **11**, 462–8.

Olverman, H. J., Jones, A. W., Mewett, K. N., and Watkins, J. C. (1988). Structure/activity relationships of *N*-methyl-D-aspartate receptor ligands as studied by their inhibition of [^{3}H]D-2-amino-5-phosphonopentanoic acid binding in rat brain membranes. *Neuroscience*, **26**, 17–31.

Ornstein, P. L., Schaus, J. M., Chambers, J. W., Huser, D. L., Leander, J. D., Wong, D. T., Paschal, J. W., Jones, N. D., and Deeter, J. B. (1989). Synthesis and pharmacology of a series of 3- and 4-(phosphonoalkyl)pyridine- and piperidine-2-carboxylic acids: potent *N*-methyl-D-aspartate receptor antagonists. *Journal of Medicinal Chemistry*, **32**, 827–33.

Patneau, D. K. and Mayer, M. L. (1990). Structure–activity relationships for amino acid transmitter candidates acting at *N*-methyl-D-aspartate and quisqualate receptors. *Journal of Neuroscience*, **10**, 2385–99.

Rang, H. P. (1966). The kinetics of action of acetylcholine antagonists in smooth muscle. *Proceedings of the Royal Society (London), Series B*, **164**, 488–510.

Sah, P. and Nicoll, R. A. (1991). Mechanisms underlying potentiation of synaptic transmission in rat anterior cingulate cortex *in vitro*. *Journal of Physiology*, **433**, 615–30.

Sah, P., Hestrin, S., and Nicoll, R. A. (1989). Tonic activation of NMDA receptors by ambient glutamate enhances excitability of neurons. *Science*, **246**, 815–18.

Silver, R. A., Traynelis, S. F., and Cull-Candy, S. G. (1992). Rapid-time course miniature and evoked excitatory currents at cerebellar synapses. *Nature*, **355**, 163–6.

Watkins, J. C. and Evans, R. H. (1981). Excitatory amino acid transmitters. *Annual Review of Pharmacology and Toxicology*, **21**, 165–204.

5 Molecular biology of NMDA receptors

P. H. SEEBURG, H. MONYER, R. SPRENGEL,
AND N. BURNASHEV

Introduction

NMDA receptors are glutamate-activated cation channels which differ from the non-NMDA classes of ionotropic glutamate receptors by several hallmark properties. These include a large single channel conductance (Nowak et al. 1984), a high Ca^{2+}/Na^+ permeability ratio (MacDermott et al. 1986), a voltage-dependent Mg^{2+} block (Mayer et al. 1984; Nowak et al. 1984), high affinity for glutamate, a requirement for glycine as coagonist (Johnson and Ascher 1987; Kleckner and Dingledine 1988), and relatively slow activation and deactivation kinetics (Johnson and Ascher 1987; Lester et al. 1990; Jahr 1992; Lester and Jahr 1992; Stern et al. 1992). Collectively, these properties underlie the specific neurophysiologic roles that glutamate-activated NMDA currents subserve (e.g. see Collingridge and Singer 1991), and explain their involvement in the phenomenon termed excitotoxicity (e.g. see Choi 1988).

The current model of the composition of NMDA receptors suggests that these receptors assemble from two distantly sequence-related subunits, the NMDAR1 (NR1) subunit (Moriyoshi et al. 1991) and an NR2 subunit of which four types (NR2A to 2D) have been characterized (Ikeda et al. 1992; Kutsuwada et al. 1992; Meguro et al. 1992; Monyer et al. 1992; Ishii et al. 1993), predicting the existence of at least four NMDA receptor subtypes. Although the primary structures of NMDA receptor subunits are known, no sound predictions can be made regarding the membrane topology of the subunits or the stoichiometry of the subunits in native or recombinant channels. The mature subunits of NMDA receptors, and of other ionotropic glutamate receptor channels, contain four hydrophobic sequence regions. On this basis, the subunits are expected to cross the lipid bilayer four times to assume a membrane topology as established for the nicotinic acetylcholine receptor (Unwin 1993) whose subunits have extracellularly located amino- and carboxy-termini. However, certain features of glutamate receptor channels (e.g. see Tingley et al. 1993) are compatible with a different topology. Here we describe the molecular components of NMDA receptors as revealed from cloned nucleotide sequences, the functional characteristics of recombinantly expressed NMDA channels, and the distribution patterns in rat brain of the mRNAs encoding the channel subunits. We also present structure–function relationships governing some of the particular properties of NMDA receptor channels.

The NR1 subunit

The NR1 subunit is the principal constituent of the NMDA receptor, being expressed at substantial levels in virtually all central neurones (Moriyoshi *et al.* 1991), including those of spinal cord (Tölle *et al.* 1993). This subunit was first characterized by S. Nakanishi and co-workers (Moriyoshi *et al.* 1991), using expression cloning in the *Xenopus* oocyte. This considerable achievement was made possible by the fact that the NR1 subunit can self-assemble to produce functional receptors having many of the properties of native NMDA receptors. These include the voltage-dependent Mg^{2+} block and a requirement for glycine to activate the channel. Homomeric NR1 channels probably have high Ca^{2+} permeability, as much as this can be deduced from measurements in the *Xenopus* oocyte where reversal potentials in high Ca^{2+} solutions cannot be accurately determined.

The NR1 gene contains 22 exons and is spread over a region of approximately 25 000 pairs (Hollmann *et al.* 1993). The primary transcript of this gene can be differentially spliced to produce at least nine mRNAs (Sugihara *et al.* 1992; Hollmann *et al.* 1993). One of these encodes a small polypeptide, with amino-terminal NR1 subunit sequences only, which is not expected to participate in channel formation. The other eight NR1 mRNAs (Fig. 5.1) differ in the presence or absence of any of three exonic sequences, one encoding a 21 amino acid stretch in the amino-terminal (extracellular) region of the NR1 subunit, the others encoding amino acid sequences in the carboxy-terminal hydrophilic region distal to TM4. Subsets of the NR1 splice variants were found by several other laboratories (Anantharam *et al.* 1992; Durand *et al.* 1992; Nakanishi *et al.* 1992). Functional differences of NR1 splice forms expressed as homo-oligomeric channels were reported for agonist and antagonist sensitivity and for the potentiating effect of spermine. Furthermore, Zn^{2+} was shown to increase agonist-activated currents in select NR1 splice variants (Hollmann *et al.* 1993). However, caution should be exercized regarding the physiological relevance of results obtained with NR1 subunit channels. Homo-oligomeric NR1 receptors may constitute artefacts of *in vitro* expression and may not contribute to NMDA currents in neurones. For example, heteromeric NR1–NR2 receptor configurations do not show the potentiation by Zn^{2+} seen with certain homomeric NR1 splice forms, but are potently inhibited by Zn^{2+} (Hollmann *et al.* 1993). Notably, carboxy-terminal splice forms of the NR1 subunit appear to differ in the presence or absence of phosphorylation sites for protein kinase C which might serve to modulate heteromeric NR1–NR2 channel activity (Tingley *et al.* 1993).

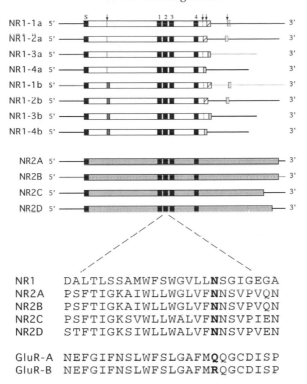

NR1   DALTLSSAMWFSWGVLL**N**SGIGEGA
NR2A   PSFTIGKAIWLLWGLVF**N**NSVPVQN
NR2B   PSFTIGKAIWLLWGLVF**N**NSVPVQN
NR2C   PSFTIGKSVWLLWALVF**N**NSVPIEN
NR2D   STFTIGKSIWLLWALVF**N**NSVPVEN

GluR-A   NEFGIFNSLWFSLGAFM**Q**QGCDISP
GluR-B   NEFGIFNSLWFSLGAFM**R**QGCDISP

Fig. 5.1 The NMDA receptor subunits and their mRNAs. The mRNAs for NR1 splice forms NR1-1a to -4b (Sugihara *et al.* 1992; Hollmann *et al.* 1993) and for the NR2 subunits (Ikeda *et al.* 1992; Kutsuwada *et al.* 1992; Meguro *et al.* 1992; Monyer *et al.* 1992; Ishii *et al.* 1993) are represented by lines. The coding regions of the different subunit mRNAs are boxed (open boxes for NR1 and shaded boxes for NR2). Filled squares within subunits denote hydrophobic regions for the amino-terminal signal sequence (S) and four transmembrane regions, TM1 to TM4 (numbered 1 to 4). The eight splice forms of the primary NR1 transcript are generated by presence or absence of several exonic sequences. One exon encodes 21 amino acids inserted amino-terminally into NR1-1b to -4b (stippled). The other exons contribute to carboxy-terminal peptide sequences distal of TM4 and to the length of the 3′ untranslated mRNA sequence. Arrows indicate locations of sequence differences between the NR1 splice forms. For the NR2 subunits, the length of carboxy-terminal extensions beyond TM4 are remarkable. These are longest in NR2A and NR2B and slightly shorter for NR2C and NR2D. The 5′ and 3′ untranslated mRNA sequences are not drawn to scale. The amino acid sequences of the putative channel forming segment TM2 of NMDA receptor subunits are listed (below the linear subunit diagrams). The N-site, shown in bold, is aligned with the Q/R-site of AMPA receptor subunits GluR-A and GluR-B (25).

The NR2 subunits

The NR2 subunits of the NMDA receptor were found by the screening of brain-derived cDNA libraries with nucleotide sequences conserved in glutamate-operated ion channels (Ikeda *et al.* 1992; Kutsuwada *et al.* 1992; Meguro *et al.* 1992; Monyer *et al.* 1992; Ishii *et al.* 1993). These subunits, termed NMDAR2 (NR2A to NR2D) for the rat, and $\varepsilon1$ to $\varepsilon4$ in mouse, are highly related to each other but only distantly related to other ionotropic glutamate receptor subunits, including the common NMDA receptor subunit NR1. Evidence that NR2 subunits are part of NMDA receptors comes from the observation that coexpression with NR1 greatly potentiates agonist-evoked currents. This suggests that NR1 and NR2 subunits enter into productive assemblies because NR2 expression alone does not generate functional channels. NR2 subunits show as a striking feature extended carboxy-terminal hydrophilic sequences (>550 amino acids) distal to TM4. These carboxy-termini are in fact larger than the amino-terminal sequences proximal of TM1 (Fig. 5.1), which are predicted to be extracellularly located. Truncation of the extended carboxy-terminal sequences does not lead to observable differences in current properties nor in ligand binding (unpublished observation). This may suggest that the NR2 carboxy-termini are located intracellularly, as proposed for the carboxy-terminus of NR1 (Tingley *et al.* 1993).

NR2 subunits share with the NR1 subunit a structural hallmark in a channel-forming region. An asparagine residue in TM2 occupies a position where the homologous subunits of AMPA and high-affinity kainate receptors carry a glutamine or arginine residue (Sommer and Seeburg 1992). As discussed below, this asparagine residue is a critical channel determinant for the particular divalent ion conductance and blocking properties of NMDA receptor channels.

Properties of heteromeric NMDA channels

Native NMDA receptors differ from AMPA and kainate receptor channels in the relatively slow onset and decline of the current response after a pulse of high glutamate concentration (Johnson and Ascher 1987; Lester *et al.* 1990; Jahr 1992; Lester and Jahr 1992; Stern *et al.* 1992). The rise time of the current evoked by fast application of 100 μM glutamate in the presence of 10 μM glycine is identical for all subunit combinations expressed in 293 cells (20% to 80% rise time of approximately 13 ms). Subunit-specific differences are, however, observed with respect to the current offset time after the fast removal of glutamate (Fig. 5.2). The offset time is considerably faster in cells expressing NR1–NR2A channels (time constant of 120 ms) than in cells expressing NR1–NR2B or NR1–NR2C channels

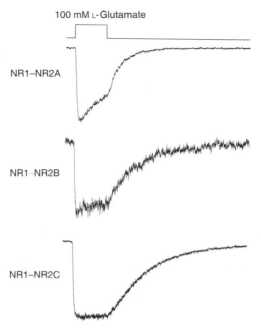

Fig. 5.2 Traces of whole-cell current responses to fast application of glutamate measured from 293 cells expressing different NMDA receptor subunits. The duration of the glutamate pulse shown in the top trace was 300 ms; the membrane potential was −60 mV. Glutamate was applied in the presence of 10 μM glycine.

(time constant of 380 ms for both) (Monyer *et al.* 1992). It is worth pointing out that NR1–NR2A channel currents show a slow but clear desensitization (time constant of 100 ms), whereas currents through NR1–NR2B and NR1–NR2C channels do not desensitize in this time range (Monyer *et al.* 1992; data for NR1–NR2B channels are unpublished).

NMDA receptors differ from other ionotropic glutamate receptors in their single-channel characteristics. In a study of recombinant NR1–NR2 subtypes using outside-out patches from *Xenopus* oocytes injected with cRNAs it was observed that the NR1–NR2A and NR1–NR2B channels have similar single-channel properties (Stern *et al.* 1992). Their main conductance level (approximately 80% of all channel openings) was 50 pS with channel openings also seen at a 38 pS subconductance level. The mean apparent open time of the 50 pS openings was approximately 2.8 ms. NR1–NR2C channels show different properties. The main conductance level (75% of all openings) was 36 pS and a subconductance level of 11 pS was observed. The mean apparent open time for the 36 pS openings was short, approximately 0.6 ms. All measurements were performed in 1 mM external Ca^{2+} solution. Due to the dependence of single-channel conductance on the external Ca^{2+} concentration, the difference seen for NR1–NR2C channels might indicate a stronger blocking action of Ca^{2+} on the Na^+ current than in NR1–NR2A or NR1–NR2B channels. As observed by Stern *et al.* (1992), the NR1–NR2A and NR1–NR2B channels have characteristics similar to those of the hippocampal CA1 channels whilst the NR1–NR2C channel has properties reminiscent of a channel found in cultured rat E17-E19 large cerebellar neurones.

Heteromeric NR1–NR2 channels show high Ca^{2+} permeability and low Mg^{2+} permeability (Fig. 5.3). The NR1 and NR2 subunits contain in their TM2 region an asparagine at a position (N-site) which is homologous to the Q/R-site of the AMPA or kainate receptor subunits (Ikeda *et al.* 1991; Kutsuwada *et al.* 1992; Meguro *et al.* 1992; Monyer *et al.* 1992; Moriyoshi *et al.* 1992; Ishii *et al.* 1993). Replacing the asparagine by glutamine in the NR1 subunit changed the reversal potential in high Ca^{2+} solution to more negative values, indicating a decrease in Ca^{2+} permeability, but did not increase the low Mg^{2+} permeability of the heteromeric channels (Burnashev *et al.* 1992). In contrast, the same substitution in the NR2 subunit considerably increased Mg^{2+} permeability but failed to change the Ca^{2+} permeability of the channel (Burnashev *et al.* 1992) (see Fig. 5.3). Introducing an arginine into the N-site of the NR1 subunit generated channels with a low Ca^{2+} permeability (not shown), suggesting that the size and charge of the amino acid present in the critical site of TM2 is important for the Ca^{2+} permeability of NMDA receptor channels (Burnashev *et al.* 1992). Qualitatively similar results were obtained with the *Xenopus* oocyte expression system (Sakurada *et al.* 1993). Engineering an asparagine into the Q/R-site of AMPA receptor subunits confers on the altered channel a high permeability of Ca^{2+} relative to Mg^{2+} (Burnashev *et al.* 1992). AMPA and NMDA receptor channels thus contain common structural motifs in their TM2 regions that are responsible for some of their divalent ion selectivity and conductance properties.

Native NMDA receptor channels are blocked in a voltage-dependent manner by extracellular Mg^{2+} ions (Mayer *et al.* 1984; Nowak *et al.* 1984). It was found that the strength of this block depends on the particular subunit combination of the channel. For NR1–NR2C channels the blocking action of Mg^{2+} is considerably weaker than for NR1–NR2A channels (Kutsuwada *et al.* 1992; Monyer *et al.* 1992). Although the structural elements determining this difference are unknown, the asparagine in the N-site seems to play a role in the control of the Mg^{2+} block. The strength of block is reduced when asparagines in TM2 of NR1 or NR2 subunits are replaced by glutamine (Burnashev *et al.* 1992; Mori *et al.* 1992; Sakurada *et al.*). However, this reduction is more significant when substituting the NR2 asparagine (Fig. 5.3). Replacement in the NR1 subunit of asparagine by arginine abolishes the blocking effect of Mg^{2+} (not shown), suggesting that when the positively charged arginine occupies the critical N-site of the NR1 subunit, divalent cations appear to be prevented from entering the channel.

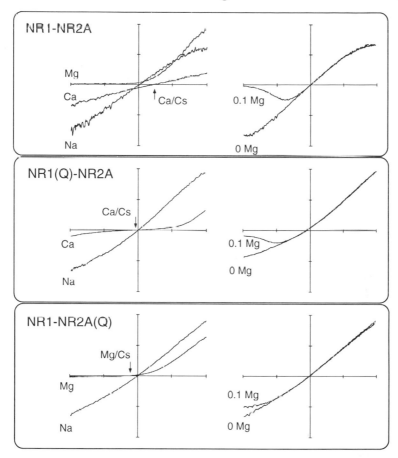

Fig. 5.3 Difference in Ca^{2+} and Mg^{2+} permeability and in Mg^{2+} block between wild-type and mutant NMDA receptor channels expressed in 293 cells. Whole-cell current–voltage relationships of glutamate-activated currents in high Na^+ (140 mM), in high Ca^{2+} (110 mM), and in high Mg^{2+} (110 mM) extracellular solutions measured during ramped changes in membrane potential (left column). Reversal potentials for divalent ions are indicated by arrows. The intracellular solution contained 140 mM CsCl. The differences in channel block by extracellular Mg^{2+} between wild-type and mutant NMDA receptor channels are shown on the right. Vertical axes correspond to current, horizontal axes to membrane potential. Voltage range ± 100 mV.

The effects of mutations on permeability and channel block suggest that the asparagines from the two subunit partners could form, at least in part, the selectivity filter of the NMDA receptor for both Mg^{2+} and Ca^{2+}.

Expression of NMDA receptor genes

The cloned nucleotide sequences encoding the NMDA receptor subunits serve as excellent probes to investigate the expression characteristics of the subunit genes in the central nervous system (CNS) of rat and mouse. Northern analysis indicated that the rat subunit transcripts are approximately 4.2 kb (NR1), 12 kb (NR2A), 15 kb (NR2B), 6 kb (NR2C), and 7 kb long (NR2D) (Moriyoshi *et al.* 1991; Ishii *et al.* 1993). The mouse subunit mRNAs are 4 kb (NR1 = ζ1), 18 kb (NR2A = ε1), 20 kb (NR2B = ε2), 4.6 and 12 kb (NR2C = ε3) (Kutsuwada *et al.* 1992; Yamazaki *et al.* 1992).

In situ hybridization (Moriyoshi *et al.* 1991; Kutsuwada *et al.* 1992; Meguro *et al.* 1992; Monyer *et al.* 1992; Tölle *et al.* 1993) documented that the NR1 gene is expressed highly and ubiquitously in virtually all neurones, including those of spinal cord. The situation is quite different for the NR2 gene transcripts whose CNS distribution is distinct but overlapping (Fig. 5.4). In the adult rat brain, NR2A mRNA is expressed in many areas, prominently in cerebral and cerebellar cortex, and in hippocampus. The NR2B mRNA is more restricted being prominent in telencephalic and thalamic areas. NR2C mRNA is very highly expressed in cerebellar granule cells. NR2D mRNA is largely restricted to diencephalic and lower brain stem regions and appears to be the only NR2 subunit in motor neurones of spinal cord (Tölle *et al.* 1993). Very low NR2D expression is observed in cortex and cerebellum. The differential distribution of the NR2 subunits is compatible with the notion that native NMDA receptors are heteromeric assemblies of NR1 and NR2 subunits. Combined with results of functional studies, this model predicts distinct NMDA receptor properties in different neuronal populations. That different functional properties are required during nervous system development is suggested by the dynamic changes in NR2 gene expression observed during CNS ontogenesis, particularly during the first two postnatal weeks (Watanabe *et al.* 1992). At early stages,

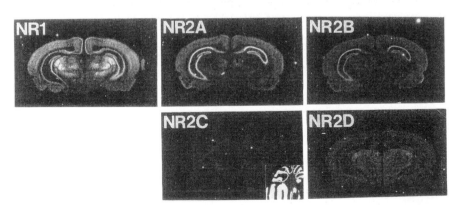

Fig. 5.4 Expression patterns of NMDA receptor mRNAs in coronal sections of P15 rat brain. (A) NR1; (B) NR2A; (C) NR2B; (D) NR2C; (E) NR2D. Inset in (D) illustrates the high NR2C gene expression in the cerebellum. Images were obtained by oligonucleotide-mediated *in situ* hybridization.

only NR2B and NR2D subunit mRNAs can be detected. NR2A and NR2C gene transcripts appear around birth and become prominent only post-natally. Changes in subunit composition of NMDA receptors could underlie the differences in NMDA receptor-mediated synaptic current properties observed during development (Carmignoto and Vicini 1992; Hestrin 1992).

Conclusion

Molecular cloning has revealed the primary structure of NMDA receptor subunits. Functional expression and CNS distribution of nucleotide sequences encoding these subunits strongly suggest that native NMDA receptors assemble from NR1 and NR2 subunits. When reconstituted in *Xenopus* oocytes or in cultured 293 cells, these receptors show properties of native NMDA receptors. These properties comprise a large single-channel conductance, high Ca^{2+} permeability, voltage-dependent Mg^{2+} block, slow gating kinetics, and a requirement for glycine. Some of these properties differ substantially depending on which of the four modulatory NR2 subunits assembles with the principal NR1 subunit. For example, NR1–NR2C channels are characterized by slower deactivation kinetics than NR1–NR2A channels. Also, conductance for monovalent ions is possibly subject to more interference by Ca^{2+} ions in NR1–NR2C channels than in NR1–NR2A channels. These data combined with the expression characteristics of NR2 genes in the developing and the mature CNS indicate that NMDA receptor properties differ in many cell populations. The data are consistent with the notion that early and late NMDA receptors may subserve different physiological functions. While a combination of molecular biology and biophysical analysis has yielded valuable results on the composition and function of NMDA receptors, several important issues remain to be addressed. These include the subunit stoichiometry, membrane topology, mechanism of Mg^{2+} block, and the nature of accessory proteins involved in processing the channel-mediated Ca^{2+} signal.

References

Anantharam, V., Panchal, R. G., Wilson, A., Kolchie, V. V., Treistman, S. N., and Bayley, H. (1992). Combinatorial RNA splicing alters the surface charge on the NMDA receptor. *FEBS Letters*, **305**, 27–30.

Burnashev, N., Monyer, H., Seeburg, P. H., and Sakmann, B. (1992). Divalent ion permeability of AMPA receptor channels is dominated by the edited form of a single subunit. *Neuron*, **8**, 189–98.

Burnashev, N., Schoepfer, R., Monyer, H., Ruppersberg, J. P., Günther, W., Seeburg, P. II., and Sakmann, B. (1992). Control by asparagine residues of calcium permeability and magnesium block in the NMDA receptor. *Science*, **257**, 1415–19.

Carmignoto, G. and Vicini, S. (1992). Activity-dependent decrease in NMDA receptor responses during development of the visual cortex. *Science*, **258**, 1007–11.

Choi, D. W. (1988). Glutamate neurotoxicity and diseases of the nervous system. *Neuron*, **1**, 623–34.

Collingridge, G. L. and Singer, W. (1991). Excitatory amino acid receptors and synaptic plasticity. In *The pharmacology of excitatory amino acids*, (ed. D. Lodge and G. L. Collingridge), a special issue of *Trends in Pharmacological Science*, pp. 42–8.

Durand, G. M., Gregor, P., Zheng, X., Bennett, M. V. L., Uhl, G. R., and Zukin, R. S. (1992). Cloning of an apparent splice variant of the rat *N*-methyl-D-aspartate receptor NMDAR1 with altered sensitivity to polyamines and activators of protein kinase C. *Proceedings of the National Academy of Science, USA*, **89**, 9359–63.

Hestrin, S. (1992). Development regulation of NMDA receptor-mediated synaptic currents at a central synapse. *Nature*, **357**, 686–9.

Hollmann, M., Boulter, J., Maron, C., Beasley, L., Sullivan, J., Pecht, G., and Heinemann, S. (1993). Zinc potentiates agonist-induced currents at certain splice variants of the NMDA receptor. *Neuron*, **10**, 943–54.

Ikeda, K., Nagasawa, H., Mori, H., Araki, K., Sakimura, K., Watanabe, M., Inoue, Y., and Mishina, M. (1992). Cloning and expression of the ε4 subunit of the NMDA receptor channel. *FEBS Letters*, **313**, 34–8.

Ishii, T., Moriyoshi, K., Sugihara, H., Sakurada, K., Kadotani, H., Yokoi, M., Akazawa, C., Shigemoto, R., Mizuno, N., Masu, M., and Nakanishi, S. (1993). Molecular characterization of the family of the *N*-methyl-D-aspartate receptor subunits. *Journal of Biological Chemistry*, **268**, 2836–43.

Jahr, C. E. (1992). High probability opening of NMDA receptor channels by L-glutamate. Fast and slow components of unitary EPSCs on stellate cells elicited by focal stimulation in slices of rat visual cortex. *Science*, **255**, 470–2.

Johnson, J. W. and Ascher, P. (1987). Glycine potentiates the NMDA response in cultured mouse brain neurons. *Nature*, **325**, 529–31.

Kleckner, N. W. and Dingledine, R. (1988). Requirement for glycine in activation of NMDA-receptors expressed in Xenopus oocytes. *Science*, **241**, 835–8.

Kutsuwada, T., Kashiwabuchi, N., Mori, H., Sakimura, K., Kushiya, E., Araki, K., Meguro, H., Masaki, H., Kumanishi, T., Arakawa, M., and Mishina, M. (1992). Molecular diversity of the NMDA receptor channel. *Nature*, **358**, 36–41.

Lester, R. A. and Jahr, C. E. (1992). NMDA channel behaviour depends on agonist affinity. *Journal of Neuroscience*, **12**, 635–43.

Lester, R. A., Clements, J. D., Westbrook, G. L., and Jahr, C. E. (1990). Channel kinetics determine the time course of NMDA receptor-mediated synaptic currents. *Nature*, **346**, 565–7.

MacDermott, A. B., Mayer, M. L., Westbrook, G. L., Smith, S. J., and Barker, J. L. (1986). NMDA receptor activation increases cytoplasmic calcium concentration in cultured spinal cord neurones. *Nature*, **321**, 519–22.

Mayer, M. L., Westbrook, G. L., and Guthrie, P. B. (1984). Voltage dependent block by Mg^{2+} of NMDA responses in spinal cord neurons. *Nature*, **309**, 261–3.

Meguro, H., Mori, H., Araki, K., Kushiya, E., Kutsuwada, T., Yamazaki, M., Kumanishi, T., Arakawa, M., Sakimura, K., and Mishina, M. (1992). Functional characterization of a heteromeric NMDA receptor channel expressed from cloned cDNAs. *Nature*, **357**, 70–4.

Monyer, H., Sprengel, R., Schoepfer, R., Herb, A., Higuchi, M., Lomeli, H., Burnashev, N., Sakmann, B., and Seeburg, P. H. (1992). Heteromeric NMDA receptors: molecular and functional distinction of subtypes. *Science*, **256**, 1217–21.

Mori, H., Masaki, H., Yamakura, T., and Mishina, M. (1992). Identification by mutagensis of a Mg^{2+}-block site of the NMDA receptor channel. *Nature*, **358**, 673–5.

Moriyoshi, K., Masu, M., Ishii, T., Shigemoto, R., Mizuno, N., and Nakanishi, N. (1991). Molecular cloning and characterization of the rat NMDA receptor. *Nature*, **354**, 31–7.

Nakanishi, N., Axel, R., and Shneider, N. A. (1992). Alternative splicing generates functionally distinct *N*-methyl-D-aspartate receptors. *Proceedings of the National Academy of Sciences, USA*, **89**, 8552–6.

Nowak, L., Bregestovski, P., Ascher, P., Herbet, A., and Prochiantz, A. (1984). Magnesium gates glutamate-activated channels in mouse central neurones. *Nature*, **307**, 462–5.

Sakurada, K., Masu, M., and Nakanishi, S. (1993). Alteration of Ca^{2+} permeability and sensitivity to Mg^{2+} and channel blockers by a single amino acid substitution in the *N*-methyl-D-aspartate receptor. *Journal of Biological Chemistry*, **268**, 410–15.

Sommer, B. and Seeburg, P. H. (1992). Glutamate receptor channels: novel properties and new clones. *Trends in Pharmacological Science*, **13**, 291–6.

Stern, P., Béhé, P., Schoepfer, R., and Colquhoun, D. (1992). Single-channel conductances of NMDA receptors expressed from cloned cDNAs: comparison with native receptors. *Proceedings of the Royal Society* (London), Series B, **250**, 271–7.

Stern, P., Edwards, F. A., and Sakmann, B. (1992). Fast and slow components of unitary EPSCs on stellate cells elicited by focal stimulation in slices of rat visual cortex. *Journal of Physiology* (London), **449**, 247–78.

Sugihara, H., Moriyoshi, K., Ishii, T., Masu, M., and Nakanishi, N. (1992). Structures and properties of seven isoforms of the NMDA receptor generated by alternative splicing. *Biochemical and Biophysical Research Communications*, **185**, 826–32.

Tingley, W. G., Roche, K. W., Thompson, A. K., and Huganir, R. L. (1993). Regulation of NMDA receptor phosphorylation by alternative splicing of the C-terminal domain. *Nature*, **364**, 70–3.

Tölle, T. R., Berthele, A., Zieglgänsberger, W., Seeburg, P. H., and Wisden, W. (1993). The differential expression of 16 NMDA and non-NMDA receptor subunits in the rat spinal cord and in periaqueductal grey. *Journal of Neuroscience*. (In press.)

Unwin, N. (1993). The nicotinic acetylcholine receptor at 9Å resolution. *Journal of Molecular Biology*, **229**, 1101–24.

Watanabe, M., Inoue, Y., Sakimura, K., and Mishina, M. (1992). Developmental changes in distribution of NMDA receptor channel subunit mRNAs. *Neuro-Report*, **3**, 1138–40.

Yamazaki, M., Araki, K., Shibata, A., and Mishina, M. (1992). Molecular cloning of a cDNA encoding a novel member of the mouse glutamate receptor family. *Biochemical and Biophysical Research Communications*, **183**, 886–92.

6 Anatomical, pharmacological, and molecular diversity of native NMDA receptor subtypes

DANIEL T. MONAGHAN AND AMY L. BULLER

N-Methyl-D-aspartate (NMDA) receptors play an important role in neurotransmission throughout the central nervous system (CNS) (Mayer and Westbrook 1987; Collingridge and Lester 1989; Monaghan *et al*. 1989; Watkins *et al*. 1990). It is now apparent that the actions of NMDA receptors are mediated by multiple receptor subtypes with differing anatomical and pharmacological properties. The molecular basis of differing NMDA receptor populations is thought to be the presence of different combinations of receptor subunits in a hetero-oligomeric receptor complex. Presumably, each receptor subtype provides the physiological and regulatory properties that are optimal for the function of the corresponding synapse. Given the distinct pharmacological properties of the NMDA receptor subtypes, it may be possible to develop therapeutics with improved specificity. Consequently, it is important to determine the relationship between individual NMDA receptor subunits and pharmacologically distinct NMDA receptor subtypes.

NMDA receptor cloning studies have shown that NMDA receptor complexes contain at least one of seven different NMDAR1 subunits (NR1A–NR1G; Sugihara *et al*. 1992) and at least one of four NMDAR2 subunits (NR2A–NR2D; Kutsuwada *et al*. 1992; Monyer *et al*. 1992; Ishii *et al*. 1993). While the NR1 subunits are generated by alternative splicing of a single gene, the NR2 subunits are the products of four highly homologous genes. Thus, there are thousands of potential subunit combinations yielding complexes of four or five subunits; however, the subunit combinations actually present in the brain remain to be determined.

In this review we will compare the anatomical and pharmacological properties of the recombinant NMDA receptor subunits with the properties of native NMDA receptor subtypes. We will first summarize the anatomical distribution of individual receptor subunits and then compare their distributions with those of NMDA receptor subtypes identified in radioligand binding studies. Radioligand binding studies indicate the presence of at least four pharmacologically distinct populations of NMDA receptors with differing regional distributions. There is substantial regional variation among members of both the NR1 and NR2 subunit families; however, the distributions of the NR2 subunits correspond much more closely to the distributions of the pharmacologically distinct NMDA receptor populations. Furthermore, there is now direct evidence that the recombinant NR2A, 2B, and 2C subunits display distinct pharmacological properties that are similar to that found in the brain regions containing these subunits. While the specific pharmacological properties of NMDA receptor subtypes may depend upon the overall subunit composition, it appears that the NR2 subunits make a greater contribution to NMDA receptor pharmacological diversity at the transmitter recognition site than the NR1 subunits.

Anatomical distributions of NMDA receptor subunits

NR1 subunits

The seven NMDAR1 subunits, NR1A–NR1G, arise from alternative splicing of three nucleotide cassettes into the NR1 sequence (Sugihara *et al.* 1992; see Fig. 6.1). Cassette 1(Anantharam *et al.* 1992; termed 'insertion 1' by Sugihara *et al.* 1992) inserts 21 amino acids after residue 190. Deletion of cassette 2 ('deletion 1'; Sugihara *et al.* 1992) removes 37 amino acids after residue 863. Deletion of cassette 3 ('deletion 2', Sugihara *et al.* 1992) removes the sequence for 38 amino acids and the stop codon, resulting in a new 22 amino acid carboxy-terminal end. The most common NR1 transcript in brain contains cassettes 2 and 3, but not cassette 1 (Anantharam *et al.* 1992; Sugihara *et al.* 1992). The seven NR1 isoforms result from the various combinations of cassettes 1, 2, and 3. Each combination has been reported, with the exception of a transcript having cassettes 1 and 2, but not cassette 3 (Anantharam *et al.* 1992; Durand *et al.* 1992; Nakanishi *et al.* 1992; Sugihara *et al.* 1992; Yamazaki *et al.* 1992).

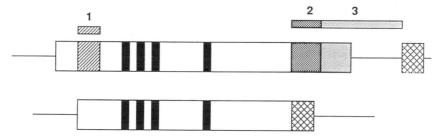

Fig. 6.1 Alternative splice variations of NMDAR1 (NR1) subunits. Seven different NR1 subunits arise from the various combinations of the alternative splicing of three nucleotide cassettes into the NR1 sequence (top panel; NR1A–NR1G; Sugihara *et al.* 1992). The first cassette (1) inserts 21 amino acids after residue 190; the second cassette (2) introduces 37 amino acids after residue 863; the third cassette (3) can be inserted immediately after cassette 2, or in the place of cassette 2. Deletion of cassette 3 results in a novel 22 amino acid carboxy-terminus. The four black bands represent the putative transmembrane domains. Bottom panel shows the NR1 subunit without the three cassettes.

In situ hybridization studies performed with oligonucleotide probes that recognize sequences common to all of the NR1 isoforms reveal a widespread distribution for NR1 subunit mRNAs (Moriyoshi *et al.* 1991; Monyer *et al.* 1992; see Fig. 6.2(A)). NR1 subunits are found in virtually every brain region. This observation is consistent with experimental evidence that NR1 subunits are essential for functional NMDA receptor expression (Kutsuwada *et al.* 1992; Meguro *et al.* 1992; Monyer *et al.* 1992; Ishii *et al.* 1993) and that most neurones are responsive to NMDA. NR1 transcripts display a wider distribution than that previously described for NMDA receptors in radioligand binding studies. In particular, significant levels of NR1 transcripts are found in the hypothalamus, ventral midbrain, ventral brain stem nuclei, and the pineal (Fig. 6.2(A)). Receptor binding studies have reported little radioligand binding in these regions (Monaghan and Cotman 1985).

Cassette 1

NR1 subunits containing cassette 1 display the most restricted regional distribution of the three cassettes (Fig. 6.2(B)). High hybridization levels are found predominantly in the cerebellar granule cells, parietal cortex, retrosplenal cortex, CA3 hippocampal pyramidal cells, dentate gyrus, and many nuclei of the lateral thalamus, midbrain, and brain stem (Fig. 6.2(B)). Within the parietal cortex, there are three distinct cell layers that display transcripts containing cassette 1. Other regions known to express NMDA receptors display relatively low levels of cassette 1 transcripts; these include the striatum, septum, nucleus accumbens, amygdala nuclei, many cortical regions, midbrain, and CA1 hippocampus.

Cassette 2

The anatomical distribution of NR1 transcripts containing cassette 2 differs significantly from that found for transcripts containing cassette 1. NR1 mRNA containing cassette 2 is found in the striatum and the lateral septum and at significantly lower levels in all regions of the thalamus and midbrain (Fig. 6.2(C)). In the cerebral cortex there is little variation in transcript density between regions or layers. Within the hippocampus, similar levels of hybridization are found in each of the cell body layers. The cerebellar granule cells contain lower signal levels.

Cassette 3

The distribution of NR1 transcripts containing cassette 3 is generally similar to the cassette 2 distribution (Fig. 6.2(D)). Transcripts containing cassette 3 are found in high concentrations throughout the cerebral cortex, hippocampus, cerebellum, striatum, and septum. While transcripts containing cassette 2 are low in diencephalic and brain stem regions, mRNA containing cassette 3 is expressed at somewhat higher levels in the thalamus,

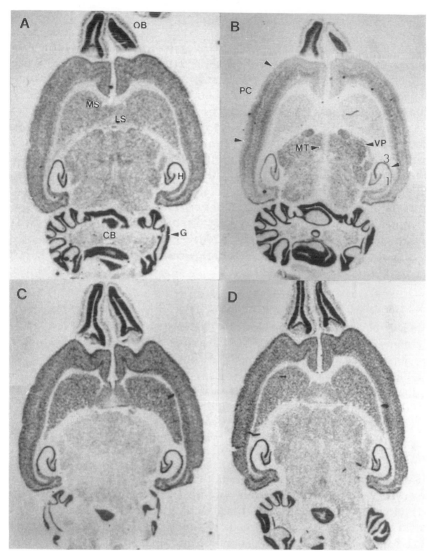

Fig. 6.2 *In situ* hybridization of NR1 subunits in horizontal sections of rat brain. In (A) a 'pan R1' oligonucleotide probe that recognizes a sequence common to all NR1 subunits labels essentially all regions of the brain. Oligonucleotide probes specific for cassette 1 (B), cassette 2 (C), and cassette 3 (D) display differing distributions. Cassette 1 is found in most brain regions, with higher levels seen in the thalamus, midbrain, parietal cortex, CA3 hippocampus, and cerebellum. Cassette 2 expression levels are high in the striatum, septum, cerebral cortex, hippocampus, and cerebellar granule cell layer, but relatively low in the thalamus and midbrain. Cassette 3 displays higher levels of expression in the striatum, septum, and cerebral cortex than in the thalamus and midbrain (D. T. Monaghan, H. Clark, and B. Schneider, unpublished observations). Abbreviations: CB, cerebellum; G, cerebellar granule cell layer; H, hippocampus; LS, lateral septum; MS, medial stratum; MT, midline thalamic nuclei; PC, parietal cortex; OB, olfactory bulb; VP, ventral posterior nucleus of thalamus; 3, CA3 hippocampus; and 1, CA1 hippocampus.

hypothalamus, midbrain, and brain stem. Within these regions there are many discrete regions expressing cassette 3 (e.g. red nucleus and ventral medial hypothalamic nucleus). NR1 transcripts that do not contain cassette 3 appear to have a widespread and generally uniform distribution (D. T. Monaghan, H. Clark, and B. Schneider, unpublished observations).

As discussed above, there are seven individual NMDA receptor NR1 subunits that have differing combinations of cassettes 1–3. Mapping these specific transcripts will probably indicate yet greater anatomical and functional diversity. For example, we find that transcripts containing cassette 2 but not cassette 3 are found in higher concentrations in the striatum than in the thalamus. Transcripts without either cassette 2 or 3 are found in higher concentrations in the thalamus than in the striatum (D. T. Monaghan, H. Clark, and B. Schneider, unpublished observations). Together, these observations suggest that there is a highly complex anatomical pattern of specific NR1 subunits in the brain.

NR2 subunits

The four NMDAR2 subunits, NR2A–NR2D (corresponding to ε1–ε4 for the mouse; Kutsuwada *et al.* 1992) display markedly different anatomical distributions (Kutsuwada *et al.* 1992; Monyer *et al.* 1992; Ishii *et al.* 1993; see Fig. 6.3). Overall, the majority of the telencephalon and diencephalon is dominated by NR2A and NR2B subunit mRNA; midline structures of the diencephalon and midbrain contain NR2D subunit mRNA; and the cerebellum and various select nuclei contain NR2C subunit mRNA.

NR2A and NR2B

NR2A and NR2B transcripts are both widely distributed in the brain; however, there are many differences in their distributions (Fig. 6.3(A) and (B)). In contrast to mRNA encoding NR2A subunits, NR2B mRNA is not found in the cerebellum (Kutsuwada *et al.* 1992; Monyer *et al.* 1992; Ishii *et al.* 1993). Low levels of NR2A subunit transcripts are found in the medial stratium and the lateral septum whereas NR2B transcripts display moderately high levels. In the cerebral cortex NR2B mRNA is distributed with a distinct lamination, with superficial layers having a greater density. In contrast, the cortical lamination pattern of NR2A mRNA is more uniform. Transcripts for both subunits are found throughout the various cortical regions but with minor variations (e.g. the levels of NR2B transcript are higher in the frontal, perirhinal, and anterior cingulate cortex than in other cortical regions; NR2A transcript displays higher levels in the parietal and superficial entorhinal cortex). Both NR2A and NR2B mRNA are expressed at moderate to high levels in most thalamic and geniculate nuclei; however, the distribution patterns within the thalamus are not identical (Fig. 6.3(A) and (B)). Hypothalamus, midbrain, and other brain stem regions generally

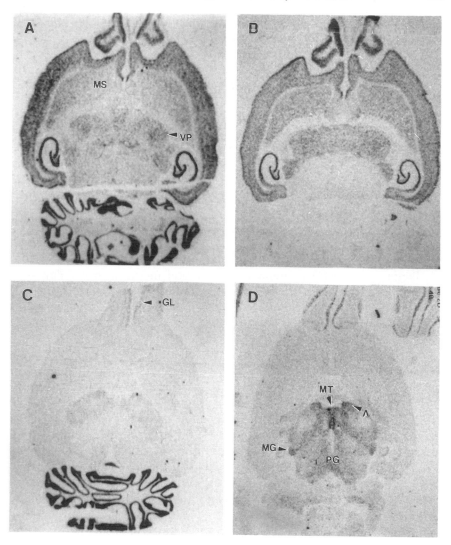

Fig. 6.3 *In situ* hybridization of oligonucleotide probes specific for NR2A (A), NR2B (B), NR2C (C), and NR2D (D) subunits are shown in horizontal sections of rat brain. While NR2A and NR2B transcripts are found throughout the telencephalon, NR2B predominates in the medial striatum (MS) and lateral septum. NR2A and NR2B transcripts also display differing distribution patterns within the cerebellum, and thalamus and between cortical layers. NR2C transcripts are found in the cerebellar granule cell layer, olfactory bulb glomerular layer, and several nuclei of the thalamus. NR2D transcripts are found in the olfactory bulb glomerular layer (GL), several midline thalamic nuclei (MT; paratenial, paraventricular, and intermediodorsal nuclei), antero-ventral nucleus (A), medial geniculate (MG), and the periaquaductal grey (PG), data from Buller *et al.*, in press).

display low levels of NR2A and NR2B message. NR2A transcripts are found in the inferior and superior colliculus.

NR2C

Transcripts encoding the NR2C subunit have a very restricted anatomical distribution (Kutsuwada *et al.* 1992; Monyer *et al.* 1992; Ishii *et al.* 1993; Fig. 6.3(C)). By far, highest levels of NR2C mRNA are found in the cerebellar granule cells. Moderate levels are also found in glomerular layer of the olfactory bulb and various nuclei of the thalamus (Fig. 6.3(C)). In addition, NR2C transcripts are found in the medial geniculate, pontine nuclei, suprachiasmatic nucleus, supraoptic nucleus, medial vestibular nucleus, and the pineal (D. T. Monaghan, H. Clark, and B. Schneider, unpublished observations).

NR2D

The recently identified NR2D subunit (whose murine homologue is called ε4; Ikeda *et al.* 1992) is predominantly found in the diencephalon and midbrain (Ishii *et al.* 1993). NR2D expression is developmentally regulated with highest levels appearing early in development (Monyer and Seeburg 1992). However, NR2D is also expressed at significant levels in select regions of the adult rat CNS (Fig. 6.3(D)).

The primary telencephalic region labelled by NR2D-specific oligo-nucleotide probes is the olfactory bulb glomerular layer (Ishii *et al.* 1993; see Fig. 6.3(D)). Low levels of NR2D transcripts are found in the cerebral cortex, hippocampus, amygdala, and striatum. Within the diencephalon, NR2D transcripts are found in midline thalamic nuclei (e.g. paraventricular, paratenial, and intermediodorsal nuclei), the anteroventral nucleus, the medial geniculate (Fig. 6.3(D)), and diffusely through the hypothalamus. NR2D mRNA is also found in the nucleus of the diagonal band. NR2D transcripts are distributed throughout the midbrain with higher concentrations in the periaqueductal grey, superior colliculi, and substantia nigra (Ishii *et al.* 1993).

Nakanishi and colleagues (Ishii *et al.* 1993) have reported that there are two forms of the NR2D subunit which differ at the carboxy-terminus, NR2D-1 and NR2D-2. The individual distributions of these forms have not yet been reported.

Receptor-radioligand binding studies

The expression of the recombinant NMDA receptor subunits has demonstrated that these subunits impart differing physiological and pharmacological properties to NMDA receptor complexes (Durand *et al.* 1992; Kutsuwada *et al.* 1992; Monyer *et al.* 1992; Nakanishi *et al.* 1992; Ishii *et al.* 1993). However, how these subunits contribute to the properties of native

NMDA receptor subtypes (of unknown subunit composition) is not known. Thus, it is important to examine the properties of native NMDA receptors and determine how regional or developmental variations in their properties may correspond to specific NMDA receptor subunits or to discrete combinations of NMDA receptor subunits.

Radioligand binding studies have also provided evidence for receptor heterogeneity. These studies have identified at least four distinct NMDA receptor subtypes in adult rat brain. These populations are best typified by the NMDA receptors found in the cerebellum (Vignon *et al.* 1986; Maragos *et al.* 1988; Ebert *et al.* 1991; Monaghan and Beaton 1991, 1992; O'Shea *et al.* 1991; Reynolds and Palmer 1991; Yoneda and Ogita 1991; Beaton *et al.* 1992), midline thalamic nuclei (Beaton *et al.* 1992; Monaghan and Beaton 1992), ventral posterior nucleus of the thalamus (Monaghan *et al.* 1988; Monaghan 1991; Sakurai *et al.* 1993), and medial striatum (Monaghan *et al.* 1988; Monaghan 1991; Sakurai *et al.* 1993). In addition to these anatomically defined NMDA receptor subpopulations, there is also radioligand binding evidence for a developmental isoform of NMDA receptors (Williams *et al.* 1993).

Cerebellar NMDA receptors

NMDA receptors in the granule cell layer of the cerebellum display a unique pharmacological profile (Monaghan and Beaton 1991; Ebert *et al.* 1991; O'Shea *et al.* 1991; Beaton *et al.* 1992; see Fig. 6.4). In contrast to NMDA, L-glutamate, L-aspartate, and other NMDA receptor agonists, the agonists quinolinate and homoquinolinate display a unique low affinity component in the inhibition of [^{3}H]L-glutamate binding to NMDA receptors (Monaghan and Beaton 1991, 1992). These results are consistent with the findings that quinolinate has a markedly low Hill coefficient as a displacer of [^{3}H]CPP ([^{3}H](+)-2-carboxypiperazin-4-yl)-propyl-1-phosphonate) binding (Porter *et al.* 1992) and that the cerebellum has a lower sensitivity to quinolinate than does the forebrain (Perkins and Stone 1983).

In general, NMDA receptor competitive antagonists bind with a lower affinity in the cerebellum than in the forebrain (Yoneda and Ogita 1991; Beaton *et al.* 1992). Additionally, certain antagonists (especially the longer chain compounds such as CPP; Fig. 6.4(D)) display a disproportionately lower affinity in the cerebellum (Beaton *et al.* 1992) due to the presence of a low affinity binding component that is not observed with forebrain NMDA receptors. Interestingly, this structure–activity relationship is similar to that reported for NMDA receptors of the red nucleus (Harris and Davies 1992). Of cerebellar NMDA receptors labelled by [^{3}H]L-glutamate, approximately 50 per cent display the atypical pharmacological properties.

Studies of the allosteric sites on the NMDA receptor complex also provide evidence for a distinct NMDA receptor subtype in the cerebellum. The pharmacological profile of the channel blocker antagonists for the

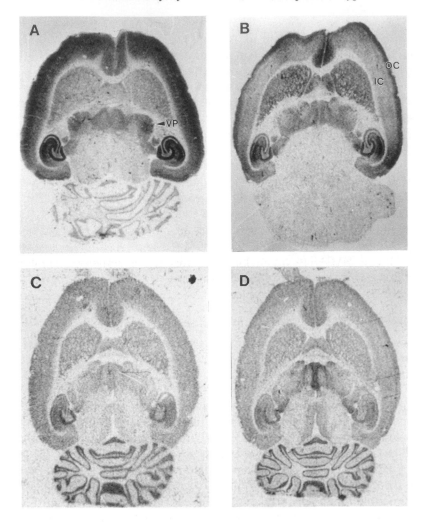

Fig. 6.4 Anatomical distributions of NMDA receptor subtypes in horizontal sections of rat brain. Autoradiographs of binding sites for (A) [^{3}H]CPP (antagonist-preferring sites, Monaghan *et al.* 1988) and (B) [^{3}H]MK-801 under conditions to label selectively 'agonist-preferring' receptors (Monaghan 1991). Note the differing distributions of NMDA receptors having higher affinity for antagonists (A) or agonists (B) in the cerebral cortex, medial striatum, lateral septum, and lateral thalamic nuclei. In (C), 50 μM of the antagonist LY 233536 inhibits NMDA-specific [^{3}H]L-glutamate binding in all brain regions except the cerebellum (cf. Fig. 6.3(C)). CPP (D) at 100 μM weakly inhibits binding to the midline thalamic nuclei as well as the cerebellum (Beaton *et al.* 1992). The difference between labelling in (C) and (D) indicates the distribution of a pharmacologically distinct population of NMDA receptors (Beaton *et al.* 1992) which has the same distribution as NR2D subunits (cf. Fig. 6.3(D)). Abbreviations: VP, ventral posterior nucleus of thalamus; IC, inner layers V–VI of parietal cortex; OC, outer layers I–III of parietal cortex.

cerebellar NMDA receptors differs from that found for forebrain NMDA receptors (Ebert *et al.* 1991; Beaton *et al.* 1992). Oocyte studies (Sekiguchi *et al.* 1990) and radioligand binding studies (O'Shea *et al.* 1991) both suggest that the glycine binding site on the cerebellar NMDA receptor may be pharmacologically distinct from that on forebrain receptors. Further-more, the binding of [^{3}H]MK-801 to NMDA receptors in the cerebellum appears to be less sensitive to the actions of polyamines and Mg^{2+} than are forebrain NMDA receptors (Yoneda and Ogita 1991; Reynolds and Palmer 1991).

Midline thalamic NMDA receptors

Another pharmacologically distinct receptor population is found in the midline nuclei of the thalamus (e.g. paraventricular and intermediodorsal nuclei), the anteroventral nucleus, medial geniculate nuclei, periaqueductal grey, and in certain other diencephalic and midbrain regions (Beaton *et al.* 1992; Fig. 6.4(D)). Pharmacologically, this site is somewhat similar to cerebellar NMDA receptors; the quinolinates and CPP display a distinctly lower affinity for both midline thalamic and cerebellar NMDA receptors. However, the antagonist LY 233536 and related compounds display a higher affinity for the midline thalamic binding sites while having a low affinity for the cerebellar NMDA receptor binding sites. The channel blocker antagonists also display a pharmacological profile in the midline thalamic nuclei that is distinct from cerebellar and forebrain NMDA receptors (Beaton *et al.* 1992).

Agonist-preferring and antagonist-preferring NMDA receptors

The majority of NMDA receptors in the rat forebrain display generally similar pharmacological profiles. Thus, the rank order of antagonist poten-cies (and agonist potencies) is similar between most forebrain regions. However, forebrain NMDA receptors can be further subdivided in quanti-tative autoradiography studies by their relative affinity for agonists and antagonists. In the lateral thalamic nuclei, NMDA receptors display a higher affinity for antagonists than do NMDA receptors in other regions such as the medial striatum. These regions display a similar rank order of antagonist potency, but all antagonists are more potent in the lateral thalamus than in the medial striatum. Conversely, NMDA receptors in the medial striatum display a higher affinity for agonists than do NMDA receptors in the lateral thalamus. Thus, these two populations have been described as 'antagonist-preferring' and 'agonist-preferring' NMDA recep-tor populations (Monaghan *et al.* 1988; Monaghan 1991; Sakurai *et al.* 1993). In addition to these populations, there may be other receptor populations; some brain regions display low affinities (or high affinities) for both agonists and antagonists. While it is conceivable that some variations in agonist and antagonist affinity are due to an unknown endogenous modulator (other than glycine, glutamate, Mg^{2+}, or polyamines; Monaghan 1991), it is now clear that the striatum and the thalamus differ in both NR1 and NR2 subunit composition and that these subunits impart differing agonist and antagonist affinities in recombinant receptor complexes.

The anatomical distributions of 'agonist-preferring' and antagonist-preferring' NMDA receptor populations is approximated by the distributions of NMDA receptors labelled with [^{3}H]L-glutamate or with ^{3}H-labelled antagonists, respectively. While radiolabelled agonists and radiolabelled antagonists will label both populations, antagonists display some specificity for the antagonist-preferring site while [^{3}H]L-glutamate displays a modest selectivity for the agonist-preferring site. The most notable difference in the distribution of these binding sites is the greater binding of [^{3}H]L-glutamate in the medial striatum and dorsal lateral septum while ^{3}H-labelled antagonist binding is higher in the lateral thalamus (especially the ventral basal complex) and deep cerebral cortex. In the cerebral cortex there are both regional and laminar differences between [^{3}H]L-glutamate and [^{3}H]CPP or [^{3}H]CGP 39653 binding sites. Antagonist binding sites display greater levels of binding in layers IV, Vb, and VI. Among cortical regions, the anterior cingulate and perirhinal cortex are predominantly agonist-preferring while the parietal, temporal and superficial entorhinal cortex are more antagonist-preferring in character. In the striatum, antagonist-preferring NMDA sites show a modest gradient, decreasing from lateral to medial. The agonist-preferring sites display high levels in the medial striatum. In contrast to radiolabelled [^{3}H]L-glutamate, [^{3}H]CPP and [^{3}H]CGP do not readily label the atypical NMDA receptor subtypes found in the cerebellum and midline thalamus.

Neonatal NMDA receptor isoforms

In addition to NMDA receptor subtypes in adult brain, there is also evidence that distinct NMDA receptor isoforms are preferentially expressed early in development. Electrophysiological studies suggest that neonatal NMDA receptors have a reduced sensitivity to Mg^{2+} (Ben-Ari *et al.* 1988; Morrisett *et al.* 1990); however, the basis for the developmental changes in Mg^{2+}-sensitivity is presently unknown. Neonatal NMDA receptors also exhibit altered sensitivity to ifenprodil, a novel NMDA antagonist (Williams *et al.* 1993). Ligand binding experiments have shown that the potency of ifenprodil decreases during development due to the delayed appearance of a lower affinity binding component (Williams *et al.* 1993). Direct evaluation of ifenprodil antagonist potency at NR1–NR2A and NR1–NR2B receptors expressed in *Xenopus* oocytes shows that NR1–NR2B receptors display significantly higher affinity for ifenprodil than NR1–NR2A receptors. The developmental changes in ifenprodil sensitivity are thus consistent with the finding that NR2A subunits are expressed later in development than NR2B subunits (Monyer *et al.* 1992). The finding that ifenprodil is subtype-selective is consistent with other studies which indicate that ifenprodil selectively protects a subpopulation of retinal neurones from NMDA receptor-mediated toxicity (Zeevalk and Nicklas 1990).

Kalb and colleagues (1992) have also identified a distinct population of NMDA receptors that are transiently expressed in the ventral horn of the spinal cord during development. This population was observed using [^{3}H]L-glutamate or [^{3}H]MK-801 as radioligands, but not with [^{3}H]CGP 39653. Thus, an early, transient expression of 'agonist-preferring' NMDA receptors was suggested (Kalb *et al.* 1992). It is also possible that this transient population is similar to the receptor population found in the midline thalamic nuclei (NR1–NR2D receptors?); this population is also labelled by [^{3}H]L-glutamate or [^{3}H]MK-801, but poorly with [^{3}H]CGP 39653.

Relationship between recombinant NMDA receptor subunits and pharmacologically distinct NMDA receptor subtypes

The properties of a native NMDA receptor complex are thought to depend on the receptor's overall subunit composition. However, many of the experimental observations of regional variations in NMDA receptor properties are consistent with the regional variation in individual subunit components. Thus, specific NMDA receptor subunits may be predominantly responsible for some of the specific properties that distinguish NMDA receptor subtypes.

NR2C and cerebellar NMDA receptors

It is likely that the NR2C subunit contributes to the distinct pharmacological properties of the cerebellum. NR2C subunits are more specific for the cerebellum than any other individual subunit. The cerebellum is also enriched in NR1 transcripts containing cassette 1 (Fig. 6.2(A); Nakanishi *et al.* 1992); however, cassette 1 transcripts are also found in high concentrations in the lateral thalamus and parietal cortex. These regions do not display the atypical cerebellar-like pharmacology. The possibility that the NR2C subunits are responsible for the distinct pharmacological properties of the cerebellum is supported by studies using *Xenopus* oocytes injected with NR1A–NR2A, NR1A–NR2B, or NR1A–NR2C RNA. Of these three combinations, oocytes injected with NR1A–NR2C RNA display a significantly lower affinity for homoquinolinate and D-CPP-ene than do the other subunit combinations (Fig. 6.5, Table 6.1). Thus, NR2C subunits display the appropriate distribution and pharmacology to account for the low affinity of cerebellar NMDA receptors for homoquinolinate and D-CPP-ene.

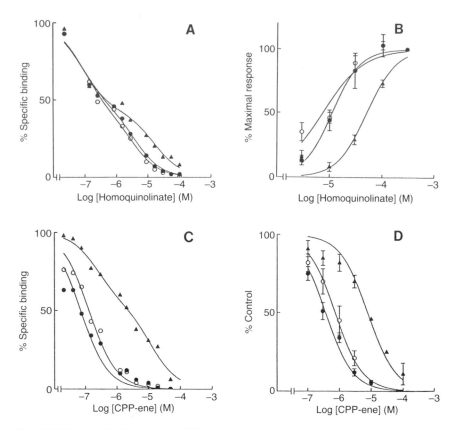

Fig. 6.5 Homoquinolinate and D-CPP-ene potencies at different native NMDA receptor populations and at recombinant NMDA receptors expressed in oocytes. Homoquinolinate (A) and D-CPP-ene (C) inhibit [³H]L-glutamate binding in the ventral posterior nucleus of the lateral thalamus (closed circles) and medial striatum (open circles) with greater potencies than in the cerebellar granule cell layer (closed triangles). Homoquinolinate (B) displays a markedly higher potency in activating NR1–NR2A (closed circles) and NR1–NR2B (open circles) receptors than in activating NR1–NRC (closed triangles) receptors expressed in *Xenopus* oocytes. D-CPP-ene (D) also displays a markedly lower potency as an antagonist of NR1–NR2C receptor complex activation by NMDA (data from Buller *et al.*, in press).

NR2D and midline thalamic NMDA receptors

NR2D subunits may account for the distinct pharmacological properties displayed by the midline thalamic nuclei. As shown in Fig. 6.3(D), the NR2D transcripts display a very specific and restricted distribution. This distribution is strikingly similar to that seen for receptors displaying the pharmacological properties typified by the midline thalamic NMDA receptors. Specifically, these NMDA receptors, as well as NR2D transcripts, are mostly limited to select structures such as thalamic midline nuclei

Table 6.1 Agonist and antagonist potencies against recombinant NMDA receptors expressed in *Xenopus* oocytes and L-[³H]glutamate binding to native NMDA receptors in brain

	Quantitative autoradiography: average K_i (μM) ± SEM			*Xenopus* oocytes: EC_{50} or IC_{50} (μM) ± SEM		
	LTH[1]	MS	CBG	NR1–R2A	NR1–R2B	NR1–R2C
Agonists						
NMDA	3.9 ± 0.22	2.8 ± 0.14	4.0 ± 0.21	31.4 ± 2.74	18.6 ± 1.7	18.6 ± 19
Homoquinolinate[2]	0.1 ± 0.09 (54%)	0.2 ± 0.1 (55%)	0.3 ± 0.18 (50%)	14.2 ± 3.9	7.4 ± 0.85	50.6 ± 67
	5.1 ± 3.14 (46%)	3.3 ± 0.67 (45%)	58 ± 9.61 (50%)			
Antagonists						
D-AP5	3.1 ± 0.31	8.1 ± 0.6	16 ± 1.3	1.1 ± 0.9	2.8 ± 0.75	9.6 ± 0.92
CPP-ene[2]	0.12 ± 0.02	0.19 ± 0.03	0.25 ± 0.06 (48%)	0.4 ± 0.07	1.1 ± 0.31	10.1 ± 1.42
			14.3 ± 3.6 (52%)			

[1] Abbreviations: LTH, lateral thalamus; MS, medial striatum; CBG, cerebellar granule cell layer.
[2] Compound displayed two affinity sites in some brain regions as shown; numbers in parentheses indicate the percentage of binding sites with high or low affinities.

(paratenial, paraventricular, and intermediodorsal nuclei), anteroventral nucleus, and medial geniculate nuclei, and periaqueductal grey (compare Fig. 6.3(D) and 6.4(D)). At present, a pharmacological characterization of recombinant NR2D subunits is not available for comparison with the midline thalamic NMDA receptor subtype.

NR2A/NR2B and antagonist-/agonist-preferring NMDA receptors

The pharmacological distinction between receptors containing NR2A and NR2B subunits is more subtle. In oocytes expressing these subunits, it is apparent that for those antagonists that have been tested, the NR2A receptors display a higher affinity for antagonists than do the NR2B subunits (Ikeda *et al.* 1992; Kutsuwada *et al.* 1992; Table 6.1). Thus, the NR2A subunit can confer 'antagonist-preferring' properties in this preparation. Consequently, it is noteworthy that the distribution of NR2A subunits (Fig. 6.3(A)) displays important parallels to that of 'antagonist-preferring' NMDA receptors as determined by [³H]CPP autoradiography (Fig. 6.4(A)). Both markers weakly label the striatum and septum while greater labelling is seen in the lateral thalamus and cerebral cortex. Furthermore, both markers display a lateral to medial gradient within the striatum, and both have minimal density variations between cortical layers and between cortical regions.

The NR2B subunit mRNA displays an anatomical distribution suggestive of 'agonist-preferring' NMDA receptors. Of the NR2 subunit family, only NR2B mRNA is expressed at high levels in the medial striatum and lateral septum, similar to the distribution of 'agonist-preferring' NMDA receptors. In addition, both the NR2B subunit and 'agonist-preferring' NMDA receptors display a distinct cortical lamination pattern (with outer cortical layers having a higher density than the deeper cortical layers), and both display relatively low levels in the olfactory bulb glomerular layer, hypothalamus, and brain stem.

In studies of NMDA receptor subunits expressed in *Xenopus* oocytes, the NR1–NR2B receptors display a slightly higher affinity for agonists than NR1–NR2A receptors (Ikeda *et al.* 1992; Kutsuwada *et al.* 1992; see Fig. 6.5 and Table 6.1). Thus NR2B subunits may contribute to the 'agonist-preferring' character of striatal NMDA receptors.

Other subunits that could potentially contribute to the 'agonist-preferring' properties of native NMDA receptors are NR1 subunits that do not contain cassette 1. The presence of cassette 1 has been reported to reduce agonist affinity (Nakanishi *et al.* 1992). Thus it is interesting that NMDA receptors in regions expressing cassette 1 often have a lower affinity for agonists (compare Fig. 6.2(B) with Fig. 6.4(A) and (B)). Since striatal and thalamic NMDA R1 subunits differ in cassettes 1, 2, and 3 (Fig. 6.2), each of these variants is also likely to contribute to some aspect of NMDA receptor heterogeneity.

Conclusions

It is now clear that there are multiple NMDA receptor subtypes that differ in several respects: anatomical distribution, pharmacological profile, regulatory properties, and physiological properties. The NR1 and NR2 subunits represent the molecular basis of NMDA receptor heterogeneity; however, the role of these subunits in generating different aspects of heterogeneity in native NMDA receptors will require further study. A large number of potential subunit combinations could form a hetero-oligomeric complex composed of four or five subunits; which combinations are present in brain is not yet known. It is thus significant that some of the properties which distinguish subtypes of native NMDA receptors correspond to the presence of identified NMDA receptor subunits. Thus, the presence of NR2C subunits appears to contribute significantly to the distinct pharmacological properties of a cerebellar NMDA receptor subtype. Given the indistinguishable anatomical patterns for NR2D subunits and another pharmacologically distinct NMDA receptor subtype, it is likely that the NR2D subunit also contributes significantly to the distinct pharmacological properties of this subtype. Anatomical and pharmacological correlations suggest that NR2A and NR2B subunits may contribute to the regional variation in 'antagonist-preferring' and 'agonist-preferring' properties of NMDA receptors, respectively. In addition, NR1 splice variants may also contribute to these properties.

The parallel anatomical and pharmacological properties of native and recombinant NMDA receptors suggest that there are at least four discrete populations of NMDA receptors of differing molecular composition that are heterogenous with regard to the glutamate binding site. The role of the NR1 and NR2 subunits in NMDA receptor heterogeneity observed at the glycine binding domain (O'Shea *et al*. 1991; Sekiguchi *et al*. 1990), the PCP channel blocking site (Vignon *et al*. 1986; Ebert *et al*. 1991; Beaton *et al*. 1992), the polyamine site (Reynolds and Palmer 1991; Yoneda and Ogita 1991), and the novel ifenprodil binding site (Williams *et al*. 1993) remains to be determined.

Acknowledgements

The authors wish to thank Drs Shigetada Nakanishi and Peter H. Seeburg for the generous gift of NR1 and NR2 cDNA clones, Dr Jeff Watkins for helpful discussions and compounds, and Anne Beaton, Heidi Clark, and Ben Schneider for excellent technical assistance. This work was supported by NIH grant NS 28966.

References

Anantharam, V., Panchal, R. G., Wilson, A., Kolchine, V. V., Treistman, S. N., and Bayley, H. (1992). Combinatorial RNA splicing alters the surface charge on the NMDA receptor. *FEBS Letters*, **305**, 27–30.

Beaton, J. A., Stemsrud, K., and Monaghan, D. T. (1992). Identification of a novel *N*-methyl-D-aspartate receptor population in the rat medial thalamus. *Journal of Neurochemistry*, **59**, 754–7.

Ben-Ari, Y., Cherubini, E., and Krnjevic, K. (1988). Changes in voltage dependence of NMDA currents during development. *Neuroscience Letters*, **94**, 88–92.

Buller, A. L., Larson, H. C., Schneider, B. E., Beaton, J. A., Morrisett, R. A., and Monaghan, D. T. The molecular basis of NMDA receptor subtypes: Native receptor diversity is predicted by subunit composition. *J. Neuroscience* (in press).

Collingridge, G. L. and Lester, R. A. J. (1989). Excitatory amino acid receptors in the vertebrate central nervous system. *Pharmacological Reviews*, **40**, 143–210.

Durand, G. M., Gregor, P., Zheng, X., Bennett, M. V. L., Uhl, G. R., and Zukin, R. S. (1992). Cloning of an apparent splice variant of the rat *N*-methyl-D-aspartate receptor NMDAR1 with altered sensitivity to polyamines and activators of protein kinase C. *Proceedings of the National Academy of Science, USA*, **89**, 9359–63.

Ebert, B., Wong, E. H. F., and Krogsgaard-Larsen, P. (1991). Identification of a novel NMDA receptor in rat cerebellum. *European Journal of Pharmacology*, **208**, 49–52.

Harris, N. C. and Davies, J. (1992). Cortically evoked excitatory synaptic transmission in the cat red nucleus is antagonised by D-AP5 but not by D-AP7. *Brain Research*, **594**, 176–80.

Ikeda, K., Nagasawa, M., Mori, H., Araki, K., Sakimura, K., Watanabe, M., Inoue, Y., and Mishina, M. (1992). Cloning and expression of the ε4 subunit of the NMDA receptor channel. *FEBS Letters*, **313**, 34–8.

Ishii, T., Moriyoshi, K., Sugihara, H., Sakurada, K., Kadotani, H., Yokoi, M., Akazawa, C., Shigemoto, R., Mizuno, N., Masu, M., and Nakanishi, S. (1993). Molecular characterization of the family of the *N*-methyl-D-aspartate receptor subunits. *Journal of Biological Chemistry*, **268**, 2836–43.

Kalb, R. G., Lidow, M. S., Halsted, M. J., and Hockfield, S. (1992). *N*-Methyl-D-aspartate receptors are transiently expressed in the developing spinal cord ventral horn. *Proceedings of the National Academy of Science, USA*, **89**, 8502–6.

Kutsuwada, T., Kashiwabuchi, N., Mori, H., Sakimura, K., Kushiya, E., Araki, K., Meguro, H., Masaki, H., Kumanishi, T., Arakawa, M., and Mishina, M. (1992). Molecular diversity of the NMDA receptor channel. *Nature*, **358**, 36–41.

Maragos, W. F., Penney, J. B., and Young, A. B. (1988). Anatomic correlation of NMDA and [³H]TCP-labelled receptors in rat brain. *Journal of Neuroscience*, **8**, 493–501.

Mayer, M. L. and Westbrook, G. L. (1987). The physiology of excitatory amino acids in the vertebrate central nervous system. *Progress in Neurobiology*, **28**, 197–276.

Meguro, H., Mori, H., Araki, K., Kushiya, E., Kutsuwada, T., Arakawa, M., Sakimura, K., and Mishina, M. (1992). Functional characterization of a heteromeric NMDA receptor channel expressed from cloned cDNAs. *Nature*, **357**, 70–4.

Monaghan, D. T. (1991). Differential stimulation of [³H]MK-801 binding to sub-populations of NMDA receptors. *Neuroscience Letters*, **122**, 21 4.

Monaghan, D. T. and Beaton, J. A. (1991). Quinolinate differentiates between forebrain and cerebellar NMDA receptors. *European Journal of Pharmacology*, **194**, 123–5.

Monaghan, D. T. and Beaton, J. A. (1992). Pharmacologically-distinct NMDA receptor populations of the cerebellum, medial thalamic nuclei, and forebrain. *Molecular Neuropharmacology*, **2**, 71–5.

Monaghan, D. T. and Cotman, C. W. (1985). Distribution of NMDA-sensitive L-[³H]-glutamate binding sites in rat brain as determined by quantitative auto-radiography. *Journal of Neuroscience*, **5**, 2909–19.

Monaghan, D. T., Olverman, H. J., Nguyen, L., Watkins, J. C., and Cotman, C. W. (1988). Two classes of NMDA recognition sites: Differential distribution and differential regulation by glycine. *Proceedings of the National Academy of Sciences, USA*, **85**, 9836–40.

Monaghan, D. T., Bridges, R. J., and Cotman, C. W. (1989). The excitatory amino acid receptors: their classes, pharmacology, and distinct properties in the function of the central nervous system. *Annual Review of Pharmacology and Toxicology*, **29**, 365–402.

Monyer, H. and Seeburg, P. (1992). Developmental expression of NMDA receptor subtypes. *Society for Neuroscience*, **18**, 395 (Abstract).

Monyer, H., Sprengel, R., Schoepfer, R., Herb, A., Higuchi, M., Lomeli, H., Burnashev, N., Sakmann, B., and Seeburg, P. H. (1992). Heteromeric NMDA receptors: Molecular and functional distinction of subtypes. *Science*, **256**, 1217–20.

Moriyoshi, K., Masu, M., Ishii, T., Shigemoto, R., Mizuno, N., and Nakanishi, S. (1991). Molecular cloning and characterization of the rat NMDA receptor. *Nature*, **354**, 31–7.

Morrisett, R. A., Mott, D. D., Lewis, D. V., Wilson, W. A., and Swartzwelder, H. S. (1990). Reduced sensitivity of the N-methyl-D-aspartate component of synaptic transmission to magnesium in hippocampal slices from immature rats. *Developmental Brain Research*, **56**, 257–62.

Nakanishi, N., Axel, R., and Shneider, N. A. (1992). Alternative splicing generates functionally distinct N-methyl-D-aspartate receptors. *Proceedings of the National Academy of Science, USA*, **89**, 8552–6.

O'Shea, R. D., Manallack, D. T., Conway, E. L., Mercer, L. D., and Beart, P. M. (1991). Evidence for heterogenous glycine domains but conserved multiple states of the excitatory amino acid recognition site of the NMDA receptor: regional binding studies with [³H]glycine and [³H]L-glutamate. *Experimental Brain Research*, **86**, 652–62.

Perkins, M. N. and Stone, T. W. (1983). Quinolinic acid: regional variations in neuronal sensitivity. *Brain Research*, **259**, 172–6.

Porter, R. H. P., Cowburn, R. F., Alasuzoff, I., Briggs, R. S. J., and Roberts, P. J. (1992). Heterogeneity of N-methyl-D-aspartate (NMDA) receptors labelled with [³H]-3-((±)2-carboxypiperazin-4-yl)propyl-1-phosphonic acid (CPP): Receptor status in Alzheimer's disease. *European Journal of Pharmacology*, **225**, 195–201.

Reynolds, I. J. and Palmer, A. M. (1991). Regional variations in [³H]MK801 binding to rat brain N-methyl-D-aspartate receptors. *Journal of Neurochemistry*, **56**, 1731–40.

Sakurai, S. Y., Penney, J. B., and Young, A. B. (1993). Regionally distinct N-methyl-D-aspartate receptors distinguished by quantitative autoradiography of [³H]MK-801 binding in rat brain. *Journal of Neurochemistry*, **60**, 1344–53.

Sekiguchi, M., Okamoto, K., and Sakai, Y. (1990). Glycine-insensitive NMDA-sensitive receptor expressed in Xenopus oocytes by guinea pig cerebellar mRNA. *Journal of Neuroscience*, **10**, 2148–55.

Sugihara, H., Moriyoshi, K., Ishii, T., Masu, M., and Nakanishi, S. (1992). Structures and properties of seven isoforms of the NMDA receptor generated by alternative splicing. *Biochemical and Biophysical Research Communications*, **185**, 826–32.

Vignon, J., Privat, A., Chaudieu, I., Thierry, A., Kamenka, J. M. and Chicheportiche, R. (1986). [³H]Thienyl-phencyclidine ([³H]TCP) binds to two different sites in rat brain. Localization by autoradiography and biochemical techniques. *Brain Research*, **378**, 133–41.

Watkins, J. C., Krogsgaard-Larsen, P., and Honoré, T. (1990). Structure–activity relationships in the development of excitatory amino acid receptor agonists and competitive antagonists. *Trends in Pharmacological Sciences*, **11**, 25–33.

Williams, K., Russell, S. L., Shen, Y. M., and Molinoff, P. B. (1993). Developmental switch in the expression of NMDA receptors occurs in vivo and in vitro. *Neuron*, **10**, 267–78.

Yamazaki, M., Mori, H., Araki, K., Mori, K. J., and Mishina, M. (1992). Cloning, expression and modulation of a mouse NMDA receptor subunit. *FEBS Letters*, **300**, 39–45.

Yoneda, Y. and Ogita, K. (1991). Heterogeneity of the *N*-methyl-D-aspartate receptor ionophore complex in rat brain, as revealed by ligand binding techniques. *Journal of Pharmacology and Experimental Therapeutics*, **259**, 86–96.

Zeevalk, G. D. and Nicklas, W. J. (1990). Action of the anti-ischemic agent ifenprodil on *N*-methyl-D-aspartate and kainate-mediated excitotoxicity. *Brain Research*, **522**, 135–9.

7 The NMDA receptor, its channel, and its modulation by glycine

P. ASCHER AND J. W. JOHNSON

Introduction

Of the glutamate receptors, the N-methyl-D-aspartate (NMDA) one is certainly the most popular choice of research scientists. This popularity is partly due to the recognition that the receptor plays a major role in a surprising variety of physiological processes (from rhythmic discharges to long-term potentiation) as well as in a number of pathological conditions (from epilepsy to neurodegenerative diseases). It is also due to the fact that the NMDA receptor, considered as a pharmacological target, can be modulated at a number of sites other than the glutamate recognition site. Among these sites, two major ones are the ionic channel itself and an 'allosteric' site through which glycine modulates the NMDA response.

The ionic channel associated with the NMDA receptor

The NMDA channel is a cationic channel

The ionic channel associated with the NMDA receptor, which will subsequently be called the 'NMDA channel', is a cationic channel which allows the passage of Na^+, K^+, and Ca^{2+}, and is blocked by Mg^{2+}.

In physiological conditions, the major current carriers are Na^+ and K^+ ions. Early attempts to establish this point (reviewed by Mayer and Westbrook (1987)) met with difficulties resulting from the voltage-dependence of the NMDA conductance change. However, when voltage-clamp methods became readily available for the study of vertebrate central neurones, it was established that in physiological solutions NMDA agonists applied at membrane voltages near resting potential induce an inward current which inverts near 0 mV. Various substitutions of internal and external monovalent cations—Na^+, K^+, and Cs^+— indicated that the reversal potential is mostly determined by the relative concentrations of these ions on each side of the membrane, suggesting that the three cations have a similar permeability. Therefore, in physiological conditions, the inward current produced by NMDA agonists is mostly carried by an influx of Na^+ ions, partially balanced by an efflux of K^+ ions (Mayer and Westbrook 1985; Ascher et al. 1988). In this respect, the NMDA channel resembles the prototypic cationic channel opened by acetylcholine at the vertebrate skeletal neuromuscular junction (Lewis 1979), the glutamate activated channel of the arthropod neuromuscular junction (Jan and Jan 1976), or the AMPA-kainate channels most frequently observed in vertebrate central neurones (Mayer and Westbrook 1986). However, a more complete analysis of the permeability to cations of the NMDA channels reveals that, when one considers *divalent* cations, the analogy stops. The NMDA channel is permeable not only to Na^+ and K^+ but also to Ca^{2+}, while it is blocked by Mg^{2+}.

The calcium permeability

The permeability to Ca^{2+} of the NMDA channel was suspected quite early, but was only unambiguously established by the experiments of MacDermott *et al.* (1986) and Mayer *et al.* (1987). These authors showed that NMDA agonists produce Ca^{2+} entry in voltage-clamped cells, i.e. in conditions excluding Ca^{2+} entry through voltage-dependent channels. The functional importance of this observation cannot be overestimated, since Ca^{2+} entry through the NMDA channel appears to trigger some of the key physiological effects of NMDA receptor activation (e.g. production of arachidonic acid, rhythmic activity, and long-term potentiation) and is also probably the main cause of the toxicity of NMDA agonists. Furthermore, the Ca^+ entry produced in physiological conditions by NMDA receptor activation is highly localized to the post-synaptic region facing the activated presynaptic terminal, contrary to the Ca^{2+} entry following the development of an action potential (Müller and Connor 1991; Regehr and Tank 1992).

The precise evaluation of how much Ca^{2+} actually enters through an open NMDA channel in physiological conditions remains to be done. In the absence of direct measurements, various attempts were made at deducing the Ca^{2+} entry in physiological conditions by using simple biophysical models to interpret the changes produced by varying the extracellular Na^+ and Ca^{2+} concentrations. Mayer and Westbrook (1987) were the first to evaluate the change of the reversal potential observed when the extracellular Na^+ was replaced by extracellular Ca^{2+}. They found that the reversal potential shifted from about 0 mV to about +30 mV. This contrasts with the fact that, after a similar ionic substitution, the reversal potential of the nicotinic receptor of the end-plate shifts from 0 to −30 mV (Lewis 1979). Many similar experiments have since been done on other cationic receptors, and although some of them have been found to be highly permeable to Ca^{2+} (in particular some AMPA-kainate receptors (Iino *et al.* 1990) and some nicotinic receptors (e.g. Mulle *et al.* 1992; Vernino *et al.* 1992)), it is still the NMDA receptor that exhibits the largest depolarizing shift in reversal potential following isotonic substitution of Ca^{2+} for Na^+.

The biophysical interpretation of this shift remains, however, tentative. Mayer and Westbrook (1987) found that their results were well described by the Goldman, Hodgkin, and Katz (GHK) equations, if they assumed a ratio of the Ca^{2+} permeability to the Na^+ permeability (P_{Ca}/P_{Na}) of 10.4. A similar calculation for the endplate nicotinic receptor leads to a P_{Ca}/P_{Na} of about 1. It is tempting to deduce from this difference a difference in the structure of the 'selectivity filter' which is usually assumed to be associated with the transmembrane segment of the receptor.

Indeed, as discussed in Chapter 5 and by Burnashev et al. (1992), site-directed mutagenesis has shown that, in mutants associating the NR1 and the NR2A (or NR2C) subunits of the NMDA receptor, the substitution in NR1 of the asparagine N598 by a glutamine (N598Q) drastically reduces the Ca^{2+} permeability. Replacing the same asparagine by an arginine abolishes the Ca^{2+} permeability. The critical amino acid is situated in the 'TMII' segment, which is presumed to be a transmembrane region, and it is therefore tempting to assume that its position identifies a component of the 'selectivity filter'.

It should not be deduced from these results, however, that the Ca^{2+} permeation is entirely controlled by a single site situated inside the transmembrane field. That the Ca^{2+} fluxes through the NMDA channel may also depend on 'surface charges' situated outside the transmembrane field was suggested by our analysis of the behaviour of NMDA single channel currents in solutions containing different Ca^{2+} concentrations. The results confirmed the reversal potentials shifts observed by Mayer and Westbrook (1987) but also revealed that, at depolarized potentials, altering the extracellular Ca^{2+} concentration causes parallel shifts in the single channel current–voltage relationship recorded at positive potentials (Ascher and Nowak 1988). This shift of the limiting slope of the current–voltage relationship can be interpreted by assuming that increasing the Ca^{2+} concentration reduces the negative surface potential at the entrance of the channel. In physiological solutions, the surface potential (ψ_o) will tend to increase the relative concentration of Ca^{2+} ions over that of Na^+ ions at the mouth of the channel, and this could contribute to an increased Ca^{2+} entry. Additional evidence in favour of a higher density of surface charges at the external mouth of the NMDA channel has recently been provided by the experiments of Gibb et al. (1993).

In a recent study, however, Zarei and Dani (1994), after a thorough analysis of the effects of various ionic substitutions on the single channel conductance and the reversal potential, have come to a different interpretation. They consider that external surface charges are present in or near the pore and create a substantial surface potential in low ionic strength solutions, but they estimate that the surface potential in physiological conditions is probably too small to significantly influence permeation. Moreover, Schneggenburger et al. (1993) have measured the amount of Ca flowing during the activation of NMDA channels in septal neurons, and calculated the fraction of the total current carried by Ca. The value obtained is smaller than the one predicted by a simple GHK model, a deviation which is opposite from that expected if there was a substantial negative surface potential. Thus a consensus has yet to be reached on the model which best describes the calcium permeability of NMDA channels.

The extracellular blockade by magnesium

The Mg^{2+} blockade of the NMDA response was first described by Ault *et al.* (1980) and identified as a 'non-competitive' antagonism. Then, in the first patch-clamp analysis of glutamate responses of cultured central neurones, Nowak *et al.* (1984) found that, in Mg^{2+}-free solution, glutamate activated large conductance (50 pS) channels. When Mg^{2+} was added at low concentrations (10–100 μM), the single channel currents changed from relatively simple openings of about 7 ms duration to bursts of shorter openings. This effect increased with hyperpolarization, and was absent at positive potentials.

Kinetic of the Mg^{2+} block at the single channel level

The effect of Mg^{2+} on single channel currents was so strikingly similar to that described by Neher and Steinbach (1978) in their classical study of the effects of QX-222 on acetylcholine-activated channels that it was immediately assumed that the effect of Mg^{2+} was due to 'channel block', Mg^{2+} plugging the channel by binding at a site situated inside the transmembrane field and experiencing a fraction δ $(0 < \delta < 1)$ of this field.

If the short openings and brief closures observed in the presence of Mg^{2+} are due to the entry and exit of Mg^{2+} into and out of the open channel, it is possible to deduce from the variation of their mean duration and the Mg^{2+} concentration the rates of association (k_+) and dissociation (k_-) of Mg^{2+} with its binding site. The simplest scheme, used by Neher and Steinbach (1978) can be written as:

$$C \underset{\alpha}{\overset{}{\rightleftharpoons}} O \underset{k_-}{\overset{k_+ \cdot [Mg^{2+}]}{\rightleftharpoons}} B \qquad \text{(Model 1)}$$

where C is the closed (resting) state, O is the open state (the C $\longleftrightarrow$ O transition is controlled by the agonist), B is the blocked state, and α is the rate of the transition from open to closed. This scheme predicts that $\bar{t}_O$, the mean duration of the short openings, is related to k_+ by

$$1/\bar{t}_O = \alpha + k_+ \cdot [Mg^{2+}]$$

while the mean duration of the short closure, $\bar{t}_C$, is related to k_- by

$$1/\bar{t}_C = k_-$$

From these relationships one can evaluate the dissociation constant of Mg^{2+}, $K_{Mg} = k_-/k_+$. The evaluation of K_{Mg} at various membrane poten-

tials (V) showed that it was an exponential function of V which could be
written, assuming a channel block model of the type proposed by
Woodhull (1973), as:

$$K_{Mg(V)} = K_{Mg(V=0)} \cdot \exp \frac{z\delta VF}{RT}$$

where $K_{Mg(V)}$ is the dissociation constant of Mg^{2+} at a potential V and
where δ represents the fraction of the transmembrane field sensed by Mg^{2+}
near the binding site. With this approach, Ascher and Nowak (1988)
evaluated $K_{Mg(V=0)}$ as 8.8 mM and δ as 1.0, which suggested that the
binding site for Mg^{2+} is close to the internal surface of the membrane. A
later study (Jahr and Stevens 1990a) led to lower values of δ (0.8) and
$K_{Mg(V=0)}$ (1.8 mM).

Model 1 is only a first approximation, and a more detailed analysis has to
take into account two additional factors: the fact that there is more than
one closed state and the fact that there is more than one pathway out of the
blocked state.

The existence of more than one closed state has been readily demonstrated by the study of the open and closed duration in the absence of
Mg^{2+}. In the simple case of a two-state equilibrium, a single time constant
would have described the duration of the closed state durations. The
analysis of the NMDA receptor single channel currents has indicated the
presence of multiple closed and open states (for example, see Jahr and
Stevens 1990a; Gibb and Colquhoun, 1992). α in Model 1 is therefore
unlikely to be a simple constant.

A second difficulty is that, in the simple 'open-channel' block model, the
duration of the bursts should increase when the Mg^{2+} concentration is
increased, so that the 'total open-time' in each burst is equal to the mean
open time in the absence of Mg^{2+} (Neher 1983). At low agonist concentrations, this implies that Mg^{2+} should not alter the total current. This was not
observed. The mean burst duration did not increase when the Mg^{2+} concentration increased (at high Mg^{2+} concentration the burst duration actually
decreased (Ascher and Nowak 1988)) and the total current was reduced by
Mg^{2+} even at low agonist concentrations (Mayer *et al.* 1984; Nowak *et al.*
1984).

Such a difficulty implies that the simple model used to describe the Mg^{2+}
block is not satisfactory and that additional steps must be considered. In
their initial report, Nowak *et al.* (1984) indicated that one way to account
for the change in burst duration was to assume that in addition to the 'fast'
channel block, there was also a 'slow' process which would block the
channel for, perhaps, seconds. In this case, the 'apparent' end of a burst
would usually correspond to the entrance into the 'long lasting' blocked
state rather than to return to the closed state. A 'slow block' has in fact
been observed for other blockers of the NMDA channel, like ketamine

(MacDonald *et al.* 1987) or MK-801 (Huettner and Bean 1988). There is good evidence that the channel can close with these antagonists inside. Model 2 is one representation of this hypothesis, in which the agonist, glutamate (Glu), can dissociate from the channel blocked by Mg^{2+} and lead to a state, E, which is 'closed' and 'blocked'.

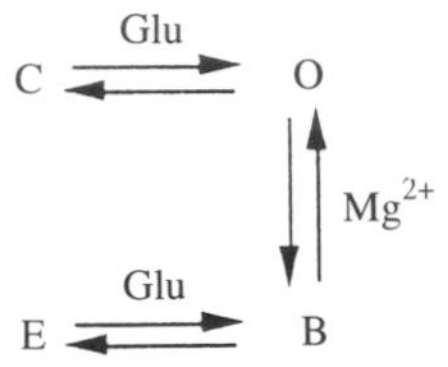

$$
\begin{array}{ccc}
C & \overset{\text{Glu}}{\underset{}{\rightleftharpoons}} & O \\
 & & \updownarrow \; Mg^{2+} \\
E & \overset{\text{Glu}}{\underset{}{\rightleftharpoons}} & B
\end{array}
\qquad \text{(Model 2)}
$$

If, in state E, Mg^{2+} is trapped into the channel, the return to state C can only occur through B and O. Another possibility is that Mg^{2+} can actually dissociate from state E as would occur if the Mg^{2+} blocking site was accessible both in the open and the closed conformation of the channel:

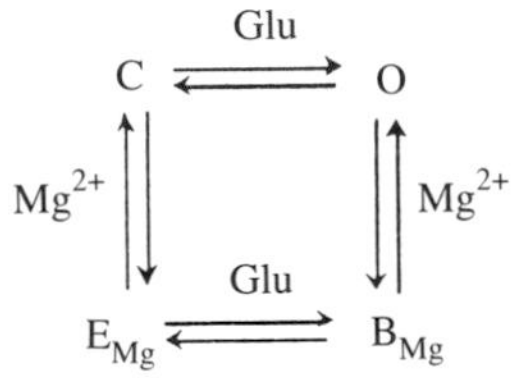

$$
\begin{array}{ccc}
C & \overset{\text{Glu}}{\underset{}{\rightleftharpoons}} & O \\
Mg^{2+} \updownarrow & & \updownarrow Mg^{2+} \\
E_{Mg} & \overset{\text{Glu}}{\underset{}{\rightleftharpoons}} & B_{Mg}
\end{array}
\qquad \text{(Model 3)}
$$

Models 2 and 3, which explicitly separate Mg^{2+} binding and glutamate binding, have not been subjected to a detailed experimental test. The only quantitative attempt at improving Model 1 to account for the behaviour of the burst duration when the Mg^{2+} concentration is increased is that of Jahr and Stevens (1990*a*) who examined whether a three-state model like Model 1 could be improved by assuming a return from the blocked state to the closed state which would bypass the open state. This model, which is illustrated below (Model 4), was found to give a good first approximation of the burst's behaviour.

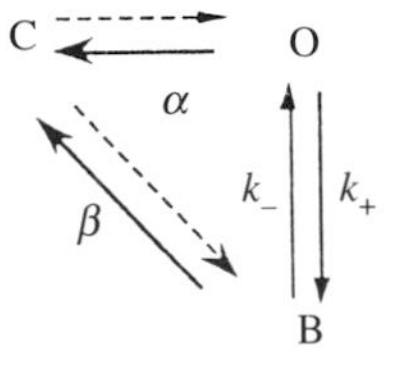

$$
\begin{array}{ccc}
C & \overset{}{\underset{\alpha}{\longleftarrow}} & O \\
 & \beta \searrow & \updownarrow \; k_- \; k_+ \\
 & & B
\end{array}
\qquad \text{(Model 4)}
$$

The values calculated for α and β were 58 s^{-1} and 45 s^{-1}. The similarity of these two values indicates that the returns to the closed state from the open and the blocked states occur at similar rates.

Model 3 can be reduced to Model 4 by making some simplifying assumptions. In the most extreme case, one can assume that the interaction of Mg^{2+} with the channel does not depend on whether the channel is open or closed, and thus that it is independent of the interaction of glutamate with the receptor. In such a case, the similarity of α and β in Model 4 implies that in model 3 the rate of transition from O to C and the rate of transition from B to C through E are similar. α and β are primarily controlled by the rate of dissociation of glutamate, which is assumed to be independent of the presence of Mg^{2+} in the channel, and slower than the rate of dissociation of Mg^{2+} from its site.

Direct entry of Mg^{2+} inside the NMDA channel is not the only possible interpretation of the Mg^{2+} blockade data. Jahr and Stevens (1990b) have explored the predictions of a model in which binding of Mg^{2+} outside of the channel pore would block the conductance by allosterically altering the voltage dependence of gating. The key difference between the predictions of this hypothesis and those of a 'channel plugging' is that when the Mg^{2+} concentration is increased the blocking rate should become saturated in the first case, and not in the second. No saturation was observed when the blocking rate was calculated over a 10 000-fold change of Mg^{2+} concentration, suggesting that the channel block mechanism is the most likely physical process to explain Mg^{2+} action.

Identification of the Mg^{2+} binding site

Site-directed mutagenesis has revealed that the asparagines of the TMII regions, which were discussed in the previous section for their role in the Ca^{2+} permeability of the NMDA channel, also play a key role in the Mg^{2+} block.

Mori et al. (1992) have mutated subunits cloned from the mouse brain. In the heteromer $\zeta_1-\varepsilon_2$, replacement of the critical asparagine by a glutamine strongly reduced the Mg^{2+} block. Substitutions done on ε_2 or ζ_1 had comparable effects. Burnashev et al. (1992) reported qualitatively similar results using rat heteromers (associating NR1 and NR2) but found a marked asymmetry between the role of the two subunits. The asparagine/ glutamine substitution in NR1 had little effect on Mg^{2+} block (as mentioned earlier, it had a marked effect on Ca^{2+} permeability). In contrast, the equivalent mutation in the NR2 subunit (e.g. N595Q for NR2A) nearly suppressed the Mg^{2+} block while having little effect on the Ca^{2+} permeability.

Variations in the Mg^{2+} blocking effect

A number of observations indicate that the Mg^{2+} block is not identical in all NMDA receptors, and, for a given receptor, may depend on the activity of intracellular kinases. That the Mg^{2+} block is not identical in all cells was initially suggested by reports that for a given cell type the amplitude of the block depended on the age of the animal, although the effect of age was not uniform (Ben Ari *et al.* 1988; Kleckner and Dingledine 1991). Two of the possible explanations of this heterogeneity can be considered: a post-translational change of the channel properties or a subunit 'switch' leading to the synthesis of new subunits and therefore of new types of receptors. Support for the first type of explanation comes from the data of Chen and Huang (1992) indicating that protein kinase C, injected intracellularly, reduces the external Mg^{2+} block of the NMDA receptor channel of trigeminal sensory neurones. Support for the second type of explanation is found in the observations showing that the various heteromeric associations of rat or mouse subunits have different Mg^{2+} sensitivities despite of the fact that they have identical 'asparagine rings'. Three heteromeric combinations (NR1–NR2A,ζ_1–ε_1, ζ_1–ε_2) have a sensitivity which resembles that described in most central neurons, while ζ_1–ε_3 and NR1–NR2C are much less sensitive to extracellular Mg^{2+} (Kutsuwada *et al.* 1992; Meguro *et al.* 1992; Monyer *et al.* 1992).

Until now, the 'variants' of Mg block (whether they correspond to different subunit assemblies or to phosphorylated–dephosphorylated states of the same receptor) have only been characterized at the whole cell level, and it is difficult to deduce from the data obtained which kinetic parameters differ. In general the blocking effect of Mg^{2+} on whole cell currents has been evaluated by fitting the data with a function

$$g = g_0 \cdot \frac{K_{Mg}^{WC}}{K_{Mg}^{WC} + [Mg^{2+}]}$$

where g and g_0 are the conductance increases in the presence and absence of Mg, and K_{Mg}^{WC} the apparent dissociation constant for whole cell currents:

$$K_{Mg}^{WC} = K_{Mg(V=0)}^{WC} \cdot \exp \frac{z\delta VF}{RT}.$$

where z is the valency of Mg^{2+}, F the Faraday's constant and T the absolute temperature.

Because of the complex relation between the total current and the structure of single channel openings, K_{Mg}^{WC} is likely to be different from K_{Mg}^{SC}, the microscopic dissociation constant deduced from single channel records. Jahr and Stevens (1990*b*) have shown that in the simple case of Model 4, at high Mg^{2+} concentration,

$$K_{Mg}^{WC} = \frac{\alpha \cdot k_-}{\beta \cdot k_+}, \text{ whereas } K_{Mg}^{SC} = \frac{k_-}{k_+}.$$

In the hippocampal neurones that they studied, α and β were similar (58 s^{-1} and 45 s^{-1} respectively) and the two values of K_{Mg} were therefore similar. However, any experimental observation of a change in K_{Mg}^{WC} (e.g. Chen and Huang 1992) should be checked at the microscopic level before one can attribute it to a change of the microscopic dissociation constant of Mg^{2+} ($K_{Mg(V=0)}^{SC}$), to a change in the 'apparent depth' (δ) of the channel binding site (which could occur via a change in the shape of the transmembrane field), or to a change in kinetics of the channel opening and closing which could be only indirectly related to Mg^{2+} block.

The blockade by intracellular Mg^{2+}

In addition to blocking the NMDA channel from the extracellular solution, Mg^{2+} also blocks the channel when present in the intracellular solution. Nowak *et al.* (1984) first reported an intracellular Mg^{2+}-dependent decrease in the NMDA single channel current at positive voltages. We have subsequently characterized the block at the single channel level (Johnson and Ascher 1990).

In contrast to the block by extracellular Mg^{2+}, the block by intracellular Mg^{2+} increases with depolarization. No apparent flickering of single channel current is associated with the blockade produced by intracellular Mg^{2+}; it is observed as a decrease in the magnitude of apparent single channel current at positive membrane voltages. At 1 mM intracellular Mg^{2+}, the block is only detectable at positive potentials, while at 10 mM Mg the block is also substantial at negative potentials (Fig. 7.1).

One possible explanation for these observations is that intracellular Mg^{2+} produces the same type of channel block as extracellular Mg^{2+}, but that the blocking and unblocking rates are too fast for 'flicker' to be resolved. If this were the case, then the fractional block of the single channel current would represent the fraction of channel open time that intracellular Mg^{2+} spends at its blocking site. The predictions of this simple model were quantified and fitted to NMDA single channel current–voltage curves measured with intracellular Mg^{2+} concentrations between 0.3 and 30 mM. The model was found to be consistent with the data. The apparent dissociation constant of Mg^{2+} from its blocking site in the NMDA channel was estimated to depend on membrane voltage according to the equation: $K_{Mg} = 8 \text{ mM} \times \exp(-V/37 \text{ mV})$. This equation can also be used to predict the shape of Mg^{2+} concentration inhibition curves at any voltage; the predicted and measured Mg^{2+} dependence of the block are illustrated at two different voltages in Fig. 7.2. If the voltage-dependence of the block, 37 mV for an e-fold change in Mg^{2+} affinity, is assumed to be due exclusively to Mg^{2+} ions moving to their blocking site through the membrane field (see Woodhull 1973), then the blocking site would be located about one third of the way through the membrane field from the inner side.

A parsimonious hypothesis that was tested is that there is a single site at which intracellular and extracellular Mg^{2+} binds. In the absence of a membrane field, the estimated apparent affinities for extracellular and

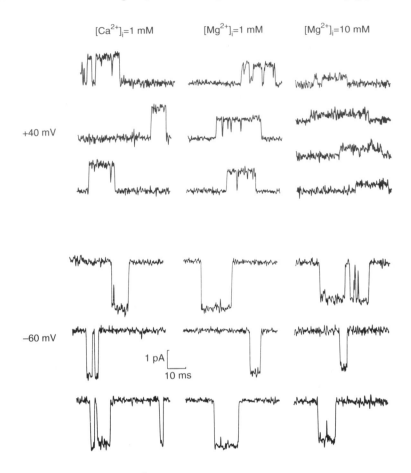

Fig. 7.1 Effects of internal Mg^{2+} on NMDA-induced single channel currents. The single channel currents produced by the addition of 10 μM NMDA + 1 μM glycine on outside-out patches were recorded at +40 mV (upper recordings) and −60 mV (lower recordings) in the presence of three different internal concentrations of divalent cations. In the first column, the internal Ca^{2+} concentration was 1 mM, and there was no Mg^{2+} in the solution. In the second and third columns, Ca^{2+} was absent from the internal solution to which had been added Mg^{2+} in the presence of 10 mM EGTA, bringing the free Mg^{2+} concentration to 1 mM (middle column) or 10 mM (right column). The external solution contained no Mg^{2+}. The recordings obtained in the presence of Ca^{2+} are similar to those recorded in the absence of internal Ca^{2+} (not shown) and, in particular, the current–voltage relationship is linear over the whole range of potentials tested (−90 mV to +90 mV). In the presence of 1 mM Mg^{2+} inside, the current size is reduced at +40 mV, while no effect is seen at −60 mV. The reduction in current size observed at +40 mV is not associated with any fast flickering, although, in the experiments illustrated, the opening of the channel showed more brief closures at +40 mV than at −60 mV. In the presence of 10 mM internal Mg^{2+} the current size was strikingly reduced at +40 mV, and some effect was detectable at −60 mV. This reduction explains the small size of the single channel currents recorded by Huettner and Bean (1988).

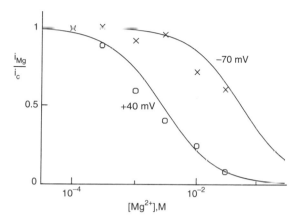

Fig. 7.2 Concentration–inhibition curves for Mg^{2+} at two different voltages. Data points are the NMDA single-channel current at each Mg^{2+} concentration and voltage (i_{Mg}) normalized to the single-channel current at the same voltage but in the absence of Mg^{2+}(i_c). Each single-channel current is based on measurements from one to four patches. The solid lines are predicted from the voltage-dependence of Mg^{2+} affinity as estimated from fits to single-channel current–voltage curves (see text). The predicted values of K_{Mg} are 53 mM and 2.7 mM at −70 and +40 mV respectively.

intracellular Mg^{2+} are similar (8.8 and 8 mM respectively), consistent with the hypothesis. A clear prediction of this hypothesis is that the Mg^{2+} dissociation rate at any voltage should be the same, regardless of the side of the origin of Mg^{2+}. If there is only one blocking site, a bound Mg^{2+} ion should not be able to 'remember' from which side of the membrane it came, and therefore should have the same mean residence time. However, this prediction was not supported by experiment. At moderately negative voltages, NMDA channel blockade by intracellular and extracellular Mg^{2+} was observed simultaneously. Under these conditions, intracellular Mg^{2+} still dissociated from its blocking site much more quickly than did extracellular Mg^{2+}. We therefore concluded that the blocks by intracellular and extracellular Mg^{2+} must take place at distinct sites.

The apparent position of the blocking sites in the membrane field presents a paradox. If the extracellular Mg^{2+} blocking site is located near the inner surface of the membrane, it does not seem possible that the intracellular Mg^{2+} blocking site could be one third of the way through the membrane field. The resolution of this conflict might be found in revising the assumptions used to deduce the blocking site location from the voltage-dependence of the block. For example, it is assumed that the movement of Mg^{2+} to and from its blocking site is independent of movement of other ions. If in fact the NMDA channel acts as a single file ion pore (see Hille and Schwarz 1978), blocking may require the co-ordinated movement of more than one ion and the blocking sites could appear to be deeper in the membrane field than they really are.

Indeed, the asparagines of the TMII sequence identified as controlling the Mg^{2+} blockade (see above) are situated quite close to the extracellular side of the TMII sequence (at least if one accepts the topology of the sequence in which the TMII sequence is a transmembrane segment in which the amino-terminal side is intracellular). This is certainly not in agreement with the predictions of a simple model of 'constant field', because the asparagine would experience only about 20 per cent of the transmembrane field.

The applicability to the block by intracellular Mg^{2+} of the models previously presented for the block by extracellular Mg^{2+} can also be tested. As already discussed, if Model 1 were correct, then the burst length in the presence of Mg^{2+} should increase. However, as was previously found to be the case with extracellular Mg^{2+}, intracellular Mg^{2+} induces a small decrease in the mean burst length (Y. Li-Smerin and J. Johnson, unpublished observations). It therefore seems likely that the NMDA channel can close when Mg^{2+} from either the inside or the outside is blocking the channel.

The physiological significance of the block by intracellular Mg^{2+} is not clear at present. The normal intracellular Mg^{2+} concentration is probably around 1 mM (for example, see Alvarez-Leefmans *et al.* 1986). At this concentration the block by intracellular Mg^{2+} would only be significant at voltages well depolarized of resting potential. In practice, the block by intracellular Mg^{2+} will reduce the shunt of the action potential produced by glutamate. This effect reinforces the analogy between the depolarizations induced by the activation of NMDA receptors and those induced by the blockade of K^+ channels. As discussed by Schulman and Weight (1976), Carew and Kandel (1976), and Brown (1983), a depolarization induced by the blockade of the K^+ channels functionally differs from a depolarization induced by the opening of (voltage independent) cationic channels in two respects: firstly, in the negative potential range it does not reduce the depolarizing effect of additional synaptic excitatory inputs, and secondly, in the positive potential range, it does not shunt the action potentials and eventually enlarges them. Both effects are also found in the case of the NMDA channel. In the negative potential range, the block by external Mg^{2+} produces a negative resistance region (which led to an initial interpretation of the NMDA effect as a K^+ conductance decrease) and will prevent the shunt of synaptic inputs. In the positive potential range, the block by internal Mg^{2+} will prevent the shunting of action potentials.

It is possible that there are other circumstances under which the block by intracellular Mg^{2+} could be significant. Following brain traumas that cause anoxic conditions, neurones probably depolarize to near 0 mV due to energy depletion and the release of glutamate into the extracellular space. The glutamate that is released during such episodes causes excitation of NMDA receptors, and thus a large Ca^+ influx that can lead to cell death (see Chapter 18). However, application of glutamate to cultured neurones can cause in addition an increase in intracellular Mg^{2+} concentration to above 10 mM (Brocard *et al.*, 1993). In a depolarized neurone, such high intracellular Mg^{2+} concentrations could cause substantial block of the NMDA channel and thereby limit Ca^{2+} influx. It is therefore possible that this effect of intracellular Mg^{2+} could play a neuroprotective role under pathophysiological conditions.

The effect of glycine

The response to NMDA is greatly augmented by low concentrations of glycine (Johnson and Ascher 1987). The augmenting effects of glycine are consistently observed only in situations in which very good control of the contents of the extracellular solution is possible, such as in experiments on cultured neurones or on *Xenopus* oocytes induced to express NMDA receptors by injection of RNA. Unusually good control of the contents of the extracellular solution is necessary because, even in the absence of added glycine, contamination of solutions by glycine is a universal problem. The high affinity of glycine for its binding site on the NMDA receptor means that even low levels of glycine contamination can result in substantial binding to the NMDA receptor. If it is not practical to lower extracellular glycine sufficiently, the action of glycine can be demonstrated in the presence of a competitive glycine antagonist, which effectively decreases glycine affinity. Using one or more of these approaches, glycine has now been shown to augment the NMDA response in a wide variety of preparations (reviewed by Thomson 1990).

When extensive efforts are made to minimize the extracellular glycine concentration, the NMDA response can be reduced to such low levels that it has been suggested that glycine binding is an absolute requirement for NMDA channel opening (Kleckner and Dingledine 1988). Numerous subsequent experiments supported this idea (see below in section entitled 'Antagonists and partial agonists of glycine'). Thus, the NMDA receptor appears to be the only ligand-gated ion channel that requires for its activation the binding of two different agonists.

Steady state action of glycine

The apparent dissociation constant of glycine for the NMDA receptor (K_{Gly}) has been measured with various experimental protocols and in numerous different preparations. The reported values range from about 100 to 700 nM (see Thomson 1990). We have estimated K_{Gly} with concentration–response curves measured in whole-cell patch-clamped mouse brain neurones in primary culture (Johnson and Ascher 1992). The value of K_{Gly} estimated from fitting the Hill equation to glycine concentration–response curves was 150 nM in the presence of 10 μM NMDA. The small response to NMDA that is always present in the absence of added glycine was subtracted from all responses to allow fitting of the Hill equation in these experiments. If this response is assumed to result from contaminating glycine, it is possible both to estimate the average concentration of contaminating glycine (in this case, 20 nM) and to correct the resulting error in the estimate of apparent affinity. Following correction, the estimated value of K_{Gly} was 130 nM. This is in the range of the lowest values reported. It seems very probable, however, that some NMDA receptors have a lower affinity for glycine, if they resemble recombinant receptors. Compared in identical conditions, the recombinant receptors formed with the subunits ε_1 and ζ_1 were found to have a K_{Gly} of 2.1 μM while those formed with the subunits ε_3 and ζ_1 had a K_{Gly} of 0.2 μM (Kutsuwada *et al.* 1992; see also Sekiguchi *et al.* 1990; Monyer *et al.* 1992; Stern *et al.* 1992).

The diversity of the values of K_{Gly}, if confirmed for native receptors, would have important consequences in the search for a functional role of glycine, and in particular for deciding whether variations of the extracellular glycine concentration may have functional consequences. Although the glycine transporter is, in principle, capable of lowering the extracellular glycine concentration to below 200 nM (Attwell and Bouvier 1992), many attempts at evaluating extracellular glycine concentration have suggested that the average value may be in the micromolar range. In this case, NMDA receptors with high affinity for glycine would always be saturated, and further increases in the glycine levels would have little effect. On the other hand, if there are native NMDA receptors with a low glycine affinity, like the ε_1–ζ_1 combination, they could be sensitive to fluctuations of the glycine levels in the μM range.

Kinetics of glycine binding

The kinetics of drug action can be studied by causing a rapid change in the concentration of the drug (a concentration jump) with a fast perfusion apparatus, and recording the change with time (or relaxation) of drug-dependent current following the concentration jump. This approach has been used extensively to study the kinetics of glycine interaction with the NMDA receptor. We have concentrated on relaxation measurements in the presence of low concentrations (10 μM or less) of NMDA to minimize possible interference from simultaneous time-dependent changes due to desensitization (Johnson and Ascher 1992).

The interpretation of kinetic experiments is particularly dependent on the use of a model of drug–receptor interaction. The simplest model for the interaction of glycine with its binding site on the NMDA receptor can be written:

$$\text{Gly} + \text{R} \underset{k_-}{\overset{k_+}{\rightleftarrows}} \text{GlyR} \tag{1}$$

where R and GlyR are the unliganded and liganded glycine receptor respectively, and k_+ and k_- the association and dissociation rate constants respectively. If this scheme is valid, then several predictions can be made. When glycine concentration is jumped from 0 to a test value in the constant presence of 10 μM NMDA, the NMDA receptor-mediated current relaxation should follow a single exponential time course. The time constant of the current relaxation (τ_{on}) should decrease as the glycine concentration increases. When the converse concentration jump from a test glycine concentration to 0 is made, the time constant of the exponential current relaxation (τ_{off}) should be independent of the starting glycine concentration. τ_{on} and τ_{off} should be related to k_+ and k_- by:

$$(\tau_{on})^{-1} = k_+ \cdot [\text{Gly}] + k_- \tag{2}$$

$$(\tau_{off})^{-1} = k_- \tag{3}$$

Finally, the ratio of the rate constants, k_-/k_+, should equal the value of K_{Gly} measured in equilibrium concentration–response curves.

The true reaction scheme must be more complicated than that written above, since the interaction of NMDA with its binding site, the conformational changes of the channel between closed and opened, and receptor desensitization have been ignored. However, if the measurements are made under conditions in which glycine binding kinetics are far slower than the kinetics of the other reactions, the current relaxations should reflect the interaction of glycine with its binding site.

Under conditions in which glycine binding kinetics should be rate limiting, we measured the values of τ_{on} and τ_{off} at a variety of glycine concentrations. The results were consistent with the above model in the following respects:

(1) the relaxations closely approximated exponentials;
(2) a linear relation was found between $1/\tau_{on}$ and glycine concentration after the concentration jump as predicted from Equation 2;
(3) the value of $1/\tau_{off}$ was independent of the glycine concentration before the concentration jump;
(4) when k_- and k_+ (estimated from Equations 2 and 3) were used to calculate K_{Gly}, its value (80 nM) was in reasonable agreement with the values estimated from concentration–response curves.

A possible artefact in these measurements could have resulted from the use of whole-cell recordings from cultured neurones. One could imagine that repetitive binding of glycine in regions where diffusion is restricted (for example, between the clamped neurone and the glial cell underneath it) could reduce in similar proportions the on and off rates of glycine binding. However, the values calculated for τ_{on} and τ_{off} from experiments in the whole-cell mode were confirmed in experiments on outside-out patches, i.e. under conditions in which regions of restricted diffusion should be minimized.

The number of glycine binding sites

Because the kinetic data described above are consistent with the simple bimolecular reaction scheme described by Equation 1, they are taken as support for the presence of only a single glycine binding site on the NMDA receptor. From concentration–response curves, the measured Hill coefficient was slightly greater than 1, weakly suggesting that glycine may act co-operatively, a possibility that would require more than one glycine binding site per NMDA receptor. However, there are other characteristics of the NMDA response that could lead to the measurement of a Hill coefficient of greater than 1, such as current-dependent desensitization. The degree of co-operativity was therefore investigated further by carefully examining the low concentration region (below 50 nM) of the concentration–response curve, a region that should both minimize potential artefacts and reveal evidence for co-operativity with maximum sensitivity. The results provided no support for there being co-operativity in the glycine concentration–response curve (Johnson and Ascher 1992).

The simplest interpretation of these data is that there is only one glycine binding site per NMDA receptor. However, there are numerous binding schemes with more than one site that would be approximately consistent with these data. For example, there could be more than one site, if the occupation of any of them were sufficient to activate the NMDA channel.

Evidence from several other studies, however, has suggested that there is more than one glycine binding site on the NMDA receptor. Thedinga *et al.* (1989) found that the density of [³H]glycine binding sites was double that of NMDA-displaceable [³H]glutamate binding sites. They suggested, however, that if NMDA binding sites can exist in either an agonist- or antagonist-preferring form (Monaghan *et al.* 1988), then the total concentration of NMDA and glycine sites may be equal. Because there is general agreement that there are at least two glutamate binding sites on the NMDA receptor (see Chapter 4), either interpretation would suggest that there is more than one glycine binding site per NMDA receptor. Other electrophysiological studies of the relaxation of NMDA- and glycine-activated currents following concentration jumps have favoured the presence of two glycine binding sites, based on firstly the time course of activation and desensitization (Benveniste *et al.* 1990*a,b*), secondly, the time course of activation in the presence of a glycine antagonist (Benveniste and Mayer 1991), and thirdly, the sigmoid character of activation (Clements and Westbrook 1991).

While the weight of evidence from fitting of kinetic models to current relaxations has fallen on the side of multiple glycine binding sites, the interpretation of kinetic experiments is highly dependent on the types of models that are chosen for comparison and the type of data that are fitted. A second source of data relevant to the number of glycine binding sites has recently become available, following the cloning of the NMDA receptor. The first demonstrated functional cloned NMDA subunit (Moriyoshi *et al.* 1991) produced NMDA-activated responses that were modulated by glycine following the injection of RNA coding for only a single subunit into the oocyte. Assuming that the NMDA receptor is composed of five subunits, as is the nicotinic acetylcholine receptor, then the most straightforward interpretation of the data would indicate that five binding sites for gluta- mate and five for glycine were present. However, subsequent studies have revealed that NMDA receptors are expressed much more efficiently when more than one type of subunit is present (Meguro *et al.* 1992; Monyer *et al.* 1992) and the characteristics of the modulation by glycine were highly dependent on the subtypes present. Both the glycine dissociation rate (Monyer *et al.* 1992) and the glycine apparent dissociation constant (Kutsu- wada *et al.* 1992) varied depending on the subunit combination, and it is even possible to activate some combinations of subunits by glycine alone (Kutsuwada *et al.* 1992; Meguro *et al.* 1992). It is not known which com- binations of subunits occur physiologically, and the effective number of functional binding sites is not necessarily equal to the number of subunits with binding sites, especially if sites with widely varying affinities are present. Therefore, a definitive determination of the number of glycine (or glutamate) binding sites has yet to be made; the numbers may vary be- tween different preparations.

Antagonists and partial agonists of glycine

Shortly after our report of the potentiation of NMDA responses by glycine, Kessler *et al.* (1987, 1989) found that kynurenate, a known antagonist of NMDA responses, displaced glycine much more effectively than it dis- placed glutamate from the NMDA receptor. This suggested that the ant- agonism was exerted through the glycine binding site, a hypothesis soon confirmed by experiments which showed that the blockade of NMDA responses by kynurenate was relieved by the addition of glycine (Monahan *et al.* 1989). At the same time, kynurenate derivatives of higher potency but with similar effects had started to appear, leading to compounds like 5- iodo-7-chloro-kynurenate, which is 1000-fold more potent than kynuren- ate, and to the even more powerful L 689 560 (see Kemp and Leeson 1993).

Soon after the first report on kynurenate, Fletcher and Lodge (1988) found that another NMDA antagonist, HA-966, was probably acting through binding to the glycine site since, again, the blockade of the NMDA responses could be reversed by the addition of glycine. However, a more detailed comparison of the effect of kynurenate (or kynurenate derivatives like 7-Cl-kynurenate) and HA-966 revealed some important differences. Foster and Kemp (1989) observed that when the concentration of 7-Cl-kynurenate was raised, a complete blockade of the NMDA response could be obtained, whereas when the HA-966 concentration was raised, a residual response always persisted. Furthermore, when NMDA was applied in the absence of glycine, the small response observed was blocked by 7-Cl-kynurenate, but not by HA-966.

These observations could be interpreted in two ways. If one assumed that NMDA was capable of opening some NMDA channels in the absence of glycine, the effect of HA-966 could be seen as that of a competitive antagonist of glycine, while 7-Cl-kynurenate would be an 'inverse agonist'. On the other hand, if, as proposed by Kleckner and Dingledine (1988), glycine is absolutely necessary for NMDA receptor activation, then the response observed in the absence of glycine has to be interpreted as a response resulting from the presence of some 'contaminating glycine', 7-Cl-kynurenate is a competitive antagonist, and HA-966 is a partial agonist. Support for the latter interpretation has come from an increasing number of experiments confirming the results of Kleckner and Dingledine (1988) and from the observation that, when all precautions are taken to minimize the glycine contamination, HA-966 actually potentiates the NMDA response (Foster and Kemp 1989; Henderson *et al.* 1990; Huettner 1990).

The use of 'concentration jumps' confirmed that the responses observed in the nominal absence of glycine are due to the presence of some contaminating glycine. This was particularly clear in the studies of the current relaxations observed when, in the presence of a steady concentration of NMDA, either kynurenate, 7-Cl-kynurenate, or HA-966 was applied suddenly. In conditions where the three drugs reduced the currents, the decrease of the current was exponential and independent of the drug concentration. If the compounds were 'inverse agonists', their rate of action should have increased when their concentration was increased. On the other hand, the observations are consistent with a model in which the antagonists have rapid access to the free glycine binding sites, but find their access to the other sites limited by their occupation by contaminating glycine. The limiting factor which fixes the rate of the current decrease is therefore the slow dissociation of glycine.

Indeed the on-rate measured was the same for both antagonists and for HA-966, and was close to the dissociation rate of glycine, even in the nominal absence of glycine (Henderson *et al.* 1990). The 'anomaly' disappears if one uses a low affinity glycine agonist: the access to the site is no longer measurably limited by the presence of the agonist, and the rate of action of kynurenate or 7-Cl-kynurenate increases with the drug concentration (Benveniste *et al.* 1990*a*).

The allosteric interaction between glycine and NMDA agonists

The kinetic description of the interaction between glycine binding and NMDA binding is still uncertain, because the available data suggest three models which are difficult to reconcile.

The model proposed by Mark Mayer and his colleagues (Mayer *et al.* 1989; Benveniste *et al.* 1990*a*; Vyklicky *et al.* 1990) derives from data gathered on hippocampal neurones recorded in the whole-cell mode. The central observation (made in a low Ca^{2+} solution to avoid Ca^{2+}-dependent desensitization) is that, in the presence of saturating concentrations of glycine, the response to the application of NMDA agonists does not show desensitization. Desensitization only appears if the glycine concentration is lowered below saturation, and becomes increasingly marked as the glycine concentration tends towards zero. The relations between the parameters of desensitization and the glycine concentration are well described by a model in which the binding of the NMDA agonist to its receptor site decreases the affinity of glycine for its binding site. The model is further supported by the fact that in the presence of a high concentration of glycine, desensitization can be produced by the addition of glycine competitive antagonists.

In our study of the interaction between glycine and the NMDA receptor (Johnson and Ascher 1992), it was found that in the absence of NMDA (Fig. 7.3) the dissociation rate of glycine was slightly but not significantly slower than in the presence of 10 μM NMDA. The observed effects of NMDA concentration on glycine binding were in the direction predicted by the model of Benveniste *et al.* (1990*a*) but they were small, and when glycine dissociation rates were measured in higher NMDA concentrations (at which much faster dissociation rates were observed by Benveniste *et al.* (1990*a*)), the time course of dissociation was similar. The simplest model with which our data are consistent is one in which glycine binding and NMDA binding are to a first approximation independent processes; their principal interaction takes place at the NMDA channel, the opening of which requires simultaneous occupation of both NMDA and glycine binding sites.

Among the possible explanations of the apparent contradiction between the two sets of data discussed above, a simple one is that the heterogeneity of NMDA receptors accounts for the observed differences in mechanism of interaction. That NMDA receptors are heterogeneous in their sensitivity to glycine has been considered by a number of authors (e.g. Monaghan *et al.* 1988; Sekiguchi *et al.* 1990; Kleckner and Dingledine 1991) and has been widely confirmed, after the cloning of a variety of NMDA receptor

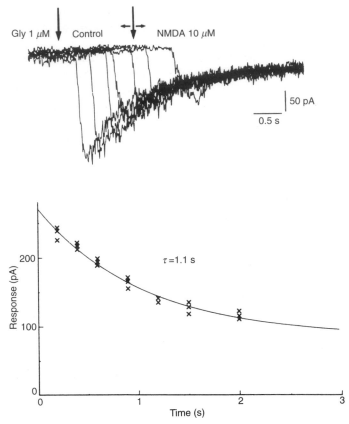

Fig. 7.3 Estimate of glycine dissociation rate in the absence of NMDA. The upper part of the figure shows superimposed, unaveraged, whole-cell current recordings from a single cell. 1 μM glycine was applied for at least 10 s before the beginning of the recording. At the time indicated by the left arrow, the extracellular solution was 'jumped' to a solution with no added agonists ('control'). After a wait of 0.2–2 s, the extracellular solution was 'jumped' to one with 10 μM NMDA but no added glycine. The relative number of NMDA receptors with glycine still bound was reflected by the size of the response to NMDA. Data from three measurements in the same cell at each 'control' duration are plotted as a function of duration in the lower plot. The time constant of glycine dissociation, τ_{off}, in the absence of NMDA was estimated from the single exponential fit to the data.

subunits, by the demonstration of the marked functional differences between the various heteromeric assemblies constructed from the different subunits. As mentioned earlier, the glycine affinity is highly variable in the various heteromers (Ikeda *et al.* 1992; Kutsuwada *et al.* 1992; Meguro *et al.* 1992; Monyer *et al.* 1992). For example, the fact that the time constants (τ_{off}) of the glycine 'off-relaxations' measured by Monyer *et al.* (1992) for recombinant receptors were 147 ms in the case of NR1–NR2A and 683 ms in the case of NR1–NR2C provides a possible parallel with the mean value of 322 ms found by Benveniste *et al.* (1990*a*) and the mean value of 1.0 s found by Johnson and Ascher (1992).

However, one cannot neglect other explanations. In the example just discussed, the cells used were different (hippocampal as compared with cortical neurones), and the experimental conditions differed both by the agonist concentrations (100 µM as compared with 10 µM NMDA or no NMDA) and by the level of internal dialysis (as discussed below). Would the difference persist if the experimental conditions were made more similar? Lester *et al.* (1993) recently analysed the dissociation of glycine in the absence of NMDA in much the same way as Johnson and Ascher (1992) had done, and found very similar time constants for the process (1.7 s instead of a mean value of 1.4 s). This suggests that differences in the experimental conditions were more important than differences in the intrinsic properties of the receptor. Among the differences in experimental conditions a key one appears to be the degree of 'wash-out' of the intracellular constituents. In general, the experiments of Mark Mayer and his colleagues were done with relatively large cells and relatively small electrodes, i.e. in conditions where the intracellular components are relatively well preserved. In our experiments, whole-cell recordings were done with smaller cells and larger electrodes, and many results were obtained in outside-out patches.

This hypothesis of a 'transformation' of receptor properties after intensive exchange of the normal cytoplasm by an artificial one is reinforced by the evolution of the 'glycine-insensitive' desensitization described in the next section.

Glycine-insensitive desensitization

The presence of desensitization during a continuous application of NMDA was first reported by Mayer and Westbrook (1985) in conditions which suggested a link with Ca^{2+} entry. The existence of a 'slow' Ca^{2+}-dependent desensitization has been widely confirmed since these initial observations (see Zorumski and Thio 1992) and it has been found that this phenomenon can be nearly eliminated by lowering the extracellular Ca^{2+} concentration to 0.2 mM (Mayer *et al.* 1989).

In such low Ca^{2+} solutions, NMDA responses show two types of desensitization. The first is the 'glycine-sensitive' desensitization discussed in the previous section, and observed in the whole-cell recording mode (Mayer *et al.* 1989; Benveniste *et al.* 1990*a*) or in oocytes (Lerma *et al.* 1990). In contrast, in outside-out patches, one finds a desensitization which depends on the concentration of the NMDA agonist, but appears independent of the glycine concentration (Sather *et al.* 1990) (Fig. 7.4). This glycine-insensitive desensitization has also been found in cells recorded in the whole-cell mode with relatively large pipettes (Sather *et al.* 1990; Shirasaki

100 μM NMDA + 10 μM Gly

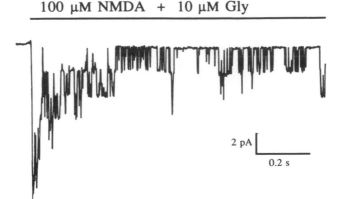

2 pA

0.2 s

Fig. 7.4 Desensitization of NMDA responses in an outside-out patch. The response illustrated was recorded at −50 mV after the application of NMDA (100 μM) and glycine (10 μM). Prior to the application of this solution, the patch was exposed to glycine (10 μM). The time constant of the desensitization, measured on the averaged sum of 17 similar records, was 320 ms.

et al. 1990; Chizhmakov *et al.* 1992). In general, a good correlation appears to exist between the presence of the glycine-independent desensitization and the extent of intracellular exchange. We have recently characterized the glycine-insensitive desensitization in a preparation that we have called 'nucleated patch', which is obtained by pulling the nucleus out of the cell while keeping it surrounded by the plasma membrane (Sather *et al.* 1992). The resulting structure behaves like a very large outside-out patch, and this size gives it an advantage over classical outside-out patches if one wants to average the behaviour of many channels after a concentration jump.

The NMDA responses of a nucleated patch change progressively after the formation of the patch. In particular, if one follows the response to a pulse of NMDA at saturating concentration in the presence of glycine at saturating concentration, the desensitization observed just after the formation of the patch is relatively slow and small; with time it accelerates and increases until it reaches a stable level. This transformation also occurs in classical outside-out patches where it develops in a few minutes after excision (Lester *et al.* 1993). In the case of nucleated patches it takes tens of minutes, possibly because the nucleus sticks to the pipette tip and slows down the exchange between the pipette and the cytoplasm. This has allowed detailed analysis of the kinetic parameters which are altered with time. A central observation has been that the peak response to a given agonist concentration is not altered during the 'wash-out' process, while the speed and the size of the desensitization increase for tens of minutes until they reach stable values. Thus the evolution does not modify the number of 'activatable' receptors under the pipette, but only alters the kinetics of their opening and closing.

The analysis of the time-dependence and concentration-dependence of the responses in nucleated patches has led us to describe the glycine-insensitive desensitization with a cyclic model derived from that proposed by Katz and Thesleff (1957) for the nicotinic acetylcholine receptor. The central assumptions of the model are that the desensitized states exist in the absence of the ligand and that they have a higher affinity for the ligand than the resting (activatable) states. To describe their data on outside-out patches, Lester *et al.* (1993) have used a sequential model which does not assume the existence of desensitized states in the absence of ligand but individualizes the transition between bound-closed and bound-open states. They find that the model also gives, to a first approximation, a satisfactory description of the main data. Both models lead to estimates of dissociation constants which confirm that a major difference between the NMDA receptor and the other best-known ionotropic receptors (the nicotinic receptor, the AMPA receptor, etc.) is the slowness of the dissociation of glutamate from the resting state. This slowness is the main reason for the slow decay of the NMDA component of glutamatergic synaptic potentials (see Lester *et al.* 1990; Lester and Jahr 1992).

More complete models will certainly be needed to account for some additional features of desensitization in outside-out patches. One of these features is the extremely slow recovery from glutamate-induced desensitization (Sather *et al.* 1992), which is predicted neither by a simple cyclic model (Sather *et al.* 1992) nor by the sequential model of Lester *et al.* (1993), but which can be accounted for by a 'double cyclic model' (Sather *et al.* 1992). There are also observations suggesting that NMDA agonists can induce desensitization when applied in the absence of glycine (Chizhmakov *et al.* 1992; Lester *et al.* 1993). These observations may require the addition of a specific step in the models (Lester *et al.* 1993). However, given the extreme difficulty that we found in eliminating all traces of glycine from the extracellular solutions, we wonder if the explanation of these observations could be found in the traces of glycine which were always present. In the 'double cyclic scheme' (Sather *et al.* 1992), in which the long-lasting desensitized state can be reached without activation, the combined action of the NMDA agonist and traces of glycine could lead to a sizeable desensitization.

During the various stages of evolution of the nucleated patches, the rates of the transitions leading from the resting state to the open state do not seem to change substantially. This suggests that the study of the channel kinetics on a classical outside-out patch, or on a 'washed-out' nucleated patch, can be used directly to characterize the activation kinetics of the NMDA receptor in an intact cell. This claim is reinforced by the recent observations of Lester *et al.* (1993) which suggest that during the evolution of the patch the glycine-sensitive desensitization does not disappear but is only masked.

While it is worthwhile looking in detail at the kinetics of the NMDA receptor in the outside-out patch, the use of the resulting models in the understanding of synaptic responses will remain a major challenge. Lester and Jahr (1992) and Lester *et al.* (1993) have tentatively suggested that the behaviour observed in an outside-patch may exist in 'synaptic' channels in the intact cells. This would certainly help with the mechanistic study of synaptic currents, but at this point there does not seem to be much experimental evidence either in favour of or against such a hypothesis. In particular, we do not know if glycine-insensitive desensitization exists at synaptic receptors in intact cells.

Conclusion

The mechanisms of action of Mg^{2+} and glycine are still somewhat controversial, in part because of conflicting experimental data. One possible resolution of these contradictions has arisen from the cloning of a series of subunits of the NMDA receptor. The striking diversity of these subunits very probably implies a diversity of channels in the living cells. This diversity poses its own problems, in particular that of identifying among all possible combinations of subunits those which are effectively built in a given cell. Concerning the kinetic and molecular models discussed in this chapter the diversity offers the possibility to rationalize the quantitative differences between experimental results by attributing them to differences in the molecular species studied. This may not be always justified but it should considerably smooth, or soothe, professional relations between colleagues with divergent results.

However, part of the contradictions between the experimental data may arise from a cause other than the intrinsic diversity of channels, such as a difference in the regulation of the channel function or a difference in experimental conditions. Indeed the marked difference observed between the kinetics of the responses in intact cells and excised patches indicate that we do not yet have at hand an experimental preparation that allows a detailed kinetic study of some of the central questions concerning the NMDA receptors. Whole-cell studies are complicated because one does not control perfectly the voltage, the ionic composition, or the drug concentrations in many regions of the cells (dendrites in particular) and because one does not have an easy access to the information provided by single channel events. Cell-attached recordings do not allow rapid concentration changes of extracellular ligands. The data from outside-out and inside-out patches are weakened by the fact that the kinetics of opening are not exactly those of 'intact' channels. One may hope that the study of the modulation of NMDA channels by intracytoplasmic constituents, which has only started, will not only lead to an understanding of this modulation but also allow the development of new preparations combining the technical advantages of the outside-out patch with more 'functional' receptor behaviour.

Acknowledgements

We thank B. Dieudonné and P. Paoletti for their comments on the manuscript. Our work was supported by grants from the CNRS, the Human Frontier Science Program and NIMH (R 29 MH 45817 and K 02 MH 00944)

References

Alvarez-Leefmans, F. J., Gamino, S. M., Giraldez, F., and Gonzales-Serratos, H. (1986). Intracellular free magnesium in frog skeletal muscle fibres measured with ion-selective microelectrodes. *Journal of Physiology*, **378**, 461–83.

Ascher, P. (1988). Divalent cations and the NMDA channel. *Biomedical Research*, **9**, 31–7.

Ascher, P. and Nowak, L. (1988). The role of divalent cations in the N-methyl-D-aspartate responses of mouse central neurones in culture. *Journal of Physiology*, **399**, 247–66.

Ascher, P., Bregestovski, P., and Nowak, L. (1988). N-methyl-D-aspartate-activated channels of mouse central neurones in magnesium-free solutions. *Journal of Physiology*, **399**, 207–26.

Attwell, D. and Bouvier, M. (1992). Cloners quick on the uptake. *Current Biology*, **2**, 541–3.

Ault, B., Evans, R. H., Francis, A. A., Oakes, D. J., and Watkins, J. C. (1980). Selective depression of excitatory amino acid induced depolarizations by magnesium ions in isolated spinal cord preparations. *Journal of Physiology*, **307**, 413–28.

Ben-Ari, Y., Cherubini, E. A., and Krnjevic, K. (1988). Changes in voltage dependence of NMDA currents during development. *Neuroscience Letters*, **94**, 88–92.

Benveniste, M. and Mayer, M. L. (1991). Kinetic analysis of antagonist action at N-methyl-D-aspartic acid receptors. Two binding sites each for glutamate and glycine. *Biophysical Journal*, **59**, 560–73.

Benveniste, M., Clements, J., Vyklicky, L., Jr, and Mayer, M. L. (1990a). A kinetic analysis of the modulation of N-methyl-D-aspartic acid receptors by glycine in mouse cultured hippocampal neurones. *Journal of Physiology*, **428**, 333–57.

Benveniste, M., Mienville, J.-M., Sernagor, E., and Mayer, M. L. (1990b). Concentration-jump experiments with NMDA antagonists in mouse cultured hippocampal neurons. *Journal of Neurophysiology*, **63**, 1373–84.

Brocard, J. B., Rajdev, S., and Reynolds, I. J. (1993). Glutamate-induced increases in intracellular free Mg^{2+} in cultured cortical neurons. *Neuron*, **11**, 751–7.

Brown, D. A. (1983). Slow cholinergic excitation—a mechanism for increasing neuronal excitability. *Trends in Neurosciences*, **6**, 302–7.

Burnashev, N., Schoepfer, R., Monyer, H., Ruppersberg, J. P., Günther, W., Seeburg, P. H., and Sakmann, B. (1992). Control by asparagine residues of calcium permeability and magnesium blockade in the NMDA receptor. *Science*, **257**, 1415–19.

Carew, T. and Kandel, E. R. (1976). Two functional effects of decreased conductance EPSP's: synaptic augmentation and increased electrotonic coupling. *Science*, **192**, 150–3.

Chen, L. and Huang, L.-Y. M. (1992). Protein kinase C reduces Mg^{2+} block of NMDA receptor channels as a mechanism of modulation. *Nature*, **356**, 521–3.

Chizhmakov, I. V., Kiskin, N. I., and Krishtal, O. A. (1992). Two types of steady-state desensitization of N-methyl-D-aspartate receptor in isolated hippocampal neurones of rat. *Journal of Physiology*, **448**, 453–72.

Clements, J. D. and Westbrook, G. L. (1991). Activation kinetics reveal the number of glutamate and glycine binding sites on the N-methyl-D-aspartate receptor. *Neuron*, **7**, 605–13.

Fletcher, E. J. and Lodge, D. (1988). Glycine reverses antagonism of N-methyl-D-aspartate (NMDA) by 1-hydroxy-3-aminopyrrolidone-2 (HA-966) but not by D-2-amino-5-phosphonovalerate (D-AP5). *European Journal of Pharmacology*, **151**, 161–3.

Foster, A. C. and Kemp, J. A. (1989). HA-966 antagonizes N-methyl-D-aspartate receptors through a selective interaction with the glycine modulatory site. *Journal of Neuroscience*, **9**, 2191–6.

Gibb, A. J. and Colquhoun, D. (1992). Activation of N-methyl-D-aspartate receptors by L-glutamate in cells dissociated from adult rat hippocampus. *Journal of Physiology*, **456**, 143–79.

Gibb, A. J., Carr, J. A., and Colquhoun, D. (1993). Inward rectification of the NMDA receptor single channel conductance in rat hippocampal cells. *Journal of Physiology*, **459**, 404P.

Henderson, G., Johnson, J. W., and Ascher, P. (1990). Competitive antagonists and partial agonists at the glycine modulatory site of the mouse N-methyl-D-aspartate receptors. *Journal of Physiology*, **430**, 189–212.

Hille, B. and Schwarz, W. (1978). Potassium channels as multi-ion single-file pores. *Journal of General Physiology*, **72**, 409–42.

Huettner, J. E. (1990). Antagonists of NMDA-activated current in cortical neurons: competition with glycine and blockade of open channels. In *Excitatory amino acids and neuronal plasticity*, (ed. Y. Ben Ari), pp. 35–43. Plenum, New York.

Huettner, J. E. and Bean, B. P. (1988). Block of N-methyl-D-aspartate-activated current by the anticonvulsant MK-801: selective binding to open channels. *Proceedings of the National Academy of Sciences, USA*, **85**, 1307–11.

Iino, M., Ozawa, S., and Tsuzuki, K. (1990). Permeation of calcium through excitatory amino acid receptor channels in cultured rat hippocampal neurones. *Journal of Physiology*, **424**, 151–65.

Ikeda, K., Nagasawa, M., Mori, H., Araki, K., Sakimura, K., Watanabe, M., Inoue, Y., and Mishina, M. (1992). Cloning and expression of the ε4 subunit of the NMDA receptor channel. *FEBS Letters*, **313**, 34–8.

Jahr, C. E. and Stevens, C. F. (1990a). A quantitative description of NMDA receptor channel kinetic behavior. *Journal of Neuroscience*, **10**, 1830–7.

Jahr, C. E. and Stevens, C. F. (1990b). Voltage dependence of NMDA-activated macroscopic conductances predicted by single-channel kinetics. *Journal of Neuroscience*, **10**, 3178–82.

Jan, L. Y. and Jan, Y. N. (1976). L-glutamate as an excitatory transmitter at the *Drosophila* larval neuromuscular junction. *Journal of Physiology*, **262**, 522–5.

Johnson, J. W. and Ascher, P. (1987). Glycine potentiates the NMDA response in cultured mouse brain neurones. *Nature*, **325**, 529–31.

Johnson, J. W. and Ascher, P. (1990). Voltage-dependent block by intracellular Mg^{2+} of N-methyl-D-aspartate-activated channels. *Biophysical Journal*, **57**, 1085–90.

Johnson, J. W. and Ascher, P. (1992). Equilibrium and kinetic study of glycine action on the N-methyl-D-aspartate receptor in cultured mouse brain neurons. *Journal of Physiology*, **455**, 339–65.

Katz, B. and Thesleff, S. (1957). A study of the 'desensitization' produced by acetylcholine at the motor end-plate. *Journal of Physiology*, **138**, 63–80.

Kemp, J. A. and Leeson, P. D. (1993). The glycine site of the NMDA receptor. Five years on. *Trends in Pharmacological Sciences*, **14**, 20–5.

Kessler, M., Baudry, M., Terramani, T., and Lynch, G. (1987). Complex interactions between a glycine binding site and NMDA receptors. *Society of Neuroscience Abstracts*, **13**, 760.

Kessler, M., Terramani, T., Lynch, G., and Baudry, M. (1989). A glycine site associated with N-methyl-D-aspartic acid receptors: characterization and identification of a new class of antagonists. *Journal of Neurochemistry*, **52**, 1319–28.

Kleckner, N. W. and Dingledine, R. (1988). Requirement for glycine in activation of NMDA receptors expressed in *Xenopus* oocytes. *Science*, **241**, 835–7.

Kleckner, N. W. and Dingledine, R. (1991). Regulation of hippocampal NMDA receptors by magnesium and glycine during development. *Molecular Brain Research*, **11**, 151–9.

Kutsuwada, T., Kashiwabuchi, N., Mori, H., Sakimura, K., Kushiya, E., Araki, K., Meguro, H., Masaki, H., Kumanishi, T., Arakawa, M., and Mishina, M. (1992). Molecular diversity of the NMDA receptor channel. *Nature*, **358**, 36–41.

Lerma, J., Zukin, R. S., and Bennett, M. V. L. (1990). Glycine decreases desensitization of N-methyl-D-aspartate (NMDA) receptors expressed in *Xenopus* oocytes and is required for NMDA responses. *Proceedings of the National Academy of Sciences, USA*, **87**, 2354–8.

Lester, R. A. J., and Jahr, C. R. (1992). NMDA channel behavior depends on agonist affinity. *Journal of Neuroscience*, **12**, 635–43.

Lester, R. A. J., Clements, J. D., Westbrook, G. L., and Jahr, C. E. (1990). Channel kinetics determine the time course of NMDA receptor-mediated synaptic currents. *Nature*, **346**, 565–7.

Lester, R. A. J. Tong, G., and Jahr, C. E. (1993). Interactions between the glycine and glutamate binding sites of the NMDA receptor. *Journal of Neuroscience*, **13**, 1088–96.

Lewis, C. A. (1979). Ion concentration dependence of the reversal potential and the single channel conductance of ion channels at the frog neuromuscular junction. *Journal of Physiology*, **286**, 417–45.

MacDermott, A. B., Mayer, M. L., Westbrook, G. L., Smith, S. J., and Barker, J. L. (1986). NMDA-receptor activation increases cytoplasmic calcium concentration in cultured spinal cord neurons. *Nature*, **321**, 519–22.

MacDonald, J. F., Miljkovic, Z., and Pennefather, P. (1987). Use dependent block of excitatory amino acid currents in cultured neurones by ketamine. *Journal of Neurophysiology*, **58**, 251–66.

Mayer, M. L., MacDermott, A. B., Westbrook, G. L., Smith, S. J., and Barker, J. L. (1987). Agonist- and voltage-gated calcium entry in cultured mouse spinal cord neurones under voltage clamp measured using arsenazo III. *Journal of Neuroscience*, **7**, 3230–44.

Mayer, M. L. and Westbrook, G. L. (1985). The action of N-methyl-D-aspartic acid on mouse spinal neurones in culture. *Journal of Physiology*, **361**, 65–90.

Mayer, M. L. and Westbrook, G. L. (1986). The physiology of excitatory amino acids in the vertebrate central nervous system. *Progress in Neurobiology*, **28**, 197–276.

Mayer, M. L. and Westbrook, G. L. (1987). Permeation and block of N-methyl-D-aspartic acid receptor channels by divalent cations in mouse cultured central neurones. *Journal of Physiology*, **394**, 501–27.

Mayer, M. L., Westbrook, G. L., and Guthrie, P. B. (1984). Voltage-dependent block by Mg^{2+} of NMDA responses in spinal cord neurones. *Nature*, **309**, 261–3.

Mayer, M. L., Vyklicky, L., Jr, and Clements, J. (1989). Regulation of NMDA receptor desensitization in mouse hippocampal neurones by glycine. *Nature*, **338**, 425–7.

Meguro, H., Mori, H., Araki, K., Kushiya, E., Kutsuwada, T., Yamazaki, M., Kumanishi, T., Arakawa, M., Sakimura, K., and Mishina, M. (1992). Functional characterization of a heteromeric NMDA receptor channel expressed from cloned cDNAs. *Nature*, **357**, 70–4.

Monaghan, D. T., Olverman, J. J., Nguyen, L., Watkins, J. C., and Cotman, C. W. (1988). Two classes of N-methyl-D-aspartate recognition sites: differential distribution and differential regulation by glycine. *Proceedings of the National Academy of Sciences, USA*, **85**, 9836–40.

Monahan, J. B., Corpus, V. M., Hood, W. F., Thomas, J. W., Compton, R. P. (1989). Characterization of a [^{3}H] glycine recognition site as a modulatory site of the N-methyl-D-aspartate receptor complex. *Journal of Neurochemistry*, **53**, 370–5.

Monyer, H., Sprengel, R., Schoepfer, R., Herb, A., Higuchi, M., Lomeli, H., Burnashev, N., Sakmann, B., and Seeburg, P. H. (1992). Heteromeric NMDA receptors: molecular and functional distinction of subtypes. *Science*, **256**, 1217–21.

Mori, H., Masaki, H., Yamakura, T., and Mishina, M. (1992). Identification by mutagenesis of a Mg^{2+}-block site of the NMDA receptor channel. *Nature*, **358**, 673–5.

Moriyoshi, K., Masu, M., Ishii, T., Shigemoto, R., Mizuno, N., and Nakanishi, S. (1991). Molecular cloning and characterization of the rat NMDA receptor. *Nature*, **354**, 31–7.

Mulle, C., Choquet, D., Korn, H., and Changeux, J. P. (1992). Calcium influx through nicotinic receptor in rat central neurons: its relevance to cellular regulation. *Neuron*, **8**, 135–43.

Müller, W. and Connor, J. A. (1991). Dendritic spines as individual neuronal compartments for synaptic Ca^{2+} responses. *Nature*, **354**, 73–6.

Neher, E. (1983). The charge carried by single-channel currents of rat cultured muscle cells in the presence of local anesthetics. *Journal of Physiology*, **339**, 663–78.

Neher, E. and Steinbach, J. H. (1978). Local anaesthetics transiently block currents through single acetylcholine-receptor channels. *Journal of Physiology*, **277**, 153–76.

Nowak, L., Bregestovski, P., Ascher, P., Herbet, A., and Prochiantz, A. (1984). Magnesium gates glutamate-activated channels in mouse central neurones. *Nature*, **307**, 462–5.

Regehr, W. G. and Tank, D. W. (1992). Calcium concentration dynamics produced by synaptic activation of CA1 hippocampal pyramidal cells. *Journal of Neuroscience*, **12**, 4202–23.

Sather, W., Johnson, J. W., Henderson, G., and Ascher, P. (1990). Glycine-insensitive desensitization of NMDA responses in cultured mouse embryonic neurones. *Neuron*, **4**, 725–31.

Sather, W., Dieudonné, S., MacDonald, J. F., and Ascher, P. (1992). Activation and desensitization of *N*-methyl-D-aspartate receptors in nucleated outside-out patches from mouse neurones. *Journal of Physiology*, **450**, 643–72.

Schneggenburger, R., Zhou, Z., Konnerth, A., and Neher, E. (1993). Fractional contribution of calcium to the cation current through glutamate receptor channels. *Neuron*, **11**, 133–43.

Schulman, J. A. and Weight, F. F. (1976). Synaptic transmission: long-lasting potentiation by a postsynaptic mechanism. *Science*, **194**, 1437–9.

Sekiguchi, M., Okamoto, K., and Sakai, Y. (1990). Glycine-insensitive NMDA-sensitive receptor expressed in *Xenopus* oocytes by guinea pig cerebellar mRNA. *Journal of Neuroscience*, **10**, 2148–55.

Shirasaki, T., Nakagawa, T., Wakamori, M., Tateishi, N., Fukuda, A., Murase, K., and Akaike, N. (1990). Glycine-insensitive desensitization of *N*-methyl-D-aspartate receptors in acutely isolated mammalian central neurons. *Neuroscience Letters*, **108**, 93–8.

Stern, P., Béhé, P., Schoepfer, R., and Colquhoun, D. (1992). Single channel conductances of NMDA receptors expressed from cloned cDNAs: comparison with native receptors. *Proceedings of the Royal Society*, (London), Series B, **250**, 271–7.

Thedinga, K. H., Benedict, M. S., and Fagg, G. E. (1989). The *N*-methyl-D-aspartate (NMDA) receptor complex: a stoichiometric analysis of radioligand binding domains. *Neuroscience Letters*, **104**, 217–22.

Thomson, A. (1990). Glycine is a coagonist at the NMDA receptor/channel complex. *Progress in Neurobiology*, **35**, 53–76.

Vernino, S., Amador, M., Luetje, C. W., Patrick, J., and Dani, J. A. (1992). Calcium modulation and high calcium permeability of neuronal nicotinic acetylcholine receptors. *Neuron*, **8**, 127–34.

Vyklicky, L., Jr, Benveniste, M., and Mayer, M. L. (1990). Modulation of *N*-methyl-D-aspartic acid receptor desensitization by glycine in mouse cultured hippocampal neurones. *Journal of Physiology*, **428**, 313–31.

Woodhull, A. M. (1973). Ionic blockage of sodium channels in nerve. *Journal of General Physiology*, **61**, 687–708.

Zarei, M. M. and Dani, J. A. (1994). Ionic permeability characteristics of the N-methyl-D-aspartate receptor channel. *Journal of General Physiology*, **103**, 231–48.

Zorumski, C. F. and Thio, L. L. (1992). Properties of vertebrate glutamate receptors: calcium mobilization and desensitization. *Progress in Neurobiology*, **39**, 295–336.

8 The time course of NMDA receptor-mediated synaptic currents

ROBIN A. J. LESTER, JOHN D. CLEMENTS,
GANG TONG, GARY L. WESTBROOK, AND
CRAIG E. JAHR

Introduction

The slowly rising, long-lasting time course of the NMDA receptor-mediated excitatory post-synaptic current (EPSC) is unusual for a response mediated by a directly gated ion channel. Although the EPSC time course has been physiologically reconciled with the role of the NMDA receptor in associative synaptic plasticity, until recently, the precise mechanisms underlying its generation remained obscure. This chapter will focus on how the interaction between synaptically released transmitter and the post-synaptic receptor gives rise to the distinctive properties of the NMDA synaptic current.

Transmitter does not rebind during the course of the NMDA EPSC

The long-lasting time course of the NMDA receptor-mediated synaptic response has been well documented by several groups (Dale and Roberts 1985; Wigstrom et al. 1985; Collingridge et al. 1988; Forsythe and Westbrook 1988; Hestrin et al. 1990; Lester et al. 1990). An example of the NMDA EPSC recorded between a pair of hippocampal neurones in culture is illustrated in Fig. 8.1(A). In order to reveal the full characteristics of the NMDA EPSC, recordings were obtained in nominally Mg^{2+}-free solutions (Ault et al. 1980; Mayer et al. 1984; Nowak et al. 1984) and in the presence of saturating concentrations of glycine (Johnson and Ascher 1987; Kleckner and Dingledine 1988) and the α-amino-3-hydroxy-5-methyl-4-isoxazole-propionic acid (AMPA) receptor antagonist, 6-cyano-7-nitroquinoxaline-2,3-dione (Blake et al. 1988; Honoré et al. 1988).

A rapidly released transmitter could induce a long synaptic response in two ways: it could either remain bound to the receptor throughout the duration of the response or linger in the synaptic cleft and continually rebind and reactivate the receptor. For NMDA receptors, the correct mechanism can be identified by making use of the fact that competitive antagonists, such as D-2-amino-5-phosphonovalerate (D-AP5) (Davies et al. 1981), can only bind to the NMDA receptor provided the transmitter

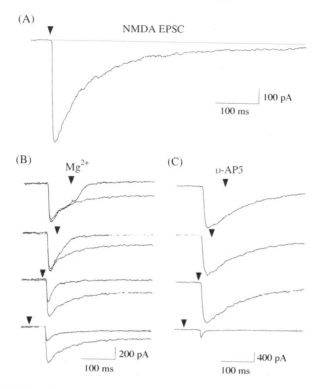

Fig. 8.1 Rebinding of transmitter does not determine the time course of the NMDA EPSC. (A) NMDA EPSC recorded between a pair of hippocampal neurons. 100 μM Mg^{2+} (B) or 100 μM D-AP5 (C) was applied before and during the NMDA EPSC at the times indicated by the arrowheads. (A, adapted from Lester *et al.* (1993) with permission; B and C, from Lester *et al.* (1990) with permission.)

itself is not bound. Thus, if the response depended on the rebinding of transmitter, and D-AP5 was introduced into the cleft during the NMDA EPSC, the response should be attenuated. Because this approach requires a rapid solution-exchange, the method was tested by using the non-competitive NMDA antagonist, Mg^{2+}, which should block the synaptic current irrespective of the activation mechanism. Figure 8.1(B) shows that Mg^{2+} blocked the NMDA synaptic response at times corresponding to its delivery into the synaptic cleft. Conversely, D-AP5 had no effect on the synaptic current (Fig. 8.1(C) top three traces) when it was applied during the decay, but blocked the NMDA EPSC, in an all-or-none manner, when it reached the synapse before stimulation (Fig. 8.1(C), lowest trace) (Lester *et al.* 1990). This result indicates that the transmitter does not rebind during the course of the NMDA synaptic response, and thereby implies that transmitter must remain bound to NMDA receptors throughout.

Further support for this view comes from considering the transient activation of NMDA receptors in membrane patches by the transmitter candidate, L-glutamate.

Glutamate remains bound to the NMDA receptor for prolonged periods

In this set of experiments, pulses of L-glutamate (henceforth called glutamate) were rapidly applied to outside-out patches containing many NMDA channels, in a manner analogous to synaptic stimulation. This 'artificial synapse' technique allows very good control of the level of free agonist (Brett *et al.* 1986; Franke *et al.* 1987).

Figure 8.2 shows examples of the NMDA channel activity that resulted from a brief application of glutamate. Channel openings outlasted the presence of free agonist by hundreds of milliseconds and confirmed that glutamate could remain bound to and activate the NMDA receptor for prolonged periods of time (Lester *et al.* 1990; see also Gibb and Colquhoun (1991)).

Channel properties define the overall time course of the NMDA EPSC

A comparison of the rise and decay of the NMDA EPSC and the currents generated by a pulse of glutamate to an outside-out patch revealed a striking similarity in the two responses. The synaptic and patch currents

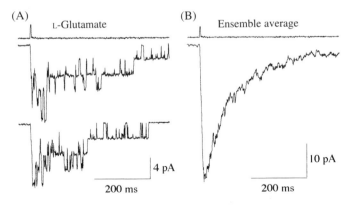

Fig. 8.2 Rapid activation of NMDA receptors in an outside-out patch. (A) Multiple openings of single NMDA channels in a hippocampal neurone outside-out patch by a 4 ms pulse of 200 μM L-glutamate (*middle and lower traces*). Time of agonist application is indicated by the open tip current (*upper trace*). (B) Ensemble average of the single channel activity resulting from a 4 ms pulse of L-glutamate in a different outside-out patch. (Adapted from Lester and Jahr (1992) with permission.)

both show two decay components with virtually identical time constants (see below for explanation of the two-component decay). Furthermore, NMDA channel activation is slow at saturating concentrations of glutamate (Fig. 8.3, *inset*), arguing that the slow rise of the NMDA EPSC results from intrinsic channel properties rather than from the diffusion of transmitter to distant sites (Hestrin *et al.* 1990; Lester *et al.* 1990). Therefore, the NMDA receptor channel properties (or more strictly the interaction between the neurotransmitter, glutamate, and the NMDA receptor) can fully account for the NMDA EPSC. Indeed, the above experiments show that a brief pulse of glutamate can reproduce all the characteristics of the NMDA EPSC and argue that the transmitter does not need to be present in the synaptic cleft for very long (Lester *et al.* 1990). However, these studies do not directly address the time course of free transmitter in the synaptic cleft. This was estimated by examining the displacement of the NMDA antagonist, D-α-aminoadipate (D-AA), from NMDA receptors by synaptically released transmitter.

Free transmitter is only transiently present in the synaptic cleft

A comparison of the equilibrium potency of two competitive NMDA receptor antagonists, D-AA (Gibb and Colquhoun 1991) and D-carboxypiperizin-propyl-phosphonic acid (D-CPP) (Davies *et al.* 1986), in whole-cell recordings from hippocampal neurones shows that they differ in

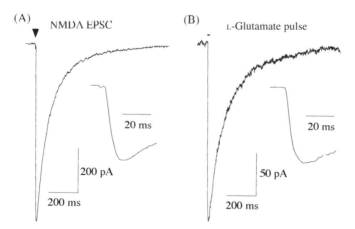

Fig. 8.3 Comparison of the NMDA EPSC and current induced by a short pulse of L-glutamate in an outside-out patch. Averages of 30 NMDA EPSCs (A) and the ensemble average of 80 outside-out patch currents induced by a 5 ms pulse of 100 μM L-glutamate (B). Both currents decay biexponentially with time constants of 71 and 272 ms for the NMDA EPSC and 83 and 323 ms for the patch current. The rise times of the currents are compared (*insets*). The rise times (10–90%) are 7.7 and 7.9 ms for the NMDA EPSC and the patch current, respectively. (Adapted from Lester *et al.* (1990) with permission.)

affinity by 100-fold (Fig. 8.4(A)). However, when these same two concentrations of drug are tested against the NMDA EPSC they are not equipotent; the lower affinity antagonist, D-AA, is less effective than D-CPP (Fig. 8.4(B)). Construction of dose–response curves for the synaptic blocking ability of these antagonists revealed that D-AA was less potent than predicted by its equilibrium dissociation constant (k_d) of approximately 30 μM (Evans *et al.* 1979; Olverman *et al.* 1988), whereas D-CPP antagonized the NMDA EPSC according to its k_d of 400 nM (Benveniste and Mayer 1991) (Fig. 8.4(C)). The reason for the apparent discrepancy lies with differences in the dissociation rates of the drugs; D-CPP unbinds slowly from NMDA receptors (Benveniste and Mayer 1991) and D-AA extremely rapidly (see Fig. 8.4(A)). Thus, even though synaptically released transmitter is presumed to be in the cleft for a very short time, it is present for long enough to bind to some of the NMDA receptors from which D-AA has dissociated, thus reducing the effectiveness of this antagonist. On the other hand,

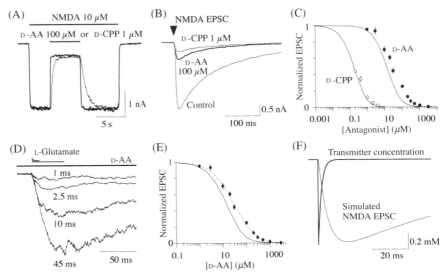

Fig. 8.4 Time course of free transmitter in the synaptic cleft. Comparison of the blocking ability of D-AA (*thick line*) and D-CPP (*thin line*) against a whole-cell NMDA current (A) and an NMDA EPSC (B). (C) Dose–response NMDA EPSC inhibition curves for D-AA (*filled circles*) and D-CPP (*open circles*). The solid lines are theoretical inhibition curves assuming two antagonist binding sites and k_ds of 30 μM and 400 nM for D-AA and D-CPP, respectively. (D) Ensemble average NMDA currents in an outside-out patch induced by various duration pulses of L-glutamate (5 mM) in the continual presence of D-AA (200 μM). Model fit of the D-AA inhibition curve of the NMDA EPSC (E, *dashed line*) assuming the instantaneous rise of neurotransmitter to a peak concentration of 1.1 mM and subsequent exponential decay with a time constant of 1.2 ms (F, *thick line*). A model-simulated NMDA EPSC is also shown (F, *thin line*). (Adapted from Clements *et al.* (1992) with permission.)

because D-CPP unbinds only slowly, transmitter must have been cleared from the cleft before a significant number of D-CPP molecules have dissociated. These observations form the basis for estimating the duration of free transmitter at glutamatergic synapses. For instance, the longer that free transmitter is present, in the continual presence of D-AA, the larger the resulting current will be. This is illustrated for different durations of glutamate applied to an outside-out patch (Fig. 8.4(D)). Since we have measured the effectiveness of D-AA as a synaptic blocker (Fig. 8.4(C)) the argument can be turned around and the transmitter time course can be calculated. Based on the estimation of the binding and unbinding rates of glutamate and D-AA, a multistate model of the NMDA receptor was used to simulate the NMDA EPSC assuming an instantaneous rise and an exponential decay in the amount of free transmitter (Clements *et al.* 1992). The peak concentration and time constant of its decay were then systematically varied until they provided the best fit for the D-AA dose–response curve (Fig. 8.4(E)). Figure 8.4(F) shows the resulting free transmitter transient with the simulated NMDA EPSC. The estimated parameters predict that the average amount of free transmitter at post-synaptic NMDA receptors peaks at 1.1 mM and decays exponentially with a time constant of 1.2 ms (Clements *et al.* 1992). These data confirm the earlier predictions that glutamate is only transiently present in the synaptic cleft.

Agonist dissociation rate limits the duration of the NMDA receptor current

Because transmitter is present only briefly relative to the time course of the NMDA EPSC, the rate of dissociation of transmitter should ultimately determine the duration of the synaptic response. Through the use of the artificial synapse it has been possible to examine the details of dissociation of agonists from NMDA receptors. Two other NMDA agonists, L-cysteate and L-aspartate, were selected because of their respective 100- and 10-fold lower affinities than glutamate (Patneau and Mayer 1990). Compared with the proposed transmitter, glutamate, brief pulses of these ligands produced NMDA currents for which the rate of decay increased as the agonist affinity decreased (Fig. 8.5). It was also apparent that the contribution of the second component of current decay decreased with agonist affinity. Indeed with L-cysteate this phase was almost completely absent (see below). Thus, it is the high affinity (slow dissociation) that gives rise to such a long-lasting synaptic response (Olverman *et al.* 1984; Lester and Jahr 1992). Moreover, since the decay of the NMDA EPSC closely resembles the patch currents produced by glutamate, this argues that the proposed transmitter, L-aspartate, is not a candidate transmitter, at least for cultured hippocampal synapses (Jahr and Lester 1992).

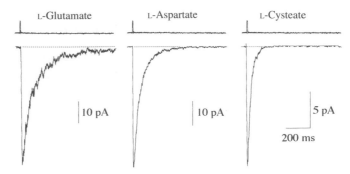

Fig. 8.5 Decay of NMDA currents is determined by the agonist affinity. Ensemble averages of the currents (*lower traces*) induced in outside-out patches by 4 ms pulses of L-glutamate (200 μM), L-aspartate (2 mM), and L-cysteate (20 mM). Open tip currents are indicated (*upper traces*). (Adapted from Lester and Jahr (1992) with permission.)

Decreasing the affinity of glutamate speeds the decay of the NMDA EPSC

Although it has not been possible to change directly the nature of the transmitter present in synaptic terminals, it is possible to decrease the affinity of the transmitter for NMDA receptors in the presence of the partial glycine site agonist, 1-hydroxy-3-amino-pyrrolidone-2 (HA-966) (Fletcher and Lodge 1988; Kemp and Priestley 1991). Such an action apparently results from the allosteric coupling of the glycine and glutamate binding sites of the NMDA receptor (Mayer *et al.* 1989; Benveniste *et al.* 1990). From the above studies a decrease in the affinity of glutamate should result in faster dissociation and shorter NMDA synaptic responses. This was confirmed either by directly evoking an NMDA EPSC between a pair of hippocampal neurones or by using the outside-out patch as an artificial synapse (Fig. 8.6). In the presence of HA-966 both patch and synaptic currents were reduced in amplitude (Fig. 8.6(A)) and had increased rates of decay (Lester *et al.* 1993). These results verify that the rate of dissociation of transmitter determines the decay of the NMDA EPSC.

Desensitization contributes to the time course of the NMDA EPSC

If simple dissociation of transmitter is completely responsible for the decay of the NMDA EPSC, a single exponential decay is the likely outcome. However, as mentioned above, the NMDA EPSC decays biexponentially (see Fig. 8.3). One explanation for this observation is that desensitization of NMDA receptors occurs during the EPSC decay and that the second decay component results from reopening of channels following recovery

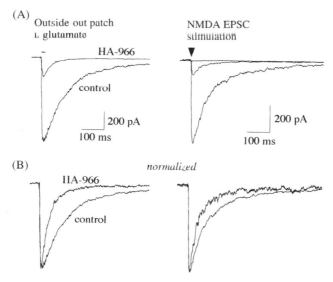

Fig. 8.6 Dissociation of transmitter determines the duration of the NMDA EPSC. (A) Comparison of the ensemble averaged outside-out patch current induced by a 10 ms pulse of 200 μM L-glutamate (*left*) and the NMDA EPSC (*right*) in the absence (*control*) and the presence (*smaller responses*) of 300 μM HA-966. The flat trace (right) shows the complete block of the NMDA EPSC by 50 μM D-AP5. (B) The control and HA-966 patch currents and NMDA EPSCs are shown normalized to highlight the increase in decay rate produced by HA-966. (Adapted from Lester *et al.* (1993) with permission.)

from desensitization. As illustrated in Fig. 8.7(A) NMDA receptors become desensitized in the continuous presence of glutamate (Sather *et al.* 1990; Chizhmakov *et al.* 1992; Lester and Jahr 1992). Because transmitter remains bound to NMDA receptors for prolonged periods following its release, it is conceivable that some synaptic receptors could become desensitized. In order to determine if desensitization of NMDA receptors occurs during brief exposure to transmitter, paired pulses of saturating concentrations of glutamate were applied at various interpulse intervals (Fig. 8.7(B)). The incomplete recovery of the second pulse confirms that some desensitization of NMDA receptors occurred, and because released transmitter is present in the synaptic cleft for a few milliseconds (see above) desensitization probably contributes to the behaviour of the NMDA EPSC. In addition, desensitization is less pronounced with lower affinity ligands (Fig. 8.7(C)) suggesting that the extent of NMDA EPSC desensitization will be related to the affinity of the transmitter. Coupled with the parallel decrease in the second decay component of the NMDA current with decreasing agonist affinity (see Fig. 8.5) these data argue that the slow phase of the NMDA EPSC is due to channel reopening from a desensitized state (Lester and Jahr 1992). Perhaps more important, in

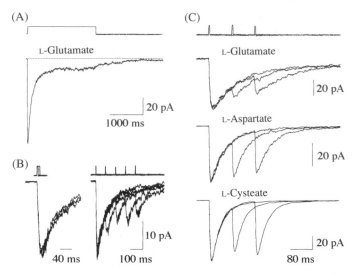

Fig. 8.7 Desensitization of NMDA receptors contributes to the decay of outside-out patch currents induced by brief pulses of agonist. (A) Ensemble averaged outside-out patch currents induced by a 2 s pulse of 200 µM L-glutamate show the rapid desensitization of NMDA receptors. (B) Ensemble averages of the NMDA patch currents in response to 4, 8, and 12 ms pulses of 200 µM L-glutamate (*left*) demonstrate that a 4 ms pulse saturates the NMDA receptors in the patch. Averaged currents induced by paired-pulse applications (4 ms) of 200 µM L-glutamate in the same patch. Interpulse intervals are 80, 160, 240, and 320 ms. (C) Comparison of paired-pulse activation of NMDA receptors in outside-out patches by different affinity agonists. Interpulse intervals are 80 and 160 ms. Open tip currents are shown in each case (*upper traces*). (A, unpublished observations of R. A. J. Lester and C. E. Jahr; B and C, adapted from Lester and Jahr (1992) with permission.)

terms of synaptic function, is the rate of recovery of NMDA receptors from desensitization. Figure 8.8 shows that even following brief activation of NMDA receptors by glutamate, recovery is extremely slow, and a comparison with L-cysteate reveals that it is also a consequence of the affinity of the agonist. These experiments argue that as a consequence of synaptic stimulation by the neurotransmitter, glutamate, NMDA receptors would not be fully available for reactivation for approximately 10 s (Lester and Jahr 1992). Overall, lower affinity agonists such as L-aspartate, if used as transmitters, would give rise to NMDA EPSCs with quite different properties.

Conclusions

The synaptic mechanisms that give rise to the generation of the NMDA EPSC are likely to be of major importance when considering the overall

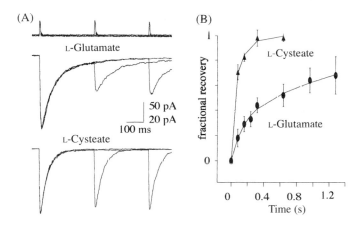

Fig. 8.8 Recovery from desensitization depends on the affinity of the NMDA agonist. (A) Ensemble averages of the outside-out patch currents induced by paired-pulse applications (4 ms) of 200 µM L-glutamate (*middle trace*) and 20 mM L-cysteate (*lower trace*). Interpulse intervals are 320 and 640 ms. Open tip currents are shown (*upper trace*). (B) Time course of the recovery of the NMDA current from desensitization expressed as the ratio of the amplitude of the second to first response plotted against the interpulse interval for L-glutamate (*circles*) and L-cysteate (*triangles*). (Adapted from Lester and Jahr (1992) with permission.)

behaviour of glutamatergic transmission and plasticity. As transmitter is present in the synaptic cleft only transiently, the low affinity post-synaptic AMPA receptor may more faithfully follow rapid presynaptic signals because any steady-state desensitization of these receptors (Trussell and Fischbach 1989) will be limited. Conversely, the slow dissociation of transmitter from NMDA receptors explains why the NMDA receptor is primed for associative depolarization hundreds of milliseconds after synaptic stimulation (Gustafsson *et al.* 1987). Furthermore, the free transmitter concentration profile in the cleft predicts that post-synaptic NMDA receptors will be saturated by glutamate from a single impulse, whereas AMPA receptors will only be about 60 per cent occupied (Clements *et al.* 1992). Thus, at individual synapses, NMDA receptors will operate in their full capacity as inducers of long-term potentiation (Collingridge *et al.* 1983; Harris *et al.* 1984) and AMPA receptors will be available to respond to the enhanced transmitter release that has been proposed to accompany long-term potentiation (Bliss *et al.* 1986; Bekkers and Stevens 1990; Malinow and Tsien 1990). In addition, the above observations suggest that regulation of the NMDA synaptic response could occur through changes in receptor desensitization and/or agonist affinity, as a result of biochemical modification (MacDonald *et al.* 1989) or differences in the molecular stoichiometry of the NMDA receptor (Monyer *et al.* 1992).

Acknowledgements

We would like to thank J. Volk for preparation of the primary cultures of hippocampal neurones. This work was supported by PHS grants NS26494 and MH46613 (G.L.W.) and NS21419 (C.E.J.).

References

Ault, B., Evans, R. H., Francis, A. A., Oakes, D. J., and Watkins, J. C. (1980). Selective depression of excitatory amino acid induced depolarizations by magnesium ions in isolated spinal cord preparations. *Journal of Physiology*, **307**, 413–28.

Bekkers, J. M. and Stevens, C. F. (1990). Presynaptic mechanism for long-term potentiation in the hippocampus. *Nature*, **346**, 724–9.

Benveniste, M. and Mayer, M. L. (1991). Structure–activity analysis of binding kinetics for NMDA receptor competitive antagonists: the influence of conformational restriction. *British Journal of Pharmacology*, **104**, 207–21.

Benveniste, M., Vyklicky, L. Jr, Mayer, M. L., and Clements, J. (1990). A kinetic analysis of the modulation of N-methyl-D-aspartate receptors by glycine in mouse cultured hippocampal neurons. *Journal of Physiology*, **428**, 333–57.

Biscoe, T. J., Evans, R. H., Francis, A. A., Martin, M. R., Watkins, J. C., Davies, J, and Watkins, J. C. (1977). D-α-aminoadipate as a selective antagonist of amino acid-induced and synaptic excitation of mammalian spinal neurones. *Nature*, **270**, 743–5.

Blake, J. F., Brown, M. W., and Collingridge, G. L. (1988). CNQX blocks acidic amino acid induced depolarizations and synaptic components mediated by non-NMDA receptors in rat hippocampal slices. *Neuroscience Letters*, **89**, 182–6.

Bliss, T. V. P., Douglas, R. M., Errington, M. L., and Lynch, M. A. (1986). Correlation between long-term potentiation and release of endogenous amino acids from dentate gyrus of anaesthetized rats. *Journal of Physiology*, **377**, 391–408.

Brett, R. S., Dilger, J. P., Adams, P. R., and Lancaster, B. (1986). A method for the rapid exchange of solutions bathing excised membrane patches. *Biophysical Journal*, **50**, 987–92.

Chizhmakov, I. V., Kiskin, N. I., and Kristal, O. A. (1992). Two types of steady-state desensitization of N-methyl-D-aspartate receptors in isolated hippocampal neurons of rat. *Journal of Physiology*, **448**, 453–72.

Clements, J. D., Lester, R. A. J., Gong, T., Jahr, C. E., and Westbrook, G. L. (1992). Time course of glutamate in the synaptic cleft. *Science*, **258**, 1498–501.

Collingridge, G. L., Kehl, S. J., and McLennan, H. (1983). Excitatory amino acids in synaptic transmission in the Schaffer collateral-commissural pathway of the rat hippocampus. *Journal of Physiology*, **334**, 33–46.

Collingridge, G. L., Herron, C. E., and Lester, R. A. J. (1988). Synaptic activation of N-methyl-D-aspartate receptors in the Schaffer collateral-commissural pathway of rat hippocampus. *Journal of Physiology*, **399**, 283–300.

Dale, N. and Roberts, A. (1985). Dual-component amino acid-mediated synaptic potentials: excitatory drive for swimming in *Xenopus* embryos. *Journal of Physiology*, **363**, 35–59.

Davies, J., Francis, A. A., Jones, A. W., and Watkins, J. C. (1981). 2-amino-5-phosphonovalerate (2APV), a potent and selective antagonist of amino acid-induced and synaptic excitation. *Neuroscience Letters*, 21, 77–81.

Davies, J., Evans, R. H., Herrling, P. L., Jones, A. W., Olverman, H. J., Pook, P., and Watkins, J. C. (1986). CPP, a new potent and selective NMDA antagonist. Depression of central neuron responses, affinity for [³H] D-AP5 binding sites on brain membranes and anticonvulsant activity. *Brain Research*, 382, 169–73.

Evans, R. H., Francis, A. A., Hunt, K., Oakes, D. J., and Watkins, J. C. (1979). Antagonism of excitatory amino acid-induced responses and of synaptic excitation in isolated spinal cord of the frog. *British Journal of Pharmacology*, 67, 591–603.

Fletcher, E. J. and Lodge, D. (1988). Glycine reverses the antagonism of N-methyl-D-aspartate (NMDA) by 1-hydroxy-3-aminopyrrolidone-2-one (HA-966) but not by D-2-amino-5-phosphonovalerate (D-AP5) on rat cortical slices. *European Journal of Pharmacology*, 151, 161–2.

Forsythe, I. D. and Westbrook, G. L. (1988). Slow excitatory postsynaptic currents mediated by N-methyl-D-aspartate receptors on cultured mouse central neurones. *Journal of Physiology*, 396, 515–33.

Franke, Ch., Hatt, H., and Dudel, J. (1987). Liquid filament switch for ultra fast exchanges of solutions at excised patches of synaptic membrane of crayfish muscle. *Neuroscience Letters*, 77, 199–204.

Gibb, A. T. and Colquhoun, D. (1991). Glutamate activation of a single NMDA receptor channel produces a cluster of openings. *Proceedings of the Royal Society* (London), Series B, 243, 39–45.

Gustafsson, B., Wigstrom, H., Abraham, W. C., and Huang, Y.-Y. (1987). Long-term potentiation in the hippocampus using depolarizing current pulses as the conditioning stimulus to single volley synaptic potentials. *Journal of Neuroscience*, 7, 774–80.

Harris, E. W., Ganong, A. H., and Cotman, C. W. (1984). Long-term potentiation in the hippocampus involves activation of N-methyl-D aspartate receptors. *Brain Research*, 323, 132–7.

Hestrin, S., Sah, P., and Nicoll, R. A. (1990). Mechanisms generating the time course of dual component excitatory synaptic currents recorded in hippocampal slices. *Neuron*, 5, 247–53.

Honoré, T., Davies, S. N., Drejer, J., Fletcher, E. J., Jacobsen, P., Lodge, D., and Nielsen, F. E. (1988). Quinoxalinediones: potent competitive non-N-methyl-D-aspartate glutamate receptor antagonists. *Science*, 241, 701–3.

Jahr, C. E. and Lester, R. A. J. (1992). Synaptic excitation mediated by glutamate-gated ion channels. *Current Opinions in Neurobiology*, 2, 270–4.

Johnson, J. W. and Ascher, P. (1987). Glycine potentiates the NMDA receptor response in cultured mouse brain neurones. *Nature*, 325, 529–31.

Kemp, J. A. and Priestley, T. (1991). Effects of (+)-HA-966 and 7-chlorokynurenic acid on the kinetics of N-methyl-D-aspartate receptor agonist responses in rat cultured cortical neurons. *Molecular Pharmacology*, 39, 666–70.

Kleckner, N. W. and Dingledine, R. (1988). Requirement for glycine ion activation of NMDA-receptors expressed in *Xenopus* oocytes. *Science*, 241, 835–7.

Lester, R. A. J. and Jahr, C. E. (1992). Behavior of NMDA channels depends on agonist affinity. *Journal of Neuroscience*, 12, 635–43.

Lester, R. A. J., Clements, J. D., Westbrook, G. L., and Jahr, C. E. (1990). Channel kinetics determine the time course of NMDA receptor-mediated synaptic currents. *Nature*, 346, 565–7.

Lester, R. A. J., Tong, G., and Jahr, C. E. (1993). Interactions between the glutamate and glycine binding sites of the NMDA receptor. *Journal of Neuroscience*, **13**, 1088–96.

MacDonald, J. F., Mody, I., and Salter, M. W. (1989). Regulation of N-methyl-D-aspartate receptors revealed by intracellular dialysis of murine neurones in culture. *Journal of Physiology*, **414**, 17–34.

Malinow, R. and Tsien, R. W. (1990). Presynaptic enhancement shown by whole-cell recordings of long-term potentiation in hippocampal slices. *Nature*, **346**, 177–80.

Mayer, M. L., Westbrook, G. L., and Guthrie, P. B. (1984). Voltage-dependent block by Mg^{2+} of NMDA responses in spinal cord neurones. *Nature*, **309**, 261–3.

Mayer, M. L., Vyklicky, L., Jr, and Clements, J. (1989). Regulation of NMDA receptor desensitization in mouse hippocampal neurons by glycine. *Nature*, **338**, 425–7.

Monyer, H., Sprengel, R., Schoepfer, R., Herb, A., Higuchi, M., Lomeli, H., Burnashev, N., Sakmann, B., and Seeberg, P. H. (1992). Heteromeric NMDA receptors: molecular and functional distinction of subtypes. *Science*, **256**, 1217–21.

Nowak, L., Bregestovski, P., Ascher, P., Herbet, A., and Prochiantz, A. (1984). Magnesium gates glutamate-activated channels in mouse central neurones. *Nature*, **307**, 462–5.

Olverman, H. J., Jones, A. W., and Watkins, J. C. (1984). L-glutamate has higher affinity than other amino acids for [^{3}H]-D-AP5 binding sites in rat brain membranes. *Nature*, **307**, 460–2.

Olverman, H. J., Jones, A. W., and Watkins, J. C. (1988). [^{3}H] D-2-amino-5-phosphopentanoate as a ligand for N-methyl-D-aspartate receptors in the mammalian central nervous system *Neuroscience*, **26**, 1–15.

Patneau, D. K. and Mayer, M. L. (1990). Structure–activity relationships for amino acid transmitter candidates acting at N-methyl-D-aspartate and quisqualate receptors. *Journal of Neuroscience*, **10**, 2385–99.

Sather, W., Johnson, J. W., Henderson, G., and Ascher, P. (1990). Glycine-insensitive desensitization of NMDA responses in cultured mouse embryonic neurons. *Neuron*, **4**, 725–31.

Trussel, L. O. and Fischbach, G. D. (1989). Glutamate receptor desensitization and its role in synaptic transmission. *Neuron*, **3**, 209–18.

Wigstrom, H., Gustafsson, B., and Huang, Y.-Y. (1985). A synaptic potential following single volleys in the hippocampal CA1 region possibly involved in the induction of long-lasting potentiation. *Acta Physiologica Scandinavica*, **124**, 475–8.

9 Activation of NMDA receptors

A. J. GIBB, B. EDMONDS, R. A. SILVER,
S. G. CULL-CANDY, AND
D. COLQUHOUN

Introduction

It is a fascinating thought that two small amino acids like glutamate and glycine are able to induce conformational changes in an enormous membrane protein like the NMDA receptor, simply by colliding with specific sites on the receptor. Understanding the processes occurring during receptor activation is of fundamental importance to pharmacology, and activation of receptors such as the NMDA receptor, which have an integral membrane ion channel, has proved to be particularly amenable to study using single channel recording techniques. The activation of muscle and *Torpedo* acetylcholine receptors (AChRs) has been studied in great detail (Colquhoun and Sakmann 1985; Sine and Steinbach 1986, 1987; Sine *et al.* 1990; Dilger and Brett 1990; Liu and Dilger 1991). Using these approaches the rates of the reactions involved in receptor activation have been estimated and for the endplate AChRs (Colquhoun and Sakmann 1985) these rates are consistent with the observed rate of synaptic transmission at the neuromuscular junction. This has led to the expectation that new insights into the processes underlying the NMDA receptor-mediated component of excitatory post-synaptic currents (NMDA EPSCs) will be obtained from studies of NMDA receptor single channels.

Studies of NMDA receptor activation have recently taken two main experimental approaches: in one, short (millisecond) pulses of a high (millimolar) glutamate concentration are applied to outside-out patches (Lester *et al.* 1990; Clements and Westbrook 1991; Edmonds and Colquhoun 1992) to mimic the process of synaptic transmission. Using this 'concentration jump' technique applied to outside-out patches or intact synapses in culture, Craig Jahr and co-workers have demonstrated elegantly that the time course of the NMDA EPSC is determined by the kinetics of NMDA receptor activation (Lester *et al.* 1990). A second approach is to record the single channel currents produced by NMDA receptor activation at very low glutamate concentrations and to use these data to identify single NMDA receptor activations (Gibb and Colquhoun 1991, 1992); the fact that these are long leads to the same conclusion.

The NMDA EPSC has a slow rising phase (Hestrin *et al.* 1990a; Lester *et al.* 1990; Silver *et al.* 1992; Stern *et al.* 1992b) and a slow decay. The 10–90 per cent rise time of the NMDA EPSC is around 7–10 ms while the decay phase has been fitted either with a single exponential with decay time constant in the range 50–100 ms (Forsythe and Westbrook 1988; Collingridge *et al.* 1988; Hestrin *et al.* 1990*a*; Lester *et al.* 1990; Silver *et al.* 1992; Stern *et al.* 1992*b*) or with two exponential components: a fast component with time constant in the range 40–100 ms and a more variable slow component with time constant in the range 100–500 ms (Hestrin *et al.* 1990*b*; Lester *et al.* 1990; Stern *et al.* 1992*b*). In some cases a slow exponential component cannot be detected.

Single activations of NMDA receptors

A single receptor activation is defined as the time from the start of the first opening after agonist binding to the receptor until the end of the last opening before dissociation of all agonist molecules from the receptor, so that the receptor returns to its resting, unoccupied state. Thus, for the entire duration of the activation, at least one agonist binding site is occupied. The time between first agonist occupancy and first channel opening obviously cannot be measured using steady-state recordings. Yet this information, along with an estimate of the transmitter concentration profile during synaptic transmission, is necessary in order to describe the time course of the NMDA EPSC. In order to get information on the times between agonist binding and channel opening, concentration jump experiments are needed (Edmonds and Colquhoun 1992; Jahr 1992). A complete description of NMDA receptor activation will require both steady-state and concentration jump recordings over a wide range of agonist concentrations.

Shut time distributions

With both inside-out patches and outside-out patches, low glutamate concentrations (20–100 nM) in combination with a high glycine concentration (1 μM) have been found to activate NMDA receptor channels (Gibb and Colquhoun 1991, 1992). Under these conditions most patches show a low level of channel activity with long closed periods of around a second in duration between each group of channel openings. In order to divide the data record into periods within or between activations, the distribution of closed times in the data is examined.

Figure 9.1(a) shows an example of the distribution of shut times observed when a low agonist concentration is used. In both inside-out and outside-out patches from hippocampal cells the shut time distributions for NMDA receptor channels activated by glutamate can generally be fitted with five exponential components in the absence of magnesium. In a study of 26 inside-out or cell-attached patches (Gibb and Colquhoun 1992) the mean time constants (and relative areas) were $\tau_1 = 68 \pm 7$ μs; $\tau_2 = 0.72 \pm 0.12$ ms $(13 \pm 1.5\%)$; $\tau_3 = 7.56 \pm 0.8$ ms $(17 \pm 2\%)$; $\tau_4 = 137 + 26$ ms $(22 \pm 4\%)$; and $\tau_5 = 922 \pm 195$ ms $(18 \pm 3\%)$. In a related study where the concentration dependence of the shut time distribution was assessed using outside-out patches, only the slowest shut time component was found to be clearly dependent on the glutamate concentration (Gibb and Colquhoun 1991). This suggests that the longest shut times in the data record reflect periods where the agonist has vacated the receptor. At the same time, it is possible to suggest from purely physical considerations that at least the first three shut time components must represent gaps which are *within* activations (i.e. closed periods where the agonist is bound to the receptor). The reason for this is that at a glutamate concentration of 20 nM, even individual bindings to the receptor (not all of which will result in receptor activation) are likely to occur only every 500 ms or so assuming a microscopic association rate constant for the agonist of 10^8 M^{-1} s^{-1}. Thus the gaps underlying the third shut time component of 8 ms duration on average must occur within activations. This is supported by the fact that the time constant of τ_3 in the shut time distribution does not change with increasing agonist concentration (Gibb and Colquhoun 1991). Such long periods within a single activation have not been reported for any other neurotransmitter receptor.

A related point to this concerns glycine binding. In these experiments the glycine concentration was fixed at 1 μM in order to effectively saturate the glycine binding site on the receptor $(K_D \approx 200$ nM). However, at 1 μM, the time between glycine bindings to the receptor could be as short as 10 ms, implying that gaps of around 8 ms duration could represent periods where glycine unbound and then rebound to the receptor. In fact this is very unlikely to be the case: a related study found that τ_3 of the shut time distribution was not sensitive to the glycine concentration (Gibb and Edwards 1991) and estimates for the dissociation rate for glycine from the receptor (Benveniste *et al.* 1990; Clements and Westbrook 1991; Sather *et al.* 1992) suggest this is in the order of 1 s^{-1} which is much too slow to account for the frequency of '8 ms gaps' in the data.

The fourth shut time $(\tau_4 = 137$ ms) component is the component for which it is most difficult to assign some physical interpretation at present. It is difficult to measure accurately because only at the lowest glutamate concentrations can it be clearly distinguished from τ_5. This time constant (τ_4) appears to change when either the glutamate or glycine concentration is changed (Gibb and Edwards 1991; Gibb and Colquhoun 1991) but the concentration dependence is not steep enough to identify clearly these gaps as representing periods when either glutamate or glycine dissociated from the receptor. It could be that it represents a short-lived desensitized state. Lester and Jahr (1992) have also suggested for different reasons that the NMDA receptor may enter a short-lived desensitized state during synaptic

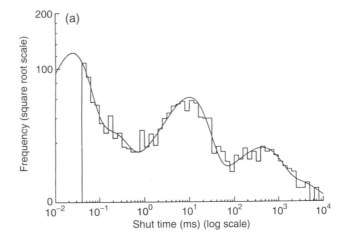

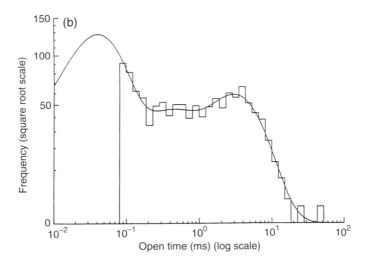

currents. If τ_4 does represent a short-lived desensitized state then each receptor activation could include closed periods of 100 ms or more (see section below on 'Clusters and super-clusters').

Open time distributions

Figure 9.1(b) shows an example of the distribution of all open times measured from an inside-out patch. Distributions of apparent open times were generally well fitted with the sum of three exponential components. These had time constants (and relative areas) of 87 ± 9 μs ($51 \pm 4\%$), 0.91 ± 0.16 ms ($31 \pm 3\%$), and 4.72 ± 0.6 ms ($18 \pm 3\%$). The distribution

Fig. 9.1 Distributions of channel closed times (a) and open times (b) from a single recording. There were 1377 gaps longer than 40 μs in duration and 1206 open times longer than 80 μs in duration. The histograms show the distribution of log time versus the square root of bin frequency on the abscissa (Blatz and Magleby 1986; Sigworth and Sine 1987). This transformation converts the normal exponential distribution into a peaked function. Thus each peak corresponds approximately to the time constant of each exponential component. The distribution is shown fitted with the sum of five exponential components with time constants (and relative areas) of: 23 μs (53%), 0.15 ms (12%), 9.89 ms (27%), 411 ms (71%), and 2.1 s (1%). The fit predicts the presence of 2579 gaps. The record was filtered at 3 kHz (-3 dB). In (b) the distribution of apparent open times between 80 μs and 20 ms long is shown fitted with the sum of three exponential components with parameters of 38 μs (57%), 0.27 ms (15%), and 2.93 ms (29%). The fit predicts that there were 2641 openings in the data record. Patches were isolated from cells dissociated from adult rat hippocampal slices after treatment with trypsin or papain for 90 min using the method described by Numann and Wong (1984). Slices were bathed in a standard Krebs–Henseleit solution of composition 118 mM NaCl, 25 mM KCl, 2.5 mM $CaCl_2$, 30 mM $NaHCO_3$, 1 mM, NaH_2PO_4, 1 mM, $MgCl_2$, and 20 mM glucose, pH 7.4, when bubbled with 95 per cent O_2 and 5 per cent CO_2. For patch-clamp recording, cells were bathed in a 'Mg-free' Krebs solution which was of the above composition, but with no added $MgCl_2$. The pipette solution contained 118 mM NaCl, 10 mM EDTA, 30 mM $NaHCO_3$, 20 mM glucose, 20–100 nM L-glutamate, and 1 μM glycine (Fluka). This was bubbled with 95 per cent O_2, 5 per cent CO_2 just before use. All recordings were made at room temperature (20–24 °C).

---

means averaged 1.22 ± 0.23 ms. The open times are clearly more complex than those for a nicotinic receptor (though the possible problems of receptor heterogeneity have yet to be examined).

The presence of three exponential components in the open time distribution and five exponential components in the shut time distribution suggests that a minimum of three distinct open states and five distinct shut states is required to describe NMDA channel gating. In fact, further open and shut states will be required to account for multiple conductance states and possible desensitized states, as well as glycine bound and unbound states.

It is clear that the distributions of open times and shut times suggest there is likely to be a substantial number of both shuttings and openings which are too short to be detected. We therefore refer to these as *apparent* open times or shut times since unresolved gaps, for example, will result in overestimation of the channel open times. In order to correct for these missed events (Hawkes *et al.* 1992) a specific mechanism for receptor activation must be postulated.

Correlations in NMDA receptor channel data

The *sequence* of open and shut times may provide information relevant to suggesting an activation mechanism. The correlations that we find in the data can, in principle, give information about the connectivity between states in the activation mechanism (Fredkin *et al.* 1985; Colquhoun and

Hawkes 1987), even when the time resolution is limited (Ball and Sansom 1988).

Significant positive correlations were found between open times and closed times, and a negative correlation was present between the length of adjacent open and closed times (Gibb and Colquhoun 1992). There was also a positive correlation between adjacent bursts and clusters. Blatz and Magleby (1989) and McManus and Magleby (1989) demonstrated the advantages of using *distributions* of adjacent intervals as a means of examining the strength of correlations in a single channel data record. Figure 9.2 shows a plot of the mean open time adjacent to different shut time ranges. It is clear that, on average, longer openings are adjacent to short gaps and vice versa, as suggested by the negative correlation coefficient calculated for adjacent open and closed times.

At first sight a correlation like this may seem paradoxical since random processes are supposed to be 'memoryless' in the sense that each opening or closing is an independent event. How then, can the length of an opening appear to be dependent on the closed periods adjacent to it? The answer lies in the fact that it is not possible to tell which state the receptor is in by looking at the data. The distributions of shut times and open times suggest there are at least five discrete shut states of the receptor and three discrete open states. However, all that is seen from the data is that the channel is either open or shut. As a result, even though the lifetimes of sojourns in

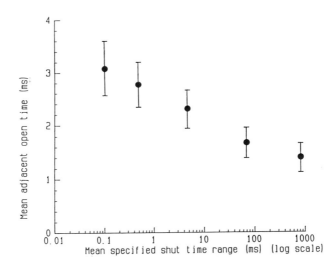

Fig. 9.2 Relationship between the mean durations of adjacent open and shut intervals. The graph plots the mean ± SEM of the mean open times in 16 different patches against the average of the mean adjacent shut time ranges used in each patch. (Reproduced from Gibb and Colquhoun 1992.)

individual states may be independent of each other (as expected for a Markov process), the *observed* open and closed times may be correlated (Fredkin *et al.* 1985; Colquhoun and Hawkes 1987). Essentially this occurs when the system can oscillate between adjacent open and closed states several times, then a transition occurs so that a different pair of open and closed states is occupied. Thus, in order to see correlations in the data, at least two open states and two shut states are needed. Whether or not correlations arise depends on the connectivity of the receptor activation mechanism. Therefore, the fact that there are correlations in the NMDA receptor gating can, in principle, be used to suggest how the proposed open and closed states are connected together.

One advantage of the adjacent interval analysis is that it allows a test to be made of the Markov assumptions (Blatz and Magleby 1989; McManus and Magleby 1989). This is done by looking not only at the *mean* duration of adjacent events but also at their distributions. In Fig. 9.3(A) the distribution of open times adjacent to gaps in the range 50 μs to 0.3 ms is shown while Fig. 9.3(B) shows the distribution of open time adjacent to gaps in the range 50 ms to 5 s. The data in Fig. 9.3 are from the same patch as illustrated in Figs 9.1 and 9.2. Each distribution is fitted with three exponential components just like the unconditional open time distribution in Fig. 9.1(B). Furthermore, the distribution time constants are similar in both cases; only the relative area of each component differs, there being more long openings and fewer short openings adjacent to short gaps, and more short openings and fewer long openings adjacent to long gaps. When the results for 16 patches analysed in this way were averaged together (Gibb and Colquhoun 1992) the time constants of the exponential components fitted to the open time distributions did not change (and were not significantly different from the unconditional distribution time constants) with changing length of adjacent gaps. This is strong evidence that the durations of sojourns in individual states are independent, and that the molecule is 'memoryless' in the sense that the chance of leaving a given state is independent of how long that state has already been in existence. This supports the idea that the receptor activation mechanism can be viewed as a discrete Markov process.

Clusters and super-clusters: how long is an activation?

Consideration of the shut time distributions at low agonist concentrations provided clear evidence that NMDA receptor activations contained much longer closed periods than those observed with endplate AChRs (Colquhoun and Sakmann, 1985). Using τ_3 and τ_4 of each shut time distribution, a critical gap length, t_c was calculated which was then used to divide the data record into groups of openings (Colquhoun and Sakmann 1985) referred to as *clusters*. In an exactly analogous way, '*super-clusters*' were calculated except that τ_4 and τ_5 from the shut time distributions were used; the super-

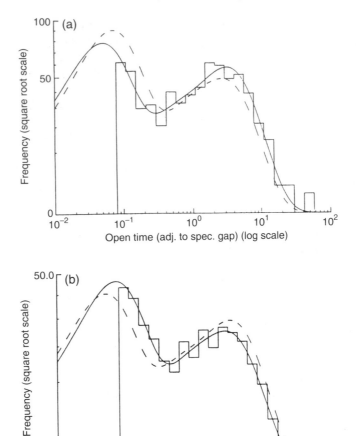

Fig. 9.3 Conditional distributions of apparent open times adjacent to brief (a) and long (b) shut times from the same patch as illustrated in Figs 9.1 and 9.2. (a) From a total of 1206 apparent open times 640 were identified as adjacent to shut times in the range 50 μs to 0.3 ms. These were fitted with the sum of three exponential components (solid curve) with parameters of 48 μs (52%), 0.36 ms (8%), and 3.21 ms (40%). The fit predicted a total of 1154 open times. (b) A total of 335 open times were identified as adjacent to shut times in the range 50 ms to 5 s. These were fitted with the sum of three exponentials (solid curve) with parameters of 68 μs (60%), 0.46 ms (5.8%), and 2.79 ms (35%). The dashed line in (a) shows the fit from (b) scaled to contain the same number of openings as in (a); in (b), the dashed line shows the fit from (a) scaled to contain the same number of openings as in (b). (Reproduced from Gibb and Colquhoun 1992.)

cluster will represent individual activations if the fourth shut time component (mean 137 ms) also occurs within activations. As discussed above, the evidence for this is less strong and rests mainly on the fact that a definite glutamate concentration-dependence for this component has not been observed.

Figure 9.4(A) and (B) show examples of the distribution of cluster lengths and super-cluster lengths respectively. In general these can be fitted with three exponential components. The mean time constants (and relative areas) for the cluster length distributions were $\tau_1 = 88 \pm 10$ μs $(45 \pm 5\%)$, $\tau_2 = 3.4 \pm 0.9$ ms $(25 \pm 4\%)$, and $\tau_3 = 32 \pm 4.3$ ms $(30 \pm 4\%)$. For super-cluster lengths these were 0.16 ± 0.05 ms $(34 \pm 6\%)$, 4 ± 0.9 ms $(16 \pm 3\%)$, and 166 ± 24 ms $(51 \pm 5\%)$.

The fraction of time that the channel is open during clusters (cluster P_{open}) was found to be 0.62 ± 0.11. The super-cluster P_{open} was 0.2 ± 0.05. Both these values are surprisingly low when compared with acetylcholine receptor channels where the P_{open} during an activation is greater than 0.9 (Colquhoun and Sakmann 1985).

When two exponential components are fitted to the NMDA EPSC decay (e.g. Lester *et al.* 1990; Stern *et al.* 1992b) the cluster lengths are similar to the time constant of the faster exponential while the super-cluster lengths are similar to, or shorter than the slow component found when two exponentials are fitted to NMDA EPSCs. However, the interpretation that the lengths of clusters and superclusters determine the time course of the NMDA EPSC is only an approximation, as shown by the results of concentration jump experiments.

Concentration jump experiments

Glutamate is thought to remain in the synaptic cleft for around a millisecond (Clements *et al.* 1992; Colquhoun *et al.* 1992; Hestrin 1992), and yet the current carried by NMDA receptors is still observed more than a second after the glutamate concentration has decayed to near zero. When a synaptic current is mimicked in an outside-out patch by a brief (1 ms) application of a saturating concentration (1 mM) of glutamate, the decay of the macroscopic current can be fitted with the sum of two exponential components, yielding time constants of 34 ms and 279 ms (Edmonds and Colquhoun 1992), similar to values reported for glutamatergic synapses (e.g. Stern *et al.* 1992b: $\tau_1 = 16$–80 ms, $\tau_2 = 108$–307 ms). Moreover, the time constants are similar to those of the slow components of the cluster (38 ms) and super-cluster (329 ms) length distributions, respectively, observed with steady-state application of a low concentration (30 nM) of glutamate (Edmonds and Colquhoun 1992).

A brief pulse (1 ms or less) of glutamate would be expected to produce (at most) only one activation of the receptor. If, as suggested above, super-

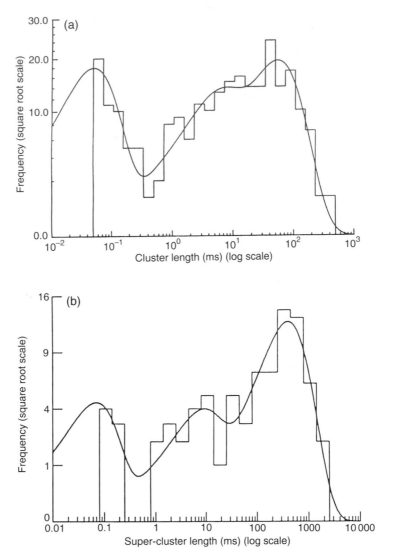

Fig. 9.4 Distribution of the length of clusters (a) and super-clusters (b) in the data record. (a) 244 clusters were identified using a critical gap length of 28.3 ms. The distribution is shown fitted with the sum of three exponential components with time constants (and areas) of 50 μs (39%), 4.6 ms (19%), and 55 ms (42%). The fit predicts that there were a total of 324 clusters in the data record. (b) 81 super-clusters were identified using a critical gap length of 400 ms. The distribution was fitted with three exponential components of 68 μs (22%), 7.6 ms (16%), and 403 ms (62%). The fit predicts a total of 95 super-clusters in the data record. (Adapted from Gibb and Colquhoun 1992.)

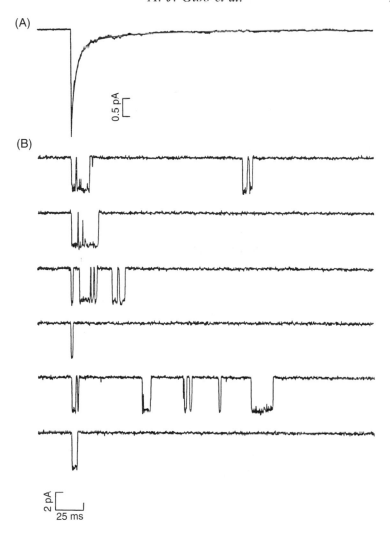

Fig. 9.5 Alignment of channel activations from a low concentration experiment. (A) Illustration of the ensemble average of 297 aligned super-clusters. Superimposed on the data is the fitted curve (τ_1 = 4.6 ms, relative amplitude 82%; τ_2 = 38 ms, relative amplitude 18%). (B) Six individual super-clusters used to construct the average in (A) are shown digitally filtered to a final calculated half-power frequency (Gaussian) of 1 kHz. Recordings were made from an outside-out patch isolated from a granule cell in a hippocampal slice from a 12 day old rat using methods as described by Edwards *et al.* (1989). Channels were activated with 30 nM glutamate and 100 nM glycine. (Reproduced from Edmonds and Colquhoun 1992.)

clusters of openings represent individual channel activations, then their long duration appears to explain the slow decay of the NMDA EPSC. However, we have found that this explanation is incomplete. In order to explain the shape of the EPSC it is necessary to consider, in addition to the duration of the activation, the length of time (the '*first latency*') from the moment the agonist is applied until the moment when the first opening (the start of the visible activation) appears. At the neuromuscular junction, the first latency is very short, so averaging of channel activations after aligning the beginnings of the first channel opening (i.e. simulating zero latency), would result in an average time course for current decay that closely resembles an endplate current. Figure 9.5 shows, however, that when super-clusters, recorded in experiments with very low glutamate concentrations, are so aligned, the average current decays far too quickly (mainly with a time constant of about 5 ms) to resemble the EPSC; slower component(s) are, of course, present but their amplitude is far smaller than for an EPSC, and is too small to be fitted reliably (Edmonds and Colquhoun 1992). This happens, in part, because the super-clusters are open for only 10–20 per cent of the time on average (compared with 99 per cent of the time for the muscle nicotinic receptor). There are at least two possible explanations for this disagreement: the first latency may well not be brief (as was assumed in the alignment method), and/or the structure of a single channel activation elicited by a 1 ms pulse of 1 mM glutamate may be different from the activation elicited by very low steady glutamate concentrations. Before considering the experimental evidence further, it will be helpful to consider the influence of the first latency on the shape of the EPSC with the help of a simplified example.

First latency, convolution, and EPSC decay

Consider a hypothetical channel which, after brief agonist application, produces an activation consisting of a single opening, after the first latency has elapsed. In Fig. 9.6(A), nine examples are shown of simulated channels with a mean first latency of 1 ms and a mean open time of 10 ms (the variability of both being described by simple exponential distributions). The average current (shown at the top), is seen, not surprisingly, to have a rising phase that can be fitted with an exponential with a time constant of about 1 ms, and the decay phase has a time constant of about 10 ms. Apart from being about 10 times too slow, this example is similar to what happens at a neuromuscular junction.

More surprising, perhaps, are the results shown in Fig. 9.6(B), in which the numbers are reversed, and simulated channels have a mean first latency of 10 ms and a mean open time of 1 ms. The averaged current shown at the top is seen to have essentially the same shape as that in Fig. 9.6(A) (though it is 10 times smaller, and considerably noisier relative to its amplitude). Thus, in this case, the rate of decay reflects the duration of the first latency,

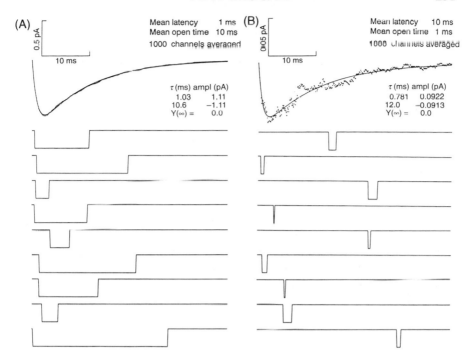

Fig. 9.6 Simulations of channels that have an exponentially distributed latency before showing a single opening (the length of which is also exponentially distributed). The opening is shown as a downward deflection of amplitude 1 pA. (A) The lower part shows examples of nine individual simulated traces for the case where the mean first latency is 1 ms, and the mean open time is 10 ms. The mean of 1000 such traces is shown at the top. It has been fitted (equally weighted least-squares) with the sum of two exponential components. The fit gave time constants of 1.03 ms (rise) and 10.6 ms (decay), which are close to the values of 1 and 10 ms used for simulation, and amplitudes of 1.11 pA and −1.11 pA, as predicted by Equation 7. The maximum is close to the t_{max} of 2.56 ms predicted by Equation 8, at which time the probability of being open is similar to the value from Equation 6, $p_{open}(t_{max}) = 0.774$. (B) This is similar to part (A) except that the mean first latency is 10 ms, and the mean open time is 1 ms. The mean of 1000 such traces is shown at the top. The fit to this gave time constants of 0.78 ms and 12.0 ms (reasonably close to the 1 and 10 ms used for simulation, given the noisiness of the trace), and amplitudes of 0.092 pA and −0.091 pA, similar to the value of 0.11 pA predicted by Equation 7. As in (A), the maximum is close to the t_{max} of 2.56 ms predicted by Equation 8, at which time the probability of being open is similar to the value from Equation 6, $P_{open}(t_{max}) = 0.077$.

whereas the rate of rise represents the mean channel open time (this case resembles observations on sodium channels: Aldrich *et al.* 1983). The reason for this result, which seems paradoxical at first sight, can be seen from the simulations (e.g. the exponential distribution of first latencies means that short latencies are more common than long ones) and from the relevant theory which, in this simple example, is both easy and informative.

Denote the mean length of the first latency as $1/\beta$, and the mean length of an opening as $1/\alpha$. Both have simple exponential distributions, so the distribution (probability density function) of the first latency is

$$f_1(t) = \beta e^{-\beta t} \tag{1}$$

and the distribution of open time is

$$f_2(t) = \alpha e^{-\alpha t} \tag{2}$$

Now consider the distribution, which will be denoted by $g(t)$, of the length of the entire event that follows the agonist pulse. This length is the sum of the length of the first latency and the length of the subsequent opening. If the total length has a specified value, t say, this could be made up either of a short first latency and a long opening, or of a long first latency and a short opening. If the length of the first latency is denoted by u, then the length of the opening must be $t - u$. For a Markov process, events that happen in non-overlapping time intervals are independent so the multiplication rule of probability can be applied to give the probability (density) of both of these events occurring as the product $f_1(u)f_2(t - u)$. Now u can clearly have any value from 0 up to t, so the summation rule of probability must be used to find the probability density for one or other of the possible values occurring. In this case the variables are continuous so the sum becomes an integral, and the final result is therefore

$$g(t) = \int_{u=0}^{u=t} f_1(u)f_2(t - u) \, du \tag{3}$$

and, in this case the integral can easily be evaluated explicitly to give

$$g(t) = \frac{\alpha\beta}{\beta - \alpha} \left(e^{-\alpha t} - e^{-\beta t} \right) \tag{4}$$

Notice that this result is identical if α and β are interchanged: whichever is the faster represents the rising phase, and the slower represents the decay phase. In other words the distribution of the sum of two intervals does not depend on whether the 'short one' or the 'long one' comes first. Equations with the form of (3) are known as a *convolution integrals*. Such equations occur whenever we consider the distribution of the sum of random variables, and are the basis for obtaining things like the distribution of burst lengths, though in cases more complex than this it is necessary to use Laplace transforms and matrix methods to obtain useful results (e.g. see Colquhoun and Hawkes 1982). (Incidentally, convolution integrals also occur in single channel work in a rather different context: in linear systems such as electronic filters, the output of the system can be found by convolving the input with the impulse response function for the system, i.e. the input is represented as a series of impulse responses the outputs for which superimpose linearly; e.g. Colquhoun and Sigworth 1983.)

In this particular simple case, though not in general, there is a very simple relationship between the distribution, $g(t)$, of the total event length, and the shape of the averaged current. The time course of the current is given, apart from a scale factor, by the probability that a channel is open at time t. Now a channel will be open at time t if the first latency is of length u, *and* if the channel stays open for a time *equal to or greater than $t - u$*. The probability that a channel stays open for a time $t - u$ or longer, is calculated from $F_2(t) = \int_0^\infty f_2(u)\,\mathrm{d}u$. Thus, $F_2(t - u) = \mathrm{e}^{-\alpha(t - u)}$, so, by an argument exactly like that used above, the probability that a channel is open at time t is

$$P_{\text{open}}(t) = \int_{u=0}^{u=t} f_1(u)\,F_2(t - u)\,\mathrm{d}u \tag{5}$$

This differs from (3) only by a factor of $1/\alpha = $ mean open lifetime, so

$$P_{\text{open}}(t) = g(t)/\alpha, \tag{6}$$

which is, apart from its amplitude, unchanged when α and β are interchanged. The amplitudes of the two exponential components are equal and opposite, being

$$\text{amp} = \beta/(\alpha + \beta), \tag{7}$$

with a maximum at

$$t_{\text{max}} = \ln(\beta/\alpha)/(\beta - \alpha). \tag{8}$$

The simulated average currents in Fig. 9.6 are indeed well-fitted by these values.

Evidence concerning the slow decay of the EPSC

As a first step in trying to assess the contributions of the first latency and of the activation structure (see above), we have calculated the distribution of first latencies that would have to be postulated to account for the slow response to a brief concentration jump *if* the activations produced by the jump were the same as those seen at low agonist concentrations. The result was that many of the first latencies would have to be long: their distribution would need two components with $\tau_1 = 15$ ms (10% of area) and $\tau_2 = 174$ ms (90% of area) (Edmonds and Colquhoun 1992). Unfortunately, it is difficult to measure experimentally the first latency distribution and the post-jump activation structure, because of the inability to determine accurately the number of channels in the patch). However, preliminary work on this problem shows that there are certainly some long latencies, and that the average latency may be quite long. It is likely, therefore, that long first latencies make a substantial contribution to the slow decay of the concentration jumps and synaptic currents. We have not yet determined, however, whether a difference in the structure of activations also contributes to the slow kinetics.

Synaptic NMDA receptor channels

To understand the involvement of individual NMDA channels in synaptic transmission in more detail it would clearly be useful to know some of the basic properties of *synaptic* NMDA channels. There are almost certainly differences in the kinetic behaviour and, possibly, in the conductance of these channels at synapses in different cell types; their properties could also vary between different types of excitatory synapse within the same cell or at a single synapse. Differences in conductances have been described for native receptors in experiments where different types of cerebellar neurones have been compared (reviewed by Cull-Candy *et al.* 1991) and in experiments comparing properties of recombinant NMDA receptors composed of various subunit combinations (Stern *et al.* 1992*a*). The possibility of heterogeneity resulting from subunit splicing variants (Anantharam *et al.* 1992; Nakanishi *et al.* 1992; Sugihara *et al.* 1992) has yet to be explored. So far, however, most of the single channel information about native receptors has been obtained from channels in somatic patches, because post-synaptic receptors are not accessible to patch electrodes. Until recently, kinetic information obtained from post-synaptic NMDA channels has been limited to that which can be obtained by analysing the decay phase of the macroscopic EPSC. Recently, two methods have been used in trying to overcome this difficulty and obtain direct information about the conductance of the post-synaptic NMDA channel:

(1) direct recording of single channels in the decay phase of the whole-cell synaptic current under conditions where the background noise is unusually low;

(2) non-stationary variance analysis of the decay phase of the synaptic NMDA component.

These approaches have been applied both to synapses formed in culture (Robinson *et al.* 1991) and to identified intact synapses in thin slices of cerebellum (Silver *et al.* 1992).

NMDA receptor channels have been examined at the rat mossy fibre–granule cell synapse (Silver *et al.* 1992) which is the only excitatory input on to these cells. This synapse is particularly suitable for examination with whole-cell recording because of the electrical properties of granule cells, which give whole-cell patch-clamp recordings of exceptionally low noise and high-temporal resolution. Furthermore, properties of somatic single non-NMDA and NMDA channels have previously been characterized in some detail in cultured granule cells (Cull-Candy *et al.* 1988; Howe *et al.* 1988, 1991; Traynelis and Cull-Candy 1991). As at many other central glutamatergic synapses, transmission is mediated by non-NMDA and NMDA receptor channels. The non-NMDA component of the evoked EPSC is exceptionally fast, with a 10–90 per cent rise time of approximately 400 μs and a decay time constant of about 1.3 ms (for monotonically rising events). By contrast, the NMDA component has a slow rise time of about 9 ms, and a monoexponential decay with a mean time constant of 52 ms. The spontaneous miniature EPSCs (MEPSCs, recorded in tetrodotoxin), which are thought to arise from the release of single transmitter packets, invariably show activation of both non-NMDA and NMDA receptor types, indicating that the receptors are co-localized at this synapse as previously observed at hippocampal synapses in culture (Bekkers and Stevens 1989).

Figure 9.7 illustrates whole-cell patch-clamp recordings of spontaneous MEPSCs in granule cells (rising phases have been aligned). Directly resolved single NMDA channels are apparent following the brief synaptic non-NMDA component. The mean conductance of these synaptic NMDA channels is about 48 pS; the slight skew to lower current values in the amplitude distribution for NMDA single channel currents (Fig. 9.7(c)) would be consistent with the presence of some lower conductance levels activated at the synapse. This value is very similar to our estimate of 50 pS that can be derived from non-stationary variance analysis of the NMDA component of evoked EPSCs in these cells (Traynelis *et al.* 1993). We have compared the conductance of the synaptic NMDA channels with the conductance change for the NMDA component of MEPSCs, which has a *mean* amplitude of only 20 pS (Silver *et al.* 1992). Clearly, the single transmitter packet opens few NMDA channels at these synapses. Calculations of the number of NMDA channels opened during the MEPSC is complicated by the likelihood that there is a long mean latency between receptor activation and NMDA channel opening (see above); channels apparently open for the first time well after the peak of the current. The average number of channels open during the MEPSC can be obtained by dividing the average charge transfer during the NMDA component by the average charge transfer per channel activation (measured at very low glutamate concentrations; see above). An estimate obtained this way suggests that, on average, only about two NMDA channels are opened by the transmitter packet.

We cannot determine precisely how many receptors are exposed to the transmitter because the *proportion* of post-synaptic receptors that open during a miniature current is unknown. If we assume that transmitter

Activation of NMDA receptors

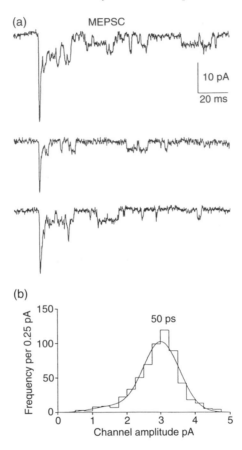

Fig. 9.7 Spontaneous miniature EPSCs were recorded in 0.5 μM TTX from cerebellar granule neurones in thin slices (Edwards *et al.* 1989). (a) Three examples of spontaneous MEPSCs consisting of an initial fast non-NMDA component followed by individually resolved ~ 50 pS NMDA channel openings ($V_m = -60$ mV). (b) Amplitude histogram for single NMDA channel transitions in the tail of MEPSCs. The main peak corresponds to 50 pS conductance level. MEPSCs were filtered to 1 kHz (-3 dB) and were included if they were preceded by 25 ms of NMDA channel free baseline. Conductance measurements were made during the 100 ms after the onset of the MEPSC. Channels were included if they had a monotonic rise and remained at one level for >0.5 ms. The amplitude histogram was fitted with several Gaussian components using the maximum likelihood method (Colquhoun and Sigworth 1983). Measurements were made in Krebs solutions containing 2 mM calcium, 3–5 μM glycine, and 10–20 μM bicuculline metho-bromide. Patch pipettes of thick-walled borosilicate glass, coated with Sylgard resin were polished to a resistance of 5–15 MΩ, and filled with 110 mM CsF, 30 mM CsCl, 4 mM NaCl, 0.5 mM CaCl$_2$, 10 mM HEPES, and 5 mM EGTA (pH 7.3). (Adapted from Silver *et al.* 1992.)

saturates the NMDA receptors, which seems reasonably likely given that the EC_{50} is 200-fold lower than for non-NMDA receptors (Patneau and Mayer 1990), and given that the proportion of granule cell NMDA receptors which open at a saturating glutamate concentration is similar to the estimate of 0.2 obtained by Jahr (1992) for hippocampal neurones, then approximately three post-synaptic NMDA receptors are exposed to each transmitter packet. This is similar to our previous estimate of five channels (Silver *et al.* 1992), which was calculated by a different approach. However, there may be many complicating factors; for example, the concentration of free protons in the synaptic cleft is expected to reduce the number of NMDA receptors that can be activated to about 50 per cent at physiological pH (7.3) in cerebellar granule cells (Traynelis and Cull-Candy 1990; see also Tang *et al.* 1990). A transient acidification of the synaptic cleft from co-release of protons and glutamate from the nerve terminal (reviewed by Chesler and Kaila 1992) could diminish the proportion of activatable NMDA receptors during transmission. This acidification is thought to occur because vesticular uptake at glutamate synapses is driven by an electrochemical proton gradient generated by a proton ATPase (Maycox *et al.* 1990; see Traynelis and Cull-Candy 1991 for discussion). Hence vesicular pH may be far from the mean extracellular value. Although the number of synaptic NMDA channels opened by a packet of transmitter at this synapse is reasonably certain, our estimate for the number of channels exposed to the transmitter packet should clearly be treated with caution as many other modulatory factors will also influence the proportion of NMDA channels that open.

Future directions

Any attempts to describe quantitatively the activation of NMDA receptors, and the synaptic currents mediated by them, must take into account the possibility that they are heterogeneous. The cloning of the receptor has shown that there are at least five subunit types (Moriyoshi *et al.* 1991; Meguro *et al.* 1992; Monyer *et al.* 1992), only two of which are needed to produce efficient channels. Furthermore, the NR1 subunit occurs in six different alternatively spliced versions (Anantharam *et al.* 1992; Nakanishi *et al.* 1992; Sugihara *et al.* 1992), though the functional importance of these variants is not yet known. The properties of native NMDA receptors in cultured cerebellar granule cells (Howe *et al.* 1991) and in hippocampal cells (Gibb and Colquhoun 1991, 1992; Edmonds and Colquhoun 1992) are strikingly similar (and they resemble closely the NR1–NR2B combination expressed in oocytes: Stern *et al.* 1992*a*). However, there are indications of NMDA receptor heterogeneity in other cell types (see Cull-Candy *et al.* 1988; Monaghan *et al.* 1988; Howe *et al.* 1991). It is certainly not yet clear whether or not the NMDA receptors are homogeneous even at a single synapse. An additional complication is that expression of cloned subunits does not necessarily result in homogeneous receptors (e.g. Gibb *et al.* 1990). There is substantial variability in the reported values for the rise and decay times of NMDA EPSCs, but it is not yet known whether these arise from heterogeneity of the NMDA receptors involved, or other factors (including differences in measurement methods). Clearly the elucidation of the extent of receptor heterogeneity, of developmental changes (Hestrin 1992), and the nature of synaptic NMDA receptors, are important topics for the future.

It seems likely that a combination of information from equilibrium measurements over a wide range of agonist concentrations, with the results from concentration jumps on one-channel patches, will soon provide enough information to allow a realistic mechanism to be postulated for the activation of the NMDA receptor. This will be greatly helped by the fact that it is now possible to do a simultaneous maximum likelihood fit of a mechanism to all the data, allowing properly for missed brief events, and taking into account the sequence of openings and shuttings so information from their correlations is used (Hawkes *et al.* 1992).

References

Aldrich, R. W., Corey, D. P., and Stevens, C. F. (1983). A reinterpretation of mammalian sodium channel gating based on single channel recording. *Nature*, **306**, 436–41.

Anantharam, V., Panchal, R. G., Wilson, A., Kolchine, V. V., Treistman, S. N., and Bayley, H. (1992). Combinatorial RNA splicing alters the surface charge on the NMDA receptor. *FEBS Letters*, **305**, 27–30.

Ball, F. G. and Sansom, M. S. P. (1988). Single channel autocorrelation functions: the effects of time interval omission. *Biophysical Journal*, **53**, 819–32.

Beckers, J. M. and Stevens, C. F. (1989). NMDA and non-NMDA receptors are co-localized at individual excitatory synapses in cultured rat hippocampus. *Nature*, **341** 230–3.

Benveniste, M. J., Clements, J. D., Vyklicky, L., Jr, and Mayer, M. L. (1990). A kinetic analysis of the modulation of N-methyl-D-aspartic acid receptors by glycine in mouse cultured hippocampal neurones. *Journal of Physiology*, **428**, 333–57.

Blatz, A. L. and Magleby, K. L. (1986). Correcting single channel data for missed events. *Biophysical Journal*, **49**, 967–80.

Blatz, A. L. and Magleby, K. L. (1989). Adjacent interval analysis distinguishes among gating mechanisms for the fast chloride channel from rat skeletal muscle. *Journal of Physiology*, **410**, 561–85.

Chesler, M. and Kailer, K. (1992). Modulation of pH by neuronal activity. *Trends in Neurosciences*, **15**, 396–402.

Clements, J. D. and Westbrook, G. L. (1991). Activation kinetics reveal the number of glutamate and glycine binding sites on the N-methyl-D-aspartate receptor. *Neuron*, **7**, 605–13.

Clements, J. D., Lester, R. A. J., Tong, G., Jahr, C. E., and Westbrook, G. L. (1992). Time course of glutamate in the synaptic cleft. *Science*, **258**, 1498–301.

Collingridge, G. L., Herron, C. E., and Lester, R. A. J. (1988). Synaptic activation of N-methyl-D-aspartate receptors in the Schaffer collateral-commissural pathway of rat hippocampus. *Journal of Physiology*, **399**, 283–300.

Colquhoun, D. and Hawkes, A. G. (1982). On the stochastic properties of bursts of single ion channel openings and of clusters of bursts. *Philosophical Transactions of the Royal Society*, Series B, **300**, 1–59.

Colquhoun, D. and Hawkes, A. G. (1987). A note on correlations in single ion channel records. *Proceedings of the Royal Society* (London), Series B, **230**, 15–52.

Colquhoun, D. and Sakmann, B. (1985). Fast events in single-channel currents activated by acetylcholine and its analogues in the frog muscle end-plate. *Journal of Physiology*, **369**, 501–57.

Colquhoun, D. and Sigworth, F. J. (1983). Fitting and statistical analysis of single-channel records. In *Single-channel recording*, (ed. B. Sakmann and E. Neher), pp. 191–263. Plenum Press, New York.

Colquhoun, D., Jonas, P., and Sakmann, P. (1992). Action of brief pulses of glutamate on AMPA/kainate receptors in patches from different neurones of rat hippocampal slices. *Journal of Physiology*, **458**, 261–87.

Cull-Candy, S. G., Howe, J. R., and Usowicz, M. M. (1988). Single glutamate receptor channels in two types of cerebellar neurones. In *Excitatory amino acids in health and disease*, (ed. D. Lodge), pp. 165–85. Wiley, Chichester, UK.

Cull-Candy, S. G., Wyllie, D. A. J., and Traynelis, S. R. (1991). Excitatory amino acid-gated channel types in mammalian neurons and glia. In *Excitatory amino acids and synaptic function*, pp. 69–89. Academic Press, London.

Dilger, J. P. and Brett, R. S. (1990). Direct measurement of the concentration- and time-dependent open probability of the nicotinic acetylcholine receptor channel. *Biophysical Journal*, **57**, 723–31.

Edmonds, B. and Colquhoun, D. (1992). Rapid decay of averaged single channel NMDA receptor activations recorded at low agonist concentration. *Proceedings of the Royal Society B*, **250**, 279–86.

Edwards, F. A., Konnerth, A., Sakmann, B., and Takahashi, T. (1989). A thin slice preparation for patch clamp recordings from synaptically connected neurones of the mammalian central nervous system. *Pflügers Archiv/European Journal of Physiology*, **414**, 600–12.

Forsythe, I. D. and Westbrook, G. L. (1988). Slow excitatory postsynaptic currents mediated by N-methyl-D-aspartate receptors on cultured mouse central neurones. *Journal of Physiology*, **396**, 515–33.

Fredkin, D. R., Motal, M., and Rice, J. A. (1985). Identification of aggregated Markovian models: application to the nicotinic acetylcholine receptor. In *Proceedings of the Berkeley conference in honor of Jerzy Neuman and Jack Kiefer*, (ed. L. M. Le Cam and R. A. Olshen), pp. 269–89. Wadsworth, Monterey, USA.

Gibb, A. J. and Colquhoun, D. (1991). Glutamate activation of a single NMDA receptor-channel produces a cluster of channel openings. *Proceedings of the Royal Society* (London), Series B, **243**, 39–45.

Gibb, A. J. and Colquhoun, D. (1992). Activation of NMDA receptors by L-glutamate in cells dissociated from adult rat hippocampus. *Journal of Physiology*, **456**, 143–79.

Gibb, A. J. and Edwards, F. A. (1991). Glycine does not influence the properties of single clusters of NMDA channel openings in inside-out patches from rat hippocampal cells. *Journal of Physiology*, **437**, 122P.

Gibb, A. J., Kojima, H., Carr, J. A., and Colquhoun, D. (1990). Expression of cloned receptor subunits produces multiple receptors. *Proceedings of the Royal Society* (London), Series B, **242**, 108–12.

Hawkes, A. G., Jalali, A., and Colquhoun, D. (1992). Asymptotic distributions of apparent open times and shut times in a single channel record allowing for the omission of brief events. *Philosophical Transactions of the Royal Society*, Series B, **337**, 383–404.

Hestrin, S. (1992). Development regulation of NMDA receptor-mediated synaptic currents at a central synapse. *Nature*, **357**, 686–9.

Hestrin, S., Nicoll, R. A., Perkel, D. J., and Sah, P. (1990a). Analysis of excitatory synaptic action in pyramidal cells using whole-cell recording from rat hippocampal slices. *Journal of Physiology*, **422**, 203–25.

Hestrin, S., Sah, P., and Nicoll, R. A. (1990b). Mechanisms generating the time course of dual component excitatory synaptic currents recorded in hippocampal slices. *Neuron*, **5**, 247–53.

Howe, J. R., Colquhoun, D., and Cull-Candy, S. G. (1988). On the kinetics of large-conductance glutamate-receptor ion channels in rat cerebellar granule neurons. *Proceedings of the Royal Society* (London), Series B, **233**, 407–22.

Howe, J. R., Cull-Candy, S. G., and Colquhoun, D. (1991). Currents through single glutamate-receptor channels in outside-out patches from rat cerebellar granule cells. *Journal of Physiology*, **432**, 143–202.

Jahr, C. E. (1992). High probability opening of NMDA receptor channels by L-glutamate. *Science*, **255**, 470–2.

Kay, A. R. and Wong, R. K. S. (1986). Isolation of neurons suitable for patch-clamping from adult mammalian central nervous systems. *Journal of Neuroscience Methods*, **16**, 227–38.

Lester, R. A. J. and Jahr, C. E. (1992). NMDA channel behavior depends on agonist affinity. *Journal of Neuroscience*, **12**, 635–43.

Lester, R. A. J., Clements, J. D., Westbrook, G. L., and Jahr, C. E. (1990). Channel kinetics determine the time course of NMDA receptor-mediated synaptic currents. *Nature*, **346**, 567–7.

Liu, Y. and Dilger, J. P. (1991). Opening rate of acetylcholine receptor channels. *Biophysical Journal*, **60**, 424–32.

McManus, O. B. and Magleby, K. L. (1989). Kinetic time constants independent of previous single-channel activity suggest Markov gating for a large conductance Ca-activated K channel. *Journal of General Physiology*, **94**, 1037–70.

Maycox, P. R., Hell, J. W., and Jahn, R. (1990). Amino acid neurotransmission: spotlight of synaptic vesicles. *Trends in Neurosciences*, **13**, 83–7.

Meguro, H., Mori, H., Araki, K., Kushiya, E., Kutsuwada, T., Yamazaki, M., Kumanishi, T., Arakawa, M., Sakimura, K., and Mishina, M. (1992). Functional characterization of a heteromeric NMDA receptor channel expressed from cloned cDNAs. *Nature*. **357**, 70–4.

Monaghan, D. T., Olverman, H. J., Nguyen, L., Watkins, J. C., and Cotman, C. W. (1988). Two classes of N-methyl-D-aspartate recognition sites: differential distribution and differential recognition by glycine. *Proceedings of the National Academy of Science, USA*, **85**, 9836–40.

Monyer, H., Sprengel, R., Schoepfer, R., Herb., A, Higuchi, M., Lomeli, H.,

Burnashev, N., Sakmann, B., and Seeburg, P. H. (1992). Heteromeric NMDA receptors: molecular and functional distinction of subtypes. *Science*, **256**, 1217–20.

Moriyoshi, K., Masu, M., Ishii, T., Shigemoto, R., Mizuno, N., and Nakanishi, S. (1991). Molecular cloning and characterization of the rat NMDA receptor. *Nature*, **354**, 31–7.

Nakanishi, N., Axel, R., and Schneider, N. A. (1992). Alternative splicing generates functionally distinct NMDA receptors. *Proceedings of the National Academy of Science, USA*, **89**, 8552–6.

Numann, R. E. and Wong, R. K. S. (1984). Voltage-clamp study of GABA response desensitization in single pyramidal cells dissociated from the hippocampus of adult guinea pigs. *Neuroscience Letters*, **47**, 289–95.

Patneau, D. and Mayer, M. L. (1990). Structure-activity relationships for amino acid transmitter candidates acting at N-methyl-D-aspartate and quisqualate receptors. *Journal of Neuroscience*, **10**, 2385–99.

Robinson, H. P. C., Sahara, Y., and Kawai, N. (1991). Non-stationary fluctuation analysis and direct resolution of single channel currents at post-synaptic sites. *Biophysical Journal*, **59**, 295–304.

Sather, W., Dieudonné, S., MacDonald, J. F., and Ascher, P. (1992). Activation and desensitization of NMDA receptors in nucleated outside-out patches of mouse neurones. *Journal of Physiology*, **450**, 643–72.

Sigworth, F. J. and Sine, S. M. (1987). Data transformation for improved display and fitting of single channel dwell time histograms. *Biophysical Journal*, **52**, 1047–54.

Silver, R. A., Traynelis, S. F., and Cull-Candy, S. G. (1992). Rapid-time-course miniature and evoked excitatory currents at cerebellar synapses. *Nature*, **355**, 163–6.

Sine, S. M. and Steinbach, J. H. (1986). Activation of acetylcholine receptors on clonal mammalian BC3H-1 cells by low concentrations of agonist. *Journal of Physiology*, **373**, 129–62.

Sine, S. M. and Steinbach, J. H. (1987). Activation of acetylcholine receptors on clonal mammalian BC3H-1 cells by high concentrations of agonist. *Journal of Physiology*, **385**, 325–59.

Sine, S. M., Claudio, T., and Sigworth, F. J. (1990). Activation of *Torpedo* acetylcholine receptors expressed in mouse fibroblasts: single channel current kinetics reveal distinct agonist binding affinities. *Journal of General Physiology*, **96**, 395–437.

Stern, P., Béhé, P., Schoepfer, R., and Colquhoun, D. (1992a). Single-channel conductances of NMDA receptors expressed from cloned cDNAs: comparison with native receptors. *Proceedings of the Royal Society* (London), Series B, **250**, 271–7.

Stern, P., Edwards, F. A., and Sakmann, B. (1992b). Fast and slow components of unitary EPSCs on stellate cells elicited by focal stimulation in slices of rat visual cortex. *Journal of Physiology*, **449**, 247–78.

Sugihara, H., Moriyoshi, K., Ishii, T., Masu, M., and Nakanishi, S. (1992). Structures and properties of seven isoforms of the NMDA receptor generated by alternative splicing. *Biochemical and Biophysical Research Communications*, **185**, 826–32.

Tang, C.-M., Dichter, M., and Morad, M. (1990). Modulation of the N-methyl-D-aspartate channel by extracellular H^+. *Proceedings of the National Academy of Science, USA*, **87**, 6445–9.

Activation of NMDA receptors

Traynelis, S. F. and Cull-Candy, S. G. (1990). Proton inhibition of NMDA receptors in cerebellar neurones. *Nature*. **345**, 347–50.

Traynelis, S. F. and Cull-Candy, S. G. (1991). Pharmacological properties and H⁺ sensitivity of excitatory amino acid receptor channels in rat cerebellar granule neurones. *Journal of Physiology*, **433**, 727–63.

Traynelis, S. F., Silver, R. A., and Cull-Candy, S. G. (1993). Estimated conductance of glutamate receptor channels activated during EPSCs at the cerebellar mossy fibre-granule cell synapse. *Neuron*, **11**, 279–89.

10 NMDA receptors and their interactions with other excitatory amino acid receptors in synaptic transmission in the mammalian central nervous system

T. E. SALT

Introduction

It is now generally accepted that there are multiple excitatory amino acid receptors. The ionotropic excitatory amino acid receptors (i.e. those which directly gate cation channels) have been classified, using a number of agonists and antagonists, into N-methyl-D-aspartate (NMDA) receptors, kainate receptors, and AMPA receptors (formerly known as quisqualate receptors) (Chapter 1). The distinction between kainate receptors and AMPA receptors is not completely clear as the agonists and antagonists which have been used to classify these receptors are not adequately select-ive. As a consequence, a 'working classification' for the ionotropic excita-tory amino acid receptors has emerged in common use: receptors are often referred to as NMDA receptors and non-NMDA (i.e. AMPA/kainate) receptors. In addition to the ionotropic excitatory amino acid receptors, there is also a family of metabotropic excitatory amino acid receptors, which are activated by agonists such as L-glutamate, ibotenate, and (1S, 3R)-ACPD (Schoepp et al. 1990). Activation of these receptors typically leads to intracellular effects such as changes in inositol phosphate or cyclic nucleotide metabolism. Recent molecular biological studies have provided data which are consistent with the pharmacological classification outlined above, but have also provided considerably more detail on the different receptor types (Gasic and Hollmann 1992).

The study of excitatory amino acid receptor involvement in central synaptic transmission has relied heavily, and continues to rely, on the development of potent and selective antagonists. A selection of antagonists with activity at the ionotropic excitatory amino acid receptors is listed in Table 10.1. Until comparatively recently, such agents existed only for the NMDA receptor, largely through the pioneering chemical work of Watkins and his collaborators. Thus, the role of NMDA receptors in synaptic transmission has been extensively studied for over a decade, some of the earliest work being carried out by John Davies, to whom this chapter is

Table 10.1 Some commonly used antagonists of ionotropic excitatory amino acid receptors

Name	Abbreviation
NMDA receptor antagonists	
D-2-Amino-5-phosphonopentanoic acid	AP5
(or D-2-amino-5-phosphonovaleric acid)	
D-2-Amino-7-phosphonoheptanoic acid	AP7
3-((R)-2-Carboxypiperazin-4-yl)-propyl-1-phosphonic acid	CPP
Ketamine (channel blocker)	Ket
non-NMDA recetor (AMPA/kainate) antagonists	
γ-D-Glutamylaminomethylsulphonic acid	GAMS
6-Cyano-7-nitroquinoxaline-2,3-dione	CNQX
6,7-Dinitroquinoxaline-2,3-dione	DNQX
2,3-Dihydroxy-6-nitro-7-sulphamoyl-benzo(F)quinoxaline	NBQX
Broad-spectrum antagonists	
Kynurenic acid	Kyn
γ-D-Glutamylglycine	DGG
cis-2,3-Piperidinedicarboxylic acid	PDA
p-Chlorobenzoyl-2,3-piperazine-dicarboxylic acid	PZDA

dedicated. This chapter seeks to review some of the electrophysiological work which has been carried out using excitatory amino acid antagonists. Space does not permit an exhaustive survey of all investigations, and thus a selection of studies of brain areas has been chosen for review in an attempt to draw out similarities in receptor function in synaptic transmission: a common feature of these areas is that they have been the subject of intensive study, often using different electrophysiological techniques.

A technique which has been widely used in studies of excitatory amino acid synaptic pharmacology, both *in vivo* and *in vitro*, is iontophoresis (and/or micro-pressure perfusion): this allows the local application of agonists and antagonists in the vicinity of the neurone whose activity is being recorded (Stone 1985). A major, well-known disadvantage of this technique is that it is impossible to know the concentrations of drugs that are reaching the receptors, and furthermore, the applied drugs will almost certainly be distributed non-uniformly in the vicinity of the neurone. It is thus particularly important that when an antagonist is used in an attempt to block a synaptic response that the effectiveness of the antagonist is tested on every neurone on which it is used, both in terms of ability to antagonize the appropriate agonist, and in terms of specificity for the receptor which is under investigation. Failure to carry out such a control procedure renders the results useless and potentially misleading. Nevertheless, when used with care, iontophoresis can be an extremely powerful technique in the study of synaptic pharmacology, as it allows the local application of drugs. The alternative to iontophoretic application, *in vitro*, is bath application of antagonists and agonists. This technique allows a more quantitative approach to the pharmacology of synapses, as the concentrations of antagonists in the medium are known. A disadvantage is that the site of action of drugs may be less clear (this may be a serious disadvantage in synaptically complex central nervous system areas, for example the spinal cord or cerebral cortex). Furthermore, the time taken for agonists and antagonists to reach appropriate concentrations in the tissue is considerably greater using bath application than with iontophoretic or micropressure application.

The peculiar biophysical and pharmacological properties of the NMDA receptor channel complex (see reviews elsewhere in this volume) have provided an additional means for the identification of NMDA receptor function in synaptic transmission. For example, many *in vitro* investigations have made use of the finding that the NMDA receptor-gated channel is blocked by Mg^{2+} ions in a voltage-dependent manner, and that this confers a non-linear voltage relationship upon excitatory post-synaptic potentials (EPSPs) which have NMDA receptor-mediated components. Thus, it is possible, by manipulating the membrane potential of a neurone and/or the extracellular Mg^{2+} concentration, to modify the magnitude of NMDA receptor-mediated EPSP components, and thus to make them more apparent in order to carry out pharmacological studies using antagonists. The approach of manipulating the Mg^{2+} levels is clearly only suitable for *in vitro* studies although local elevation of Mg^{2+} concentration has been shown to reduce NMDA responses *in vivo* (Davies and Watkins 1977; Eaton and Salt 1991). The few *in vivo* intracellular recording experiments where attempts have been made to reveal the voltage dependence of putative NMDA receptor-mediated EPSP components (assuming some degree of tonic Mg^{2+}-blockade of the ion channel) have produced inconclusive results (Lo and Sherman 1989; Salt and Eaton 1990). Although the *in vivo* approach suffers from considerable disadvantages in terms of recording stability, resolution, and ability to control and manipulate experimental variables (e.g. membrane potential, concentrations of ions and modulators), it does have several advantages: firstly, it is possible to study the synaptic pharmacology of long, functionally identified projection pathways, and in many instances to stimulate these in a physiologically appropriate manner. The latter has been especially relevant in the study of sensory pathways. A second advantage of the *in vivo* approach is that it is more likely to approximate to 'normal physiological' conditions. This is of course of great relevance when the host of modulatory and regulatory factors (both known and unknown) which may affect synaptic transmission is considered.

General characteristics of excitatory amino acid-mediated EPSPs

Intracellular recordings from neurones in many brain regions, either *in vivo* or *in vitro*, have revealed that excitatory amino acid-mediated EPSPs are often composed of both non-NMDA (i.e. AMPA/kainate) and NMDA receptor-mediated components (Tables 10.2–10.4). The excitatory synapses impinging upon CA1 pyramidal cells of the hippocampus have been extensively studied in terms of their excitatory amino acid synaptic pharmacology (e.g. Herron *et al.* 1986; Collingridge *et al.* 1988; Forsythe and Westbrook 1988; Bekkers and Stevens 1989; Hestrin *et al.* 1990*a*; Konnerth *et al.* 1990; Thomson and Radpour 1991); this is discussed elsewhere in this volume. The findings have, however, been generalized and in many ways have been considered as a model for how excitatory amino acid-mediated synaptic transmission may operate at other central synapses. Generally, the non-NMDA receptor-mediated component, characterized by its insensitivity to NMDA antagonists such as AP5 and its sensitivity to non-NMDA antagonists such as CNQX, has a faster rise time and fall time than the NMDA receptor-mediated component. The NMDA receptor-mediated component can typically be characterized by it sensitivity to antagonists such as AP5 or CPP, and its sensitivity to blockade by Mg^{2+} ions at relatively hyperpolarized membrane potentials, giving rise to a non-linear current-voltage relationship. Furthermore, this component generally displays a longer rising and falling phase than the AMPA/kainate receptor component. It is likely that these differences in time course are due to differences in channel kinetics between NMDA-gated channels and AMPA/kainate-gated channels (Hestrin *et al.* 1990*b*; Lester *et al.* 1990), and that a single presynaptic action potential can evoke a post-synaptic response which is mediated by both NMDA receptors and non-NMDA receptors (Forsythe and Westbrook 1988; Thomson *et al.* 1989). It is unclear how widely applicable the preceding generalization is, but it is likely that in many cases, an apparent lack of an NMDA receptor-mediated synaptic component may be due to inappropriate experimental conditions or inability of the recording technique to resolve such components (see below). However, there also appear to be well-documented examples of synaptic transmission without any apparent involvement of NMDA receptors.

Excitatory amino acid pathways

Spinal cord

Some of the earliest data which suggested an involvement of NMDA receptors in synaptic transmission were obtained by Davies and Watkins from extracellular, single-neurone recordings in the cat spinal cord, using

Table 10.2 Sample of published data on some examples of spinal excitatory amino acid pathways, studied *in vivo* or *in vitro*

Region	Pathway	Preparation	Rec.	Receptor(s)	Antagonist(s)	Appl'n	References
Dorsal horn	monosynaptic, Group I muscle afferents	cat, *in vivo*	e.c.	non-NMDA	GAMS, DGG, PDA, CNQX, AP5, CPP	ionto.	Davies and Watkins (1983, 1985); Davies (1988)
	monosynaptic, Group II muscle afferents	cat, *in vivo*	e.c.	NMDA	CPP, GAMS, PZDA	ionto.	Davies (1988)
	polysynaptic, myelinated afferents	cat, *in vivo*	e.c.	non-NMDA/NMDA	CNQX, PZDA, AP5, CPP	ionto.	Davies and Watkins (1983, 1985); Davies (1988)
	non-nociceptive and nociceptive afferents	cat/rat, *in vivo*	e.c.	non-NMDA	Ket, PDA	ionto./i.v.	Headley *et al.* (1987)
	myelinated afferents	hamster, *in vitro*	e.c.fd.	non-NMDA	CNQX, CPP	bath	Morris (1989)
	primary afferents	rat, *in vitro*	i.c.	NMDA	AP5	bath	Jeftinija (1989)
	primary afferents	rat, *in vitro*	v.c.	non-NMDA/NMDA	CNQX, AP5	bath	Gerber and Randic (1989)
Ventral horn	polysynaptic, primary afferents	cat, *in vivo*	e.c.	NMDA/non-NMDA	AP5, PDA, DGG	ionto.	Davies and Watkins (1982, 1983)
	non-nociceptive and nociceptive afferents	cat/rat, *in vivo*	e.c.	non-NMDA/NMDA	Ket, PDA	ionto./i.v.	Headley *et al.* (1987)
	primary afferents	rat, *in vitro*	e.c.	non-NMDA	CNQX	bath	Long *et al.* (1990)
	Group 1A afferents	rat, *in vitro*	i.c.	non-NMDA	Kyn, AP5	bath	Jahr and Yoshioka (1986)
	primary afferents	rat, *in vitro*	i.c.	NMDA/non-NMDA	Kyn, AP5, CNQX	bath	Ziskind-Conhaim (1990)
	primary afferents	rat, *in vitro*	i.c.	non-NMDA/NMDA	CNQX, AP5	bath	King *et al.* (1992)
	primary afferents	rat, *in vitro*	p.c.	non-NMDA/NMDA	CNQX, CPP	bath	Konnerth *et al.* (1991)
Spinal cord co-culture	primary afferents	mouse, *in vitro*	p.c.	NMDA/non-NMDA	AP5	bath	Forsythe and Westbrook (1988)

Abbreviations: Rec., recording technique; e.c., extracellular; single neurone; e.c.fd., extracellular, field potential; i.c., intracellular; v.c., voltage clamp; or p.c., patch-clamp. Appl'n, antagonist application method: ionto., micro-ion-ophoresis; i.v., intravenous; or bath, bath application.

iontophoretic applications of the then newly synthesized NMDA antagonists (Davies and Watkins 1979, 1982, 1983). In these studies, the (presumed) polysynaptic excitation of various groups of dorsal horn and ventral horn neurones by electrical stimulation of myelinated peripheral nerves was found to be susceptible to antagonism by these compounds. In contrast, the monosynaptic excitation of these neurones evoked by stimulation of such afferents was resistant to NMDA antagonists, but could be ant- agonized by broad-spectrum excitatory amino acid antagonists such as PDA or DGG, and was thus presumed to be mediated by non-NMDA excitatory amino acid receptors (Davies and Watkins 1979, 1982, 1983, 1985; Davies *et al.* 1982). Since then, various workers, using *in vitro* electrophysiological methods ranging from field potential recordings to patch-clamp techniques, have provided data which are broadly consistent with this view, both in the dorsal horn (Gerber and Randic 1989; Jeftinija 1989; Morris 1989) and ventral horn (Jahr and Yoshioka 1986; Long *et al.* 1990; King *et al.* 1992). A notable exception to the above generalization is the (presumed) monosynaptic excitation evoked by group II muscle spindle afferents: this response, recorded extracellularly from single neurones *in vivo*, was found to be antagonized by iontophoretically applied CPP (Davies 1988). This would clearly warrant further investigation with intracellular recording techniques. Detailed analysis of EPSPs and EPSCs recorded *in vitro* has also revealed that monosynaptic EPSPs may have an NMDA receptor-mediated component in addition to a non-NMDA receptor-mediated component, and that the NMDA receptor-mediated component has a slower time course than the non-NMDA receptor- mediated component (Forsythe and Westbrook 1988; Ziskind-Conhaim 1990; Konnerth *et al.* 1991). How these *in vitro* findings relate to the situation which is found *in vivo* upon physiological activation of afferents is not entirely clear. It is noteworthy that the responses of dorsal horn neurones to non-noxious and noxious sensory stimuli are resistant to iontophoretically applied NMDA antagonists (Headley *et al.* 1987; Dougherty and Willis 1991) and intravenously administered ketamine (Headley *et al.* 1987), a non- competitive NMDA antagonist: this would argue strongly against a role for NMDA receptors in responses of dorsal horn neurones to acute sensory inputs. In contrast, there is evidence for an involvement of non-NMDA re- ceptors in synaptic responses to a variety of sensory stimuli via myelinated and/or unmyelinated afferents in the dorsal horn of the spinal cord and medulla (Hill and Salt 1982; Headley *et al.* 1987). In the ventral horn, how- ever, responses of neurones to noxious sensory stimuli appear to involve both NMDA receptors and non-NMDA receptors (Headley *et al.* 1987).

Supraspinal brain areas

The pharmacology of excitatory amino acid transmission has been ex- tensively studied in various specific thalamic relay nuclei, both *in vitro* and *in vivo*, using both electrical and natural stimulation of sensory afferent pathways. The various studies are summarized in Table 10.3. Taken together, all of these studies point to a consistent role for both NMDA and non-NMDA receptors in synaptic transmission in the thalamic relay nuclei. The involvement of NMDA receptors becomes more apparent upon repetitive stimulation of afferents: the responses evoked either by prolonged natural stimulation or by electrical stimulation with a train of pulses with a frequency in excess of 10 Hz, can be readily antagonized by a variety of competitive and non-competitive NMDA antagonists, applied either iontophoretically or systemically in *in vivo* studies (Salt 1986, 1987; Salt *et al.* 1988; Salt and Eaton 1989; Sillito *et al.* 1990; Funke *et al.* 1991), or in the bathing medium *in vitro* (Soltesz *et al.* 1989). With single pulse electrical stimuli or short duration physiological stimuli, there is apparently considerably less NMDA receptor involvement in transmission, to such an extent that it may not be seen, especially with extracellular recording techniques (Crunelli *et al.* 1987; Davies and Sheardown 1988; Salt 1986, 1987; Salt and Eaton 1989). However, careful analysis of intracellular recordings indicates that there is an NMDA receptor component to sensory EPSPs which appears to have a slower time course than the initial non-NMDA receptor component (Scharfman *et al.* 1990; Salt and Eaton 1991; Esguerra *et al.* 1992; Leresche 1992). It is noteworthy that in the thalamus *in vivo*, following application of the AMPA receptor antagonist CNQX, it is possible to see an EPSP component which is sensitive to the NMDA antagonist CPP (Salt and Eaton 1991): this indicates that the occurrence of NMDA receptor-mediated transmission under physiological conditions is not dependent upon the prior occurrence of an AMPA receptor-mediated EPSP (Figure 10.1).

The dual nature NMDA/non-NMDA synaptic response does not seem to be universally present in all subcortical brain structures. For example, *in vivo* intracellular recording studies in cats have indicated that both the cortico-striatal (Herrling 1985) and interposito-rubral (Davies and Sheardown 1988) pathways appear to be mediated by non-NMDA receptors, as the EPSPs evoked by stimulation of the respective pathways are resistant to iontophoretically applied NMDA antagonists, but are sensitive to broad-spectrum excitatory amino acid antagonists (Fig. 10.2). Neurones in these nuclei clearly have functional NMDA receptors, as they are depolarized by iontophoretically applied NMDA, and indeed, the responses of neurones in the red nucleus in the same preparation to stimulation of the cortico-rubral pathway are sensitive to NMDA antagonists (Davies *et al.* 1986; Harris and Davies 1992). It is of course possible that the resistance to antagonists of the cortico-striatal and interposito-rubral EPSPs merely reflects an inability of the iontophoretically applied NMDA antagonists to penetrate the synaptic cleft of perhaps more distally located NMDA receptor-operated synapses. This seems to be unlikely in the case of the

Table 10.3 Sample of published data on some examples of brain sub-cortical excitatory amino acid pathways, studied *in vivo* or *in vitro*

CNS region	Pathway	Preparation	Rec.	Receptor(s)	Antagonist(s)	Appl'n	References
Cerebellum							
Purkinje cell	parallel fibre	rabbit, *in vivo*	e.c.	non-NMDA	AP5, Kyn	ionto.	Kano and Kato (1987)
		rat, *in vitro* (culture)	p.c.	non-NMDA	AP5, Kyn	bath	Hirano and Hagiwara (1988)
		rat, *in vitro*	p.c.	non-NMDA	CPP, CNQX	bath	Llano et al. (1991)
Purkinje cell	climbing fibre	rat, *in vitro*	p.c.	non-NMDA	CPP, CNQX	bath	Llano et al. (1991)
		guinea pig, *in vitro*	i.c.	non-NMDA/NMDA	AP5, DGG	ionto.	Kimura et al. (1985)
granule cell	mossy fibre	rat, *in vitro*	p.c.	non-NMDA/NMDA	AP5, CNQX	bath	D'Angelo et al. (1990); Silver et al. (1992)
Striatum	cortico-caudate	cat, *in vivo*	i.c.	non-NMDA	AP7, Kyn	ionto.	Herrling (1985)
	cortico-caudate/local	rat, *in vitro*	i.c.	non-NMDA/NMDA	AP7, Kyn	bath	Cherubini et al. (1988)
Thalamus							
ventrobasal	lemniscal afferents	rat, *in vivo*	e.c.	non-NMDA/NMDA	AP5, CPP, Kyn, CNQX, GAMS	ionto.	Salt (1986, 1987); Eaton and Salt (1989)
lateral geniculate	optic nerve	rat, *in vivo*	i.c.	non-NMDA/NMDA	CPP, CNQX	ionto.	Salt and Eaton (1991)
		cat, *in vivo*	e.c.	NMDA/non-NMDA	AP5, CPP, CNQX, Kyn	ionto.	Sillito et al. (1990); Funke et al. (1991)
		rat, *in vitro*	i.c.	non-NMDA	AP5, DGG	bath	Crunelli et al. (1987)
		cat/rat, *in vitro*	i.c.	NMDA/non-NMDA	AP5, CNQX	bath	Soltesz et al. (1989); Scharfman et al. (1990)
		ferret, *in vitro*	i.c.	NMDA/non-NMDA	AP5, CNQX	bath	Esguerra et al. (1992)
		rat, *in vitro*	p.c.	NMDA/non-NMDA	CNQX	bath	Leresche (1992)
ventrolateral	interposito-thalamic	cat, *in vivo*	e.c.	non-NMDA	CPP, GAMS, PZDA	ionto.	Davies and Sheardown (1988)
Red nucleus	interposito-rubral	cat, *in vivo*	e.c.	non-NMDA	AP5, CPP, GAMS, PZDA	ionto.	Davies et al. (1986)
		cat, *in vivo*	i.c.	non-NMDA	AP5, CPP, PZDA, Ket	ionto.	Davies and Sheardown (1988)
	cortico-rubral	cat, *in vivo*	e.c.	non-NMDA/NMDA	CPP, AP5, AP7, PZDA, NBQX	ionto.	Davies et al. (1986); Harris et al. (1992); Harris and Davies (1992)

Abbreviations are as for Table 10.2

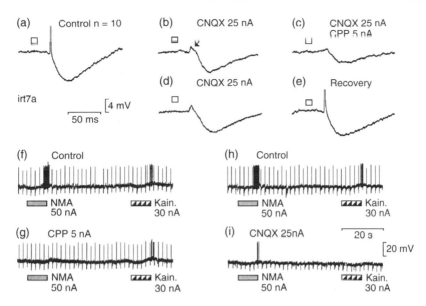

Fig. 10.1 Intracellular recordings from a rat ventrobasal thalamus neurone, *in vivo* (resting membrane potential = −60 mV), showing the effects of the NMDA receptor antagonist CPP and the non-NMDA receptor antagonist CNQX on sensory (air-jet stimulus) EPSPs ((a)–(e)) and agonist-evoked responses ((f–i)). (a) Average of 10 responses to air-jet stimulation (open box above record). Note that the action potential that was evoked by each stimulus in (a) and (e) is truncated. The occurrence of the action potential obscures the sensory EPSP, which is followed by a large hyperpolarizing IPSP (b) Similar records to that in (a) but obtained during the iontophoresis of CNQX. CNQX antagonized the sensory EPSP to such an extent that action potentials were no longer evoked, leaving a residual EPSP component (arrow). (c) When CPP was applied in addition to CNQX, the sensory EPSP that remained during iontophoresis of CNQX alone was reduced to a large extent. (d) Termination of CPP ejection while the CNQX ejection was continued resulted in an increase in EPSP amplitude. (e) When the CNQX ejection was terminated, the responses to sensory stimulation recovered. (f)–(i) Responses of the same neurone to iontophoresis of NMA and kainate (bars beneath the records). (f) and (h) are control records taken prior to ejection of either CPP or CNQX. CPP and CNQX selectively reduced responses to either NMA (g) or kainate (i), respectively. The neuronal activity seen between ejections of the two agonists is that evoked by sensory stimulation (repeated at 0.5 Hz). Note that this is reduced during CNQX ejection. (Reproduced from Salt and Eaton (1991).)

interposito-rubral pathway, as these EPSPs were also found to be resistant to intravenously administered ketamine (Davies and Sheardown 1988). Furthermore, *in vivo*, the cortico-rubral pathway appears to use both NMDA receptors and non-NMDA receptors (Davies *et al.* 1986; Harris *et al.* 1992). An alternative, or additional, possibility is that the NMDA receptor population is heterogeneous, and that the antagonists used in the above studies were inappropriate for NMDA receptors which may be

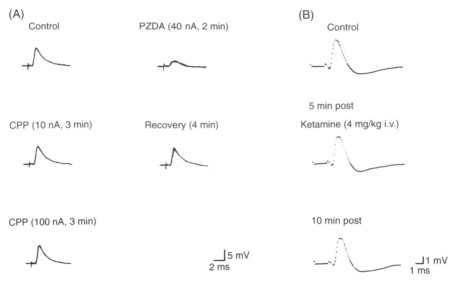

Fig. 10.2 Influence of excitatory amino acid antagonists on interpositus nucleus-evoked monosynaptic EPSPs in rubrospinal neurones of the anaesthetized cat. (A) Superimposed oscilloscope records of the EPSP before and during the ejection of CPP (with 10 nA and then 100 nA) followed by the broad spectrum excitatory amino antagonist PZDA (40 nA) and subsequent recovery. Only PZDA reduced the monosynaptic EPSP. (B) Records of computer-averaged EPSPs from another rubrospinal neurone illustrating the lack of effect of an intravenous injection of ketamine (4 mg/kg) on the interpositus nucleus-evoked synaptic response. (Resting membrane potential of the cells in A and B was −58 and − 64 mV, respectively; stimulus strengths employed to evoke EPSPs were subthreshold for action potential generation.) (Reproduced from Davies (1989).)

synaptic in the interposito-rubral pathway. In this respect it is noteworthy that the 5-carbon chain NMDA antagonist AP5 will antagonize the cortico-rubral pathway, whereas 7-carbon chain antagonists (such as AP7 and CPP) will not block this pathway (Harris and Davies 1992). However, given that both AP5 and CPP have been used in unsuccessful attempts to block the interposito-rubral pathway, this possibility seems remote. The possibility remains, then, that this EPSP is mediated by non-NMDA receptors, with no detectable NMDA receptor component. Further, *in vitro* experiments may shed more light on this matter, as have *in vitro* experiments on the cortico-striatal pathway. In *in vitro* experiments in the rat striatum, an EPSP component has been found which is sensitive to bath-applied AP7, albeit under conditions of reduced Mg^{2+} concentration and membrane depolarization in order to reveal the NMDA component (Cherubini *et al*. 1988). In these latter experiments it was, however, not possible to exclude the possibility that the stimulation protocol activated local circuits rather than, or in addition to, terminals of cortical afferents.

The situation seems to be somewhat clearer in the case of cerebellar Purkinje cells. These neurones are somewhat unusual, in that they possess virtually no NMDA receptors in the adult rat, although NMDA receptors are transiently expressed during development (Crepel *et al.* 1983; Dupont *et al.* 1987; Llano *et al.* 1988; Audinat *et al.* 1990; Krupa and Crepel 1990; Farrant and Cull-Candy 1991), and may be also present in adults of other species (e.g. the guinea pig) (Sekiguchi *et al.* 1987). The two pathways on to Purkinje cells, the parallel fibres arising from cerebellar granule cells, and the climbing fibres arising from the inferior olive, have been extensively studied with extracellular, intracellular, and patch-clamp recording techniques, both *in vivo* and *in vitro* (see Table 10.3). There now seems little doubt, at least in the rat, that EPSPs/EPSCs evoked by electrical stimulation of either of these pathways are mediated by non-NMDA receptors, with no involvement of NMDA receptors (Kano and Kato 1987; Hirano and Hagiwara 1988; Garthwaite and Beaumont 1989; Llano *et al.* 1991). However, in the guinea pig, the climbing-fibre response in Purkinje cell dendrites is sensitive to the NMDA antagonist, AP5. In contrast, granule cells and basket cells appear to have functional NMDA receptors, and the mossy fibre pathway on to rat cerebellar granule cells *in vitro* appears to involve both non-NMDA and NMDA receptors (D'Angelo 1990; Silver *et al.* 1992).

Cortical excitatory amino acid pathways

The first detailed documentation of an intracellularly recorded EPSP with an NMDA receptor-mediated component was obtained in layer II/III neurones of the rat sensorimotor cortex slice preparation. In these studies, an EPSP component was evoked by electrical stimulation of the white matter which had the unconventional voltage-dependence and Mg^{2+} sensitivity which would be predicted for an NMDA receptor-mediated EPSP; this synaptic response was sensitive to both competitive and non-competitive NMDA antagonists, applied iontophoretically in the vicinity of the neurone with appropriate currents (Thomson *et al.* 1985; Thomson 1986). Subsequently, Thomson and her colleagues (1989) were able to show that such EPSPs were dual component non-NMDA/NMDA receptor EPSPs, and that they could be evoked in one layer II/III pyramidal cell by stimulation of another layer II/III pyramidal cell (Fig. 10.3). In the visual cortex slice preparation, similar results have been obtained, in that the output of layer II/III pyramidal cells on to layer V pyramidal cells also seems to evoke a dual non-NMDA/NMDA receptor-mediated EPSP (Jones and Baughman 1988). It is noteworthy in both of these groups of studies that, although the NMDA receptor-mediated EPSP components were sensitive to blockade by Mg^{2+} ions and were increased in amplitude by membrane depolarization, it was possible to see these components clearly at resting potential with Mg^{2+} present in the medium. Other

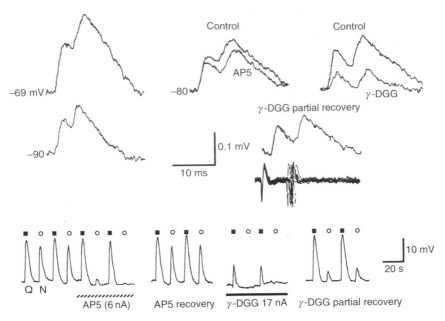

Fig. 10.3 Spike-triggered averages of an EPSP of a layer III cortical neurone recorded at three membrane potentials (−69, −80, and −90 mV) under control conditions, and during electrophoretic ejection of AP5 (6 nA) and DGG (17 nA) at −80 mV. Each record is an average of 512 sweeps. Ten superimposed sweeps of the extracellular recording from the presynaptic neurone are shown and demonstrate that this cell fired pairs of spikes, at short intervals, evoking a double EPSP in the post-synaptic cell. All averaged sweeps were triggered by spike pairs. The variability in the latency and rise time of the second EPSP is due to inevitable small changes in the duration and constancy of the interspike interval during the 3 h recording period. Although AP5 reduced the EPSP amplitude, it had little effect on the early rising phase. In contrast, DGG reduced all phases of the EPSP. The lower records illustrate the responses of the post-synaptic neurone to NMDA (N: 14 nA, 1 s) and quisqualate (Q: 60 nA, 1 s) and their sensitivity to AP5 (6 nA) and DGG (17 nA). Similar reductions in both the response to NMDA and the EPSP are seen during application of AP5 and during partial recovery following DGG. More complete blockade of the EPSP, particularly its rising phase, was always associated with blockade of responses to quisqualate. (Reproduced, with permission, from Thomson *et al.* (1989).)

groups, making intracellular recordings *in vitro* from neurones from various cortical areas, have reported EPSPs which are also dual-component in nature (Table 10.4). More recently, a patch-clamp investigation in the visual cortex slice, recording from layer IV neurones with stimulation of nearby layer IV neurones, has also revealed a dual non-NMDA/NMDA receptor-mediated EPSC (Stern *et al.* 1992). A novel *in vitro* approach has been the development of the mouse thalamo-cortical slice preparation: this allows the recording of somatosensory cortical neurones and their responses to stimulation of the thalamus. In this

Table 10.4 Sample of published data on some examples of cortical excitatory amino acid pathways, studied *in vivo* or *in vitro*

Cortical region	Cortical layer	Preparation	Rec.	Receptor(s)	Antagonist(s)	Appl'n	References
Somatosensory/motor	II/III	rat, *in vitro*	i.c.	non-NMDA/NMDA	AP5, Ket, DGG	ionto.	Thomson et al. (1985, 1989); Thomson (1986)
	IV	mouse, *in vitro*	p.c.	non-NMDA/NMDA	AP5, CNQX	bath	Agmon and O'Dowd (1992)
		cat, *in vivo*	e.c.	non-NMDA/NMDA	AP5, PDA, DNQX, Kyn	ionto.	Hicks et al. (1991)
	IV	rat, *in vivo*	e.c.	non-NMDA/NMDA	AP5, DNQX	ionto.	Armstrong-James et al. (1993)
Visual	V	cat, *in vivo*	i.c.	non-NMDA/NMDA	AP7, CPP, CNQX	ionto.	Herring et al. (1990)
	V	rat, *in vitro*	i.c.	non-NMDA/NMDA	AP5, Kyn	bath	Jones and Baughman (1988)
	II/III	cat/rat, *in vitro*	i.c.	non-NMDA/NMDA	AP5, Kyn, CNQX	bath	Shirokawa et al. (1989); Nishigori et al. (1990)
	IV	rat, *in vitro*	p.c.	non-NMDA/NMDA	AP5, CNQX	bath	Stern et al. (1992)
	II–VI	cat, *in vivo*	e.c.	non-NMDA/NMDA	AP5, Kyn, CNQX	ionto.	Fox et al. (1989, 1990)
	II–VI	cat, *in vivo*	e.c.	non-NMDA/NMDA	AP5, Kyn	ionto.	Tsumoto et al. (1986); Hagihara et al. (1988)
Auditory	II–VI	rat/guinea pig, *in vitro*	i.c.	non-NMDA/NMDA	AP5, DNQX	bath	Cox et al. (1992)
Entorhinal	IV/V	rat, *in vitro*	i.c.	non-NMDA/NMDA	AP5	bath	Jones (1987)
Olfactory	Olfactory tract	rat/mouse, *in vitro*	e.c./i.d.	non-NMDA/NMDA	AP5, PDA, Kyn, DNQX	bath	Collins (1991); Collins and Howlett (1988)

Abbreviations are as for Table 10.2

preparation, stimulation of the thalamus has been shown to evoke an EPSC in cortical neurones with a substantial NMDA receptor-mediated component in immature tissue where inhibitory synaptic mechanisms are incompletely developed (Agmon and O'Dowd 1992).

Cortical excitatory amino acid transmission has also been investigated in several *in vivo* studies, using extracellular recording and iontophoresis. In such studies, as in many *in vitro* studies, it is difficult to know precisely which pathways are activated, following either electrical stimulation of the thalamus or natural sensory stimulation (either visual or somatosensory), as both types of stimuli are likely to recruit additional local circuit pathways in addition to the direct thalamo-cortical projection. Nevertheless, the data obtained in these various studies point to an involvement of both NMDA receptors and non-NMDA receptors in cortical synaptic transmission (Tsumoto *et al.* 1986; Hagihara *et al.* 1988; Fox *et al.* 1989, 1990; Hicks *et al.* 1991; Armstrong-James *et al.* 1993), and it has been suggested that NMDA receptors have a more prominent synaptic role in local cortical circuits than in direct thalamic input (Hagihara *et al.* 1988; Armstrong-James *et al.* 1993). This would be consistent with the *in vitro* data discussed above. Recently, intracellular recording from physiologically identified cat motor cortex pyramidal tract neurones, *in vivo*, has indicated that EPSPs evoked by thalamic stimulation show little or no NMDA receptor involvement, but that recurrent cortical EPSPs show substantial NMDA receptor-mediated components (Fig. 10.4) (Herrling *et al.* 1990). It is also noteworthy that such cortico-cortical EPSPs are of longer duration than EPSPs evoked by thalamic stimulation.

Physiological considerations

The possible role(s) of the NMDA receptor in processes such as learning and memory, epilepsy, and neurodegeneration are described in detail elsewhere in this volume. The preceding discussion has indicated that at many, but not all, central synapses there is dual non-NMDA/NMDA receptor-mediated transmission, although this may be to varying degrees. Furthermore, although the NMDA component of transmission may be difficult to reveal in some experimental situations, it appears that the NMDA receptor does play an important role in transmission under physiological conditions at many central synapses. Under physiological conditions, that is with Mg^{2+} ions present in the extracellular medium, the NMDA receptor channel complex is likely to be in a partially blocked state, thus effectively conferring voltage-dependency on NMDA receptor-mediated responses (Mayer *et al.* 1984; Nowak *et al.* 1984). This makes them eminently suitable for both temporal and spatial integrative functions. The involvement of NMDA receptors in temporal integration upon repetitive neuronal synaptic input has been proposed in both the hippo-

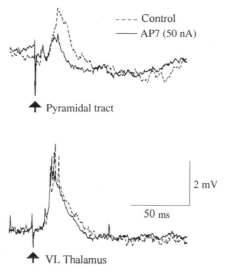

Fig. 10.4 Effects of excitatory amino acid antagonists on EPSPs evoked in a pyramidal tract neurone in the motor cortex of the anaesthetized cat by stimulation of either the ventrolateral thalamus or the pyramidal tract. This latter stimulus activates recurrent collaterals within Layer V of the motor cortex. (a) Superimposed synaptic potentials evoked by stimulation (arrow) of the pyramidal tract (average of 20 sweeps) under control conditions and during iontophoresis of the NMDA antagonist AP7. Note that AP7 reduced the peak of the EPSP and the late phase, with little effect on the early rising phase of the EPSP. (b) EPSPs (average of 15 sweeps) evoked by stimulation of the ventrolateral (VL) thalamus of the same neurone under control conditions and during AP7 ejection. Note that the antagonist had little effect on the EPSP evoked by thalamic stimulation. The same ejection current of AP7 (50 nA) was found to antagonize responses to iontophoretically applied NMDA but not AMPA. (Previously unpublished observations of P. L. Herrling and T. E. Salt.)

campus (Herron *et al.* 1986) and the thalamus (Salt 1986), and is likely also to occur in other locations. The finding that NMDA receptors and non-NMDA receptors are co-localized at the same synapses (Bekkers and Stevens 1989; Jones and Baughman 1991) would provide an anatomical substrate for such mechanisms. The possibilities of NMDA receptor involvement in spatial integrative mechanisms have not been the subject of explicit studies. However, the responses of visual cortical neurones, *in vivo*, to natural stimuli such as moving bars of light are the result of both temporal and spatial cortical integration, and such responses are susceptible to NMDA antagonists (Fox *et al.* 1989, 1990).

Given that there is substantial co-activation of NMDA and non-NMDA receptors at many synapses, it seems likely that other excitatory amino acid receptors are also involved in synaptic processes. The metabotropic excitatory amino acid receptor family has received considerable attention recently, and these receptors have been localized in many brain areas

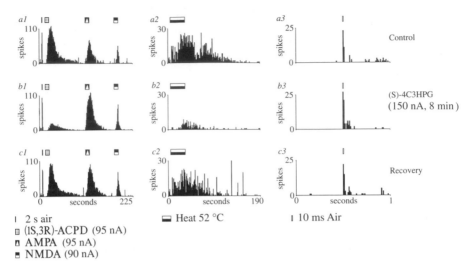

I 2 s air	⌷ Heat 52 °C I 10 ms Air
⊞ (1S,3R)-ACPD (95 nA)	
⬠ AMPA (95 nA)	
▪ NMDA (90 nA)	

Fig. 10.5 The selective antagonism, by (S)-4-carboxy-3-hydroxyphenylglycine [(S)-4C3HPG], of (1S,3R)-ACPD-induced neural firing and antagonism of the nociceptive response of a ventrobasal thalamus neurone responsive to air-jet stimulation and to noxious thermal stimulation in the anaesthetized rat. Each record is a histogram of action potential spikes counted into successive 1 s (records a1–c1 and a2–c2) or 10 ms (records a3–b3) epochs. In all records, the bars above the records indicate the timing and duration of iontophoretic agonist application or sensory stimulation. (a1) Control responses to an air jet (2 s) directed at the receptive field, (1S,3R)-ACPD, AMPA, and NMDA. (a2) Control response to noxious thermal stimulation. (a3) Control responses to 10 successive 10 ms air-jet stimuli, as a cumulative histogram. (b1–b3) The same sequences of stimuli and agonists as in the control records, but during the concurrent iontophoresis of (S)-4C3HPG. Note that the responses to (1S, 3R)-ACPD and to noxious stimulation are reduced selectively. (c1–c3) The effects of the antagonist were reversible, as shown in these records, taken 5 min after the end of the antagonist ejection. (Reproduced from Eaton *et al.* (1993).)

(Masu *et al.* 1991; Martin *et al.* 1992). The selective agonist (1S, 3R)-ACPD has been shown to have a variety of effects on neurones in various regions (Schoepp *et al.* 1990; Miller 1991). Some of these actions are likely to be mediated via changes in inositol phosphate metabolism, whilst others appear to be mediated via cyclic nucleotides. Synaptic events have been isolated which resemble (1S,3R)-ACPD-evoked responses, and thus have been suggested to be metabotropic receptor-mediated responses (Glaum and Miller 1992; McCormick and Von Krosigk 1992). However, studies of the possible synaptic role(s) of these receptors have been hampered by the lack of suitably selective antagonists. Recently, Watkins and his colleagues have developed a series of compounds, some of which are effective antagonists of (1S,3R)-ACPD-stimulated inositol phosphate turnover and (1S,3R)-ACPD-evoked depolarizations, and excitations (Birse *et al.* 1993). These compounds have now been used in a study of synaptic pharmacology in the thalamus, and it has been found that the responses of thalamic neurones, *in vivo*, to noxious sensory stimulation were sensitive to these (1S,3R)-ACPD antagonists, applied iontophoretically (Fig. 10.5) (Eaton *et al*. 1992, 1993). Given the high density of mGluR1, post-synaptically, in the thalamus (Martin *et al*. 1992), it is tempting to speculate that there is metabotropic involvement in the responses of thalamic neurones to noxious stimuli. It is of interest that previous work from the same laboratory had shown that these responses also showed substantial NMDA receptor involvement (Eaton and Salt 1990). The possibility that there is a functional interaction between NMDA receptors and metabotropic receptors is intriguing (Challiss *et al*. 1993), and will no doubt be the subject of much future work.

Acknowledgements

This chapter is dedicated to the memory of John Davies, one of the pioneers in the field of excitatory amino acid synaptic pharmacology. I would like to thank Dr P. L. Herrling for helpful discussions and comments on the manuscript.

References

Agmon, A. and O'Dowd, D. K. (1992). NMDA receptor-mediated currents are prominent in the thalamocortical synaptic response before maturation of inhibition. *Journal of Neurophysiology*, **68**, 345–9.

Armstrong-James, M., Welker, E., and Callahan, C. A. (1993). The contribution of NMDA and non-NMDA receptors to fast and slow transmission of sensory information in the rat S1 barrel cortex. *Journal of Neuroscience*, **13**, 2149–60.

Artola, A. and Singer, W. (1987). Long-term potentiation and NMDA receptors in rat visual cortex. *Nature*, **330**, 649–52.

Audinat, E., Knöpfel, T., and Gähwiler, B. H. (1990). Responses to excitatory amino acids of Purkinje cells and neurones of the deep nuclei in cerebellar slice cultures. *Journal of Physiology*, **430**, 297–313.

Bekkers, J. M. and Stevens, C. F. (1989). NMDA and non-NMDA receptors are co-localized at individual excitatory synapses in cultured rat hippocampus. *Nature*, **341**, 230–3.

Birse, E. F., Eaton, S. A., Jane, D. E., Jones, P. L. S. J., Porter, R. H. P., Pook, P. C.-K., Sunter, D. C., Udvarhelyi, P. M., Wharton, B., Roberts, P. J., Salt, T. E., and Watkins, J. C. (1993). Phenylglycine derivatives as new pharmacological tools for investigating the role of metabotropic glutamate receptors in the central nervous system. *Neuroscience*, **52**, 481–8.

Challiss, R. A. J., Mistry, R., Gray, D. W., and Nahorski, S. R. (1993). Effect of NMDA on 1S,3R-ACPD-stimulated phosphoinositide hydrolysis in neonatal rat cerebral cortex slices. *British Journal of Pharmacology*, **108**, 85.

Cherubini, E., Herrling, P. L., Lanfumey, L., and Stanzione, P. (1988). Excitatory amino acids in synaptic excitation of rat striatal neurones in vitro. *Journal of Physiology*, **400**, 677–90.

Collingridge, G. L., Herron, C. E., and Lester, R. A. J. (1988). Synaptic activation of N-methyl-D-aspartate receptors in the Schaffer collateral-commissural pathway of rat hippocampus. *Journal of Physiology*, **399**, 283–300.

Collins, G. G. S. (1991). Pharmacological evidence that NMDA receptors contribute to mono- and di-synaptic potentials in slices of mouse olfactory cortex. *Neuropharmacology*, **30**, 547–55.

Collins, G. G. S. and Howlett, S. J. (1988). The pharmacology of excitatory transmission in the rat olfactory cortex slice. *Neuropharmacology*, **27**, 697–705.

Cox, C. L., Metherate, R., Weinberger, N. M., and Ashe, J. H. (1992). Synaptic potentials and effects of amino acid antagonists in the auditory cortex. *Brain Research Bulletin*, **28**, 401–10.

Crepel, F., Dupont, J.-L., and Gardette, R. (1983). Voltage clamp analysis of the effect of excitatory amino-acids and derivatives on Purkinje cell dendrites in rat cerebellar slices maintained in vitro. *Brain Research*, **279**, 311–15.

Crunelli, V., Kelly, J. S., Leresche, N., and Pirchio, M. (1987). On the excitatory postsynaptic potential evoked by stimulation of the optic tract in the rat lateral geniculate nucleus. *Journal of Physiology*, **384**, 603–18.

D'Angelo, E., Rossi, P., and Garthwaite, J. (1990). Dual-component NMDA receptor currents at a single central synapse. *Nature*, **346**, 467–70.

Davies, J. (1988). A reappraisal of the role of NMDA and non-NMDA receptors in neurotransmission in the cat dorsal horn. In *Frontiers in excitatory amino acid research*, (ed. E. Cavalheiro, J. Lehman, and L. Turski), pp. 355–62. Alan R. Liss Inc., New York.

Davies J. (1989). NMDA receptors in synaptic pathways. In *The NMDA receptor*, (ed. J. C. Watkins and G. L. Collingridge), pp. 77–91. Oxford University Press.

Davies, J. and Sheardown, M. J. (1988). Which excitatory amino acid receptors mediate interpositus afferent-evoked monosynaptic excitation in the red nucleus and thalamus? In *Frontiers in excitatory amino acid research*, (ed. E. Cavalheiro, J. Lehman, and L. Turski), pp. 137–44. Alan R. Liss Inc., New York.

Davies, J. and Watkins, J. C. (1977). Effect of magnesium ions on the responses of spinal neurones to excitatory amino acids and acetylcholine. *Brain Research*, **130**, 364–8.

Davies, J. and Watkins, J. C. (1979). Selective antagonism of amino acid-induced and synaptic excitation in the cat spinal cord. *Journal of Physiology*, **297**, 621–35.

Davies, J. and Watkins, J. C. (1982). Actions of D and L forms of 2-amino-5-phosphonovalerate and 2-amino-4-phosphonobutyrate in the cat spinal cord. *Brain Research*, **235**, 378–86.

Davies, J. and Watkins, J. C. (1983). Role of excitatory amino acid receptors in mono- and polysynaptic excitation in the cat spinal cord. *Experimental Brain Research*, **49**, 280–90.

Davies, J. and Watkins, J. C. (1985). Depressant actions of γ-D-glutamylaminomethyl sulfonate (GAMS) on amino acid-induced and synaptic excitation in the cat spinal cord. *Brain Research*, **327**, 113–20.

Davies, J., Evans, R. H., Jones, A. W., Smith, D. A. S., and Watkins, J. C. (1982). Differential activation and blockade of excitatory amino acid receptors in the mammalian and amphibian central nervous systems. *Comparative Biochemistry and Physiology*, **72C**, 211–24.

Davies, J., Miller, A. J., and Sheardown, M. J. (1986). Amino acid receptor mediated excitatory synaptic transmission in the cat red nucleus. *Journal of Physiology*, **376**, 13–29.

Dougherty, P. M. and Willis, W. D. (1991). Modification of the responses of primate spinothalamic neurons to mechanical stimulation by excitatory amino acids and an *N*-methyl-D-aspartate antagonist. *Brain Research*, **542**, 15–22.

Dupont, J. L., Gardette, R., and Crepel, F. (1987). Postnatal development of the chemosensitivity of rat cerebellar Purkinje cells to excitatory amino acids. An in vitro study. *Developmental Brain Research*, **34**, 59–68.

Eaton, S. A. and Salt, T. E. (1990). Thalmic NMDA receptors and nociceptive sensory synaptic transmission. *Neuroscience Letters*, **110**, 297–302.

Eaton, S. A. and Salt, T. E. (1991). Membrane and action potential responses evoked by excitatory amino acids acting at *N*-methyl-D-aspartate receptors and non-*N*-methyl-D-aspartate receptors in the rat thalamus in vivo. *Neuroscience*, **44**, 277–86.

Eaton, S. A., Salt, T. E., Sunter, D. C., Udvarhelyi, P. M., and Watkins, J. C. (1992). Antagonism of nociceptive responses of rat thalamic neurones in vivo by novel antagonists of (1S,3R)-ACPD. *British Journal of Pharmacology*, **107**, 244P.

Eaton, S. A., Birse, E. F., Wharton, B., Sunter, D. C., Udvarhelyi, P. M., Watkins, J. C., and Salt, T. E. (1993). Mediation of thalamic sensory responses in vivo by ACPD-activated excitatory amino acid receptors. *European Journal of Neuroscience*, **5**, 186–9.

Esguerra, M., Kwon, Y. H., and Sur, M. (1992). Retinogeniculate EPSPs recorded intracellularly in the ferret lateral geniculate nucleus in vitro: Role of NMDA receptors. *Visual Neuroscience*, **8**, 545–55.

Farrant, M. and Cull-Candy, S. G. (1991). Excitatory amino acid receptor-channels in Purkinje cells in thin cerebellar slices. *Proceedings of the Royal Society* (London), Series B, **244**, 179–84.

Forsythe, I. D. and Westbrook, G. L. (1988). Slow excitatory postsynaptic currents mediated by *N*-methyl-D-aspartate receptors on cultured mouse central neurones. *Journal of Physiology*, **396**, 515–33.

Fox, K., Sato, H., and Daw, N. (1989). The location and function of NMDA receptors in cat and kitten visual cortex. *Journal of Neuroscience*, **9**, 2443–54.

Fox, K., Sato, H., and Daw, N. (1990). The effect of varying stimulus intensity on NMDA-receptor activity in cat visual cortex. *Journal of Neurophysiology*, **64**, 1413–28.

Funke, K., Eysel, U. T., and FitzGibbon, T. (1991). Retinogeniculate transmission by NMDA and non-NMDA receptors in the cat. *Brain Research*, **547**, 229–38.

Garthwaite, J. and Beaumont, P. S. (1989). Excitatory amino acid receptors in the parallel fibre pathway in rat cerebellar slices. *Neuroscience Letters*, **107**, 151–6.

Gasic, G. P. and Hollmann, M. (1992). Molecular neurobiology of glutamate receptors. *Annual Review of Physiology*, **54**, 507–36.

Gerber, G. and Randic, M. (1989). Excitatory amino acid-mediated components of synaptically evoked input from dorsal roots to deep dorsal horn neurons in the rat spinal cord slice. *Neuroscience Letters*, **106**, 211–19.

Glaum, S. R. and Miller, R. J. (1992). Metabotropic glutamate receptors mediate excitatory transmission in the nucleus of the solitary tract. *Journal of Neuroscience*, **12**, 2251–8.

Hagihara, K., Tsumoto, T., Sato, H., and Hata, Y. (1988). Actions of excitatory amino acid antagonists on geniculo-cortical transmission in the cat's visual cortex. *Experimental Brain Research*, **69**, 407–16.

Harris, N. C. and Davies, J. (1992). Cortically evoked excitatory synaptic

262   *Synaptic transmission in the mammalian central nervous system*

transmission in the cat red nucleus is antagonised by D-AP5 but not by D-AP7. *Brain Research*, **594**, 176–80.

Harris, N. C., Qune, M., and Davies, J. (1992). Involvement of NMDA and non-NMDA receptors in monosynaptic excitatory transmission in the cat red nucleus in vivo. *British Journal of Pharmacology*, **104**, 386P.

Headley, P. M., Parsons, C. G., and West, D. C. (1987). The role of *N*-methylaspartate receptors in mediating responses of rat and cat spinal neurones to defined sensory stimuli. *Journal of Physiology*, **385**, 169–88.

Herrling, P. L. (1985). Pharmacology of the corticocaudate excitatory post-synaptic potential in the cat: evidence for its mediation by quisqualate- or kainate-receptors. *Neuroscience*, **14**, 417–26.

Herrling, P. L., Meier, C. L., Salt, T. E., and Seno, N. (1990). Involvement of NMDA receptors and non-NMDA receptors in cortico-cortical and thalamo-cortical excitatory postsynaptic potentials in the anaesthetized cat. *Journal of Physiology*, **425**, 89P.

Herron, C. E., Lester, R. A. J., Coan, E. J., and Collingridge, G. L. (1986). Frequency-dependent involvement of NMDA receptors in the hippocampus: a novel synaptic mechanism. *Nature*, **322**, 265–7.

Hestrin, S., Nicoll, R. A., Perkel, D. J., and Sah, P. (1990a). Analysis of excitatory synaptic action in pyramidal cells using whole-cell recording from rat hippo-campal slices. *Journal of Physiology*, **422**, 203–25.

Hestrin, S., Sah, P., and Nicoll, R. A. (1990b). Mechanisms generating the time course of dual component excitatory synaptic currents recorded in hippocampal slices. *Neuron*, **5**, 247–53.

Hicks, T. P., Kaneko, T., Metherate, R., Oka, J.-I., and Stark, C. A. (1991). Amino acids as transmitters of synaptic excitation in neocortical sensory pro-cesses. *Canadian Journal of Physiology and Pharmacology*, **69**, 1099–114.

Hill, R. G. and Salt, T. E. (1982). An ionophoretic study of the responses of rat caudal trigeminal nucleus neurones to non-noxious mechanical sensory stimuli. *Journal of Physiology*, **327**, 65–78.

Hirano, T. and Hagiwara, S. (1988). Synaptic transmission between rat cerebellar granule and Purkinje cells in dissociated cell culture: Effects of excitatory amino acid transmitter antagonists. *Proceedings of the National Academy of Sciences, USA*, **85**, 934–8.

Jahr, C. E. and Yoshioka, K. (1986). 1a afferent excitation of motoneurones in the in vitro new-born rat spinal cord is selectively antagonized by kynurenate. *Journal of Physiology*, **370**, 515–30.

Jeftinija, S. (1989). Excitatory transmission in the dorsal horn is in part mediated through APV-sensitive NMDA receptors. *Neuroscience Letters*, **96**, 191–6.

Jones, K. A. and Baughman, R. W. (1988). NMDA- and non-NMDA-receptor components of excitatory synaptic potentials recorded from cells in layer V of rat visual cortex. *Journal of Neuroscience*, **8**, 3522–34.

Jones, K. A. and Baughman, R. W. (1991). Both NMDA and non-NMDA sub-types of glutamate receptors are concentrated at synapses on cerebral cortical neurons in culture. *Neuron*, **7**, 593–603.

Jones, R. S. G. (1987). Complex synaptic responses of entorhinal cortical cells in the rat to subicular stimulation in vitro: demonstration of an NMDA receptor-mediated component. *Neuroscience Letters*, **81**, 209–14.

Kano, M. and Kato, M. (1987). Quisqualate receptors are specifically involved in cerebellar synaptic plasticity. *Nature*, **325**, 276–9.

Kimura, H., Okamoto, K., and Sakai, Y. (1985). Pharmacological evidence for L-aspartate as the neurotransmitter of cerebellar climbing fibres in the guinea-pig. *Journal of Physiology*, **365**, 103–19.

King, A. E., Lopez-Garcia, J. A., and Cumberbatch, M. (1992). Antagonism of synaptic potentials in ventral horn neurones by 6-cyano-7-nitroquinoxaline-2,3-dione: a study in the rat spinal cord in vitro. *British Journal of Pharmacology*, **107**, 375–81.

Konnerth, A., Keller, B. U., Ballanyi, K., and Yaari, Y. (1990). Voltage sensitivity of NMDA-receptor mediated postsynaptic currents. *Experimental Brain Research*, **81**, 209–12.

Konnerth, A., Keller, B. U., and Lev-Tov, A. (1991). Patch clamp analysis of excitatory synapses in mammalian spinal cord slices. *Pflüger's Archiv/European Journal of Physiology*, **417**, 285–90.

Krupa, M. and Crepel, F. (1990). Transient sensitivity of rat cerebellar Purkinje cells to N-methyl-D-aspartate during development. A voltage clamp study in in vitro slices. *European Journal of Neuroscience*, **2**, 312–16.

Leresche, N. (1992). Synaptic currents in thalamo-cortical neurons of the rat lateral geniculate nucleus. *European Journal of Neuroscience*, **4**, 595–602.

Lester, R. A. J., Clements, J. D., Westbrook, G. L., and Jahr, C. E. (1990). Channel kinetics determine the time course of NMDA receptor-mediated synaptic currents. *Nature*, **346**, 565–7.

Llano, I., Marty, A., Johnson, J. W., Ascher, P., and Gähwiler, B. H. (1988). Patch-clamp recording of amino-acid activated responses in 'organotypic' slice cultures. *Proceedings of the National Academy of Sciences, USA*, **85**, 3221–5.

Llano, I., Marty, A., Armstrong, C. M., and Konnerth, A. (1991). Synaptic and agonist-induced excitatory currents of Purkinje cells in rat cerebellar slices. *Journal of Physiology*, **434**, 183–213.

Lo, F. S. and Sherman, S. M. (1989). Dependence of retinogeniculate transmission on membrane voltage in the cat. Differences between X and Y cells. *European Journal of Neuroscience*, **1**, 204–9.

Long, S. K., Smith, D. A. S., Siarey, R. J., and Evans, R. H. (1990). Effect of 6-cyano-2,3-dihydroxy-7-nitro-quinoxaline (CNQX) on dorsal root-, NMDA-, kainate- and quisqualate-mediated depolarization of rat motoneurones in vitro. *British Journal of Pharmacology*, **100**, 850–4.

McCormick, D. A. and Von Krosigk, M. (1992). Corticothalamic activation modulates thalamic firing through glutamate 'metabotropic' receptors. *Proceedings of the National Academy of Sciences, USA*, **89**, 2774–8.

Martin, L. J., Blackstone, C. D., Huganir, R. L., and Price, D. L. (1992). Cellular localization of a metabotropic glutamate receptor in rat brain. *Neuron*, **9**, 259–70.

Masu, M., Tanabe, Y., Tsuchida, K., Shigemoto, R., and Nakanishi, S. (1991). Sequence and expression of a metabotropic glutamate receptor. *Nature*, **349**, 760–5.

Mayer, M. L., Westbrook, G. L., and Guthrie, P. B. (1984). Voltage-dependent block by Mg^{2+} of NMDA responses in spinal cord neurones. *Nature*, **309**, 261–3.

Miller, R. J. (1991). Metabotropic excitatory amino acid receptors reveal their true colors. *Trends in Pharmacological Sciences*, **12**, 365–7.

Morris, R. (1989). Responses of spinal dorsal horn neurones evoked by myelinated primary afferent stimulation are blocked by excitatory amino acid antagonists acting at kainate/quisqualate receptors. *Neuroscience Letters*, **105**, 79–85.

Nishigori, A., Tsumoto, T., and Kimura, F. (1990). Contribution of quisqualate/kainate and NMDA receptors to excitatory synaptic transmission in the rat's visual cortex. *Visual Neuroscience*, **5**, 591–604.

Nowak, L., Bregestovski, P., Ascher, P., Herbet, A., and Prochiantz, A. (1984). Magnesium gates glutamate-activated channels in mouse central neurones. *Nature*, **307**, 462–5.

Sah, P., Hestrin, S., and Nicoll, R. A. (1990). Properties of excitatory postsynaptic currents recorded in vitro from rat hippocampal interneurones. *Journal of Physiology*, **430**, 605–16.

Salt, T. E. (1986). Mediation of thalamic sensory input by both NMDA and non-NMDA receptors. *Nature*, **322**, 263–5.

Salt, T. E. (1987). Excitatory amino acid receptors and synaptic transmission in the rat ventrobasal thalamus. *Journal of Physiology*, **391**, 499–510.

Salt, T. E. and Eaton, S. A. (1989). Function of non-NMDA receptors and NMDA receptors in synaptic responses to natural somatosensory stimulation in the ventrobasal thalamus. *Experimental Brain Research*, **77**, 646–52.

Salt, T. E. and Eaton, S. A. (1990). Postsynaptic potentials evoked in ventro-basal thalamus neurones by natural sensory stimuli. *Neuroscience Letters*, **114**, 295–9.

Salt, T. E. and Eaton, S. A (1991). Sensory excitatory postsynaptic potentials mediated by NMDA and non-NMDA receptors in the thalamus in vivo. *European Journal of Neuroscience*, **3**, 296–300.

Salt, T. E., Wilson, D. G., and Prasad, S. K. (1988). Antagonism of *N*-methylaspartate and synaptic responses of neurones in the rat ventrobasal thalamus by ketamine and MK-801. *British Journal of Pharmacology*, **94**, 443–8.

Scharfman, H. E., Lu, S.-M., Guido, W., Adams, P. R., and Sherman, S. M. (1990). *N*-methyl-D-aspartate receptors contribute to excitatory postsynaptic potentials of cat lateral geniculate neurons recorded in thalamic slices. *Proceedings of the National Academy of Sciences, USA*, **87**, 4548–52.

Schoepp, D., Bockaert, J., and Sladeczek, F. (1990). Pharmacological and functional characteristics of metabotropic excitatory amino acid receptors. *Trends in Pharmacological Sciences*, **11**, 508–15.

Sekiguchi, M., Okamoto, K., and Sakai, Y. (1987). NMDA receptors on Purkinje cell dendrites in guinea pig cerebellar slices. *Brain Research*, **437**, 402–6.

Shirokawa, T., Nishigori, A., Kimura, F., and Tsumoto, T. (1989). Actions of excitatory amino acid antagonists on synaptic potentials of layer II/III neurons of the cat's visual cortex. *Experimental Brain Research*, **78**, 489–500.

Sillito, A. M., Murphy, P. C., and Salt, T. E. (1990). The contribution of the non-*N*-methyl-D-aspartate group of excitatory amino acid receptors to retinogeniculate transmission in the cat. *Neuroscience*, **34**, 273–80.

Silver, R. A., Traynelis, S. F., and Cull-Candy, S. G. (1992). Rapid-time-course miniature and evoked excitatory currents at cerebellar synapses in situ. *Nature*, **355**, 163–6.

Soltesz, I., Haby, M., Jassik-Gerschenfeld, D., Leresche, N., and Crunelli, V. (1989). NMDA and non-NMDA receptors mediate both high and low frequency synaptic potentials in the rat lateral geniculate nucleus. *Society for Neuroscience Abstracts*, **15**, 1310.

Stern, P., Edwards, F. A., and Sakmann, B. (1992). Fast and slow components of unitary EPSCs on stellate cells elicited by focal stimulation in slices of rat visual cortex. *Journal of Physiology*, **449**, 247–78.

Stone, T. W. (1985). *Microiontophoresis and pressure ejection*. IBRO Handbook Series, *Methods in Neurosciences*, Vol. 8. John Wiley & Sons, Chichester.

Thomson, A. M. (1986). A magnesium-sensitive post-synaptic potential in rat cerebral cortex resembles neuronal responses to N-methylaspartate. *Journal of Physiology*, **370**, 531–49.

Thomson, A. M. and Radpour, S. (1991). Excitatory connections between CA1 pyramidal cells revealed by spike triggered averaging in slices of rat hippocampus are partially NMDA receptor mediated. *European Journal of Neuroscience*, **3**, 587–601.

Thomson, A. M., West, D. C., and Lodge, D. (1985). An N-methylaspartate receptor-mediated synapse in rat cerebral cortex: a site action of ketamine? *Nature*, **313**, 479–81.

Thomson, A. M., Girdlestone, D., and West, D. C. (1989). A local circuit neocortical synapse that operates via both NMDA and non-NMDA receptors. *British Journal of Pharmacology*, **96**, 406–8.

Tsumoto, T., Masui, H., and Sato, H. (1986). Excitatory amino acid transmitters in neuronal circuits of the cat visual cortex. *Journal of Neurophysiology*, **55**, 469–83.

Ziskind-Conhaim, L. (1990). NMDA receptors mediate poly-and monosynaptic potentials in motoneurons of rat embryos. *Journal of Neuroscience*, **10**, 125–35.

11 The importance of NMDA receptors in the processing of spinal primary afferent input

R. H. EVANS

Introduction

This chapter covers the following aspects which are relevant to the role of N-methyl-D-aspartate (NMDA) receptors in spinal neurotransmission:

(1) the involvement of NMDA receptors and the co-agonist glycine site in long duration spinal reflexes elicited from dorsal roots;

(2) the relationship between glutamatergic and peptidergic transmission from primary afferent C fibres;

(3) the selective depression of NMDA-receptive excitatory pathways by analgesic and myorelaxant drugs.

Long duration spinal reflexes

The absence of Mg^{2+} from the frog Ringer's solution used to bathe isolated spinal cord preparations led to the discovery of the NMDA receptor as a pharmacological entity (Evans *et al.* 1977*a*) and ultimately to the discovery of the special interaction between Mg^{2+} and the NMDA receptor channel (Nowak *et al.* 1984). Although the extracellular fluids of frogs and rats contain similar levels of Mg^{2+} (see Conway 1957), for traditional reasons Mg^{2+} ions are not added to Ringer's solution. In bathing media containing physiological levels of Mg^{2+} (approximately 1 mM) isolated spinal preparations of frog or rat show much reduced spontaneous synaptic activity but considerable enhancement of synaptic reflexes elicited following electrical stimulation of a dorsal root. Such reflexes elicited by a single shock to a dorsal root in medium containing 1–2 mM Mg^{2+} are sustained for many seconds. The shorter lasting components of EPSPs evoked monosynaptically from primary afferent fibres are mediated at non-NMDA receptors whereas longer-lasting components are mediated at NMDA receptors (Yoshimura and Jessell 1990). This finding is consistent with the first observations on monosynaptic EPSPs evoked from sensory nerves of *Xenopus* embryo spinal cord (Dale and Roberts 1985). A similar pharmacological profile is seen in other regions of the central nervous system (CNS) (see Collingridge and Lester 1989).

In particular, synaptic potentials evoked at relatively high stimulus intensities show components that have durations in excess of 30 s. Such long-lasting events in ventral roots following stimulation of an ipsilateral dorsal root were first reported by Evans (1986). More recently similar events have been recorded as EPSPs from substantia gelatinosa neurones following stimuli appropriate for activation of Aδ afferent fibres (Yoshimura and Jessell 1989). Long duration reflexes can under appropriate circumstances be completely abolished by NMDA receptor antagonists (Fig. 11.1) (Evans 1986; Siarey *et al.* 1992). Because they depend upon the presence of Mg^{2+}, the enduring character of these reflexes could be explained by positive feedback resulting from the unblocking of NMDA receptor channels as

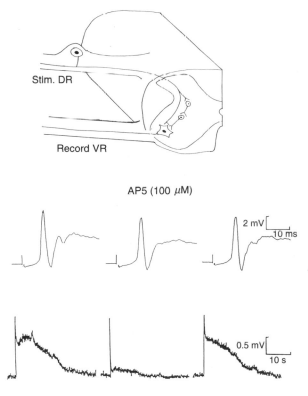

Fig. 11.1 Effect of the NMDA receptor antagonist on synaptic potentials recorded across a grease gap over the ventral root (VR) of a 5 day old rat *in vitro* spinal cord preparation. The synaptic responses were evoked by stimulation of a dorsal root (DR), as depicted in the diagram, at 90 s intervals. The NMDA receptor antagonist AP5 (100 μM) had little or no effect on the early part of the response (upper traces). However, the long lasting VR response (lower traces) was almost abolished at this concentration. Records are shown, from left to right, 5 min before introduction, 15 min after introduction, and 20 min after washout of AP5. The upper and lower records are of the same evoked response. Data from experiments of Siarey *et al.* (1992).

suggested by Collingridge *et al.* (1988) for EPSPs in the hippocampus. The voltage-dependent unblocking of the NMDA receptor channel at spinal cord neurones could provide the central basis for an intensity-related coding of sensory modality (see Cervero and Janig 1992). Evidence for a role of NMDA receptors in long-term modulation of primary afferent input has been provided by the observation that wind-up of peripherally evoked synaptic excitation in the dorsal horn was prevented by an NMDA receptor antagonist. (Davies and Lodge 1987). Indeed, a key role for NMDA receptors in the central processing of nociception is to be expected following discovery of them by sensory physiologists (see Berinaga 1992).

It has been reported that long duration synaptic potentials in spinal preparations are a property of early development because in rats older than 10 days, synaptic potentials are of much shorter duration than in younger rats (Gibbs and Kendig 1992). However, such comparisons between spinal root recordings from animals of different ages should be cautiously interpreted. Myelination of spinal root fibres may be more significant than developmental changes in pharmacological receptor distribution as a cause of the apparent decrease in duration of synaptic response. Certainly, increased myelination is likely to explain the apparent loss in sensitivity to substance P (Gibbs and Kendig 1992).

The role of the glycine co-agonist site of the NMDA receptor complex in spinal transmission

Enhancement by D-serine of excitation induced by NMDA (Birch *et al.* 1988; Brugger *et al.* 1990; Siarey *et al.* 1991) or electrical stimulation of dorsal roots (Siarey *et al.* 1991) was seen only in the presence of an antagonist (CNQX) of the glycine site (Fig. 11.2).

Relationship between tachykinin and NMDA receptors

Because they are evoked at stimulus intensities sufficient to activate primary afferent C fibres, long duration spinal reflexes have been attributed to synaptic transmission from these fibres and more specifically to release of substance P (Akagi and Yanagisawa 1987) and the calcitonin gene-related peptide (Woodley and Kendig 1991) from their central terminals. It is difficult to activate C fibres electrically in the absence of activation of A and/or A, Aβ, and Aδ fibres. In particular there is the problem of repetitive firing of A fibres which can occur following a single high intensity shock. This phenomenon can be seen in Figure 1 of Thompson *et al.* (1990). Therefore it cannot be stated with certainty that reflexes evoked by stimulation of a mixed nerve at high intensity are a sole consequence of the activation of C fibres.

However, capsaicin at concentrations up to 1 μM can be used selectively

(A)   CNQX (10 μM)

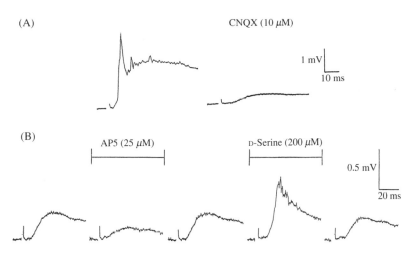

Fig. 11.2 Involvement of the co-agonist glycine site in NMDA receptor-mediated spinal transmission recorded as shown in Fig. 11.1. The synaptic response on the upper right was depressed following introduction of CNQX (10 μM) which was then present throughout. The lower traces show depression by AP5 (25 μM) and potentiation by the glycine site agonist D-serine (200 μM). D-Serine had no significant action when applied in the absence of CNQX (not illustrated). The observation is consistent with maximal operation of the glycine site under control conditions. Data from the experiments of Siarey et al. 1991. Other details as for Fig. 11.1.

to activate primary afferent C fibres (Brugger et al. 1990). The excitation of motoneurones following application of capsaicin or bradykinin to *in vitro* spinal cord preparations is depressed by antagonists of both NMDA and non-NMDA receptors (Bhoola et al. 1987; Brugger et al. 1990). Such observations have been refined to demonstrate that these algesic agents activate NMDA receptors on spinal neurones following their local application to primary afferent fibres (Dray and Perkins 1987; Urban and Dray 1992). Yoshimura and Jessell (1990) approached the problem of separation of C and A fibre input to spinal cord slice preparations by using a low concentration of tetrodotoxin to selectively block conduction in Aδ fibres. They found composite monosynaptic EPSPs from C fibres with all components depressed by the non-NMDA antagonist CNQX and later components depressed by AP5.

The above experiments provide strong evidence that an excitatory amino acid, probably glutamate, is released synaptically from primary afferent C fibres and acts at post-junctional NMDA receptors.

Spinal C fibre primary afferent terminals appear to utilize both neuropeptides and excitatory amino acids as excitatory transmitters. The neuropeptides may serve to modulate the gain of glutamatergic transmission as proposed by Woolf and Wiesenfeld-Hallin (1986). Administration of tachykinin or electrical stimulation of C fibres has been shown to enhance polysynaptic reflexes from A fibres (Woolf and Wiesenfeld-Hallin 1986), reflexes which are known to utilize predominantly NMDA receptors. The latter effect was blocked by a tachykinin NK2 receptor antagonist (Xu *et al.* 1991). Co-activation of NMDA and tachykinin NK1 receptors by C fibre transmitters has been implicated in the central sensitization of nociception at the spinal level (Xu *et al.* 1992). Such a mechanism of sensitization implies either that there is separate control of tachykinin and glutamate release from single C fibre terminals or that there are separate glutamatergic and tachykininergic C fibre primary afferent nerves. Substance P has been shown to facilitate NMDA-induced excitation of frog motoneurones (Holohean *et al.* 1992). Interactions between tachykinins and amino acids released from different nerves need not require synaptic connection of both types of nerve with the post-junctional neurone. It has been shown that in frog sympathic ganglion, a neuropeptide can act on neurones which are 200 μm away from the peptidergic terminals (Jan *et al.* 1980). The hypothetical relationship between NMDA and tachykinin receptors is summarized in Fig. 11.3.

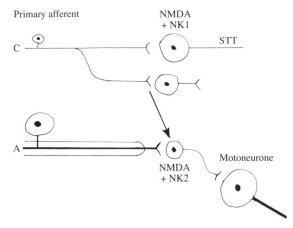

Fig. 11.3 Diagram depicting possible relationships between tachykinin and NMDA receptors. Primary afferent transmission from A and C fibres is sensitive to NMDA antagonists (see text). Tachykinin-induced enhancement of polysynaptic reflexes from primary afferent A fibre is antagonized by NK2-selective receptor antagonist (Xu *et al.* 1991), but spinal sensitization of nociceptive transmission from primary afferent C fibres is antagonized by NK1-selective receptor antagonist (Xu *et al.* 1992). Thus amino acid transmitter released from low threshold A fibres is depicted as being released at interneurones that possess predominantly NK2 as well as NMDA receptors. These neurones, because they are unlikely to be directly innervated by primary afferent C fibres, would experience the effects of tachykinin by diffusion from C fibre primary afferent terminals. Tachykinin and amino acid transmitters from primary afferent C fibres which innervate spinothalamic tract (STT) neurones are depicted as acting at a predominant population of NK1 as well as NMDA receptors.

Modulation of the effects of NMDA at central neurones has been reported previously to occur with serotonin (Reynolds *et al.* 1988; Nedergaard *et al.* 1986). Such interactions lead on to the possibility of selective depression of NMDA-receptive pathways by CNS depressants acting at non-amino acid excitatory transmitter receptors as described below.

Modulation of NMDA-receptive pathways by analgesic and myorelaxant drugs

As described above, the later components of synaptic transmission between segmental spinal nerves are mediated at NMDA receptors. The potent depressant action of the myorelaxant $GABA_B$ agonist, baclofen, against all components of segmental transmission was first described almost 20 years ago (Davidoff and Sears 1974). Thus baclofen is a potent presynaptic depressant of EPSPs mediated at non-NMDA and NMDA receptors (Siarey *et al.* 1992*a*). However, in contrast, diazepam and α_2 adrenoceptor agonists which have analgesic and myorelaxant activity appear to depress selectively only those components of spinal reflexes which are mediated through pathways which utilize NMDA receptors (Siarey *et al.* 1992) (Fig. 11.4). Indeed, the efficacy of diazepam as a depressant of NMDA-receptive synaptic excitation is considerably greater than its efficacy for enhancement of $GABA_A$ receptor-mediated primary afferent depolarization (Siarey *et al.* 1992). Opiates also have the property of selectively depressing the later components of spinal reflexes (Yanagisawa *et al.* 1984) or responses to algesic drugs (Dray and Perkins 1987) which are mediated via NMDA-receptive synapses.

It is necessary to stress that these non-amino acid related depressant drugs are not directly affecting the activity of NMDA receptor complexes as can happen when very high concentrations are applied (Evans *et al.* 1977*b*). They are acting at their own receptor types as indicated by the pA_2 values obtained using, for example, a selective benzodiazepine antagonist (Siarey *et al.* 1992*a*). Presumably benzodiazepine and other receptors are distributed in such a manner that there is functional coincidence between them and NMDA receptors. There are several possibilities for interaction between NMDA-receptive excitatory synaptic transmission and other processes. For example, non-steroid anti-inflammatory drugs have been shown to antagonize the aversive behaviour produced following spinal administration of glutamate, suggesting that the effects of excitatory transmitter can be augmented by prostaglandins (Malmberg and Yaksh 1992).

The way forward?

The technique of recording d.c. shifts from spinal roots has provided many interesting observations over the past two decades. It is likely that, in the

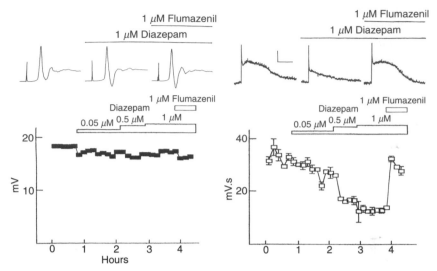

Fig. 11.4 Selective interaction of diazepam with spinal pathways which utilize NMDA receptors. The three traces on the left at the top are monosynaptic reflexes which, as Fig. 11.1 shows, do not involve NMDA receptors. Diazepam had no significant effect on these responses. However, in the same preparation, the long-lasting ventral root reflex shown to be mediated largely by NMDA receptors (see Fig. 11.1) is very susceptible to diazepam. The depressant effect of diazepam was reversed by the benzodiazepine antagonist flumazenil (1 μM). Diazepam was applied in cumulative increasing concentrations of 0.05, 0.5, and 1 μM as indicated. The time courses of each effect are plotted below. Other details as for Fig. 11.1.

right hands, this technique will continue, despite the demands of high fashion, to provide still more useful information on the mechanism of action of novel neuroactive amino acids and other compounds. However, with the exception of the α-motoneurone, it is not possible to record primary afferent nerve-induced monosynaptic post-junctional responses from spinal nerves. Again, with the exception of motoneurones, it is not possible to compare the effects of bath-applied and synaptically released agonists. In order to investigate the synaptic mechanisms which operate at synapses between different classes of primary afferent nerve and dorsal horn neurones, it is necessary to have a method of recording the ionic currents and potentials at single dorsal horn neurones. It is possible that the patch-clamp technique may be the way forward for examination of the role of NMDA and other channels in synaptic mechanisms of the dorsal horn. Figure 11.5 (unpublished work from this laboratory) is an example of a synaptic current evoked in a patch-clamped (Blanton *et al.* 1989) dorsal horn neurone following high intensity stimulation of primary afferent fibres in the dorsal root. It can be seen that a large component of the inward current is depressed by the competitive NMDA receptor antagonist

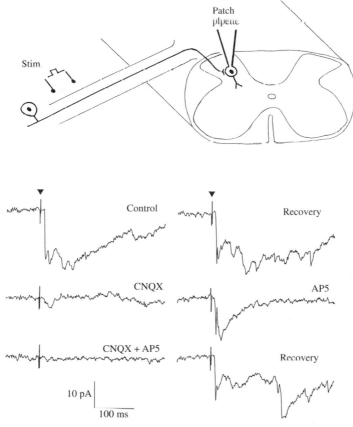

Fig. 11.5 Effect of excitatory amino acid antagonists on dorsal root-evoked (8T) synaptic currents recorded from a dorsal horn neurone (S. T. Alford, G. L. Collingridge, and R. H. Evans, unpublished data). Records are consecutive from top to bottom of left to right hand columns. Application of the AMPA receptor antagonist CNQX (10 μM, shown on the left) left a small inward current followed by an outward one. Then application of the NMDA receptor antagonist AP5 (100 μM) removed abolished the remaining synaptic response. The response recovered after washout of the antagonists (top right). Then the subsequent application of AP5 (100 μM) selectively blocked later components of the inward current. The times of dorsal root stimulation are indicated by the triangles above each column.

(Alford *et al.* 1991). It will be interesting in future experiments to compare the actions of NMDA and tachykinin in receptor antagonists at these synapses.

Acknowledgements

R. H. Evans is helped by The Medical Research Council, The Wellcome Trust, and The Taberner Trust.

References

Akagi, H. and Yanagisawa, M. (1987). GABAergic modulation of a substance P-mediated reflex of slow time course in the isolated rat spinal cord. *British Journal of Pharmacology*, **91**, 189–97.

Alford, S. T., Collingridge, G. L., and Evans, R. H. (1990). Application of whole cell patch clamp techniques to dorsal horn neurones of the hemisected rat spinal cord. *Society of Neuroscience Abstracts*, **16**, 174–5.

Berinaga, M. (1992). Neuroscience comment: playing 'telephone' with the body's message of pain. *Science*, **258**, 1085.

Bhoola, K. D., Evans, R. H., and Forster, M. R. (1987). Excitatory effect of bradykinin on spinal neurones. *British Journal of Pharmacology*, **90**, 15P.

Birch, P. J., Grossman, C. J., and Hayes, A. G. (1988). Kynurenic acid antagonises responses to NMDA via an action at the strychnine-insensitive glycine receptor. *European Journal of Pharmacology*, **156**, 177–80.

Blanton, M., Lo Turco, J. J., and Kriegstein, A. R. (1989). Whole cell recording from neurons in slices of reptilian and mammalian cerebral cortex. *Journal of Neuroscience Methods*, **30**, 203–10.

Brugger, F., Evans, R. H., and Hawkins, N. S. (1990). Effects of N-methyl-D-aspartate antagonists and spantide on spinal reflexes and responses to substance P and capsaicin in isolated spinal cord preparations from mouse and rat. *Neuroscience*, **36**, 611–22.

Brugger, F., Wicki, U., Nassenstein-Elton, D., Fagg, G. E., Olpe, H.-R., and Pozza, M. (1990). Modulation of the NMDA receptor by D-serine in the cortex and the spinal cord in vitro. *European Journal of Pharmacology*, **191**, 29–38.

Cervero, F. and Jänig, W. (1992). Visceral nociceptors: A new world order. *Trends in Neuroscience*, **15**, 374–78.

Collingridge, G. L. and Lester, R. A. J. (1989). Excitatory amino acid receptors in the vertebrate central nervous system. *Pharmacological Reviews*, **40**, 143–210.

Collingridge, G. L., Herron, C. E., and Lester, R. A. J. (1988). Synaptic activation of N-methyl-D-aspartate receptors in the Schaffer collateral-commissural pathway of rat hippocampus. *Journal of Physiology* (London), **399**, 301–12.

Conway, E. J. (1957). Nature and significance of concentration relations of potassium and sodium ions in skeletal muscle. *Physiological Reviews*, **37**, 84–132.

Dale, N. and Roberts, A. (1985). Dual component amino-acid-mediated synaptic potentials: excitatory drive for swimming in Xenopus embryos. *Journal of Physiology* (London), **363**, 35–60.

Davidoff, R. A. and Sears, M. D. (1974). The effects of lioresal on synaptic activity in the isolate spinal cord. *Neurology*, **24**, 957–63.

Davies, S. N. and Lodge, D. (1987). Evidence for involvement of N-methylaspartate receptors in 'wind-up' of class 2 neurones in the dorsal horn of the rat. *Brain Research*, **424**, 402–6.

Dray, A. and Perkins, M. N. (1987). Blockade of nociceptive responses in the neonatal rat spinal cord in vitro by excitatory amino acid antagonists. *Journal of Physiology* (London), **382**, 177P.

Evans, R. H. (1986). A slow spinal synaptic response mediated at NMA receptors. *British Journal of Pharmacology*, **88**, 269P.

Evans, R. H., Francis, A. A., and Watkins, J. C. (1977*a*). Selective antagonism by Mg^{2+} of amino acid-induced depolarization of spinal neurones. *Experientia*, **33**, 246–8.

Evans, R. H., Francis, A. A., and Watkins, J. C. (1977*b*). Differential antagonism by chlorpromazine and diazepam of frog motoneurone depolarization induced by glutamate-related amino acids. *European Journal of Pharmacology*, **44**, 325–30.

Gibbs, L. M. and Kendig, J. J. (1992). Substance P and NMDA receptor-mediated slow potentials in neonatal rat spinal cord: age-related changes. *Brain Research*, **595**, 236–41.

Holohean, A. M., Hackman, J. C., Shope, S. B., and Davidoff, R. A. (1992). Serotonin 1$_A$ facilitation of frog motoneurone responses to afferent stimuli and to *N*-methyl-D-aspartate. *Neuroscience*, **48**, 469–77.

Jan, L. Y., Jan, Y. N., and Brownfield, M. S. (1980). Peptidergic transmitters in synaptic boutons of sympathetic ganglia. *Nature*, **288**, 380–1.

Malmberg, A. B. and Yaksh, T. L. (1992). Hyperalgesia mediated by spinal glutamate or substance P receptor blocked by spinalcyclooxygenase inhibition. *Science*, **257**, 1276–9.

Nedergaard, S., Engberg, I., and Flatman, J. A. (1986). Serotonin facilitates NMDA responses of cat neocortical neurones. *Acta Physiologica Scandinavica*, **128**, 323–5.

Nowak, L., Bregostovski, P., Ascher, P., Herbet, A., and Proschiantz, A. (1984). Magnesium gates glutamate-activated channels in mouse central neurones. *Nature*, **307**, 462–5.

Reynolds, J. N., Baskys, S., and Carlen, P. L. (1988). The effects of serotonin on *N*-methyl-D-aspartate and synaptically evoked depolarizations in rat neocortical neurons. *Brain Research*, **456**, 286–92.

Siarey, R. J., Long, S. K., and Evans, R. H. (1991). Potentiation of synaptic reflexes by D-serine in the rat spinal cord in vitro. *European Journal of Pharmacology*, **195**, 241–4.

Siarey, R. J., Long, S. K., and Evans, R. H. (1992). A comparison of the effect of diazepam and tizanidine on synaptically-evoked primary afferent depolarization in the rat spinal cord in vitro. *Journal of Physiology* (London), **452**, 200P.

Thompson, S. W. N., King, A. E., and Woolf, C. J. (1990). Activity-dependent changes in rat ventral horn neurons in vitro: summation of prolonged afferent evoked postsynaptic depolarizations produce a D-2-amino-5-phosphonovaleric acid sensitive windup. *European Journal of Neuroscience*, **2**, 638–49.

Urban, L. and Dray, A. (1992). Synaptic activation of dorsal horn neurons by selective C-fibre excitation with capsaicin in the mouse spinal cord in vitro. *Neuroscience*, **47**, 693–702.

Woodley, S. J. and Kendig, J. J. (1991). Substance p and NMDA receptors mediate a slow nociceptive ventral root potential in neonatal rat spinal cord. *Brain Research*, **559**, 17–21.

Woolf, C. J. and Wiesenfeld-Hallin, Z. (1986). Substance P and calcitonin-gene-related peptide synergistically modulate the gain of the nociceptive flexor withdrawal reflex in the rat. *Neuroscience Letters*, **66**, 226–30.

Xu, X.-J., Maggi, C. A., and Wiesenfeld-Hallin, Z. (1991). On the role of NK-2 tachykinin receptors in the mediation of spinal reflex excitability in the rat. *Neuroscience*, **44**, 483–90.

Xu, X.-J., Dalsgaard, C.-J., and Wiesenfeld-Hallin, Z. (1992). Spinal substance P and N-methyl-D-aspartate receptors are coactivated in the induction of central sensitization of the nociceptive flexor reflex. *Neuroscience*, **51**, 641–8.

Yanagisawa, M., Murakoshi, T., Tumai, S., and Otsuka, M. (1984). Tail-pinch method in vitro and the effects of some antinociceptive compounds. *European Journal of Pharmacology*, **106**, 231–9.

Yoshimura, M. and Jessell, T. (1989). Primary afferent-evoked synaptic responses and slow potential generation in rat substantia gelatinosa neurons in vitro. *Journal of Neurophysiology*, **62**, 96–108.

Yoshimura, M. and Jessell, T. (1990). Amino acid-mediated EPSPs at primary afferent synapses with substantia gelatinosa neurones in the rat spinal cord. *Journal of Physiology* (London), **430**, 315–35.

12 The role of NMDA receptors in synaptic integration and the organization of motor patterns

SIMON ALFORD AND LENNART BRODIN

Introduction

The ubiquity of the *N*-methyl-D-aspartate (NMDA) receptor throughout much of the vertebrate central nervous system (CNS), coupled with its unique properties, discussed elsewhere in this book, result not only in its functional implication in many complex integrative systems of the CNS, but have also ensured that neuroscientists will study it. Consequently, the NMDA receptor has been implicated in the organization of all sensory modalities in addition to many aspects of motor output. Much of the range of these functions has been treated in a recent review (Daw *et al*. 1993). They include, but are by no means limited to, the processing of visual information (Fox *et al*. 1990), auditory information, and the central sensitization of nociceptive responses (Dickenson and Sullivan 1990). In this chapter it is our intention to discuss in some detail the contribution of NMDA receptors to the control of motor activity. It should be added at this point, however, that the features of the NMDA receptor that makes its contribution to motor output so special, namely its voltage sensitivity (Nowak *et al*. 1984), slow kinetics (Lester *et al*. 1990), and permeability to Ca^{2+} (Mayer *et al*. 1987), are of equal importance in the integration of sensory information gathered with those sensory modalities mentioned above.

The NMDA receptor and locomotion

The most visible functional motor output of animals is that of locomotion. This motor function is perhaps the most accessible for the study of the integrative properties of CNS motor output. The mechanisms by which animals are able to generate this form of activity has been a subject of investigation for most of this century. It is only in the last 15 years, however, that the cellular and pharmacological mechanisms underlying vertebrate locomotor output have started to be unravelled.

The basic neural activity of locomotion, which consists of an alternating activation of the muscle groups on the two sides of the body, is generated by networks of interneurones located in the spinal cord (Grillner 1985).

These networks are often referred to as the central pattern generators (CPGs) of locomotion. The network activity is controlled by descending systems, primarily reticulospinal pathways, and it is also modulated by sensory input at the segmental level. The importance of the activation of NMDA receptors in the control of vertebrate locomotor activity has been clear since the work of Roberts and colleagues (Dale and Roberts 1985) first demonstrated the role of these receptors in synaptic transmission. Parallel studies in the lamprey (Grillner *et al.* 1981; Brodin and Grillner 1985; Brodin *et al.* 1985; Dale and Grillner 1986) demonstrated the key role of this receptor subtype in the control of locomotion across the vertebrates and has subsequently demonstrated much of the mechanism of action of NMDA receptors in controlling spinal motor output. Many of the rather special features of the NMDA receptor discussed in detail elsewhere in this book are utilized in the spinal cord to contribute to the rhythmicity and stability of the spinal central pattern generator.

Dale and Roberts (1985) demonstrated that the slow kinetics of this receptor contributes to maintenance of motor output in the *Xenopus* embryo. In addition, the combination of the permeability of the receptor ion channel to Ca^{2+}, coupled with its voltage dependent block by Mg^{2+}, are vital to the generation of pacemaker-like oscillations in neurones of the lamprey spinal motor system (Grillner and Wallén 1985; Sigvardt *et al.* 1985; Wallén and Grillner 1987) and to the generation of rhythmic activity in the absence of glycinergic inhibition in the *Xenopus* embryo (Soffe and Roberts 1989). The NMDA receptor has also been shown to provide an important function in the control of motor output in adult frogs (McClellan and Farel 1985), salamanders, and turtles (Currie and Stein 1992), though it is not always clear whether NMDA receptor activation occurs at the level of sensory input or motor pattern generation (Stein and Schild 1989). Other preparations that have been demonstrated to utilize NMDA receptors in the control of motor activity include spontaneous motor output in the embryonic chick (Barry and O'Donovan 1987), swallowing in the neonatal rat (Kessler and Jean 1991), and generation of respiratory activity in the neonatal rat (Feldman and Smith 1989). Also in the neonate rat spinal cord NMDA receptor activation occurs during the generation of fictive locomotion (Kudo and Yamada 1987; Smith *et al.* 1988; Cazalets *et al.* 1990). More recent data indicate that the activation of NMDA receptors in the adult rabbit spinal cord (Fenaux *et al.* 1991) is involved in motor co-ordination and in the cat spinal cord is sufficient to initiate and maintain locomotor output in the absence of inputs from higher centres (Douglas *et al.* 1993).

The role of NMDA receptor activation in lamprey locomotion

A great deal of what we know of the cellular properties responsible for the control of spinal motor output has been achieved in somewhat simple model vertebrate preparations. The lamprey spinal cord has proved to be an ideal preparation for the study of the properties of motor control from the systems to the cellular level using the isolated CNS (Grillner *et al.* 1987). In this preparation the neuronal correlate of locomotion 'fictive locomotion' may be studied in isolation (Cohen and Wallén 1980; Poon 1980). In the lamprey spinal cord, locomotion comprises an alternate activation of bursts in ventral roots on opposite sides of the spinal cord at each segmental level (Fig. 12.1(A) and (B)). This activity is driven by mutually inhibitory hemisegments of the spinal cord (Grillner and Wallén 1980; Alford and Williams 1989) each of which also possesses circuitry and cellular properties capable of causing rhythmic activity. The activation of NMDA receptors is important in this rhythm generation (Brodin and Grillner 1985; Brodin *et al.* 1985; Sigvardt *et al.* 1985).

To gain an understanding of the role that NMDA receptors play in the control of locomotion, it is necessary to understand their role in glutamatergic synaptic transmission. Paired cell recordings between neurones of the *Xenopus* embryo (Dale and Roberts 1985) and the lamprey (Dale and Grillner 1986) spinal motor systems has demonstrated that glutamatergic synaptic transmission comprises two electrogenic components. A rapidly rising and falling α-amino-3-hydroxy-5-methyl-4-isoxazolepropionic acid (AMPA) receptor-mediated component and a more slowly rising and falling NMDA receptor-mediated component. At normal resting membrane potentials and in the presence of Mg^{2+} in the cerebrospinal fluid, the NMDA receptor-mediated component is masked by the voltage-dependent block of Mg^{2+} of the NMDA receptor ion channel (Alford and Grillner 1990; Fig. 12.2). Work in other systems has demonstrated that these features of synaptic transmission are true in many other areas of the CNS and as discussed elsewhere in this book contribute to many important physiological mechanisms (Hestrin *et al.* 1990). It is also agreeable that these features of the NMDA receptor-mediated excitatory post-synaptic potential (EPSP) are readily predicted from the properties of NMDA receptors studied in isolation. These features include their slow kinetics, voltage sensitivity in the presence of extracellular Mg^{2+}, permeability to Ca^{2+}, and reversal potential.

Rhythmic oscillations and the NMDA receptor

Within the spinal motor system the generation of rhythmic locomotor output results from a complex interplay between the connectivity of both excitatory and inhibitory neurones which comprise the network and some of the special properties of the cells themselves. As an example it is perhaps worthwhile considering some of the features of the lamprey spinal locomotor pattern generator in detail, as this system is relatively well understood.

In the absence of synaptic transmission, after blockade of regenerative

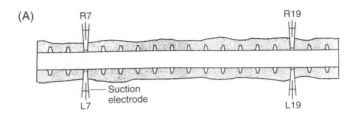

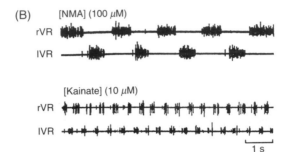

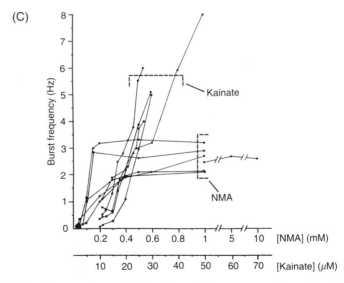

Fig. 12.1 Fictive locomotion evoked by *N*-methyl-D,L-aspartate (NMA) and kainate in lamprey. (A) Schematic illustration of the *in vitro* preparation of the lamprey spinal cord. Suction electrodes are used to record ventral root activity in a rostral and a caudal pair of roots. (B) Recordings of the activity in a pair of ventral roots in the presence of 100 μM NMA (upper traces) and 10 μM kainate (lower traces). Note the difference in burst rate (see Brodin and Grillner 1985). (C) Dose–frequency response curves for fictive locomotion induced by NMA and kainate respectively. The frequency of the NMA-evoked activity starts at very low values and reaches a plateau at 2–3 Hz, while the frequency of the kainate-induced activity has a higher frequency range.

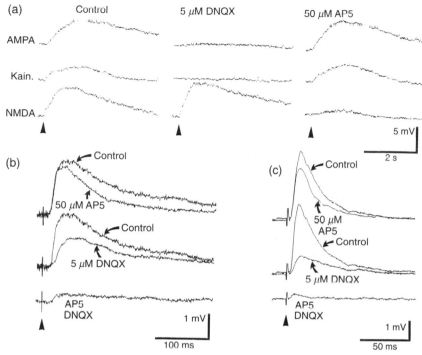

Fig. 12.2 Excitatory amino acid inputs to motoneurones in the lamprey spinal cord (see Alford and Grillner 1990). (a) Responses of a motoneurone to pressure ejection of amino acid agonists in a spinal cord bathed in 1 μM TTX and low Mg^{2+}. Drugs were applied by a brief pressure pulse at the arrow. The response to AMPA and kainate was blocked by bath application of 5 μM 6,7-dinitroquinoxaline-2,3-dione (DNQX) but that to NMDA was left unaffected. The response to NMDA was blocked by application of 50 μM 2-amino-5-phosphonopentanoate (AP5) but those to AMPA and kainate were left unaffected. (b) The effect of bath application of 5 μM DNQX and 50 μM AP5 on monosynaptic compound EPSPs recorded in a motoneurone in low Mg^{2+} Ringer's solution. (c) As for (b) but in Ringer's solution containing a normal concentration of Mg^{2+}.

Na^+ spikes with tetrodotoxin (TTX), the application of NMDA to the medium bathing the spinal cord initiates a rhythmic fluctuation in the membrane potential of moto- and premoto-neurones (Sigvardt *et al.* 1985). In the last few years the mechanisms behind this phenomenon have been largely revealed (Fig. 12.3). The activation of NMDA receptors at hyper-polarized membrane potentials will cause the activation of only a small inward conductance. However, under the influence of this conductance and the buffering of Ca^{2+}, and thus reduction of Ca^{2+}-activated outward conductances, the neurone will slowly depolarize. Depolarization forces Mg^{2+} from its ion channel binding site (Nowak *et al.* 1984) increasing the amplitude of the NMDA receptor-mediated inward current, which thus

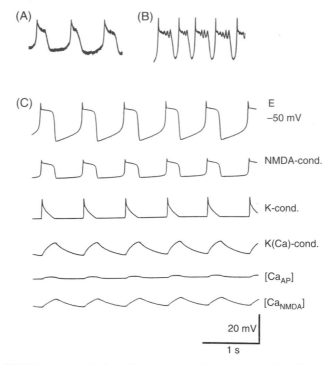

Fig. 12.3 NMDA receptor-induced inherent membrane potential oscillations in lamprey spinal neurones. (A) and (B) show examples of oscillations recorded in spinal neurones in the presence of NMA and TTX. (C) Computer simulations of oscillations in an electrical neurone model equipped with NMDA conductances and other voltage-gated conductances (see Brodin *et al.* 1991). The top trace shows the membrane potential (E), and the traces below show the change of the NMDA conductance (cond.), the calcium level in the common voltage-gated calcium pool and the calcium level in the NMDA-gated calcium pool, respectively. Note that the two latter have been given different time constants to account for the different effects of calcium entering during action potentials and during NMDA receptor activation.

leads to a 'feed-forward' increase in amplitude of this current and a spike-like event. This rapid depolarization initiates the entry of Ca^{2+} into the neurone both through the NMDA receptor ionophore and through low voltage-operated Ca^{2+} channels. This entry of Ca^{2+} activates Ca^{2+}-dependent K^+ channels and thus a hyperpolarizing outward conductance. As the neurone hyperpolarizes under the influence of this outward conductance Mg^{2+} is driven into its NMDA receptor ion channel binding site, limiting the NMDA receptor-mediated inward current and hastening the hyperpolarizing of the neurone, again in a feed forward manner (a form of reverse spike). With the neurone hyperpolarized, Ca^{2+} no longer enters and is taken up into internal stores, and/or extruded. This inactivates the

Ca^{2+} dependent K^+ conductance so once more under the influence of a small NMDA receptor-mediated conductance the neurone restarts this cycle by slowly depolarizing (Wallén and Grillner 1987). It is interesting to note that strikingly similar properties are seen elsewhere in the vertebrate brain (Tell and Jean 1991; Hu and Bourque 1992).

Oscillations and the control of locomotion

It is instructive to consider how a mechanism such as this will contribute to locomotion in the intact animal. During locomotion NMDA receptors are activated by the periodic release of glutamate by excitatory cells of the spinal cord (Buchanan *et al.* 1987) and by the release of glutamate from descending fibres from the brain stem (Buchanan and Grillner 1987). These reticulospinal neurones in turn receive oscillatory efference copy from the spinal cord (Kasicki and Grillner 1986) as well as sensory and central information from the brain (Orlovsky *et al.* 1990). Consequently, the neurones of the spinal cord do not receive a constant infusion of glutamate activating the NMDA receptor. However, three observations point to this crude estimation to be a reasonable starting point for the function of NMDA receptor mediated oscillations in the spinal cord. Firstly, NMDA receptor-mediated synaptic responses are very slow (Dale and Roberts 1985; Lester *et al.* 1990), indeed in the rapidly swimming *Xenopus* embryo these potentials sum to a stable plateau from cycle to cycle. In the lamprey, NMDA receptor-mediated synaptic potentials often outlast the duration of the cycle (Dale 1986). Secondly, the application of kainate (Brodin *et al.* 1985) or AMPA (Alford and Grillner 1990) to the preparation causes a rapid fictive locomotion in contrast to the slower activity generated by application of NMDA and dominated in frequency by the time course of NMDA induced oscillations. This phenomenon may be imitated by a realistic computer simulation of the spinal circuitry if it incorporates NMDA receptor-type oscillatory behaviour of the neurones (Brodin *et al.* 1991). Finally, synaptic activation of NMDA receptors is capable of initiating bursting behaviour in neurones of the spinal cord with remarkably similar properties to those seen following the bath application of NMDA (Alford and Sigvardt 1989).

To gain a more complete understanding of the role that NMDA receptors play in the control of spinal motor output a more sophisticated analysis is necessary. The time course of spinal and descending input activated glutamate release must be considered. Such a model has been developed (Tråvén *et al.* 1993) and will be considered, particularly because it points to some interesting future avenues of research in the role of factors modulating the activation of NMDA receptors during locomotion. Information obtained from such simulations suggests that if the bursting of the network is driven by NMDA-mediated synapses, the burst rate is dominated by the intrinsic frequency of the NMDA-induced oscillations.

The burst rate of the network could, however, be considerably altered by variations in the relative contributions to excitation between AMPA and NMDA receptors.

Modulation of NMDA receptor activation

Variations in relative contributions of AMPA and NMDA receptors to spinal excitation could be brought about by variations in the relative strengths of the two synaptic responses in different pairs of neurones in the spinal cord. Consequently, a control of the firing rate of neurones that give rise to synaptic responses with varying NMDA components would provide for the observed variations in burst frequency. Alternatively, activation of NMDA receptors might be differentially controlled by the concentration of glycine in proximity to NMDA receptors (Johnson and Ascher 1987; Grillner *et al.* 1991). If glycine concentrations were controlled in the spinal cord to the extent that reduced glycine concentrations impaired NMDA receptor activation then the relative contributions of AMPA and NMDA receptor activation to spinal excitation would be readily controlled. It remains difficult to postulate under what circumstances cerebrospinal fluid concentrations of glycine would fall to sufficiently low concentrations to effect this response, although a local regulation of the glycine level in the synaptic cleft cannot be excluded.

The degree of NMDA receptor activation could also be controlled by a differentiated use-dependent short-term plasticity. It is well established that the degree of synaptic depression and facilitation during repetitive stimulation varies markedly between synapses (Zucker 1989). This variability is true for individual synapses made from one presynaptic neurone on to different target cells (Koerber and Mendell 1991; Brodin *et al.* 1994) as well as for different input synapses made from different neurones on to the same target cell (Bower and Haberly 1986; Fig. 12.4). While experimental data are as yet lacking, it is tempting to postulate that reticulospinal drive synapses with large NMDA receptor-mediated components exhibit a more pronounced synaptic depression at high firing rates relative to reticulospinal synapses with small relative NMDA components and large AMPA components. If so, this mechanism could provide a predominantly NMDA-receptor mediated synaptic drive when the reticulospinal system has a low activity level. When a faster locomotor rhythm is required, the same reticulospinal neurones could fire at higher rates, resulting in a reduced NMDA receptor activation relative to that of AMPA receptors.

Finally, some NMDA receptor subunits are susceptible to modulation by second messengers. Such a mechanism could implicate NMDA receptor-mediated Ca^{2+} entry in the modulation of NMDA receptor activation. NMDA receptors show 'rundown' under conditions of dephosphorylation (MacDonald *et al.* 1989). Protein kinase C-(PKC) mediated phosphorylation of NMDA receptors has been shown to enhance NMDA receptor-

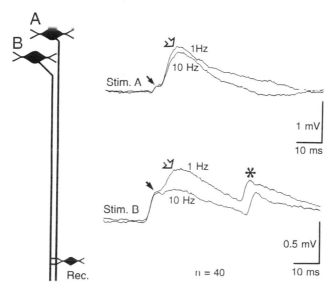

Fig. 12.4 Differential use-dependent modulation of individual glutamatergic EPSPs. Two different EPSPs were recorded in a single spinal cord neurone in lamprey, during subsequent intracellular stimulation of different (A and B) reticulospinal cells (Brodin *et al.* 1992). In each case the averaged (n = 40) responses to 1 Hz and 10 Hz repetitive stimulation, respectively, have been superimposed. In both cases the monosynaptic chemical EPSP (open arrow) is preceded by an electrotonic EPSP (small arrow), due to gap junctions. Note that the chemical EPSP in B shows a marked depression, while that in A is little affected. A polysynaptic component in B is indicated with an asterisk. As the recordings were made in the presence of 1.8 mM Mg^{2+} the NMDA components of the chemical EPSPs were suppressed.

mediated currents (Kelso *et al.* 1992), particularly of the $\varepsilon_1-\zeta$ and $\varepsilon_2-\zeta$ channels (Kutsuwada *et al.* 1992) which, like those in the spinal cord, are most sensitive to Mg^{2+} channel block. Indeed preliminary data indicate that such a mechanism may occur in the lamprey spinal cord (Alford *et al.* 1990). This hypothesis for modulation of NMDA receptor activation is perhaps not the most attractive, however, because under conditions of increasing synaptic drive, PKC activation following NMDA receptor activation would enhance NMDA receptor sensitivity where the converse effect is sought. This does not rule out other types of second messenger modulation of NMDA receptor activation, particularly dephosphorylation of the receptor and a decrease in sensitivity with increasing glutamatergic synaptic input. Indeed, PKC activation has also been reported to depress NMDA receptor-mediated conductances in the hippocampus (Markram and Segal 1992). Similarly, the enhancement of AMPA receptors by second messenger system (Wang *et al.* 1991; Shaw and Lanius 1992) could alter the balance between relative contributions of these receptors to synaptic transmission.

Presynaptic inhibition

A number of receptor systems have been implicitly or explicitly implicated in the control of NMDA receptor activation. GABA receptor activation is necessary for stability of locomotion in the lamprey spinal cord (Alford *et al.* 1991). GABA receptors may influence locomotion by acting at either pre- (Alford and Grillner 1991) or post-synaptic loci (Tegnér *et al.* 1993). First, to consider the presynaptic locus, we must return to early demonstrations of glutamatergic post-synaptic potentials (PSPs). Using paired recordings in both *Xenopus* embryos and lamprey stimulation of the presynaptic cell may activate pure AMPA receptor-mediated responses, pure NMDA receptor-mediated responses, or a mixture of the two (Dale and Grillner 1986; Dale and Roberts 1985). These observations indicate that NMDA and AMPA receptors are not always co-localized to the same synaptic site. Indeed, evidence points to the fact that in many cases AMPA and NMDA receptors may very well be located on different synaptic sites (Sillar and Roberts 1991). Recently, it has been demonstrated that presynaptic GABA receptors inhibit glutamate release in the spinal cord (Fig. 12.5;

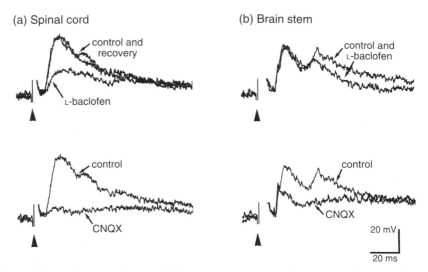

Fig. 12.5 Application of the GABA$_B$ receptor agonist baclofen to the spinal cord selectively depresses EPSPs evoked from within the spinal cord but not those from the brain stem (see Alford and Grillner 1991). (a) EPSPs were evoked by stimulation of the spinal cord ipsilateral to the impaled neurone. Application of baclofen depressed this compound EPSP. The EPSP was also abolished by the application of 6-cyano-7-nitro-quinoxaline-3-dione (CNQX) indicating that it was mediated by glutamate receptors. (b) Compound EPSPs were evoked in the same neurone by stimulation of reticulospinal fibres in the brain stem. The early part of this response, known to be carried by monosynaptic reticulospinal connections, is unaffected by the same application of baclofen as in (a). This response is also sensitive to CNQX application.

Alford and Grillner 1991). Should some glutamate synapses of the spinal cord specifically activate AMPA or NMDA receptors, presynaptic inhibition of glutamate release by GABA might specifically control relative contributions of NMDA or AMPA receptors to spinal excitation. This might occur regardless of whether the presynaptic excitatory neurone was capable of releasing glutamate on to terminals of both NMDA receptor or AMPA receptors. Presynaptic GABAergic inhibition might also affect the relative contributions of NMDA and AMPA receptors to locomotor output by controlling the presynaptic sensitivity of neurones which impinge on synapses with predominantly NMDA or AMPA receptor activity, as discussed above for short-term plastic effects of transmission. Indeed GABAergic presynaptic inhibition has been demonstrated to be synapse-specific even between inputs converging on the same neurone (Fig. 12.5; Alford and Grillner 1991). 5-hydroxytryptamine (5-HT) has been shown to be released in the spinal cord and, as for GABA, may also act presynaptically to inhibit release of glutamate (Buchanan and Grillner 1991). As for GABA this transmitter could alter the relative contributions of AMPA and NMDA receptors to spinal excitation.

Post-synaptic receptors and modulation of NMDA receptor activation

$GABA_B$ receptors located on spinal motoneurone and premotoneurone somata may also modulate the contribution of NMDA receptors to spinal locomotor drive. $GABA_B$ receptors, as described in neurones of the mammalian dorsal root ganglion (Dunlap and Fischbach 1981), depress voltage-operated Ca^{2+}channel (VOCC) activity in these spinal cells (Tegnér *et al.* 1993). The activation of VOCCs, particularly T-type channels, contributes to Ca^{2+} entry and the activation of K^+ conductances in these neurones. Without, or with a reduced contribution of, this hyperpolarizing influence on spinal neurones, the activation of NMDA receptors is likely to lead to increased excitation and less time-dependent phasic activity.

5-HT has a profound influence on the activity of the locomotor pattern generator and, in addition to its presynaptic actions, it has been shown to exert much of its effects post-synaptically. 5-HT receptor activation is able to alter the activation of Ca^{2+}-activated K^+ channels (Van Dongen *et al.* 1986). This appears to interfere directly with the activation of the K^+ conductance rather than with entry of Ca^{2+} as seen for $GABA_B$ receptors (Wallén *et al.* 1989). Consequently, application of 5-HT to the spinal cord causes an increase in the duration of the depolarized phase of NMDA-induced oscillations discussed above.

Dopamine acts in a manner complementary to that of 5-HT and similarly to post-synaptic $GABA_B$ receptors as it inhibits depolarization-induced entry of Ca^{2+}. Such a property of dopamine may also significantly alter the function of NMDA receptor-mediated membrane potential oscillations. The contribution of these components to locomotion and the role that

NMDA receptors play in the control of locomotion has not yet been elucidated. It is likely that one or more of these mechanisms may contribute to the means by which NMDA receptors contribute to locomotor stability and frequency regulation (Srinivasan *et al.* 1993).

Higher animal locomotion and NMDA receptors

We have dealt in some detail with the known cellular mechanisms of action of NMDA receptors in the generation of locomotion in simple systems, principally the lamprey spinal cord. It has become clear, though, that NMDA receptors provide a similar role in the generation of locomotion in higher vertebrate preparations. That synaptic transmission in the mammalian spinal cord utilizes NMDA receptors has been known from the very earliest research defining the variety of carboxylic amino acid agonist and antagonists in the vertebrates (Curtis *et al.* 1972; Watkins and Evans 1981).

Spanning vertebrate groups that have been separated phylogenetically for some 400 million years, NMDA receptors are known to play a role in the control of chelonid scratch mechanisms, in amphibian locomotor (Dale and Roberts 1985) and wipe (McClellan and Farel 1985) mechanisms, in bird locomotion (Barry and O'Donovan 1987), and in the generation of locomotion in the mammal (Fenaux *et al.* 1991; Douglas *et al.* 1993). Taking the mammalian preparation as perhaps the clinically most pertinent it is useful to draw a number of functional similarities between the role that NMDA receptors play in lamprey and mammalian locomotion. Isolated neonatal rat spinal cord preparations will generate fictive locomotor output. This output may be elicited by the application of NMDA or amino acid uptake inhibitors to the preparation (Cazalets *et al.* 1990; Kudo and Yamada 1987; Smith *et al.* 1988). It has also been demonstrated that antagonism of NMDA receptors with MK801 in the decerebrate or spinal rabbit causes disruption of motor output in a manner consistent with a role for NMDA receptors in the generation of locomotor patterns (Fenaux *et al.* 1991).

Application of a number of pharmacological agents to neurones of the cat spinal cord *in vivo* is capable of eliciting plateau properties remarkably similar to those reported in the lamprey (Hounsgaard *et al.* 1984). Recently it has been reported that the intrathecal injection of NMDA to the ventral horn of the cat spinal cord is capable of initiating locomotor burst activity both in the presence and absence of peripheral feedback (Douglas *et al.* 1993). These data strongly implicate NMDA receptors as an integral component of the mammalian locomotor pattern generator. An understanding of the role that NMDA receptors play in the initiation and maintenance of spinal locomotor pattern generation may have profound significance in the alleviation of suffering following spinal trauma and dysfunction.

In this light, perhaps the understanding of the role that other transmitters play as modulators of NMDA receptor function during locomotor activity is of equal importance. It has been known for some time that dopamine, 5-HT, and noradrenaline play important modulatory roles in the cat central pattern generator (Barbeau and Rossignol 1990; Rossignol *et al.* 1986). Little, however, is known of their cellular mechanisms of action. The recent realization that these transmitters may profoundly alter the functioning of NMDA receptors, and the related burst activity of spinal neurones during locomotion in simple vertebrate preparations, may go some way towards clarifying our understanding of their mechanisms in the mammalian spinal cord. The study of such mechanisms, be they in the *in vivo* mammalian, or *in vitro* simple system, should prove fruitful.

References

Alford, S. and Grillner, S. (1990). CNQX and DNQX block non-NMDA synaptic transmission but not NMDA-evoked locomotion in lamprey spinal cord. *Brain Research*, **506**, 297–302.

Alford, S. and Grillner, S. (1991). The involvement of GABA$_B$ receptors and coupled G proteins in spinal GABAergic presynaptic inhibition. *Journal of Neuroscience*, **11**, 3718–26.

Alford, S. and Sigvardt, K. A. (1989). Excitatory neurotransmission activates voltage-dependent properties in neurons in spinal motor system of lamprey. *Journal of Neurophysiology*, **62**, 334–41.

Alford, S. and Williams, T. L. (1989). Endogenous activation of glycine and NMDA receptors in lamprey spinal cord during fictive locomotion. *Journal of Neuroscience*, **9**, 2792–800.

Alford, S., Sigvardt, K. A., and Williams, T. L. (1990). NMDA receptor-mediated synaptic transmission activates a kinase-dependent outward conductance in neurones of the spinal cord. *Neuroscience Letters*, Suppl. 38, S24 (Abstract).

Alford, S., Christenson, J., and Grillner, S. (1991). Presynaptic GABA$_A$ and GABA$_B$ receptor-mediated phasic modulation in axons of spinal motor interneurons. *European Journal of Neuroscience*, **3**, 107–17.

Barbeau, H. and Rossignol, S. (1990). The effects of serotonergic drugs on the locomotor pattern and on cutaneous reflexes of the adult chronic spinal cat. *Brain Research*, **514**, 55–67.

Barry, M. A. J. and O'Donovan, M. J. (1987). The effects of excitatory amino acids and their antagonists on the generation of motor activity in the isolated chick spinal cord. *Developmental Brain Research*, **36**, 271–6.

Bower, J. M. and Haberly, L. B. (1986). Facilitating and non-facilitating synapses on pyramidal cells: a correlation between physiology and morphology. *Proceedings of the National Academy of Science, USA*, **83**, 1115–19.

Brodin, L. and Grillner, S. (1985). The role of putative excitatory amino acid neurotransmitters in the initiation of locomotion in the lamprey spinal cord. I. The effects of excitatory amino acid antagonists. *Brain Research*, **360**, 139–48.

Brodin, L., Grillner, S., and Rovainen, C. M. (1985). *N*-methyl-D-aspartate (NMDA), kainate and quisqualate receptors and the generation of fictive locomotion in the lamprey spinal cord. *Brain Research*, **325**, 302–6.

Brodin, L., Tråvén, H. G. C., Lansner, A., Wallén, P., Ekeberg, O., and Grillner,

S. (1991). Computer simulations of *N*-methyl-D-aspartate receptor-induced membrane properties in a neuron model. *Journal of Neurophysiology*, **66**, 473–84.

Brodin, L., Shupliakov, O., Hellgren, J., Pierbone, V., and Hill, R. (1994). The reticulospinal glutamate synapse in lamprey: plasticity and presynaptic variability *Journal of Neurophysiology* (In press).

Buchanan, J. T. and Grillner, S. (1987). Newly identified 'glutamate interneurons' and their role in locomotion in the lamprey spinal cord. *Science*, **236**, 312–14.

Buchanan, J. T. and Grillner, S. (1991). 5-hydroxytryptamine depresses reticulospinal excitatory post synaptic potentials in motoneurons of the lamprey. *Neuroscience Letters*, **112**, 71–4.

Buchanan, J. T., Brodin, L., Dale, N., and Grillner, S. (1987). Reticulospinal neurones activate excitatory amino acid receptors. *Brain Research*, **408**, 321–5.

Cazalets, J. R., Grillner, P., Menard, I., Cremieux, J., and Clarac, F. (1990). Two types of motor rhythm induced by NMDA and amines in an in vitro spinal cord preparation of neonatal rat. *Neuroscience Letters*, **111**, 116–21.

Cohen, A. H. and Wallén, P. (1980). The neuronal correlation of locomotion in fish. 'Fictive swimming' induced in an in vitro preparation of the lamprey spinal cord. *Experimental Brain Research*, **41**, 11–18.

Currie, S. N. and Stein, P. S. G. (1992). Glutamate antagonists applied to midbody spinal cord segments reduce the excitability of the fictive rostral scratch reflex in the turtle. *Brain Research*, **581**, 91–100.

Curtis, D. R., Duggan, A. W., Felix, D., Johnston, G. A., Tebecis, A. K., and Watkins, J. C. (1972). Excitation of mammalian central neurones by acidic amino acids. *Brain Research*, **41**, 283–301.

Dale, N. (1986). Excitatory synaptic drive for swimming mediated by amino acid receptors in the lamprey. *Journal of Neuroscience*, **6**, 2662–75.

Dale, N. and Grillner, S. (1986). Dual component synaptic potentials in the lamprey mediated by excitatory amino acid receptors. *Journal of Neuroscience*, **6**, 2653–61.

Dale, N. and Roberts, A. (1985). Dual-component amino-acid-mediated synaptic potentials: excitatory drive for swimming in *Xenopus* embryos. *Journal of Physiology*, **363**, 35–59.

Daw, N. W., Stein, P. S. G., and Fox, K. (1993). The role of NMDA receptors in information processing. *Annual Review of Neuroscience*, **16**, 207–22.

Dickenson, A. H. and Sullivan, A. F. (1990). Differential effects of excitatory amino acid antagonists on dorsal horn nociceptive neurones in the rat. *Brain Research*, **506**, 31–9.

Douglas, J. R., Noga, B. R., Dai, X., and Jordan, L. M. (1993). The effects of intrathecal administration of excitatory amino acid agonists and antagonists on the initiation of locomotion in the adult cat. *Journal of Neuroscience*, **13**, 990–1000.

Dunlap, K. and Fischbach, G. D. (1981). Neurotransmitters decrease the calcium conductance activated by depolarization of embryonic chick sensory neurones. *Journal of Physiology* (London), **317**, 519–35.

Feldman, J. L. and Smith, J. C. (1989). Cellular mechanisms underlying modulation of breathing pattern in mammals. *Annals of the New York Academy of Science*, **563**, 114–30.

Fenaux, F., Corio, M., Palisses, R., and Viala, D. (1991). Effects of an NMDA-receptor antagonist, MK801, on central locomotor programming in the rabbit. *Experimental Brain Research*, **86**, 393–401.

Fox, K , Sato, H., and Daw, N. (1990). The effect of varying stimulus intensity on NMDA receptor activity in cat visual cortex. *Journal of Neurophysiology*, 64, 1413–28.

Grillner, S. (1985). Neurobiological bases of rhythmic motor acts in vertebrates. *Science* 228, 143–9.

Grillner, S. and Wallén, P. (1980). Does the central pattern generation for locomotion in the lamprey depend on glycine inhibition? *Acta Physiologica Scandinavica*, 110, 103–5.

Grillner, S. and Wallén, P. (1985). The ionic mechanisms underlying *N*-methyl-D-aspartate receptor-induced, tetrodotoxin-resistant membrane potential oscillations in lamprey neurons active during locomotion. *Neuroscience Letters*, 60, 289–94.

Grillner, S., McClellan, A., Sigvardt, K., Wallén, P., and Wilén, M. (1981). Activation of NMDA-receptors elicits 'fictive locomotion' in lamprey spinal cord in vitro. *Acta Physiologica Scandinavica*, 113, 549–51.

Grillner, S., Wallén, P., Dale, N., Brodin, L., Buchanan, J. T., and Hill, R. (1987). Transmitters, membrane properties and network circuitry in the control of locomotion in lamprey. *Trends in Neuroscience*, 10, 34–41.

Grillner, P., Hill, R., and Grillner, S. (1991). 7-chlorokynurenic acid blocks NMDA receptor-induced fictive locomotion in lamprey-evidence for a physiological role of the glycine site. *Acta Physiologica Scandinavica*, 141, 131–2.

Hestrin, S., Nicoll, R. A., Perkel, D. J., and Sah, P. (1990). Analysis of excitatory synaptic action in pyramidal cells using whole-cell recording from rat hippocampal slices. *Journal of Physiology* (London), 422, 203–25.

Hounsgaard, J., Hultborn, H., Jespersen, B., and Kiehn, O. (1984). Intrinsic membrane properties causing a bistable behaviour of a-motoneurones. *Experimental Brain Research*, 55, 391–4.

Hu, B. and Bourque, C. W. (1992). NMDA receptor-mediated rhythmic bursting activity in rat supraoptic nucleus neurones in vitro. *Journal of Physiology*, (London), 458, 667–87.

Johnson, J. W. and Ascher, P. (1987). Glycine potentiates the NMDA response in cultured mouse brain neurons. *Nature*, 325, 529–31.

Kasicki, S. and Grillner, S. (1986). Müller cells and other reticulospinal neurones are phasically active during fictive locomotion in the isolated nervous system of the lamprey. *Neuroscience Letters*, 69, 239–43.

Kelso, S. R., Nelson, T. E., and Leonard, J. P. (1992). Protein kinase C-mediated enhancement of NMDA currents by metabotropic glutamate receptors in *Xenopus* oocytes. *Journal of Physiology* (London), 449, 705–18.

Kessler, J. P. and Jean, A. (1991). Evidence that activation of *N*-methyl-D-aspartate (NMDA) and non-NMDA receptors within the nucleus tractus solitarii triggers swallowing. *European Journal of Pharmacology*, 201, 59–67.

Koerber, H. R. and Mendell, L. M. (1991). Modulation of synaptic transmission at Ia-afferent fiber connections on motoneurons during high frequency stimulation: role of postsynaptic target. *Journal of Neurophysiology*, 65, 590–7.

Kudo, N. and Yamada, T. (1987). *N*-methyl-D-aspartate induced locomotor activity in a spinal cord-hind limb muscles preparation of the newborn rat studied in vitro. *Neuroscience Letters*, 75, 43–8.

Kutsuwada, T., Kashiwabuchi, N., Mori, H., Sakimura, K., Kushiya, E., Araki, K., Meguro, H., Masaki, H., Kumanishi, T., Arakawa, M., and Mishina, M. (1992). Molecular diversity of the NMDA receptor channel. *Nature*, 358, 36–41.

Lester, R. A. J., Clements, J. D., Westbrook, G. L., and Jahr, C. E. (1990). Channel kinetics determine the time course of NMDA receptor-mediated synaptic currents. *Nature*, **346**, 565–7.

McClellan, A. D. and Farel, P. B. (1985). Pharmacological activation of locomotor patterns in larval and adult frog spinal cords. *Brain Research*, **332**, 119–30.

MacDonald, J. F., Mody, I., and Salter, M. W. (1989). Regulation of *N*-methyl-D-aspartate receptors revealed by intracellular dialysis of murine neurones in culture. *Journal of Physiology* (London), **414**, 17–34.

Markram, H. and Segal, M. (1992). Activation of protein kinase C suppresses responses to NMDA in rat CA1 hippocampal neurones. *Journal of Physiology* (London), **457**, 491–501.

Mayer, M. L., MacDermott, A. B.,Westbrook, G. L., Smith, S. J., and Barker, J. L. (1987). Agonist- and voltage-gated calcium entry in cultured mouse spinal cord neurons under voltage clamp measured using arsenazo III. *Journal of Neuroscience*, **7**, 3230–44.

Nowak, L., Bregetovski, P., Ascher, P., Herbet, A., and Prochiantz, A. (1984). Magnesium gates glutamate activated channels in mouse central neurons. *Nature*, **307**, 462–5.

Orlovsky, G. N., Deliagina, T. G., Grillner, S., and Wallén, P. (1990). Natural vestibular stimulation evokes static and dynamic responses in lamprey reticulospinal neurons. *Acta Physiologica Scandinavica*, **138**, 13A.

Poon, M. (1980). Induction of swimming in lamprey by L-DOPA and amino acids. *Journal of Comparative Physiology*, **136**, 337–44.

Rossignol, S., Barbeau, H., and Julien, C. (1986). Locomotion of the adult chronic spinal cat and its modification by monoaminergic agonists and antagonists. In *Development and plasticity*, (ed. M. E. Goldberger, A. Gorio, and M. Murray), pp. 323–45. Liviana Press, Padova.

Shaw, C. A. and Lanius, R. A. (1992). Reversible kinase and phosphatase regulation of brain amino acid receptors in postnatal development. *Developmental Brain Research*, **70**, 153–61.

Sigvardt, K. A., Grillner, S., Wallén, P., and Van Dongen, P. A. M. (1985). Activation of NMDA receptors elicits fictive locomotion and bistable membrane properties in the lamprey spinal cord. *Brain Research*, **336**, 390–5.

Sillar, K. and Roberts, A. (1991). Segregation of NMDA and non-NMDA receptors at separate synaptic contacts: evidence from spontaneous EPSPs in *Xenopus* embryo spinal neurones. *Brain Research*, **545**, 24–32.

Smith, J. C., Feldman, J. L., and Schmidt, B. J. (1988). Neural mechanisms generating locomotion studied in mammalian brain stem-spinal cord in vitro. *FASEB Journal*, **2**, 2283–8.

Soffe, S. R. and Roberts, A. (1989). The influence of magnesium ions on the NMDA mediated responses of ventral rythmic neurones in the spinal cord of *Xenopus* embryos. *European Journal of Neuroscience*, **1**, 507–15.

Srinivasan, M., Schotland, J., Shupliakov, O., Brodin, L., Hökfelt, T., and Grillner, S. (1993). Intraspinal neurons co-localizing monoamines regulate neuronal firing in the lamprey spinal cord via complementary mechanisms. *European Journal of Neuroscience*, Suppl. **6**: 655 (abstract.)

Stein, P. S. G. and Schild, C. P. (1989). *N*-methyl-D-aspartate antagonist applied to the spinal cord hindlimb enlargement reduces the amplitude of flexion reflex in the turtle. *Brain Research*, **479**, 379–83.

Tegnér, J., Matsushima, T., El Manira, A., and Grillner, S. (1993). The spinal

GABA system modulates burst frequency and intersegmental coordination in the lamprey. Differential effects of GABA$_A$ and GABA$_B$ receptors. *Journal of Neurophysiology*, **69**, 647–57.

Tell, F. and Jean, A. (1991). Activation of *N*-methyl-D-aspartate receptors induces endogenous rhythmic bursting activities in nucleus tractus solitarii neurons: an intracellular study on adult brainstem slices. *European Journal of Neuroscience*, **3**, 1353–65.

Tråvén, H. G. C., Brodin, L., Lansner, A., Ekeberg, Ö., Wallén, P., and Grillner, S. (1993). Computer simulations of NMDA and non-NMDA receptor-mediated synaptic drive: sensory and suprapinal modulation of neurons and small networks. *Journal of Neurophysiology*, **70**. (In press.)

Van Dongen, P. A., Grillner, S., and Hökfelt, T. (1986). 5-Hydroxytryptamine (serotonin) causes a reduction of the afterhyperpolarization following the action potential in lamprey motoneurons and premotor interneurons. *Brain Research*, **366**, 320–5.

Wallén, P. and Grillner, S. (1987). *N*-methyl-D-aspartate receptor-induced, inherent oscillatory activity in neurons active during fictive locomotion in the lamprey. *Journal of Neuroscience*, **7**, 2745–55.

Wallén, P., Buchanan, J. T., Grillner, S., Hill, R. H., Christenson, J., and Hökfelt, T. (1989). Effects of 5-hydroxytryptamine on the after-hyperpolarisation, spike frequency regulation and excitatory membrane properties in lamprey spinal cord neurons. *Journal of Neurophysiology*, **61**, 759–68.

Wang, L.-Y., Salter, M. W., and MacDonald, J. F. (1991). Regulation of kainate receptors by cAMP-dependent protein kinases and phosphatases. *Science*, **253**, 1–3.

Watkins, J. C. and Evans, R. H. (1981). Excitatory amino acid transmitters. *Annual Review of Pharmacology and Toxicology*, **21**, 165–204.

Zucker, R. S. (1989). Short-term plasticity. *Annual Review of Neuroscience*, **12**, 13–31.

13 NMDA receptors and long-term potentiation in the hippocampus

ZAFAR I. BASHIR, NICOLA BERRETTA,
ZUNER A. BORTOLOTTO, KATH CLARK,
CERI H. DAVIES, BRUNO G. FRENGUELLI,
JENNI HARVEY, BRIGITTE POTIER, AND
GRAHAM L. COLLINGRIDGE

Introduction

N-methyl-D-aspartate (NMDA) receptors have been shown to have two important physiological roles in the vertebrate central nervous system; they are mediators of synaptic transmission in many pathways in the brain (see Chapters 10–12) and they are critically involved in neuronal plasticity. This chapter considers long-term potentiation (LTP) in the hippocampus, the first identified and most extensively investigated form of plasticity involving NMDA receptors. The involvement of NMDA receptors in synaptic transmission in the hippocampus is also considered in detail in view of the inextricable link between synaptic transmission and plasticity that NMDA receptors confer upon a synapse.

   Following the identification of their role in hippocampal LTP, NMDA receptors have been strongly implicated in several other forms of neuronal plasticity, including learning and memory (Chapter 15), LTP in the neocortex and in developmental plasticity (Chapter 14), and kindling and kindling-like models of epilepsy (Chapter 17).

LTP as a model of learning and memory

LTP in the hippocampus (Bliss and Collingridge 1993) has been widely studied since it is popularly believed that the mechanisms involved in its induction, expression, and maintenance are fundamental to learning and memory in vertebrates. The reasons for this are numerous and, for the type of LTP considered in this chapter, include the following:

1. LTP is an enhancement of synaptic efficiency (Fig. 13.1) that can be induced by conditioning stimuli within the physiological range. Typically a brief tetanus of the afferent pathway is used (e.g. 100 Hz, 1 s)

A

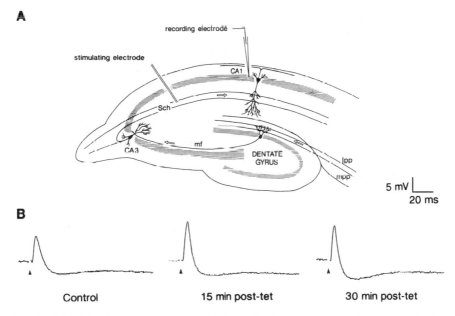

B

Control   15 min post-tet   30 min post-tet

Fig. 13.1 LTP in the hippocampus. (A) Schematic diagram of the rat hippocampal slice preparation illustrating the major excitatory pathways: lateral (lpp) and medial (mpp) perforant paths, mossy fibres (mf), and Schaffer collateral-commissural (Sch) pathway. Typical electrode placements for activating the Sch are shown. (B) An example of LTP recorded intracellularly. EPSP–IPSP sequences were recorded in response to 0.033 Hz stimulation of the Sch pathway and LTP was induced by a tetanus (tet) (100 Hz, 1 s).

although more modest parameters are effective (e.g. four shocks at 100 Hz delivered at the theta frequency).

2. LTP can last a long time (up to a few weeks *in vivo*).

3. It is most prominent in those regions of the brain (e.g. neocortex and hippocampus) that are strongly implicated in learning and memory.

4. LTP is specific to tetanized inputs; non-tetanized inputs, even those converging on the same dendritic region, are not potentiated.

5. There is the requirement for co-operativity amongst afferent fibres (i.e. an intensity threshold) to induce LTP.

6. Associativity amongst afferents can also be demonstrated, i.e. a tetanus too weak to elicit LTP will do so if paired with a strong tetanus.

7. LTP has Hebbian-like properties in that it requires conjoint pre- and post-synaptic activity for its generation.

8. As discussed in Chapter 15, drug treatments that selectively block the induction of LTP also selectively impair learning.

NMDA receptors and the induction of LTP

In the first study designed to investigate the role of the subtypes of excitatory amino acid receptors in hippocampal synaptic transmission and plasticity (Collingridge *et al*. 1983) the following observations were made:

1. The broad spectrum antagonist γ-D-glutamylglycine (DGG) but not the specific NMDA antagonist D-2-amino-5-phosphonopentanoate (AP5 or APV) depressed synaptic transmission evoked by low frequency stimulation of the Schaffer collateral-commissural (Sch) pathway in normal physiological medium.

2. AP5 reversibly prevented the induction of LTP (Fig. 13.2(B)).

3. AP5 had no effect on the potentiated response (i.e. on pre-established LTP).

4. Brief application of NMDA potentiated the synaptic response (Fig. 13.2(A)).

The simplest interpretation of these results is that excitatory amino acid

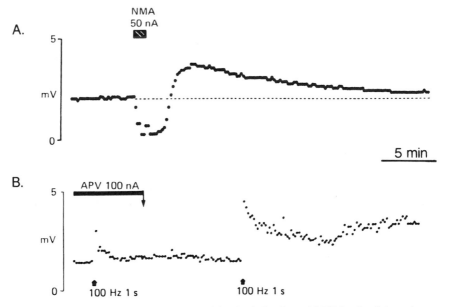

Fig. 13.2 NMDA receptors are involved in the induction of LTP in the Sch pathway. (A) Brief application of *N*-methyl-D,L-aspartate (NMA) causes a brief depression followed by potentiation of the synaptic response. (B) D,L-2-amino-5-phosphonopentanoate (AP5) prevents the induction of LTP. Graphs plot the amplitude of successive responses of the field EPSP (A) or population spike (B) and drugs were applied by iontophoresis into the terminal region of the stimulated fibres for the times indicated by bars. (Adapted from Collingridge *et al*. (1983).)

receptors of a non-NMDA type (hereafter referred to as AMPA (α-amino-3-hydroxy-5-methyl-4-isoxazolepropionic acid) receptors) mediate low frequency transmission before and after the generation of LTP while NMDA receptors mediate the induction of LTP.

Subsequent studies have extended these observations. In particular, it has been shown that the ability of a series of homologues of AP5 to block the induction of LTP correlates with their potency as NMDA antagonists (Harris *et al.* 1984); blockers of the NMDA receptor-gated ion channel (hereafter referred to as the NMDA channel) prevent the induction of LTP (Stringer and Guyenet 1983; Coan *et al.* 1987); 7-chlorokynurenic acid blocks the induction of LTP via an action at the allosteric glycine site on the NMDA receptor (Bashir *et al.* 1990); AP5 blocks LTP induced by brief tetani delivered at the theta frequency (Diamond *et al.* 1988; Larson and Lynch 1988) or by pairing low frequency shocks with depolarization of the post-synaptic cell (Gustafsson *et al.* 1987); late phases of LTP (at least 8 h *in vitro*) require NMDA receptor activation during the tetanus (Reymann *et al.* 1989); AP5 blocks LTP in the perforant pathway input to the dentate gyrus *in vivo* (Errington *et al.* 1987; Morris *et al.* 1986); and AP5 blocks LTP in the associational/commissural innervation but does not block LTP of the mossy fibre innervation of CA3 neurones (Harris and Cotman 1986; Zalutsky and Nicoll 1990). The latter observation is interesting in that mossy fibres innervate a region sparse in NMDA receptors and LTP in this pathway is non-associative. Conversely the other regions, where LTP is both AP5-sensitive and associative in nature, innervate regions rich in NMDA receptors. Only this latter form of LTP will be considered further.

NMDA receptors in hippocampal synaptic transmission

The initial stages of the mechanism by which LTP is initiated have been deduced from studies designed to determine the conditions under which NMDA receptors contribute to synaptic transmission in the Sch pathway. During low frequency transmission, NMDA receptors contribute very little to a subthreshold excitatory post-synaptic potential (EPSP) recorded from a cell at its resting membrane potential in standard physiological medium (Herron *et al.* 1986) (Fig. 13.3(A)). However, NMDA receptors contribute to the synaptic response provided that one of the following conditions is met (Fig. 13.3B):

(1) Mg^{2+} is omitted from the perfusate (Herron *et al.* 1985a);

(2) the cell is strongly depolarized (Collingridge *et al.* 1988a);

(3) synaptic inhibition is depressed by, for example, the γ-aminobutyric acid $(GABA)_A$ antagonist bicuculline (Herron *et al.* 1985b);

(4) the hyperpolarizing aspect of the inhibitory post-synaptic potential (IPSP) is reduced by voltage-clamp techniques (Collingridge *et al.* 1988a).

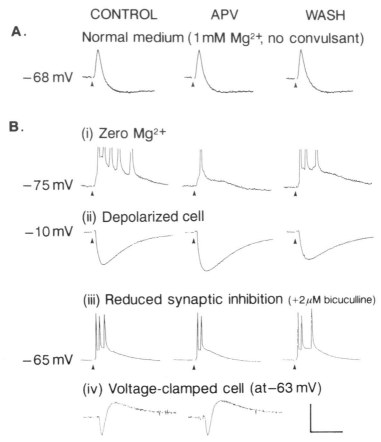

Fig. 13.3. The contribution of NMDA receptors to synaptic responses evoked by low frequency (0.033 Hz) stimulation of the Sch pathway. (A) NMDA receptors do not contribute noticeably to the response of a cell near its resting membrane potential recorded in normal physiological medium. (B) NMDA receptors do, however, contribute substantially to the synaptic response under certain experimental conditions, designed to reduce the level of the voltage-dependent block of NMDA channels by Mg^{2+}. Responses are intracellular recordings from CA1 neurones in response to electrical stimulation of the Sch pathway. Calibration (mV/ms): A, 8/40; B(i) 20/30; (ii), 20/40; (iii), 40/30; (iv), 1 nA/30. (Adapted from Herron *et al.* (1985*a,b*, 1986) and Collingridge *et al.* (1988*a*).)

These observations can be explained on the basis of the voltage-dependent block by Mg^{2+} of NMDA channels (see Chapter 7).

Relative to the AMPA receptor-mediated component, the NMDA receptor-mediated component rises slowly and lasts a long time (Collingridge *et al.* 1988*a*). However, the threshold and latency to onset of the two

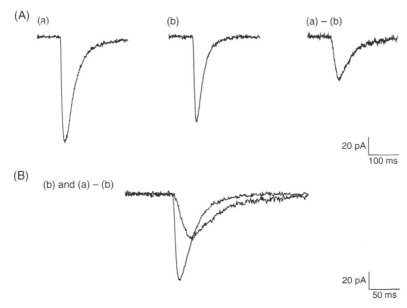

Fig. 13.4 A comparison of the time-course of AMPA and NMDA receptor-mediated EPSCs. (A) A dual-component EPSC, recorded at -60 mV, under control conditions (a) and in the presence of 50 μM D-AP5 (b). $GABA_A$ and $GABA_B$ receptor-mediated IPSCs were eliminated pharmacologically. (B) The pure AMPA receptor-mediated component (b) and the NMDA receptor-mediated component derived by subtraction (a)−(b) are superimposed to illustrate their different time courses.

components are similar (Fig. 13.4), suggesting that they are both mono-synaptic in origin and may be mediated by neurotransmitter released from the same afferent fibres. Thus, it seems that the neurotransmitter (prob-ably L-glutamate) released from terminals of the Sch pathway acts 'simul-taneously' on both AMPA and NMDA receptors. During low frequency transmission NMDA receptors contribute little to the synaptic response since this component activates fairly slowly and the cell is quite quickly hyperpolarized by the IPSP into a region where Mg^{2+} substantially blocks NMDA channels. During high frequency stimulation the cell remains at a depolarized level for much longer, thus enabling activation of the NMDA receptor system (Collingridge *et al.* 1988*b* (Fig. 13.5(A)). Since the NMDA receptor-mediated component has the potential to last a long time (>100 ms) and since it increases in size with membrane depolarization (Fig. 13.5(B)) it summates very effectively at frequencies of 10 Hz and higher (Fig. 13.5(C)). The slow nature of the NMDA receptor-mediated response, which is critical to its function in the induction of LTP, is due to the kinetic properties of NMDA channels (see Chapters 8 and 9).

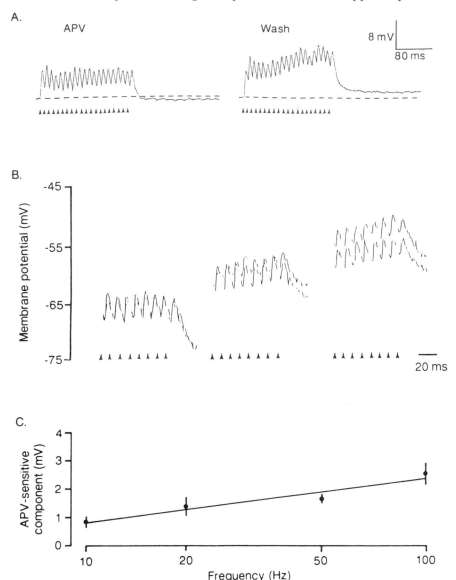

Fig. 13.5 NMDA receptors contribute to high frequency transmission. The Sch was tetanized firstly in the presence of AP5 and then following wash. (A) Responses to 100 Hz stimulation for 200 ms. (B) Records of the last eight shocks in 100 Hz, 200 ms trains for AP5 and wash are superimposed for a cell held at different membrane potentials. Note the increase in the AP5-sensitive component size with depolarization. (C) Mean (±SEM) size of the component for four cells where 20 shocks were applied at different frequencies. Note the increase in size with increasing tetanus frequency. Responses are intracellular recordings from CA1 neurones in response to electrical stimulation of the Sch pathway. (Adapted from Collingridge *et al.* (1988*b*).)

GABA$_B$ autoreceptors and the induction of LTP

The primary reason that cells remain depolarized during high frequency stimulation is because synaptic inhibition is depressed (Fig. 13.6). The depression of inhibition is a property of the GABAergic neurones them-selves since pronounced depression is exhibited by monosynaptic IPSPs and inhibitory post-synaptic currents (IPSCs), which can be evoked in the hippocampus after blockade of excitatory synaptic transmission (Davies *et al.* 1990). The depression of inhibition can most easily be investigated by delivering two shocks of identical strength and recording the resultant monosynaptic IPSCs. At intervals of between approximately 20 and 500 ms the second IPSC is markedly depressed, the maximum depression occur-ring at between 100 and 200 ms. The depression is caused by GABA feeding back and inhibiting its own release via an action on GABA$_B$ autoreceptors (Davies *et al.* 1990). This effect can be blocked by GABA$_B$ antagonists such as 3-amino-propyl(diethoxymethyl)-phosphinic acid (CGP 35348) (Davies *et al.* 1991) and 3-*N*[1-(S)-(3,4-dichlorophenyl) ethyl]amino-2-(S)-hydroxypropyl-*P*-benzyl-phosphinic acid (CGP 55845A) (Davies *et al.* 1993). Depression of inhibition, mediated by GABA$_B$ auto-receptors, also occurs during 'theta' type patterns of activity. For example, the inhibition during a burst of four stimuli delivered at 100 Hz is depressed if this burst is preceded by a single 'priming' stimulus. In slices where synaptic excitation has not been blocked pharmacologically, this depress-ion of inhibition enables the NMDA receptor system to be activated sufficiently to induce LTP. Thus, when 'priming' type stimuli are used to induce LTP, then GABA$_B$ antagonists can block the induction of LTP by preventing the depression of GABA$_A$ receptor-mediated synaptic inhibi-tion and the resultant transient activation of the NMDA receptor system (Davies *et al.* 1991).

It should be noted that GABA$_B$ antagonists do not prevent the induction of LTP when long, high frequency trains are delivered (Olpe and Karlsson 1990). This is because the GABA$_B$ autoreceptor-mediated depression of inhibition is compensated for physiologically, and other factors, such as changes in ionic equilibria, come into play (Davies and Collingridge 1993). The significance of GABA$_B$ autoreceptors, however, is that they permit the synaptic activation of NMDA receptors during the sorts of patterns of activity that are thought to occur naturally in the animal (brief, high frequency, synchronized discharges). Thus, from a physiological perspect-ive, GABA$_B$ autoreceptors are primary regulators of the induction of LTP.

Metabotropic glutamate receptors and the induction of LTP

Although the activation of NMDA receptors by the brief application of NMDA induces a synaptic potentiation (Fig. 13.2(A)) the effect does not normally persist for more than 30–60 min. This has led to the suggestion

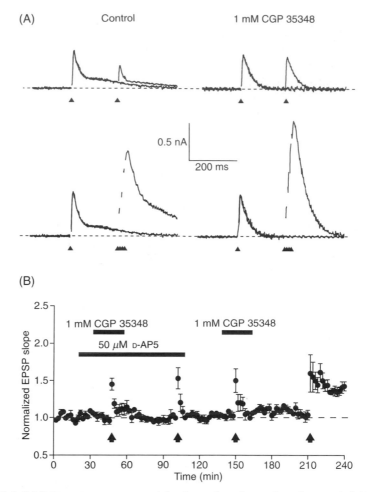

Fig. 13.6 GABA$_B$ autoreceptors, activity-dependent depression of synaptic inhibition, and the induction of LTP. (A) The GABA$_B$ antagonist CGP 35348 reverses the depression of monosynaptic IPSCs induced by a stimulus delivered 200 ms earlier to the same population of inhibitory neurones. The upper records show reversal of depression of a single IPSC (i.e. paired-pulse depression) and the lower traces show reversal of the depression of the IPSC evoked by four stimuli delivered at 100 Hz. (CGP 35348 also blocks post-synaptic GABA$_B$ receptors and so the GABA$_B$ receptor-mediated IPSC is eliminated by this treatment.) Responses to single shock stimulation are superimposed on the records to aid visualization of the extent of the depression. (B) Shows that CGP 35348, like AP5, blocks the induction of LTP induced by a 'primed-burst' protocol (four shocks at 100 Hz delivered 200 ms after a single priming stimulus—the same stimulus protocol as above—delivered at the times indicated by arrows). The graph plots pooled data (n = 4) of field EPSP slope versus time. (Adapted and expanded from Davies *et al*. (1991).)

that an additional factor may be required for the induction of LTP (Kauer *et al.* 1988). Recently, evidence has accumulated that the activation of metabotropic glutamate receptors (mGluRs) may also be involved in the induction of LTP.

The activation of mGluRs with 1-aminocyclopentane-1S,3R-dicarboxy-late (ACPD) facilitates tetanus-induced induction of LTP (McGuinness *et al.* 1991). Indeed, as shown in Fig. 13.7, ACPD is able to convert a sub-threshold tetanus into an effective one. There are at least two con-sequences of mGluR activation that can account for this facilitation.

ACPD potentiates acutely responses to NMDA (Fig. 13.8). This effect is similar to, for example, potentiation of NMDA responses by muscarinic receptor stimulation (Markram and Segal 1992). We believe that the ability of ACPD to potentiate responses to NMDA is not mediated by the activa-tion of protein kinase C (PKC) since the effect persists in the presence of protein kinase inhibitors (staurosporine and K-252b). Indeed, we find that activation of PKC by a phorbol ester inhibits (rather than mimics) the effect of ACPD, possibly by causing feedback inhibition. We also feel that the effect of ACPD does not depend on release of Ca^{2+} from intracellular stores since the effect persists in the presence of thapsigargin (Harvey and Collingridge 1993), a compound which leads to store depletion by prevent-ing their re-filling.

ACPD also induces a slow-onset potentiation (Bortolotto and Colling-ridge 1993). This effect is independent of the action of NMDA receptors, since it can be induced in the presence of AP5 (Fig. 13.9(A)). We consider, however, that it is most likely that ACPD-induced slow-onset potentiation and tetanus-induced LTP are equivalent and that ACPD is somehow able to induce LTP by obviating the need for the NMDA receptor activation

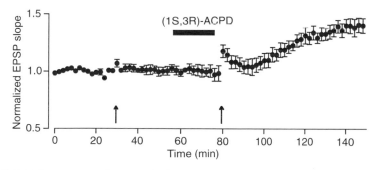

Fig. 13.7 Enhancement of tetanus-induced LTP by (1S,3R)-ACPD. The graph plots normalized pooled data (n = 7) of the slope of the field EPSP as a function of time. A low intensity tetanus was delivered at the time indicated by the first arrow and led to little or no potentiation. A second tetanus of identical strength was then delivered in the presence of 10 μM (1S,3R)-ACPD and resulted in a greater initial enhancement (i.e. larger STP) and a sustained potentiation (i.e. LTP). (Adapted from Collingridge *et al.* (1991).)

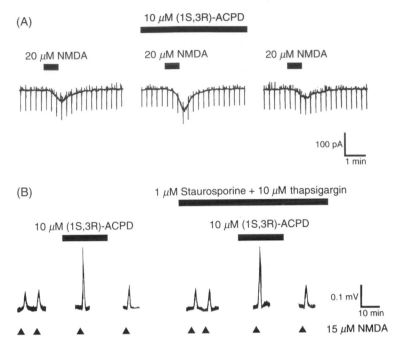

Fig. 13.8 Reversible potentiation of NMDA responses by (1S,3R)-ACPD. (A) (1S,3R)-ACPD produces a reversible potentiation of the inward currents induced in a CA1 neurone by bath application of NMDA. The cell was voltage-clamped at −60 mV using whole-cell recording techniques. The negative deflections are the current steps required to hyperpolarize the membrane by 10 mV. (B) (1S,3R)-ACPD produces reversible potentiation of NMDA responses even in the presence of high concentrations of staurosporine and thapsigargin. Recordings were obtained using a grease-gap technique. Data from unpublished experiments (A) and experiments reported in Harvey and Collingridge (1993) (B).

stage. One line of evidence for this is that the two forms of potentiation are mutually exclusive, since saturation of one form prevents the induction of the other (Fig. 13.9(B) and (C)). ACPD-induced, slow-onset potentiation is prevented by thapsigargin. One possibility, then, is that ACPD can release sufficient Ca^{2+} from intracellular stores that the NMDA receptor-mediated Ca^{2+} flux is no longer required. ACPD-induced, slow-onset potentiation is also prevented by the kinase inhibitors staurosporine and K-252b. Since these agents inhibit PKC (albeit non-specifically) and since ACPD, via activation of certain of the mGluR family, can activate phosphoinositide-specific phospholipase C (PLC), which in turn will lead to the activation of PKC, we suspect that this enzyme system is also involved in the slow-onset potentiation. Our best guess is that both limbs of the phosphoinositide signalling pathway are necessary for ACPD-induced, slow-onset potentiation.

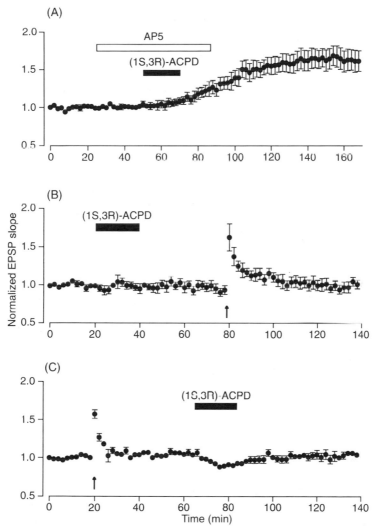

Fig. 13.9 (1S,3R)-ACPD induces, via an NMDA receptor-independent mechanism, a slow-onset potentiation that occludes with tetanus-induced LTP. (A) (1S,3R)-ACPD induces a slow-onset potentiation in the presence of 50 μM D-AP5. (B) Repeated applications of (1S,3R)-ACPD results in saturation of the effect. Following the last (fourth or fifth) application of (1S,3R)-ACPD, a tetanus induces STP but not LTP. (C) (1S,3R)-ACPD does not induce potentiation when applied for the first time following saturation of LTP (obtained by delivering three to five periods of tetanic stimulation). Each graph plots normalized data from six experiments. (1S,3R)-ACPD was applied for 20 min at a concentration of 10 μM. (Modified from Bortolotto and Collingridge (1993).)

The above experiments show that activation of mGluRs by ACPD can both modulate and substitute for tetanus-induced LTP. They do not tell, however, whether mGluRs are actually involved in the induction of LTP physiologically. For this antagonists are needed. The first studies (Reymann and Matthies 1989; Izumi *et al.* 1991) were performed with aminophosphonobutanoate (AP4) and aminophosphonopropionate (AP3), but these are weak, non-specific mGluR antagonists and so the results are difficult to interpret. More recently, α-methyl-4-carboxyphenylglycine (MCPG) was shown to be a specific, competitive mGluR antagonist (Eaton *et al.* 1993). This compound eliminates both ACPD-induced, slow-onset potentiation and tetanus-induced LTP, in an entirely specific manner (Bashir *et al.* 1993). In the presence of MCPG, tetanic stimulation elicits a decremental potentiation, known as short-term potentiation (STP). The time course of STP complements that of ACPD-induced, slow-onset potentiation, such that if they are added together the result is similar to that induced by a tetanus under control conditions. From these results it can be concluded that mGluRs, like NMDA receptors, are necessary triggers for the induction of LTP by tetanic stimulation. Thus, LTP involves two distinct trigger mechanisms; the possible roles and inter-relationships between these receptors during the induction of LTP are shown schematically in Fig. 13.10 (see also Bortolotto *et al.* 1994).

NMDA receptors and Ca^{2+} signalling in hippocampal neurones

An issue of current interest is to determine precisely what signal the activation of NMDA receptors provides with respect to the induction of LTP. Since NMDA channels are permeable to Ca^{2+} (see Chapter 7) and since the intracellular application of Ca^{2+} chelators prevents the induction of LTP (Lynch *et al.* 1983; Malenka *et al.* 1988) it is reasonable to assume that the key signal is Ca^{2+} flux through NMDA channels. Indeed, it is widely assumed that Ca^{2+} entry, localized within the spines of activated inputs, confers the property of input specificity. Such signals are not easy to study, however, since when NMDA receptors are activated the cell depolarizes and Ca^{2+} enters through voltage-gated Ca^{2+} channels. By the combination of intracellular dialysis and voltage-clamp techniques we have been able to detect the Ca^{2+} which, in response to tetanic stimulation, enters into dendrites and dendritic spines by permeating through NMDA channels (Fig. 13.11). It seems that this signal is boosted, approximately three-fold, by the release of Ca^{2+} from intracellular stores (Alford *et al.* 1993). Recently, we have obtained some preliminary evidence that MCPG reduces, but unlike AP5 does not eliminate, the tetanus-induced Ca^{2+} rise (Frenguelli *et al.* 1993). We suspect, therefore, that activation of mGluRs may also be involved, at least under certain circumstances, in the release of Ca^{2+} from intracellular stores in response to tetanic stimulation. It is possible that to access these stores it is necessary for NMDA receptors to

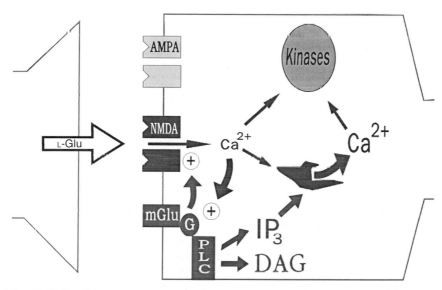

Fig. 13.10 Possible interactions between NMDA receptors and mGluRs in the induction of LTP. In this scheme the Ca^{2+} which enters through NMDA channels, is involved in the activation of kinases, releases additional Ca^{2+} from intracellular stores, and facilitates the activation of mGluRs. Stimulation of mGluRs, and the resulting formation of inositol-1,4,5-trisphosphate (IP_3) and diacylglycerol (DAG), is also involved in the activation of kinases. In addition, activation of mGluRs facilitates the activation of the NMDA receptor system.

provide a Ca^{2+} signal and for mGluRs to provide inositol trisphosphate ($InsP_3$) and that the two messengers act synergistically.

NMDA receptors and the disabling and reversing of LTP

With respect to synaptic plasticity, NMDA receptors do not act simply as triggers for the induction of LTP. To induce LTP it is necessary for there to be a brief activation of the NMDA receptor system. Presumably a certain level of activation needs to be reached to provide a transient Ca^{2+} signal of sufficient magnitude to activate the enzyme systems involved in the induction of LTP. If the level of activation is too low, not only is LTP not induced but the induction of LTP by a normally supra-threshold tetanus can be inhibited. In other words, inappropriate activation of the NMDA receptor system can 'disable' the induction process. This disabling was first shown by bathing slices in a nominally Mg^{2+}-free medium, such that the NMDA receptor system is activated both tonically and by low frequency stimulation (Coan *et al.* 1989). Under these conditions, the addition of sufficient AP5 to inhibit NMDA receptor activation at all times except during the tetanus *enables* LTP to be induced in Mg^{2+}-free medium.

Disabling can also be obtained by applying NMDA either before or after the tetanus (Izumi *et al.* 1992) or by delivering a subthreshold tetanus (Huang *et al.* 1992). This latter observation is interesting since it suggests that this disabling process could occur physiologically.

NMDA receptors have also been shown to be involved in the form of long-term depression (LTD) of synaptic transmission in the hippocampus, which can be induced by a prolonged period of stimulation (e.g. 15 min) at frequencies of about 1–2 Hz (Dudek and Bear 1992). In our experiments, this type of stimulation usually only induces LTD in slices in which LTP has previously been induced. In other words, the LTD is a depotentiation phenomenon (Barrionuevo *et al.* 1980; Fujii *et al.* 1991).

NMDA receptors and the expression of LTP

LTP is usually studied under conditions where AMPA receptors mediate the vast majority of the synaptic response. Thus, LTP is seen as an increase in the AMPA receptor-mediated component of synaptic transmission (Fig. 13.1). The locus of expression of LTP, as expressed in this manner, is the subject of much controversy (Bliss and Collingridge 1993), and is outside the scope of this chapter.

Most laboratories would agree, however, that it is also possible to induce LTP of the NMDA receptor-mediated component of synaptic transmission (Tsien and Malinow 1990; Bashir *et al.* 1991; Berretta *et al.* 1991; Asztely *et al.* 1992; Xie *et al.* 1992). We find LTP of the pharmacologically isolated NMDA receptor-mediated current which resembles LTP of AMPA receptor-mediated synaptic responses (Fig. 13.12(A)). When we compare the size of the potentiation of the AMPA and NMDA receptor-mediated components of dual-component EPSCs we see little or no difference, followed for up to 30 min following the tetanus (Fig. 13.12(B)). This could be because the synaptic potentiation is expressed by an increase in L-glutamate release or because there are post-synaptic modifications which involve both AMPA and NMDA receptors. At the present time little is known about the mechanisms which underlie LTP of the NMDA receptor-mediated component. However, the fact the induction mechanism is itself potentially plastic has profound implications for physiological and pathological processes.

Concluding remarks

The mechanisms responsible for enabling the transient activation of the NMDA receptor system during tetanic stimulation are fairly well understood. What we now need to know is precisely what happens following NMDA receptor activation to lead to the expression of LTP. Related to this question is the manner in which the activation of mGluRs contributes to the induction of LTP. This system, through its coupling to several intracellular signalling pathways, may add extra levels of complexity to the induction process. A final topic about which we know very

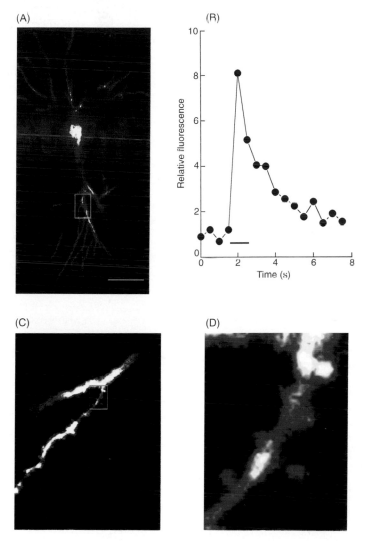

Fig. 13.11 Ca^{2+} signalling associated with the synaptic activation of NMDA receptors. (A) A confocal image of a fluo-3-loaded CA1 pyramidal neurone in a hippocampal slice. The scale bar represents 50 μm. (B) The increase in fluorescence measured over a length of dendrite within the box shown in (A) plotted *versus* time. The rise in fluorescence is due to a single period of tetanic stimulation (100 Hz, 1 s) delivered, at the time indicated by the bar, to the Schaffer collateral-commissural pathway. The neurone was voltage-clamped at −35 mV using a patch electrode. The increase in fluorescence reflects an increase in Ca^{2+} and is dependent upon the synaptic activation of NMDA receptors (Alford *et al.* 1993). (C) A higher power image, obtained with a 60× oil immersion objective, of a dendritic region of the neurone in a focal plane closer to the objective. The image is an on-line average of 15 sweeps. (D) A digital enlargement of the area within the box illustrated in (C). Note the dendritic spines. The box in (C) is approximately 5 μm wide.

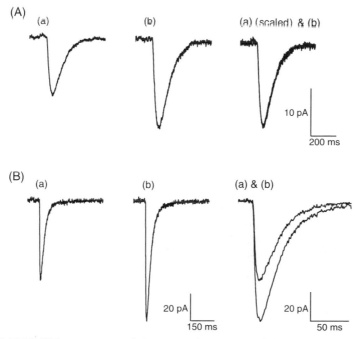

Fig. 13.12 NMDA receptors and the expression of LTP. (A) LTP of a pure NMDA receptor-mediated EPSC. The traces show responses before (a) and 30 min following (b) the induction of LTP. In the superimposed trace (a & b) the control response has been scaled to the same peak amplitude as the potentiated response to show that the LTP does not alter the time course of the EPSCs. (B) LTP of a dual-component EPSC. Responses were obtained before (a) and 30 min following (b) the induction of LTP. The cell was voltage-clamped at −60 mV. Note the increase in slope of the rising phase of the EPSC and in the amplitude of the EPSC at times exceeding 100 ms post-stimulus. These parameters measure predominantly the AMPA and NMDA receptor-mediated component of the EPSC, respectively. Data adapted from Bashir *et al.* (1991) (A) and Clark and Collingridge (1994) (B).

little concerns the mechanisms by which LTP of the NMDA receptor-mediated component is expressed.

Acknowledgements

We thank our former colleagues from the laboratory for their contributions to the work referred to here. In particular, we thank Stephen Davies who was co-author of the chapter in the first edition from which this chapter developed. The work described here has been supported by the MRC and The Wellcome Trust.

References

Alford, S., Frenguelli, B. G., Schofield, J. G., and Collingridge, G. L. (1993). Characterisation of Ca^{2+} signals induced in hippocampal CA1 neurones by the synaptic activation of NMDA receptors. *Journal of Physiology* (London), **469**, 693–716.

Asztely, F., Wigström, H., and Gustafsson, B. (1992). The relative contribution of NMDA receptor channels in the expression of long-term potentiation in the hippocampal CA1 region. *European Journal of Neuroscience*, **4**, 681–90.

Barrionuevo, G., Schottler, F., and Lynch, G. (1980). The effects of repetitive low frequency stimulation on control and 'potentiated' synaptic responses in the hippocampus. *Life Science*, **27**, 2385–91.

Bashir, Z. I., Tam, B., and Collingridge, G. L. (1990). Activation of the glycine site on the NMDA receptor is necessary for the induction of LTP. *Neuroscience Letters*, **108**, 261–6.

Bashir, Z. I., Alford, S., Davies, S. N., Randall, A. D., and Collingridge, G. L. (1991). Long-term potentiation of NMDA receptor-mediated synaptic transmission in the hippocampus. *Nature*, **349**, 156–8.

Bashir, Z. I., Bortolotto, Z. A., Davies, C. H., Berretta, N., Irving, A. J., Seal, A. J., Henley, J. M., Jane, D. E., Watkins, J. C., and Collingridge, G. L. (1993). Induction of LTP in the hippocampus needs synaptic activation of glutamate metabotropic receptors. *Nature*, **363**, 347–50.

Berretta, N., Berton, F., Bianchi, R., Brunelli, M., Capogna, M., and Francesconi, W. (1991). Long-term potentiation of NMDA receptor-mediated EPSP in guinea-pig hippocampal slices. *European Journal of Neuroscience*, **3**, 850–4.

Bliss, T. V. P. and Collingridge, G. L. (1993). A synaptic model of memory: Long-term potentiation in the hippocampus. *Nature*, **361**, 31–9.

Bortolotto, Z. A., Bashir, Z. I., Davies, C. H., and Collingridge, G. L. (1994). A molecular switch activated by metabotropic glutamate receptors regulates induction of long-term potentiation. *Nature*, **368**, 740–3.

Bortolotto, Z. A. and Collingridge, G. L. (1993). Characterisation of LTP induced by the activation of glutamate metabotropic receptors in area CA1 of the hippocampus. *Neuropharmacology*, **32**, 1–9.

Clark, K. A. and Collingridge, G. L. (1994). Synaptic potentiation of dual-component excitatory postsynaptic currents in the rat hippocampus. *J. Physiol.* (Lond.). In press.

Coan, E. J., Saywood, W., and Collingridge, G. L. (1987). MK 801 blocks NMDA receptor-mediated synaptic transmission and long term potentiation in rat hippocampal slices. *Neuroscience Letters*, **80**, 111–14.

Coan, E. J., Irving, A. J., and Collingridge, G. L. (1989). Low-frequency activation of the NMDA receptor system can prevent the induction of LTP. *Neuroscience Letters*, **105**, 205–10.

Collingridge, G. L., Kehl, S. J., and McLennan, H. (1983). Excitatory amino acids in synaptic transmission in the Schaffer-collateral commissural pathway of the rat hippocampus. *Journal of Physiology* (London), **334**, 33–46.

Collingridge, G. L., Herron, C. E., and Lester, R. A. J. (1988*a*). Synaptic activation of *N*-methyl-D-aspartate receptors in the Schaffer collateral-commissural pathway of rat hippocampus. *Journal of Physiology* (London), **399**, 283–300.

Collingridge, G. L., Herron, C. E., and Lester, R. A. J. (1988*b*). Frequency-dependent *N*-methyl-D-aspartate receptor-mediated synaptic transmission in rat hippocampus. *Journal of Physiology* (London), **399**, 301–12.

Collingridge, G. L., Harvey, J., Frenguelli, B. G., Bortolotto, Z. A., Bashir, Z. I., and Davies, C. H. (1991). Amino acid receptors and long term potentiation. *International Academy for Biomedical and Drug Research*, **2**, 41–9.

Davies, C. H. and Collingridge, G. L. (1993). The physiological regulation of synaptic inhibition by GABA_B autoreceptors in rat hippocampus. *Journal of Physiology* (London), **472**, 245–65.

Davies, C. H., Davies, S. N., and Collingridge, G. L. (1990). Paired-pulse depression of monosynaptic GABA-mediated inhibitory postsynaptic responses in rat hippocampus. *Journal of Physiology* (London), **424**, 513–31.

Davies, C. H., Starkey, S. J., Pozza, M. F., and Collingridge, G. L. (1991). GABA_B autoreceptors regulate the induction of LTP. *Nature*, **349**, 609–11.

Davies, C. H., Pozza, M. F., and Collingridge, G. L. (1993). CGP 55845A: A potent antagonist of GABA_B receptors in the CA1 region of rat hippocampus. *Neuropharmacology*, **32**, 1071–3.)

Diamond, D. M., Dunwiddie, T. V., and Rose, G. M. (1988). Characteristics of hippocampal primed burst potentiation in vitro and in the awake rat. *Journal of Neuroscience*, **8**, 4079–88.

Dudek, S. M. and Bear, M. F. (1992). Homosynaptic long-term depression in area CA1 of hippocampus and effects of N-methyl-D-aspartate receptor blockade. *Proceedings of the National Academy of Science, USA*, **89**, 4363–7.

Eaton, S. A., Jane, D. E., Jones, P. L. St. J., Porter, R. H. P., Pook, P. C.-K., Sunter, D. C., Udvarhelyi, P. M., Roberts, P. J., Salt, T. E., and Watkins, J. C. (1993). Competitive antagonism at metabotropic glutamate receptors by (S)-4-carboxyphenylglycine and (RS)-α-methyl-4-carboxyphenylglycine. *European Journal of Pharmacology and Molecular Pharmacology*, **244**, 195–7.

Errington, M. L., Lynch, M. A., and Bliss, T. V. P. (1987). Long-term potentiation in the dentate gyrus: induction and increased glutamate release are blocked by D(−)aminophosphonovalerate. *Neuroscience*, **20**, 279–84.

Frenguelli, B. G., Potier, B., Slater, N. T., Alford, S., and Collingridge, G. L. (1993). Metabotropic glutamate receptors and calcium signalling in dendrites of hippocampal CA1 neurones. *Neuropharmacology*, **32**, 1229–37.

Fujii, S., Saito, K., Miyakawa, H., Ito, K., and Kato, H. (1991). Reversal of long-term potentiation (depotentiation) induced by tetanus stimulation of the input to CA1 neurons of guinea pig hippocampal slices. *Brain Research*, **555**, 112–22.

Gustafsson, B., Wigström, H., Abraham, W. C., and Huang, Y.-Y. (1987). Long-term potentiation in the hippocampus using depolarizing current pulses as the conditioning stimulus to single volley synaptic potentials. *Journal of Neuroscience*, **7**, 774–80.

Harris, E. W. and Cotman, C. W. (1986). Long-term potentiation of guinea pig mossy fiber responses is not blocked by N-methyl-D-aspartate antagonists. *Neuroscience Letters*, **70**, 132–7.

Harris, E. W., Ganong, A. H., and Cotman, C. W. (1984). Long term potentiation in the hippocampus involves activation of N-methyl-D-aspartate receptors. *Brain Research*, **323**, 132–7.

Harvey, J. and Collingridge, G. L. (1993). Signal transduction pathways involved in the acute potentiation of NMDA responses by 1S,3R-ACPD in rat hippocampal slices. *British Journal of Pharmacology*, **109**, 1085–90.

Herron, C. E., Lester, R. A. J., Coan, E. J., and Collingridge, G. L. (1985a). Intracellular demonstration of an N-methyl-D-aspartate receptor mediated component of synaptic transmission in the rat hippocampus. *Neuroscience Letters*, **60**, 19–23.

Herron, C. E., Williamson, R., and Collingridge, G. L. (1985b). A selective N-methyl-D-aspartate antagonist depresses epileptiform activity in rat hippocampal slices. *Neuroscience Letters*, **61**, 255–60.

Herron, C. E., Lester, R. A. J., Coan, E. J., and Collingridge, G. L. (1986).

Frequency-dependent involvement of NMDA receptors in the hippocampus: a novel synaptic mechanism. *Nature*, **322**, 265–8.

Huang, Y.-Y., Colino, A., Selig, D. K., and Malenka, R. C. (1992). The influence of prior synaptic activity on the induction of long-term potentiation. *Science*, **255**, 730–3.

Izumi, Y., Clifford, D. B., and Zorumski, C. F. (1991). 2-Amino-3-phosphonopropionate blocks the induction and maintenance of long-term potentiation in rat hippocampal slices. *Neuroscience Letters*, **122**, 187–90.

Izumi, Y., Clifford, D. B., and Zorumski, C. F. (1992). Low concentrations of N-methyl-D-aspartate inhibit the induction of long-term potentiation in rat hippocampal slices. *Neuroscience Letters*, **137**, 245–8.

Kauer, J. A., Malenka, R. C., and Nicoll, R. A. (1988). NMDA application potentiates synaptic transmission in the hippocampus. *Nature*, **334**, 250–2.

Larson, J. and Lynch, G. (1988). Role of N-methyl-D-aspartate receptors in the induction of synaptic potentiation by burst stimulation patterned after the hippocampal θ-rhythm. *Brain Research*, **441**, 111–18.

Lynch, G., Larson, J., Kelso, S., Barrionuevo, G., and Schottler, F. (1983). Intracellular injections of EGTA block induction of hippocampal long-term potentiation. *Nature*, **305**, 719–21.

McGuinness, N., Anwyl, R., and Rowan, M. (1991). Trans-ACPD enhances long-term potentiation in the hippocampus. *European Journal of Pharmacology*, **197**, 231–2.

Malenka, R. C., Kauer, J. A., Zucker, R. S., and Nicoll, R. A. (1988). Postsynaptic calcium is sufficient for potentiation of hippocampal synaptic transmission. *Science*, **242**, 81–4.

Markram, H. and Segal, M. (1992). The inositol 1,4,5-trisphosphate pathway mediates cholinergic potentiation of rat hippocampal neuronal responses to NMDA. *Journal of Physiology* (London), **447**, 513–33.

Morris, R. G. M., Anderson, E., Lynch, G. S., and Baudry, M. (1986). Selective impairment of learning and blockade of long-term potentiation by an N-methyl-D-aspartate receptor antagonist, AP5. *Nature*, **319**, 774–6.

Olpe, H.-R. and Karlsson, G. (1990). The effects of baclofen and two GABA$_B$-receptor antagonists on long-term potentiation. *Naunyn Schmiedebergs Archives of Pharmacology*, **342**, 194–7.

Reymann, K. G. and Matthies, H. (1989). 2-Amino-4-phosphonobutyrate selectively eliminates late phases of long-term potentiation in rat hippocampus. *Neuroscience Letters*, **98**, 166–71.

Reymann, K. G., Matthies, H. K., Schulzeck, K., and Matthies, H. (1989). N-methyl-D-aspartate receptor activation is required for the induction of both early and late phases of long-term potentiation in rat hippocampal slices. *Neuroscience Letters*, **96**, 96–101.

Stringer, J. L. and Guyenet, P. G. (1983). Elimination of long-term potentiation in the hippocampus by phencyclidine and ketamine. *Brain Research*, **258**, 159–64.

Tsien, R. W. and Malinow, R. (1990). Long-term potentiation: Presynaptic enhancement following postsynaptic activation of calcium-dependent protein kinases. *Cold Spring Harbor Symposium on Quantitative Biology*, **55**, 147–59.

Xie, X., Berger, T. W., and Barrionuevo, G. (1992) Isolated NMDA receptor-mediated synaptic responses express both LTP and LTD. *Journal of Neurophysiology*, **67**, 1009–13.

Zalutsky, R. A. and Nicoll, R. A. (1990). Comparison of two forms of long-term potentiation in single hippocampal neurons. *Science*, **249**, 1619–24.

14 NMDA receptors and developmental plasticity in visual neocortex

ALAIN ARTOLA AND WOLF SINGER

Learning can be considered as a stimulus- and, hence, activity-dependent neuronal process that leads to a lasting change of stimulus–response relationships. The formation of a memory trace may thus be considered as a modification of the neuronal program that specifies input–output functions. This program is contained in the architecture of neuronal connectivity and in the transfer functions of these connections. Thus, any activity-dependent process that modifies, in a sufficiently stable and long-lasting way, the interactions between pairs of neurones could serve as a mechanism of learning.

Activity-dependent modifications of synaptic connections play a crucial role in the self-organization of the developing brain. Most of our knowledge on these modifications comes from investigations of the *developing* visual system of mammals. In these highly developed brains, experience-dependent shaping of neuronal architecture is a necessary prerequisite for the acquisition of normal perceptual functions. The most dramatic evidence for this comes from patients who suffered from congenital opacities of the eyes during early childhood and therefore were unable to perceive contours. With the development of lens transplants the optical media of these patients' eyes could be restored but, unexpectedly, these patients were unable to recover visual functions when operated on as juveniles or adults. Experiments in visually deprived animals have revealed that these functional deficits are primarily due to abnormalities in the visual centres of the cerebral cortex. The reason is that certain cortical functions can only be developed if visual experience is available.

Activity-dependent, long-term changes of synaptic connections can also be produced experimentally in the *adult* brain. Since the initial demonstration by Bliss and Lömo (1973) that high frequency stimulation of monosynaptic excitatory pathways in the hippocampus causes a long-term potentiation (LTP) of synaptic transmission (for review see Bliss and Collingridge 1993) this phenomenon has been uncovered, both *in vivo* and *in vitro*, in a variety of other telencephalic structures such as the motor cortex (Baranyi and Feher 1981*a,b*; Bindman *et al.* 1988; Iriki *et al.* 1989), the visual cortex (Komatsu *et al.* 1981, 1988; Artola and Singer 1987, 1990; Perkins and Teyler 1988; Berry *et al.* 1989; Kimura *et al.* 1989), the prefrontal cortex

(Sutor and Hablitz 1989; Hirsch and Crépel 1990), the cingulate cortex (Sah and Nicoll 1991), the entorhinal cortex (de Curtis and Llinas 1993), and the striatum (Calabresi *et al.* 1992*b*). More recently, evidence has also been obtained for a use-dependent, long-term decrease of synaptic efficacy that is commonly called homosynaptic long-term depression (LTD) (for taxonomy of LTD see Artola and Singer (1993)). It has been found to occur in the cerebellum (Ito and Kano 1982; Ito *et al.* 1982; Sakurai 1987), in the hippocampus (Dunwiddie and Lynch 1978; Chattarji *et al.* 1989; Stanton and Sejnowski 1989; Dudek and Bear 1992; Mulkey and Malenka 1992), the sensori-motor cortex (Bindman *et al.* 1988), the visual cortex (Artola *et al.* 1990; Kimura *et al.* 1990), the prefrontal cortex (Hirsch and Crépel 1990), and the striatum (Calabresi *et al.* 1992*a*).

Although obvious differences exist with respect to the consequences of synaptic modifications in the developing and mature visual cortex (during early development use-dependent modifications of synaptic coupling lead to extensive changes in the architecture of connections) the induction mechanisms share a number of similarities. *In vivo* and *in vitro* studies support the notion that the *N*-methyl-D-aspartate (NMDA) receptor has a key function both in developmental reorganization of cortical connections and in synaptic plasticity in the mature cortex.

Experience-dependent modifications of ocular dominance as a model of developmental plasticity

Activity-dependent consolidation and disruption of functional binocularity

As Hubel and Wiesel (1965) demonstrated in their pioneering studies, the connections between the two eyes and the cells in striate cortex are malleable during early postnatal development and subject to use-dependent modifications. After birth and before visual experience becomes effective in influencing the ocularity of cortical neurones, most cells in the visual cortex of cats are functionally connected to both eyes and respond to stimulation of either eye. At this developmental stage the terminal arborizations of the afferents from the two eyes are exuberant and show a considerable overlap. During the first postnatal weeks this overlap gets reduced, the terminals segregate to form the characteristic ocular dominance columns, and the neurones develop well delineated receptive fields in both eyes. This pruning process depends on visual signals. When the animals are kept in the dark or when retinal activity is blocked, the segregation of thalamo-cortical afferents fails to occur and the receptive fields remain poorly delineated (Cynader *et al.* 1976; Mower *et al.* 1984; Stryker and Harris 1986). The crucial role that retinal signals have in this pruning process becomes particularly obvious when visual experience is available but manipulated. If, for example, one eye is deprived of contour vision while the other is allowed to view normally, the large majority of cortical cells rapidly lose the ability to respond to the deprived eye (Wiesel and Hubel 1965; Blakemore *et al.* 1978). When induced early in development, at times when segregation of thalamic afferents is not yet completed, these functional changes go in parallel with the retraction and expansion of the territories occupied by the thalamic afferents from the two eyes. In part, the ocularity changes are thus due to selective consolidation and disruption of connections between thalamic afferents and their cortical target cells. However, the modifications of ocular dominance are also associated with changes in the efficacy of intracortical synaptic connections. This latter mechanism becomes more prominent at later stages of development when axonal segregation is already in an advanced stage. This has to be inferred from the evidence that marked changes in the ocularity of cortical neurones can occur without or with only minor modifications of the termination patterns of thalamic afferents in layer IV. One example is the late change of ocular dominance in dark-reared kittens. In normally reared kittens monocular deprivation is only effective during a critical period that lasts about 3 months (Dews and Wiesel 1970; Olson and Freeman 1980). In dark-reared kittens, by contrast, monocular deprivation induces changes of ocular dominance even after the end of this period (Cynader 1983). These late changes of ocularity are, however, not associated with changes of columnar patterns in layer IV (Mower and Christen 1985; Mower *et al.* 1985). Another example for such a dissociation is the modification occurring with strabismus. Here the morphological pattern of ocular dominance columns in layer IV is nearly unchanged (Levay *et al.* 1978), while the functional ocularity of cortical neurones is drastically altered. Most cells become monocular and excitable only either by the right or the left eye (Hubel and Wiesel 1965). In addition, tangential connections between cortical territories innervated by afferents from different eyes become removed (Löwel and Singer 1992). Finally, there is evidence from single cell recording and deoxyglucose mapping in monocularly deprived cats that activity is still present within the deprived eye's columns but is confined to layer IV, indicating transmission failure at the level of intracortical connections (Schatz and Stryker 1978; Bonds *et al.* 1980). It is these latter changes in excitatory transmission rather than the macroscopic rearrangements of columnar patterns that will be dealt with in the following sections.

Coherence of pre- and post-synaptic activity as criterion for input selection

An important step in the analysis of mechanisms underlying ocularity changes has been the discovery that deprivation-induced changes in ocular dominance do not depend solely on the relative level of activity in the afferents from the two eyes (Cynader and Mitchell 1977; Singer *et al.* 1977; Wilson *et al.* 1977; Rauschecker and Singer 1979; Greuel *et al.* 1987).

Other critical variables are the state of activation of the post-synaptic neurone and in particular the degree of temporal correlation between pre- and post-synaptic activity (Rauschecker and Singer 1979, 1981; Frégnac *et al*. 1988; Greuel *et al*. 1988). The use-dependent modifications of excitatory transmission in fact seem to follow rules which closely resemble those postulated by Hebb for adaptive neuronal connections in order to account for associative learning (Hebb 1949; Stent 1973; Rauschecker and Singer 1979; Singer 1990; Stryker *et al*. 1990). The direction of the change—increase or decrease of efficacy—depends on the correlation between pre- and post-synaptic activation. The efficacy of excitatory transmission increases if the probability is high that the presynaptic afferents and the post-synaptic cell are active in temporal contiguity and it decreases when the post-synaptic target is active while the presynaptic terminal is silent. These rules, when applied to circuits where two (or more) afferent pathways converge on to a common post-synaptic target cell, have the effect of selectively stabilizing and hence associating pathways that convey correlated activity. The probability of such afferents being active in temporal contiguity with the common target cell is high and therefore they consolidate. Likewise, these modification rules lead to competition between converging pathways if these pathways convey uncorrelated activity. In that case one subset of afferents is always inactive while the other drives the post-synaptic cell and vice versa. Hence the active subset increases its gain while the other weakens and these conditions alternate. Eventually, the subset of afferents which wins is the one that has the highest probability of being active in temporal contiguity with the post-synaptic target cell.

Thus, according to these modification rules the converging pathways arriving from the two eyes only remain connected to a common cortical cell if their activities are sufficiently correlated. If their responses are too asynchronous they compete with each other. In that case only one pathway consolidates and the other becomes repressed. The cut-off point beyond which asynchrony leads to disruption of binocularity has been determined by alternating occlusion of the two eyes with high speed solid state shutters (Altmann *et al*. 1987). The maximal interval of asynchrony still compatible with the maintenance of binocular connections was found to be in the order of 200–400 ms and thus relatively long. This excludes individual action potentials as a basis for contingency matching since the neuronal signals used for contingency matching have to persist for a few hundred milliseconds. Likely candidates for such persisting events are long-lasting post-synaptic conductance changes, second messenger cascades, or reverberation of neuronal activity in coupled cell assemblies.

The control of local circuit modifications by global gating systems

Selective stabilization of convergent pathways by contingency matching appears well adapted to ensure that only those afferents from the two eyes remain connected to common cortical target cells that come from retinal loci that have similar disparities. When the animal fixates a visual target with both eyes, corresponding loci on the two retinae are stimulated by the same parts of the visual target. Hence, the activity patterns conveyed by the ganglion cells on corresponding retinal loci resemble each other; they are correlated. However, selection by contingency matching will only lead to such specific retino-cortical connections if it is restricted to moments when the animal actually fixates a non-ambiguous target with both eyes. Pruning must not take place when the visual axes of the two eyes are not properly aligned. If the images processed by the two eyes are too different and cannot be fused, all signals from the two eyes—including those originating from retinal loci with similar disparity—are uncorrelated. If selection occurred under such conditions, all afferents from the two eyes would compete with each other and the consequence would be complete disruption of binocular connections. The same would be the case if the spontaneously produced bursts of activity that occur, for example in the geniculate afferents during certain sleep stages, were capable of inducing changes in circuitry. Moreover, to assure a sufficient degree of overlap of the images in the two eyes prior to pruning, the direction of gaze needs to be optimized. This requires some evaluation of the best match between the activity patterns in the coarsely prespecified retinotopic representations of the two eyes. This in turn necessitates preprocessing and control of eye movements. Selection of binocular connections must therefore be gated by non-retinal control systems which enable use-dependent modifications only when the necessary conditions are fulfilled. In agreement with this postulate it has been found that non-retinal afferents to striate cortex play a crucial role in gating ocular dominance plasticity.

Even when contour vision is unrestricted and retinal signals readily elicit responses in the neurones of the visual cortex, vision-dependent modifications of excitatory transmission fail to occur in a variety of rather different conditions. Thus, neurones of the kitten's striate cortex may remain binocular despite monocular deprivation when the proprioceptive input from extraocular muscles is disrupted (Buisseret and Singer 1983), when the open eye is surgically rotated within the orbit (Singer *et al.* 1982), when large angle squint is induced in both eyes (Singer *et al.* 1979), or when strasbismus is induced by bilateral cyclotorsion (Crewther *et al.* 1980). In these cases contour vision *per se* is unimpaired but the abnormal eye position and motility lead to massive disturbances of the kitten's visuo-motor co-ordination. Initially the inappropriate retinal signals cause abnormal visuo-motor reactions and during this period are effective in influencing cortical ocular dominance. Subsequently, however, the kittens rely less and less on visual cues and develop a near complete neglect of the visual modality. In this phase, retinal signals no longer modify ocular dominance and they also fail to support the development of feature-selective receptive fields.

These results suggest that retinal signals only influence the development of cortical functions when the animal uses them for the control of behaviour. Indeed, retinal signals do not lead to changes of cortical functions when the kittens are anaesthetized and/or paralysed while exposed to visual patterns (Buisseret *et al.* 1978; Freeman and Bonds 1979; Singer 1979; Singer and Rauscheker 1982). Vision-dependent modifications also failed to occur in kittens in which a sensory hemi-neglect was induced by unilateral surgical lesions in the diencephalon which affected the intralaminar nuclear complex of the thalamus and the fornix (Singer 1982). Following monocular deprivation, neurones in the visual cortex of the normal hemisphere had become monocular as is usual with monocular deprivation. However, neurones in the visual cortex of the hemisphere with the lesion had remained binocular. Thus, although both hemispheres had received identical signals from the open eye, these signals induced the expected modifications only in the normal hemisphere and remained rather ineffective in the hemisphere which—because of the diencephalic lesion— 'attended' less to retinal stimulation. Recent experiments have revealed that these effects of the thalamic lesion cannot be attributed solely to the projections originating from the intralaminar nuclei (Bear *et al.* 1988). Cortical plasticity was found unimpaired when the intralaminar lesions were made by injection of the cytotoxin NMDA, which selectively destroys neurones but leaves fibres of passage intact. This suggests that the surgical lesions were effective because they comprised both thalamic neurones and nearby fibre systems such as the fornix hippocampi and the connections between the frontal eye fields and the tectum which traverse the intralaminar nuclei.

The chemical nature of permissive gating signals

Neurones of the kitten striate cortex also remain binocular despite monocular deprivation when cortical norepinephrine (NE) is depleted by local infusion of the neurotoxin 6-hydroxydopamine (6-OHDA) (Kasamatsu and Pettigrew 1979). Since microperfusion of the depleted cortical tissue with NE reinstalls ocular dominance plasticity (Kasamatsu *et al.* 1979), it was proposed that normal NE levels are a necessary prerequisite for ocular dominance plasticity. Subsequently, however, several independent investigations challenged this conclusion by demonstrating that ocular dominance changes can be induced despite NE depletion. In these investigations, either 6-OHDA was injected prior to monocular deprivation or the noradrenergic input to cortex was blocked by means other than local 6-OHDA application (Bear and Daniels 1983; Bear *et al.* 1983; Daw *et al.* 1984*a,b*; Adrien *et al.* 1985). This apparent controversy has subsequently been resolved by the finding that ocular dominance plasticity is strongly influenced also by cholinergic mechanisms (Bear and Singer 1986). Ocular dominance plasticity was abolished if both the noradrenergic pathway from the locus coeruleus and the cholinergic projection from the basal forebrain were lesioned. Disruption of either system alone was not sufficient to arrest plasticity. The reason why 6-OHDA was so effective in blocking ocularity changes has to do with an unexpected pharmacological side effect. The drug not only destroys noradrenergic terminals but also is a potent blocker of muscarinic receptors, thus affecting both the noradrenergic and the cholinergic system (Furness 1971; Bear and Singer 1986). Subsequent investigations revealed that ocular dominance plasticity is controlled by at least three modulatory projections as it can be blocked by local application of receptor blockers of the noradrenergic β-receptors (Shirokawa and Kasamatsu 1986), the cholinergic receptor M1 (Gu and Singer 1993), and the serotonin receptors S1 and S2 (Gu and Singer 1991).

Involvement of NMDA receptor activation and Ca^{2+} fluxes in use-dependent plasticity

The experiments reported above indicate that use-dependent modifications of synaptic transmission require a certain amount of co-operativity between retinal input and additional, internally generated signals. This suggests that the process mediating cortical plasticity has a threshold which is reached only when retinal signals are coincident with additional facilitatory input. A likely substrate for such a threshold process is voltage-dependent Ca^{2+} channels and/or receptor-gated Ca^{2+} conductances, which have a higher activation threshold than the Na^+ channels which mediate the action potential. Measurements with Ca^{2+}-sensitive electrodes revealed that stimulus combinations which induce lasting changes in neuronal response properties lead to a transient decrease of the extracellular Ca^{2+} concentration. This suggests an activation of Ca^{2+} fluxes from extracellular to intracellular compartments. Such Ca^{2+} fluxes were measurable only when visual stimuli were paired with electrical activation of the brain stem reticular core or of the intralaminar nuclei (Geiger and Singer 1986), stimulation conditions that are suitable for the induction of ocularity changes (Singer and Rauschecker 1982). Moreover, these Ca^{2+} fluxes were much more pronounced in 4–5 week old kittens than in adult cats, which is compatible with the hypothesis that the respective Ca^{2+} conductances are related to mechanisms involved in developmental plasticity (Singer 1987).

Supporting evidence for this possibility comes from experiments in which lasting changes of neuronal response properties were induced by combining retinal stimulation with direct pharmacological modulation of the excitability of cortical neurones (Greuel *et al.* 1988). In anaesthetized, paralysed kittens, cortical cells were activated from the retina with light while at the same time they were exposed to iontophoretically applied pulses of the excitatory amino acids NMDA and glutamate and/or the neuromodulators acetylcholine (ACh) and NE. In more than half of the neurones, 30 min of conditioning with combined light and pharmacological stimulation was sufficient to induce a selective enhancement of the responses to the light stimulus used for conditioning and/or to produce a depression of responses to non-conditioned stimuli. Thus, with appropriate light stimulation, drastic changes in ocular dominance and/or orientation and direction preference could be obtained that outlasted the end of the conditioning sequence by more than 30 min. These results support the notion that induction of use-dependent, long-term modifications of response properties requires co-operativity between retinal input and further, internally generated, facilitatory influences. This co-operativity seems necessary to attain a critical level of post-synaptic depolarization. This depolarization in turn appears to be required to reach the threshold for use-dependent synaptic modifications.

Recent evidence indicates that the threshold for use-dependent synaptic modifications is only reached if NMDA receptor-gated conductances are activated and contribute to excitatory transmission. Infusion of DL-2-amino-5-phosphonopentanoate (AP5), a selective antagonist of the NMDA receptor, completely blocks any experience-dependent modifications of striate cortex functions such as can be induced with monocular deprivation (Kleinschmidt *et al.* 1987) and reverse suture (Gu *et al.* 1989). This blockade of plasticity is not simply a consequence of disrupted excitatory transmission because cortical cells continue to respond to light stimuli even after blockade of NMDA receptors (Bear *et al.* 1990). The fact that blockade of NMDA receptors prevents not only the disconnection of the deprived afferents (Kleinschmidt *et al.* 1987) but also the functional recovery of previously weakened connections in the case of reverse suture (Gu *et al.* 1989) indicates that NMDA receptor activation is necessary both for the use-dependent heterosynaptic weakening of deprived afferents and for the activity-dependent strengthening of active synaptic connections.

The NMDA receptor is coupled to an ionophore which is permeable to Ca^{2+} ions. A special property of this receptor-gated channel is its additional voltage-dependence. It becomes permeable to Ca^{2+} ions only when the receptor is occupied by its endogenous ligand *and* when the receptor is sufficiently depolarized (see Chapters 7–9). Thus, this mechanism has a dual function: firstly, once that activation threshold is reached it greatly amplifies the depolarizing response of the post-synaptic neurone to a given presynaptic input, and secondly, it allows for a strong influx of Ca^{2+} into the post-synaptic compartment. The NMDA receptor mechanism could therefore contribute in several ways to use-dependent synaptic plasticity: firstly, by enhancing depolarization, it could contribute to the induction of heterosynaptic depression, i.e. the weakening of inactive synapses, that occurs when the post-synaptic neurone is strongly activated. Secondly, by sensing the temporal correlation between pre- and post-synaptic activation, it could contribute to the selective stabilization of inputs whose activity is correlated with the activity of the post-synaptic neurone. The

Ca^{2+} entry mediated by activated NMDA receptors could serve as the required consolidation signal.

Recently, these conjectures have received direct support from *in vitro* studies of cortical slices in which it is possible to follow use-dependent modifications of identified synaptic connections, to control the depolarization of the post-synaptic neurone, to influence levels of intracellular Ca^{2+}, and to block transmitter receptors selectively.

Long-term potentiation and long-term depression in the neocortex

Evidence for LTP and LTD in the neocortex has been obtained both with field potential and intracellular recordings. However, field potentials which reflect the summed activity of a population of neuronal elements in the immediate vicinity of the recording electrode are difficult to interpret in neocortex. Unlike in the hippocampus, electrical activation of afferent projections to neocortex usually elicits a mixture of mono- and polysynaptic responses in virtually every layer, and these responses are further complicated by inhibitory interactions with different synaptic delays. This makes it notoriously difficult to determine whether an increase of the field response is due to an increase of synaptic gain in mono- or polysynaptic pathways, whether it results from increased excitability of the post-synaptic target cells, or whether it reflects a reduction of efficacy of the multiple inhibitory pathways. Therefore, this review will include mainly results obtained with intracellular recordings.

Induction of long-term potentiation

The requirements for the induction of neocortical LTP closely resemble those of LTP in the CA1 area of the hippocampus (for review see Bliss and Collingridge 1993). Firstly, presynaptic activation has to occur in conjunction with strong post-synaptic depolarization and secondly, a surge of intracellular $[Ca^{2+}]$ has to occur as LTP is blocked by chelating intracellular Ca^{2+} (Kimura *et al.* 1990; Hirsch and Crépel 1992). In the neocortex the level of depolarization required for LTP induction is reached only if GABAergic inhibition is reduced (Artola and Singer 1987, 1990; Kimura *et al.* 1989; Hirsch and Crépel 1990; Sah and Nicoll 1991; Bear *et al.* 1992), or if the post-synaptic neurone is depolarized with current injection during presynaptic activation (Bindman *et al.* 1988; Artola *et al.* 1990; Kossel *et al.* 1990; Frégnac *et al.* 1990; Gilbert *et al.* 1990), or when strong stimuli are applied very close to the recorded neurone (Kirkwood *et al.* 1992). Accordingly, continuously hyperpolarizing the post-synaptic neurone during conditioning stimulation prevents LTP induction (Baranyi and Szente 1987; Keller *et al.* 1991).

In most cases induction of LTP is also abolished by pharmacological blockade of NMDA receptors (Artola and Singer 1987, 1990; Kimura *et al.* 1989; Sah and Nicoll 1991). This is to be expected since activation of NMDA receptors enhances both the depolarizing responses of cortical neurones and the consecutive rise of intracellular $[Ca^{2+}]$. Indeed, in slice of the neocortex, NMDA receptors participate in monosynaptic (Artola and Singer 1987, 1990; Jones and Baughman 1988; Hirsch and Crépel 1990) and polysynaptic (Sutor and Hablitz 1989) transmission. However, with certain stimulation regimes, LTP can be induced even when NMDA receptors are blocked (Komatsu *et al.* 1991; Bear *et al.* 1992). What these stimulation regimes and preparations have in common is that they guarantee strong post-synaptic responses and/or activation of voltage-gated Ca^{2+} conductances even when NMDA receptors do not contribute to excitatory transmission (Komatsu and Iwakiri 1992). Finally, a property shared by both neocortical LTP and hippocampal LTP is that both the AMPA and the NMDA receptor-mediated evoked post-synaptic potential (EPSP) component can undergo LTP (Artola and Singer 1990; de Curtis and Llinas 1993), whereby the induction threshold for the potentiation of the NMDA receptor-mediated EPSP is lower than that of the AMPA receptor-mediated component (Artola and Singer 1990).

Cholinergic and noradrenergic agonists facilitate LTP induction in the mature cortex in the same *synergistic* way as they facilitate developmental changes. Indeed, either cholinergic or noradrenergic agonists have little effect on the induction of LTP if they are bath-applied to neocortical slices alone (Bröcher *et al.* 1992*b*; Nowicky *et al.* 1992), but they strongly increase the probability of obtaining LTP when they are applied together (Bröcher *et al.* 1992*b*). This synergy suggests action through different mechanisms. First, the modulators reduce a variety of K^+ conductances, some of them being Ca^{2+}-dependent, others voltage-gated. This action increases the amplitude of depolarizing responses and thereby enhances activation of voltage- and NMDA receptor-gated Ca^{2+} conductances (Bröcher *et al.* 1992*b*). Second, ACh has been shown in hippocampus to enhance directly the activity of NMDA receptors by an inositol-1,4,5-trisphosphate- and Ca^{2+}-dependent mechanism (Markram and Segal 1992). Third, it is possible that the neuromodulators directly influence, via their G-protein-mediated effects, the second messenger cascades which eventually translate the activity-induced Ca^{2+} surge into modifications of synaptic transmission.

Developmental changes in the susceptibility to long-term potentiation

Both in kittens and rats, the threshold for the induction of LTP is lower in slices of young than of adult animals (Komatsu *et al.* 1981; Perkins and Teyler 1988; Kato *et al.* 1991). In superficial layers of the rat visual cortex the probability of inducing LTP decreases rapidly from 2 to 4 weeks of age (Fig. 14.1). The period of enhanced LTP susceptibility coincides roughly with the critical period for developmental changes in each species. The

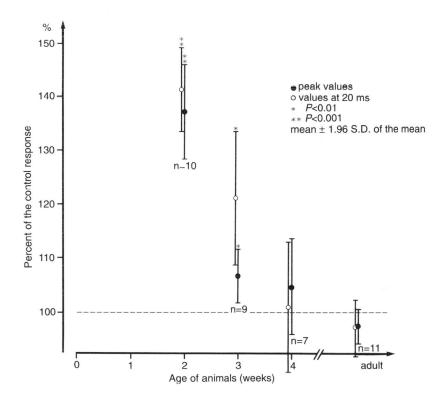

Fig. 14.1 Developmental changes in LTP amplitudes. Values represent averaged post-synaptic potential (PSP) amplitudes from the different age groups measured 15 min after tetanus and expressed in percent of pre-tetanic control values (n = number of cells). Filled and open symbols refer to early and late PSP components, respectively. These values were compared with corresponding values measured previously in slices of adult rats which were investigated under identical conditions and showed no post-tetanic response modifications (Artola and Singer 1990). In these experiments post-tetanic amplitudes of early and late PSP components were 97.5 ± 5.5% and 97.1 ± 9.3% of pretetanic controls, respectively. This comparison reveals that amplitude changes differ significantly ($P < 0.001$ or 0.01) from those in the adult controls in 2 and 3 week old but not in 4 week old animals (from Kato *et al.* 1991).

greater susceptibility of young cortices to undergo LTP is most likely due to the greater contribution of NMDA receptor-gated conductances to excitatory transmission in young animals (Tsumoto *et al.* 1987; Fox *et al.* 1989; Kato *et al.* 1991). First, the duration of evoked NMDA receptor-mediated EPSPs (Kato *et al.* 1991) and EPSCs (Hestrin 1992; Carmignoto and Vicini 1992) is several times longer at early developmental stages than that measured in older animals. Interestingly, this decrease in NMDA receptor-mediated EPSC duration is delayed in the visual cortex when animals are reared in the dark (Carmignoto and Vicini 1992), a condition that prolongs developmental plasticity (see above). Second, NMDA receptors are more numerous early in life (Bode-Greuel and Singer 1989). Another contributing factor may be the higher density of voltage-gated Ca^{2+} channels in young animals (Bode-Greuel and Singer 1988). $[Ca^{2+}]$ measurements have revealed that stimulation-dependent Ca^{2+} fluxes from extracellular to intracellular space are stronger in young visual cortex than in mature visual cortex (Bode-Greuel and Singer 1991).

Induction of long-term depression

Induction of homosynaptic LTD in neocortex requires a minimum post-synaptic depolarization since it can be blocked by continuously hyperpolarizing the post-synaptic neurone during the inducing tetanus (Artola *et al.* 1990). It also appears to require a surge of intracellular $[Ca^{2+}]$ since induction of LTD is blocked by buffering intracellular Ca^{2+} (Bröcher *et al.* 1992a; Hirsch and Crépel 1992) and is facilitated by increasing extracellular $[Ca^{2+}]$ (Artola *et al.* 1992).

Recent evidence obtained in slices of the rat visual cortex suggests that an appropriate rise of intracellular $[Ca^{2+}]$ in the post-synaptic dendrite is sufficient to trigger LTD. A transient increase of extracellular $[Ca^{2+}]$ from 2 to 4 mM for 10 min can produce a marked and long-lasting depression of synaptic transmission (Artola *et al.* 1992). This Ca^{2+}-induced LTD is voltage-dependent since it is prevented by hyperpolarizing the post-synaptic neurone, but it is independent of synaptic activation since it occurs in the absence of stimulation. The processes mediating this Ca^{2+}-induced depression appear to be similar to those involved in tetanus-induced homosynaptic LTD because Ca^{2+}-induced LTD occludes tetanus-induced LTD (Artola *et al.* 1992). Similar conditions have been reported for CA1. Here, too, depression of non-activated synaptic inputs can be obtained if the post-synaptic neurone is strongly depolarized either by antidromic activation or by current injection and this depression is blocked if $[Ca^{2+}]_o$ is low (Christofi *et al.* 1993).

The hypothesis that cortical synapses can undergo LTD irrespective of whether they are active or inactive if $[Ca^{2+}]_i$ in the post-synaptic compartment reaches a critical level, is compatible with the occurrence of stimulation-induced heterosynaptic LTD in the prefrontal cortex (Hirsch *et al.* 1993) and in the visual cortex (A. Artola and W. Singer, submitted). In both structures strong synaptic activation of a neurone can lead to depression of other, inactive inputs converging on to the same neurone (for review see Artola and Singer 1993).

Relationship between the induction of long-term depression and long-term potentiation

The requirements for LTD induction, post-synaptic depolarization, and a sufficient increase of $[Ca^{2+}]_i$ within the post-synaptic dendrite, closely resemble those for the induction of associative LTP. A major difference is that LTP induction requires a stronger post-synaptic depolarization. Results obtained in slices of the rat visual cortex (Fig. 14.2) (Artola *et al.* 1990) have led to the notion of two voltage-dependent thresholds, one for the induction of LTD and one for LTP (Fig 14.3). If the first threshold (Θ^-) is reached, the activated synapses depress, and if the second threshold (Θ^+) is reached, which requires stronger depolarization, the activated synapses potentiate. Accordingly, there are two ranges of membrane potential (V_m) where the synapses will not display any long-term modification: first, when V_m remains below the threshold for LTD (Θ^-) and, second, when V_m is around the second threshold (Θ^+) which separates the two ranges of V_m leading to LTD and LTP, respectively.

Evidence is now available that these two thresholds for the induction of LTD and LTP exist also in other brain areas such as the prefrontal cortex, the striatum, and the hippocampus. In slices of the prefrontal cortex a tetanic stimulus that would normally elicit LTP induces LTD when the depolarizing response to the tetanus is reduced by blocking NMDA receptors (Hirsch and Crépel 1991). In the striatum, the same tetanus, which produces LTP in Mg^{2+}-free medium, induces LTD in the presence of 1.2 mM $[Mg^{2+}]_o$ and no modification when the post-synaptic cell is hyperpolarized during the conditioning tetanus (Calabresi *et al.* 1992*a,b*). Thus the induction of LTD and LTP in the striatum shows the same voltage-dependence as that in the visual cortex. In the CA1 area of the hippocampus, low frequency (around 1 Hz) stimulation induces LTD while high frequency stimulation (>10 Hz) induces LTP (Dunwiddie and Lynch 1978; Dudek and Bear 1992). This is also consistent with there being different thresholds for the induction of LTD and LTP as post-synaptic depolarization increases with stimulation frequency. Furthermore, it is also possible in CA1 neurones to change the direction of the synaptic modification by modifying V_m with current injection during application of a tetanus of intermediate frequency. A 5–10 Hz tetanus which alone has no long-term effect on synaptic transmission (Dunwiddie and Lynch 1978; Dudek and Bear 1992) induces LTD if it is paired with hyperpolarizing current injection and LTP if it is paired with depolarizing current injection (Stanton and Sejnowski 1989; Xie *et al.* 1992). This result can be accounted for if one assumes that stimulation with 5–10 Hz, which is intermediate between the frequencies suitable for the induction of LTD and LTP, produces a post-synaptic depolarization around the Θ^+ threshold. Finally, there is also evidence for the Θ^- threshold in the hippocampus as low frequency tetani which normally induce LTD (see above) are no longer effective if cells are continuously hyperpolarized during stimulation (Mulkey and Malenka 1992).

It is now possible to relate these two voltage-dependent thresholds for LTD and LTP to corresponding changes of $[Ca^{2+}]_i$. That the induction of

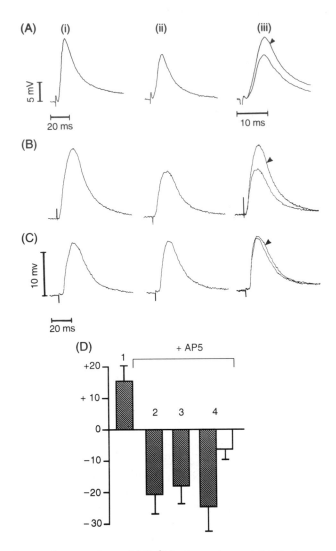

LTP requires a larger rise of $[Ca^{2+}]_i$ than that of LTD is supported by several observations. First, in neocortex, partial buffering of intracellular Ca^{2+} prevents induction of LTP but not that of LTD (Bröcher *et al.* 1992*a*). Second, in CA1 a 20 Hz tetanus normally induces LTP but when $[Ca^{2+}]_o$ is lowered from 2.5 to 0.5 mM it leads to LTD (Mulkey and Malenka 1992). The recently published finding that Ca^{2+} buffering in neocortex blocks LTP but not LTD does not contradict this result as there are reasons to believe that Ca^{2+} buffering was incomplete in these experiments (Kimura *et al.* 1990; Yoshimura *et al.* 1991).

For the induction of LTP, a very high $[Ca^{2+}]_i$ has to be reached and for

Fig. 14.2 Effect of white matter (w.m.) tetanic stimulation on synaptic responses in slices treated with either 0.3 μM bicuculline ((A) and (D)) or 0.3 μM bicuculline and 25–100 μM AP5 ((B)–(D)). (A) Synaptic responses to w.m. stimulation in a cell treated with 0.3 μM bicuculline. $V_{mr} = -71$ mV. (B) and (C) Synaptic responses to w.m. (B) and intra-cortical (i.c.) (C) stimulation in a cell treated with both 0.3 μM bicuculline and 25 μM AP5. $V_{mr} = -70$ mV. Responses (i) and (ii) were recorded before and 20 min after tetanus, respectively, and are superimposed (at expanded time scale) in (iii). Arrows indicate the pretetanic response. Note that only the response to w.m. (tetanized pathway) is modified. (D) Amplitude changes observed in responses to w.m. stimulation 20–30 min after w.m. tetanus in slices treated with 0.3 μM bicuculline (group 1: n = 20), 0.3 μM bicuculline plus 25 μM AP5 (group 2: n = 10) and 0.3 μM bicuculline plus 100 μM AP5 (group 3: n = 3). In seven (group 4) out of the 11 cells of group 2, responses to w.m. (filled bar) and to i.c. (empty bar) were recorded. The amplitude change in the tetanized pathway differs significantly ($P < 0.05$) from that in the non-tetanized pathway. Tetanus consisted of five, 2 s long stimulation trains (50 Hz) delivered at 10 s intervals. Stimulus intensity during tetanus was twice the test intensity. (Adapted from Artola *et al.* (1990).)

most stimulation protocols this requires activation of NMDA receptor-gated Ca^{2+} conductances. Indeed, direct measurements of $[Ca^{2+}]_i$ in hippocampus indicate that NMDA receptor-gated Ca^{2+} conductances are the most effective source for the Ca^{2+} surge in post-synaptic spines (Müller and Connor 1991). Homosynaptic LTD, by contrast, appears to be readily inducible with lower $[Ca^{2+}]_i$ increases (Fig. 14.4(C)) such as probably occur when only voltage-gated Ca^{2+} channels are activated or when Ca^{2+} is released from intracellular stores. Whether the Ca^{2+} provided by the NMDA receptor-gated conductances contributes to induction of homosynaptic LTD will thus depend on the strength of the conditioning stimulus. When the tetanus is strong, i.e. suitable for LTP induction, NMDA receptors need to be blocked to prevent LTP and to unmask LTD (Fig. 14.2; Artola *et al.* 1990; Hirsch and Crépel 1991). On the other hand, when very low frequencies are applied, NMDA receptor activation seems necessary to raise $[Ca^{2+}]_i$ to the level required for the induction of homosynaptic LTD both in hippocampal CA1 (Dudek and Bear 1992; Mulkey and Malenka 1992) and in the visual cortex (Kirkwood *et al.* 1992). Under such stimulation conditions LTD is prevented by blockade of NMDA receptors. Because ligand-gated Ca^{2+} conductances are usually not required to reach the Ca^{2+} concentrations necessary for LTD, depression can readily occur at inactive synapses as for example in heterosynaptic LTD. In this case it is likely that either voltage-gated Ca^{2+} channels are activated in the vicinity of the synapses that get depressed or that Ca^{2+} concentrations increase due to propagating Ca^{2+} waves. The fact that the induction of heterosynaptic LTD is prevented by blockade of NMDA receptors in the neocortex (Artola and Singer 1994) as well as in the hippocampus (Abraham and Wickens 1991; Desmond *et al.* 1991) is probably due to the reduced

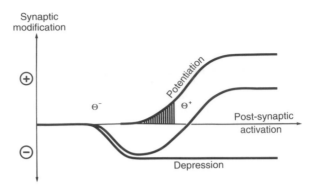

Fig. 14.3 Schematic representation of the two different voltage-dependent thresholds (Θ^- and Θ^+) for the induction of homosynaptic LTD and LTP. The ordinate indicates the direction of the synaptic gain change and the abscissa the *membrane potential level of the post-synaptic neurone* that is maintained during presynaptic activation. If the first threshold, Θ^-, is reached a mechanism is activated which leads to a long-lasting depression of synaptic efficacy, and if the second threshold, Θ^+, is reached another process is triggered which leads to the potentiation of the synapse.

Fig. 14.4 (right) Schematic representation of the suggested role of intracellular Ca^{2+} in use-dependent synaptic modifications. (A) Summary of ligand- and voltage-gated mechanisms which modulate $[Ca^{2+}]$ in the post-synaptic dendritic compartment. (B–E) Homo- and heterosynaptic modifications of synaptic transmission for two inputs terminating on spines of the same dendritic segment. Mechanisms influencing intracellular $[Ca^{2+}]$ are indicated by symbols in (A). Arrows indicate Ca^{2+} fluxes and their number the amplitude of the flux. The density of the hatching in the post-synaptic compartment is meant to reflect the expected concentration increase of intracellular Ca^{2+}. In (B)–(D) only the lower input is assumed to be active while in (E) both inputs are simultaneously active. The four conditions differ in addition by the amplitude of the depolarizing responses of the post-synaptic dendrite. It is assumed that this amplitude is determined both by the activity of the modifiable synapses and by the state of the many other excitatory, inhibitory and modulatory inputs to the same dendritic compartment (not shown). (B) AMPA, NMDA, and metabotropic quisqualate receptors are only moderately activated, voltage-gated Ca^{2+} conductances are inactive. There is no substantial rise of the intracellular $[Ca^{2+}]$ and no lasting modification of synaptic transmission at the active synapse. (C) In addition to the activation conditions in (B), voltage-gated Ca^{2+} conductances in the dendritic spine are also activated. Post-synaptic $[Ca^{2+}]$ rises to an intermediate level and induces long-term depression of the active synapse. There is only little spread of Ca^{2+} from the active spine to other dendritic compartments. (D) Activation causes more post-synaptic depolarization as in (B) and (C); accordingly, NMDA receptor-gated conductances and voltage-gated Ca^{2+} channels are strongly activated. The massive increase of $[Ca^{2+}]$ in the activated spine leads to LTP. Moreover, depolarization spreads to other compartments of the dendrite where it activates voltage-gated conductances. This leads to an intermediate rise of $[Ca^{2+}]$ also at the post-synaptic side of the inactive synapses which therefore undergo heterosynaptic depression. (E) The second input is now activated as well. It no longer undergoes LTD but becomes potentiated as well because the rise of $[Ca^{2+}]$ in the post-synaptic compartment is now sufficient for the induction of LTP.

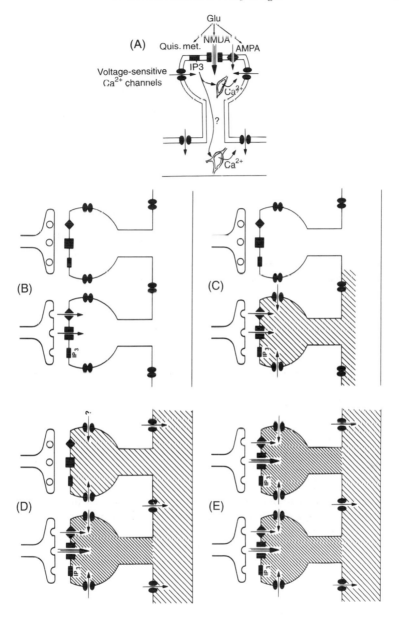

excitatory drive at the active synapses and the resulting decrease of post-synaptic depolarization of the inactive synapses (Fig. 14.4(D)).

Thus, the level rather than the origin of the Ca^{2+} surge in the vicinity of the modifiable synapse appears to be the critical variable determining whether the synapse potentiates or depresses. A mechanism by which different Ca^{2+} concentrations could exert opposite effects on synaptic efficacy has been proposed by Lisman (1989). He suggested that low $[Ca^{2+}]_i$ could lead to a selective activation of enzyme systems with high Ca^{2+} affinity while high $[Ca^{2+}]_i$ could activate preferentially enzymes with low affinity. However, these considerations do not imply that the origin of Ca^{2+} is also irrelevant under physiological activation conditions. The NMDA receptor-gated Ca^{2+} channels, the voltage-controlled Ca^{2+} channels, and the intracellular release sites are associated with different cellular compartments and probably not distributed homogeneously. Thus, if what matters is the absolute concentration of Ca^{2+} at a particular effector enzyme, the effect of the various Ca^{2+} sources will depend very much on the relative locations of release and effector sites.

In summary, available evidence on cortical LTP and LTD suggests that both modifications require a surge of post-synaptic Ca^{2+} whereby the amplitude of the surge rather than its cause determines the sign of the synaptic change. This predicts that all the signalling systems which can influence ligand- and voltage-gated Ca^{2+} conductances and the release of intracellular Ca^{2+} should contribute to the regulation of the thresholds for LTD and LTP induction. These signalling systems include both excitatory and inhibitory synaptic inputs as well as a host of modulatory transmitter systems. But none of these appear to be specific for the induction of either LTP or LTD. However, depending on the relative efficacy with which they contribute to the Ca^{2+} surge, some signalling cascades may turn out to be more effective for the induction of LTP, such as the NMDA receptor, while others—such as voltage-gated Ca^{2+} channels—may be more suitable for the induction of LTD.

Concluding remarks

The results reviewed in this chapter reveal a high degree of use-dependent plasticity in the mature neocortex. This agrees with the commonly accepted notion that the neocortex serves functions such as memory and learning and that corticalization is one of the major reasons for the increase of adaptivity of highly developed organisms. However, it was less expected that such a high degree of plasticity would be found already at the level of primary sensory areas. For a long time it has been held that these areas are malleable only during early development and do not support adaptive functions such as learning in the adult. However, more recent models on cortical processing no longer consider primary sensory cortices as relay stations with fixed properties. Rather, they emphasize the distributed nature of cortical operations and the importance of reciprocal bottom-up and top-down interactions, and assign similar functions to all cortical areas. This agrees with recent psychophysical evidence which revealed forms of perceptual learning that imply adaptivity as early as in the primary visual cortext (Poggio *et al.* 1992; Karni and Sagi 1991).

The *in vitro* analysis of use-dependent synaptic modifications in the visual cortex has revealed the coexistence of mechanisms for homosynaptic LTD and LTP in the same neurone and probably in the same synapses. Post-synaptic depolarization and $[Ca^{2+}]_i$ have been identified as the most important control parameters for the direction of the gain change. These variables depend on the state of other converging excitatory and inhibitory inputs and, because of the involvement of the NMDA receptor, also on the temporal coincidence between pre- and post-synaptic activation. Therefore, the modifications are associative and depend on the co-operativity of converging inputs. But they differ substantially in their effect from modifications predicted by the classical rule proposed by Hebb (1949) in that they include a negative term. On theoretical grounds Bienenstock *et al.* (1982) postulated a synaptic modification rule, the 'BCM rule', to account for experience-dependent developmental changes in the visual cortex. This rule assumes weakening of synapses with weak activation and strengthening of synapses with strong activation and thus, in its essential aspects (but see below), is supported by the *in vitro* data of Artola *et al.* (1990; see Fig. 14.3). This is interesting because the BCM rule was inspired by experience-dependent modifications and in fact accounts very well for most of the published developmental data (Clothiaux *et al.* 1991). This then suggests that the induction mechanisms for use-dependent synaptic modifications are similar in the developing and mature visual cortex. Recently, the conditions identified by Artola *et al.* (1990) (see Fig. 14.3) for the induction of LTD and LTP have been formalized and implemented as synaptic modification rule (the 'ABS rule'; for the differences between the ABS and the BCM rules see Artola and Singer (1993)) in an associative neuronal network (Hancock *et al.* 1991). These simulations revealed that the ABS rule is more powerful than previously implemented Hebbian rules because it allows for error correction, for the learning of exceptions, and for a very effective orthogonalization of representations in associative neuronal networks.

Comparison between the use-dependent synaptic modifications observed during early development *in vivo* and those induced *in vitro* exhibits similarities that go beyond the analogies of the formal level of rules:

1. LTP and LTD can be induced more easily in young than in adult animals.

2. Both the developmental modifications and the *in vitro* changes have a high threshold which is associated with post-synaptic activation.

3. In both cases ACh and NE have a facilitatory action.

4. In both cases induction of modifications involves NMDA receptors and the progressive shortening of NMDA receptor-mediated EPSCs parallels the rise of the induction threshold.

It thus appears likely that homosynaptic LTD and LTP and heterosynaptic LTD (Fig. 14.4) not only support use-dependent synaptic plasticity in the mature cortex but also constitute the initial steps in the chain of events which eventually lead to the experience-dependent modifications of the functional architecture of neocortex during development.

References

Abraham, W. C. and Wickens, J. R. (1991). Heterosynaptic long-term depression is facilitated by blockade of inhibition in area CA1 of the hippocampus. *Brain Research*, **546**, 336–40.

Adrien, J., Blanc, G., Buisseret, P., Frégnac, Y., Gari-Bobo, E., Imbert, M., Tassin, J. P., and Trotter, Y. (1985). Noradrenaline and functional plasticity in kitten visual cortex: a reexamination. *Journal of Physiology*, **367**, 73–98.

Altmann, L., Luhmann, H. J., Greuel, J. M., and Singer, W. (1987). Functional and neuronal binocularity in kittens raised with rapidly alternating monocular occlusion. *Journal of Neurophysiology*, **16**, 965–80.

Artola, A. and Singer, W. (1987). Long-term potentiation and NMDA receptors in rat visual cortex. *Nature*, **330**, 649–52.

Artola, A. and Singer, W. (1990). The involvement of *N*-methyl-D-aspartate receptors in induction and maintenance of long-term potentiation in rat visual cortex. *European Journal of Neuroscience*, **2**, 254–69.

Artola, A. and Singer, W. (1993). Long-term depression of excitatory synaptic transmission and its relationship to long-term potentiation. *Trends in Neuroscience*, **16**, 480–87.

Artola, A. and Singer, W. (1994). Heterosynaptic long-term depression is prevented by blockade of NMDA receptors in rat visual cortex. *Journal of Neurophysiology*, submitted.

Artola, A., Bröcher, S., and Singer, W. (1990). Different voltage-dependent thresholds for inducing long-term depression and long-term potentiation in slices of rat visual cortex. *Nature*, **347**, 69–72.

Artola, A., Hensch, T., and Singer, W. (1992). A rise of $[Ca^{++}]_i$ in the postsynaptic cell is necessary and sufficient for the induction of long-term depression (LTD) in neocortex. *Society for Neuroscience Abstracts*, **18**, 567.30.

Baranyi, A. and Feher, O. (1981*a*). Long-term facilitation of excitatory synaptic transmission in single motor cortical neurones of the cat produced by repetitive pairing of synaptic potentials and action potentials following intracellular stimulation. *Neuroscience Letters*, **23**, 303–8.

Baranyi, A. and Feher, O. (1981*b*). Synaptic facilitation requires paired activation of convergent pathways in the neocortex. *Nature*, **290**, 413–15.

Baranyi, A. and Szente, M. B. (1987). Long-lasting potentiation of synaptic transmission requires postsynaptic modifications in the neocortex. *Brain Research*, **423**, 378–84.

Bear, M. F. and Daniels, J. D. (1983). The plastic response to monocular deprivation persists in kitten visual cortex after chronic depletion of norepinephrine. *Journal of Neuroscience*, **3**, 407–16.

Bear, M. F. and Singer, W. (1986). Modulation of visual cortical plasticity by acetylcholine and noradrenaline. *Nature*, **320**, 172–6.

Bear, M. F., Paradiso, M. A., Schwartz, M., Nelson, S. B., Carnes, K. M., and Daniels, J. D. (1983). Two methods of catecholamine depletion in kitten visual cortex yield different effects on plasticity. *Nature*, **302**, 245–7.

Bear, M. F., Kleinschmidt, A., and Singer, W. (1988). Experience-dependent modifications of kitten striate cortex are not prevented by thalamic lesions that include the intralaminar nuclei. *Experimental Brain Research*, **70**, 627–31.

Bear, M. F., Kleinschmidt, A., Gu, Q., and Singer, W. (1990). Disruption of experience-dependent synaptic modifications in striate cortex by infusion of an NMDA receptor antagonist. *Journal of Neuroscience*, **10**, 909–25.

Bear, M. F., Press, W. A., and Connors, B. W. (1992). Long-term potentiation in slices of kitten visual cortex and the effects of NMDA receptor blockade. *Journal of Neurophysiology*, **67**, 841–51.

Berry, R., Teyler, T. J., and Taizhen, H. (1989). Induction of LTP in rat primary visual cortex: tetanus parameters. *Brain Research*, **481**, 221–7.

Bienenstock, E., Cooper, L. N., and Munro, P. (1982). Theory for the development of neuron selectivity: orientation specificity and binocular interaction in visual cortex. *Journal of Neuroscience*, **2**, 23–48.

Bindman, L. J., Murphy, K. P. S. J., and Pockett, S. (1988). Postsynaptic control of the induction of long-term changes in efficacy of transmission at neocortical synapses in slices of rat brain. *Journal of Neurophysiology*, **60**, 1053–65.

Blakemore, C., Garey, L. J., and Vital-Durand, F. (1978). The physiological effects of monocular deprivation and their reversal in the monkey's visual cortex. *Journal of Physiology*, **282**, 223–62.

Bliss, T. V. P. and Collingridge, G. L. (1993). A synaptic model of memory: long-term potentiation in hippocampus. *Nature*, **361**, 31–9.

Bliss, T. V. P. and Lömo, T. (1973). Long-lasting potentiation of synaptic transmission in the dentate area of the anaesthetized rabbit following stimulation of the perforant path. *Journal of Physiology*, **232**, 331–56.

Bode-Greuel, K. M. and Singer, W. (1988). Developmental changes of the distribution of binding sites for organic Ca^{2+}-channel blockers in cat visual cortex. *Experimental Brain Research*, **70**, 266–75.

Bode-Greuel, K. M. and Singer, W. (1989). The development of N-methyl-D-aspartate receptors in cat visual cortex. *Developmental Brain Research*, **46**, 197–204.

Bode-Greuel, K. M. and Singer, W. (1991). Developmental changes of calcium currents in the visual cortex of the cat. *Experimental Brain Research*, **84**, 311–18.

Bonds, A. M., Silverman, M. S., Sclar, G., and Tootell, R. B. (1980). Visually evoked potentials and deoxyglucose studies of monocularly deprived cats. Association for Research in Vision and Ophtalmology Meeting Abstracts, 225.

Bröcher, S., Artola, A., and Singer, W. (1992a). Intracellular injection of Ca^{++} chelators blocks induction of long-term depression in rat visual cortex. *Proceedings of the National Academy of Science, USA*, **89**, 123–7.

Bröcher, S., Artola, A., and Singer, W. (1992b). Agonists of cholinergic and noradrenergic receptors facilitate synergistically the induction of long-term potentiation in slices of rat visual cortex. *Brain Research*, **573**, 27–36.

Buisseret, P. and Singer, W. (1983). Proprioceptive signals from extraocular muscles gate experience-dependent modifications of receptive fields in the kitten visual cortex. *Experimental Brain Research*, **51**, 443–50.

Buisseret, P., Gary-Bobo, E., and Imbert, M. (1978). Ocular motility and recovery of orientational properties of visual cortical neurones in dark-reared kittens. *Nature*, **272**, 816–17.

Calabresi, P., Maj, R., Pisani, A., Mercuri, N. B., and Bernardi, G. (1992*a*). Long-term synaptic depression in the striatum: physiological and pharmacological characterization. *Journal of Neuroscience*, **12**, 4224–33.

Calabresi, P., Maj, R., Pisani, A., Mercuri, N. B., and Bernardi, G. (1992*b*). Long-term potentiation in the striatum is unmasked by removing the voltage-dependent magnesium block of NMDA receptor channels. *European Journal of Neuroscience*, **4**, 929–35.

Carmignoto, G. and Vicini, S. (1992). Activity-dependent decrease in NMDA receptor responses during development of the visual cortex. *Science*, **258**, 1007–11.

Chattarji, S., Stanton, P. K., and Sejnowski, T. J. (1989). Commissural synapses, but not mossy fiber synapses, in hippocampal field CA3 exhibit associative long-term potentiation and depression. *Brain Research*, **495**, 145–50.

Christofi, G., Nowicki, A. V., Bolsover, S. R., and Bindman, L. J. (1993). The postsynaptic induction of nonassociative long-term depression of excitatory synaptic transmission in rat hippocampal slices. *Journal of Neurophysiology*, **69**, 219–29.

Clothiaux, E. E., Bear, M. F., and Cooper, L. M. (1991). Synaptic plasticity in visual cortex: comparison of theory with experiment. *Journal of Neurophysiology*, **66**, 1785–804.

Crewther, S. G., Crewther, D. P., Peck, C. K., and Pettigrew, J. D. (1980). Visual cortical effects of rearing cats with monocular or binocular cyclotorsion. *Journal of Neurophysiology*, **44**, 97–118.

Cynader, M. (1983). Prolonged sensitivity to monocular deprivation in dark-reared cats: effects of age and visual exposure. *Developmental Brain Research*, **8**, 155–64.

Cynader, M. and Mitchell, D. E. (1977). Monocular astigmatism effects on kitten visual cortex development. *Nature*, **270**, 177–8.

Cynader, M., Berman, N., and Hein, A. (1976). Recovery of function in cat visual cortex following prolonged deprivation. *Experimental Brain Research*, **25**, 139–56.

Daw, N. W., Robertson, T. W., Rader, R. K., Videen, T. O., and Cosica, C. J. (1984*a*). Substantial reduction of cortical noradrenaline by lesions of adrenergic pathway does not prevent effects of monocular deprivation. *Journal of Neuroscience*, **4**, 1354–60.

Daw, N. W., Videen, T. O., Parkinson, D., and Rader, R. K. (1984*b*). DSP-4 depletes noradrenaline in kitten visual cortex without altering the effects of monocular deprivation. *Journal of Neuroscience*, **5**, 1925–33.

de Curtis, M. and Llinas, R. R. (1993). Entorhinal cortex long-term potentiation evoked by theta-patterned stimulation of associative fibers in the isolated in vitro guinea pig. *Brain Research*, **600**, 327–30.

Desmond, N. L., Colbert, C. M., Zhang, D. X., and Levy, W. B. (1991). NMDA receptor antagonists block the induction of long-term depression in the hippocampal dentate gyrus of the anesthetized rat. *Brain Research*, **552**, 93–8.

Dews, P. B. and Wiesel, T. N. (1970). Consequences of monocular deprivation in visual behaviour in kittens. *Journal of Physiology*, **206**, 437–55.

Dudek, S. M. and Bear, M. F. (1992). Homosynaptic depression in area CA1 of hippocampus and effects of *N*-methyl-D-aspartate receptor blockade. *Proceedings of the National Academy of Science, USA*, **89**, 4363–7.

Dunwiddie, T. and Lynch, G. (1978). Long-term potentiation and depression of synaptic responses in the rat hippocampus: localization and frequency dependency. *Journal of Physiology*, **276**, 353–67.

Fox, K., Sato, H., and Daw, N. (1989). The location and the function of NMDA receptors in cat and kitten visual cortex. *Journal of Neuroscience*, **9**, 2443–54.

Freeman, R. D. and Bonds, A. B. (1979). Cortical plasticity of monocularly deprived immobilized kittens depends on eye movement. *Science*, **206**, 1093–5.

Frégnac, Y., Schulz, D., Thorpe, S., and Bienenstock, E. (1988). A cellular analogue of visual cortical plasticity. *Nature*, **333**, 367–70.

Frégnac, Y., Smith, D., and Friedlander, M. J. (1990). Postsynaptic membrane potential regulates synaptic potentiation and depression in visual cortical neurons. *Society for Neuroscience Abstracts*, **16**, 798.

Furness, J. B. (1971). Some actions of 6-hydroxydopamine which affect autonomic neuromuscular transmission. In *6-Hydroxydopamine and catecholamine neurons*, (ed. T. Malmfors and H. Thoene), pp. 205–14. North Holland, Amsterdam.

Geiger, H. and Singer, W. (1986). A possible role of calcium currents in developmental plasticity. *Experimental Brain Research*, **14**, 256–70.

Gilbert, C. D., Hirsch, J. A., and Wiesel, T. N. (1990). Lateral interactions in visual cortex. *Cold Spring Harbor Symposium on Quantitative Biology*, **55**, 663–77.

Greuel, J. M., Luhmann, H. J., and Singer, W. (1987). Evidence for a threshold in experience-dependent long-term changes of kitten visual cortex. *Developmental Brain Research*, **34**, 141–9.

Greuel, J. M., Luhmann, H. J., and Singer, W. (1988). Pharmacological induction of use-dependent receptive field modifications in the visual cortex. *Science*, **242**, 74–7.

Gu, Q. and Singer, W. (1991). Involvement of serotonin in neuronal plasticity of kitten visual cortex. *International Brain Research Organization Meeting Abstract*, **3**, 47.7

Gu, Q. and Singer, W. (1993). Effects of intracortical infusion of anticholinergic drugs on neuronal plasticity in kitten striate cortex. *European Journal of Neuroscience*, **5**, 475–85.

Gu, Q., Bear, M. F., and Singer, W. (1989). Blockade of NMDA-receptors prevents ocularity changes in kitten visual cortex after reversed monocular deprivation. *Developmental Brain Research*, **47**, 281–8.

Hancock, P. J. B., Smith, L. S., and Philips, W. A. (1991). A biologically supported error correcting learning rule. *Neural Computation*, **3**, 201–12.

Hebb, D. O. (1949). *The Organization of Behavior*. John Wiley and Sons, New York.

Hestrin, S. (1992). Developmental regulation of NMDA receptor-mediated synaptic currents at a central synapse. *Nature*, **357**, 686–9.

Hirsch, J. C. and Crépel, F. (1990). Use-dependent changes in synaptic efficacy in rat prefrontal neurons *in vitro*. *Journal of Physiology*, **427**, 31–49.

Hirsch, J. C. and Crépel, F. (1991). Blockade of NMDA receptors unmasks a long-term depression in synaptic efficacy in rat prefrontal neurons *in vitro*. *Experimental Brain Research*, **85**, 621–4.

Hirsch, J. C. and Crépel, F. (1992). Postsynaptic calcium is necessary for the induction of LTP and LTD of monosynaptic EPSPs in prefrontal neurons. An *in vitro* study in the rat. *Synapse*, **10**, 173–5.

Hirsch, J., Barrionuevo, G., and Crépel, F. (1992). Homo- and heterosynaptic changes in synaptic efficacy are expressed in prefrontal neurons: an in-vitro study in the rat. *Synapse*, **12**, 82–85.

Hubel, D. H. and Wiesel, T. N. (1965). Binocular interaction in striate cortex of kittens reared with artificial squint. *Journal of Neurophysiology*, **28**, 1041–59.

Iriki, A., Pavlides, C., Keller, A., and Asanuma, H. (1989). Long-term potentiation in the motor cortex. *Science*, **245**, 1385–7.

Ito, M. and Kano, M. (1982). Long-lasting depression of parallel fiber–Purkinje cell transmission induced by conjunctive stimulation of parallel fibers and climbing fibers in the cerebellar cortex. *Neuroscience Letters*, **33**, 253–8.

Ito, M., Sakurai, M., and Tongroach, P. (1982). Climbing fibre induced depression of both mossy fibre responsiveness and glutamate sensitivity of cerebellar Purkinje cells. *Journal of Physiology*, **324**, 113–34.

Jones, K. A. and Baughman, R. W. (1988). NMDA- and non-NMDA-receptor components of excitatory synaptic potentials recorded from cells in layer V of rat visual cortex. *Journal of Neuroscience*, **8**, 3521–34.

Karni, A. and Sagi, D. (1991). Where practice makes it perfect in texture discriminations: Evidence for primary visual cortex plasticity. *Proceedings of the National Academy of Science, USA*, **88**, 4966–70.

Kasamatsu, T. and Pettigrew, J. D. (1979). Preservation of binocularity after monocular deprivation in the striate cortex of kittens treated with 6-hydroxydopamine. *Journal of Comparative Neurology*, **185**, 139–62.

Kasamatsu, T., Pettigrew, J. D., and Ary, M.-L. (1979). Restoration of visual cortical plasticity by local microperfusion of norepinephrine. *Journal of Comparative Neurology*, **185**, 163–82.

Kato, N., Artola, A., and Singer, W. (1991). Developmental changes in the susceptibility to long-term potentiation of neurones in rat visual cortex slices. *Developmental Brain Research*, **60**, 43–50.

Keller, A., Miyashita, E., and Asanuma, H. (1991). Minimal stimulus parameters and the effects of hyperpolarizaton on the induction of long-term potentiation in the cat motor cortex. *Experimental Brain Research*, **87**, 295–302.

Kimura, F., Nishigori, A., Shirokawa, T., and Tsumoto, T. (1989). Long-term potentiation and N-methyl-D-aspartate receptors in the visual cortex of young rats. *Journal of Physiology*, **414**, 125–44.

Kimura, F., Tsumoto, T., Nishigori, A., and Yoshimura, Y. (1990). Long-term depression but not potentiation is induced in Ca^{2+}-chelated visual cortex neurons. *NeuroReport*, **1**, 65–8.

Kirkwood, A., Aizemann, C. D., and Bear, M. F. (1992). Common forms of plasticity in hippocampus and visual cortex *in vitro*. *Society for Neuroscience Abstracts*, **18**, 628.33.

Kleinschmidt, A., Bear, M. F., and Singer, W. (1987). Blockade of 'NMDA' receptors disrupts experience-dependent plasticity of kitten striate cortex. *Science*, **238**, 355–8.

Komatsu, Y. and Iwakiri, M. (1992). Low-threshold Ca^{2+} channels mediate induction of long-term potentiation in kitten visual cortex. *Journal of Neurophysiology*, **67**, 401–10.

Komatsu, Y., Toyama, K., Maeda, J., and Sakaguchi, H. (1981). Long-term potentiation investigated in a slice preparation of striate cortex of young kittens. *Neuroscience Letters*, **26**, 269–74.

Komatsu, Y., Fujii, K., Maeda, J., Sakaguchi, H., and Toyama, K. (1988). Long-term potentiation of synaptic transmission in kitten visual cortex. *Journal of Neurophysiology*, **59**, 124–41.

Komatsu, Y., Narajima, X., and Toyama, K. (1991). Induction of long-term potentiation without the participation of N-methyl-D-aspartate receptors in kitten visual cortex. *Journal of Neurophysiology*, **65**, 20–32.

Kossel, A., Bonhoeffer, T., and Bolz, J. (1990). Non-Hebbian synapses in rat visual cortex. *NeuroReport*, **1**, 115–18.

Levay, S., Stryker, M. P., and Shatz, C. J. (1978). Ocular dominance columns and their development in layer IV of the cat's visual cortex: a quantitative study. *Journal of Comparative Neurology*, **179**, 223–44.

Lisman, J. (1989). A mechanism for the Hebb and the anti-Hebb processes underlying learning and memory. *Proceedings of the National Academy of Science, USA*, **86**, 9574–8.

Löwel, S. and Singer, W. (1992). Selection of intrinsic horizontal connections in the visual cortex by correlated neuronal activity. *Science*, **255**, 209–12.

Markram, R. and Segal, M. (1992). The inositol 1,4,5-triphosphate pathway mediates cholinergic potentiation of rat hippocampal neuronal responses to NMDA. *Journal of Physiology*, **447**, 513–33.

Mower, G. D. and Christen, W. G. (1985). Role of visual experience in activating critical period in cat visual cortex. *Journal of Neurophysiology*, **53**, 572–89.

Mower, G. D., Christen, W. G., and Caplan, C. J. (1984). Absence of ocular dominance columns in binocularly deprived cats. *Investigative Ophtalmology and Visual Science*, **25**, 214 (ARVO Abstr.).

Mower, G. D., Caplan, C. J., Christen, W. G., and Duffy, F. H. (1985). Dark rearing prolongs physiological but not anatomical plasticity of the cat visual cortex. *Journal of Comparative Neurology*, **235**, 448–66.

Mulkey, R. M. and Malenka, R. C. (1992). Mechanisms underlying induction of homosynaptic long-term depression in area CA1 of the hippocampus. *Neuron*, **9**, 967–75.

Müller, W. and Connor, J. A. (1991). Dendritic spines as individual compartments for synaptic Ca^{2+} responses. *Nature*, **354**, 73–6.

Nowicky, A. V., Christofi, G., and Bindman, L. J. (1992). Investigation of beta-adrenergic modulation of synaptic transmission and postsynaptic induction of associative LTP in layer V neurones in slices of rat sensorimotor cortex. *Neuroscience Letters*, **137**, 270–4.

Olson, C. R. and Freeman, R. D. (1980). Profile to the sensitive period for monocular deprivation in kitten. *Experimental Brain Research*, **39**, 17–21.

Perkins, A. T., IV and Teyler, T. J. (1988). A critical period for long-term potentiation in the developing rat visual cortex. *Brain Research*, **439**, 222–9.

Poggio, T., Fahle, M., and Edelman, S. (1992). Fast perceptual learning in visual hyperacuity. *Science*, **256**, 1018–21.

Rauschecker, J. P. and Singer, W. (1979). Changes in the circuitry of the kitten visual cortex are gated by postsynaptic activity. *Nature*, **280**, 58–60.

Rauschecker, J. P. and Singer, W. (1981). The effects of early visual experience on the cat's visual cortex and their possible explanation by Hebb synapses. *Journal of Physiology*, **310**, 215–39.

Sah, P. and Nicoll, R. A. (1991). Mechanisms underlying potentiation of synaptic transmission in rat anterior cingulate cortex *in vitro*. *Journal of Physiology*, **433**, 615–30.

Sakurai, M. (1987). Synaptic modification of parallel fibre–Purkinje cell transmission in *in vitro* guinea-pig cerebellar slices. *Journal of Physiology*, **394**, 463–80.

Shatz, C. J. and Stryker, M. P. (1978). Ocular dominance in layer IV of the cat's visual cortex and the effects of monocular deprivation. *Journal of Physiology*, **281**, 267–83.

Shirokawa, T. and Kasamatsu, T. (1986). Concentration-dependent suppression by beta-adrenergic antagonists of the shift in ocular dominance following monocular deprivation in kitten visual cortex. *Neuroscience*, **18**, 1035–46.

Singer, W. (1979). Central-core control of visual cortex function. In *The neurosciences, fourth study program*, (eds. F. O. Schmitt and F. G. Worden), pp. 1093–109. MIT Press, Cambridge, MA.

Singer, W. (1982). Central core control of developmental plasticity in the kitten visual cortex: I. Diencephalic lesions. *Experimental Brain Research*, **47**, 209–22.

Singer, W. (1987). Activity-dependent self-organization of synaptic connections as a substrate for learning. In *The neural and molecular basis of learning*, (ed. J.-P. Changeux and M. Konishi), pp. 301–36. Wiley, Chichester.

Singer, W. (1990). The formation of cooperative cell assemblies in the visual cortex. *Journal of Experimental Biology*, **153**, 177–90.

Singer, W. and Rauschecker, J. P. (1982). Central core control of developmental plasticity in the kitten visual cortex: II. Electrical activation of mesencephalic and diencephalic projections. *Experimental Brain Research*, **47**, 223–33.

Singer, W., Rauschecker, J., and Werth, R. (1977). The effect of monocular exposure to temporal contrasts on ocular dominance in kittens. *Brain Research*, **134**, 568–72.

Singer, W., von Grünau, M., and Rauschecker, J. P. (1979). Requirements for the disruption of binocularity in the visual cortex of strabismic kittens. *Brain Research*, **171**, 536–40.

Singer, W., Tretter, F., and Yinon, U. (1982). Evidence for long-term functional plasticity in the visual cortex of adult cats. *Journal of Physiology*, **324**, 239–48.

Stanton, P. K. and Sejnowski, T. J. (1989). Associative long-term depression in the hippocampus induced by hebbian covariance. *Nature*, **339**, 215–18.

Stent, G. S. (1973). A physiological mechanism for Hebb's postulate of learning. *Proceedings of the National Academy of Science, USA*, **70**, 997–1001.

Stryker, M. P. and Harris, W. (1986). Binocular impulse blockade prevents the formation of ocular dominance columns in cat visual cortex. *Neuroscience*, **6**, 2117–33.

Stryker, M., Chapman, B., Miller, K. D., and Zahs, K. R. (1990). Experimental and theoretical studies of the organization of afferents to single orientation columns in visual cortex. *Cold Spring Harbor Symposium on Quantitative Biology*, **55**, 515–27.

Sutor, B. and Hablitz, J. J. (1989). Long-term potentiation in frontal cortex: role of NMDA-modulated polysynaptic excitatory pathways. *Neuroscience Letters*, **91**, 111–17.

Tsumoto, T., Hagihara, K., Sato, H., and Hata, Y. (1987). NMDA receptors in the visual cortex of young kittens are more effective than those of adult cats. *Nature*, **327**, 513–14.

Wiesel, T. N. and Hubel, D. H. (1965). Comparison of the effects of unilateral and bilateral eye closure on cortical unit response in kittens. *Journal of Neurophysiology*, **28**, 1029–40.

Wilson, J. R., Webb, S. V., and Sherman, S. M. (1977). Conditions for dominance of one eye during competitive development of central connections in visually deprived cats. *Brain Research*, **136**, 277–87.

Xie, X., Berger, T. J., and Barrionuevo, G. (1992). Isolated NMDA receptor-mediated synaptic responses express both LTP and LTD. *Journal of Neurophysiology*, **67**, 1009–13.

Yoshimura, Y., Tsumoto, T., and Nishigori, A. (1991). Input-specific induction of long-term depression in Ca^{2+}-chelated visual cortical neurons. *NeuroReport*, **2**, 393–6.

15 The role of NMDA receptors in learning and memory

R. G. M. MORRIS AND M. DAVIS

Introduction

Research on the possible role of N-methyl-D-aspartate (NMDA) receptors in certain kinds of learning began following the discovery by Collingridge *et al.* (1983) that NMDA receptor activation is a crucial step in the induction of the associative form of hippocampal long-term potentiation (LTP). Given the longstanding idea that synaptic alterations could underly memory (Cajal 1911; Hebb 1949; Kandel and Schwartz 1982), selective NMDA antagonists such as AP5 seemed to offer an ideal pharmacological tool with which to block this form of LTP *in vivo* and so investigate the effects upon learning and memory of disrupting at least one type of synaptic plasticity. An early finding was that AP5 appeared to impair spatial learning (Morris *et al.* 1986a), a type of learning known to be dependent upon the integrity of the very structure, the hippocampus (O'Keefe and Nadel 1978), in which LTP was first discovered and is usually investigated (Bliss and Lømo 1973). Over the past decade, our understanding of the biophysics, neuropharmacology, and molecular biology of NMDA receptors has developed considerably and this book is testament to that progress. Knowledge about their role in several kinds of learning and memory has also advanced over this time and our aim in this chapter is to illustrate three principal aspects of how research in this field has developed.

First, experiments testing the putative link between NMDA receptor-dependent hippocampal LTP and hippocampal-dependent learning have been conducted so as to incorporate more exacting neuropharmacological observations. These include, for example, monitoring LTP and behaviour in the same animal, and measuring the extracellular level of competitive NMDA antagonists in the hippocampus *in vivo*. In this way, several studies have been better able to address the key issue of whether AP5-induced impairments of learning occur by virtue of the disruption of LTP or are only incidentally linked to it (Morris 1989; Morris *et al.* 1990a). Second, behavioural research using various excitatory amino acid antagonists has now been extended to other types of learning, such as fear conditioning, for which our ability to achieve stimulus control is far more precise and for which we have a better understanding of the neural circuit mediating the behavioural change (Davis 1992b). Third, in parallel with developing interest in the principle of experience-dependent self-organization of the nervous system (Constantine-Paton 1990; see also Chapter 14), work using NMDA antagonists has also been conducted on types of learning that are preferentially expressed during development, such as filial imprinting (Horn 1985). This latter approach contributes to a body of other work pointing to a commonality between the neural mechanisms underlying the postnatal development of the nervous system and those responsible for learning.

In selecting these three topics, we are acutely aware that this leaves no space to discuss the wider range of learning phenomena in which NMDA receptor activity has now been implicated. A more comprehensive review would, for example, cover such diverse topics as olfactory learning in young (Lincoln *et al*. 1988) and adult (Brennan and Keverne 1989; Staubli *et al*. 1989) animals, the development of tolerance to ethanol and opiates (Khanna *et al*. 1991; Trujillo and Akil 1991) and the striking and potentially important effect of prenatal ethanol exposure to pregnant animals in down-regulating NMDA receptor sensitivity in their subsequent offspring (Morrisett *et al*. 1989). Some readers may also be disappointed that we do not offer a comprehensive review of the now extensive behavioural pharmacology literature on the effects of systemic administration of competitive and non-competitive NMDA antagonists in both learning and drug-discrimination tasks. We justify their exclusion below on the grounds that our research interests focus on the role of NMDA receptors in specific neuronal circuits. However, the interested reader may wish to consult Willetts *et al*. (1990) for a very different perspective from that offered here. Our aim is to provide a critical review of the three approaches we have selected, illustrating the principles, key discoveries, and outstanding problems of each.

NMDA receptor-dependent hippocampal long-term potentiation is necessary for certain kinds of learning in which the hippocampus is involved

Since its first detailed description by Bliss and Lømo (1973), there has been widespread suspicion that hippocampal LTP might engage some of the same neural mechanisms as those used normally to store information during certain kinds of learning. Fuelling this so-called 'LTP and learning' hypothesis has been the recognition that several of the major properties of hippocampal LTP are very pertinent to a candidate learning or memory mechanism (Morris *et al*. 1990*a*). These include its presence in a brain structure intimately associated with certain kinds of long-term memory, its persistence over time, the synapse specificity of its expression, and the role of associativity between pre- and post-synaptic activity in its induction. However, while these physiological properties are suggestive, they are far from conclusive. For example, LTP occurs in many other brain structures including several not obviously linked to memory, its persistence over time in hippocampus is, arguably, anachronistic given that the long-term storage of hippocampal-dependent learning is almost certainly in neocortex, and the rate at which associative LTP develops seems appreciably faster than the rate at which many types of learning develop. In short, LTP might be wholly unrelated to learning. One alternative suggestion is that LTP could be a form of synaptic homeostasis which enables the neural circuits to compensate for alterations in signal throughput (J. A. Movshon, personal communication) rather than, as the LTP and learning hypothesis implies, a means of storing information. Given these uncertainties, a key experiment for testing the LTP and learning hypothesis was to block LTP in a behaving animal and examine whether learning was compromised.

NMDA antagonists block LTP *in vivo* and impair spatial learning

Morris *et al.* (1986*a*) examined the effects of chronic intraventricular infusion of the selective NMDA antagonist AP5 upon both LTP *in vivo* and the learning of two distinct behavioural tasks. The drug or vehicle solution was infused continuously over 2 weeks into the lateral ventricle from subcutaneously implanted minipumps. At a drug concentration shown to be sufficient to block LTP without effect upon baseline dentate gyrus field-potentials, spatial learning in a water maze (Morris 1981, 1984) was impaired while acquisition of a visual discrimination in the same apparatus was unaffected (Fig. 15.1). The spatial task involved searching for an escape platform hidden at one place in the pool, while the visual discrimination task involved discriminating between a black-and-white platform providing escape from the water and a grey one which did not (or vice versa). This selectivity of the AP5-induced behavioural impairment first indicated that the drug was not impeding behavioural performance by virtue of some gross sensorimotor disturbance (such as severely impaired vision), and second established a parallel between the effects of NMDA receptor blockade and those of hippocampal lesions (Morris *et al.* 1982, 1986*b*, 1990*b*; Sutherland *et al.* 1983). Such lesions impair learning of the spatial task but not the visual discrimination task. Thus, the most straightforward interpretation of this drug-induced behavioural dissociation is that AP5 impairs spatial learning because such learning depends upon activation of NMDA receptor dependent synaptic plasticity in hippocampus.

However, this interpretation has, properly, not gone unchallenged. Three main objections have been raised, concerning:

(1) the validity of the behavioural dissociation;
(2) the possibility that the apparent learning impairments are due to side effects of the drug outside the hippocampus;
(3) the possibility that AP5 alters the system properties of hippocampal neurones in addition to blocking LTP.

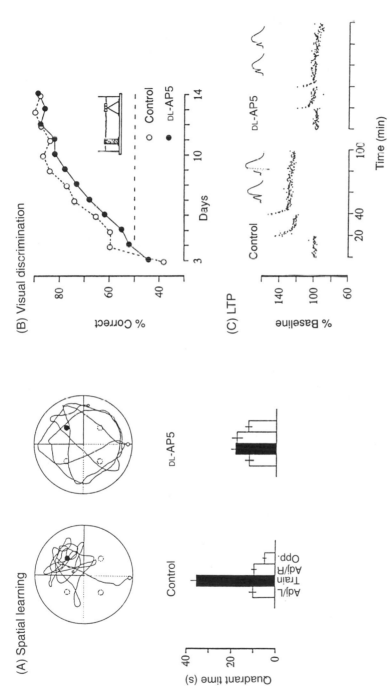

Fig. 15.1 Chronic infusion of AP5 causes a behaviourally selective impairment of learning. (A) Rats trained in a water maze for 15 trials were given a probe test in which the hidden platform was removed from the pool and the animals allowed to swim for 60 s. Control animals (infused with saline) swam persistently in the vicinity of the platform, while AP5-treated rats did not. (B) AP5 and control animals learned a visual discrimination task at an equivalent rate. This task is also unimpaired by hippocampal lesions. (C) This behavioural dissociation is obtained at a concentration sufficient to block LTP *in vivo*. (After Morris *et al.* (1986*a*).)

The validity of the behavioural dissociation

Goddard (1986) wondered whether the apparent dissociation between spatial and visual discrimination learning reflected differential diffusion of AP5 from the lateral ventricle. To examine this possibility, Butcher *et al.* (1991) measured drug levels *in vivo* and found that the diffusion of AP5 was actually quite uniform. They also infused AP5 bilaterally via two minipumps directly into occipital area 2 (i.e. just anterior to visual cortex, Zilles (1985)) and again found that learning of the visual discrimination task was unimpaired, despite a whole-tissue concentration of AP5 in visual cortex (occipital area 1) comparable to the hippocampal concentration which impairs spatial learning. The implication of this result is that NMDA receptor-dependent plasticity in cortex is not involved in visual discrimination learning in the way that, in hippocampus, it seems to be for spatial learning.

To explain this behavioural dissociation, Morris (1990*a*) proposed that LTP in the hippocampus, although not necessarily elsewhere, might be involved in those forms of associative learning in which the nature of the associative relationship between stimulus elements is itself represented. In spatial learning, it is not sufficient to learn only that one landmark is 'associated' with another; it is also necessary to encode their spatial relationship, i.e. to learn where one landmark is relative to another. In visual discrimination learning, on the other hand, the animal need only learn that one stimulus is paired with reward and that the other stimulus is not. It has to be said, however, that although there is evidence that the hippocampus is involved in contextual rather than simple associative learning (Hirsh 1974; Good and Honey 1991; Kim and Fanselow 1992; Phillips and LeDoux 1992), there is yet no direct evidence for Morris' (1990*a*) proposal. Moreover, evidence to be reviewed below indicated that NMDA receptor activation is, in the amygdala, critically involved in associative fear conditioning whose acquisition conforms to conventional principles.

A further reason why the lack of an effect of AP5 on visual discrimination learning is puzzling is because of observations that neural throughput on the geniculo-striate pathway to visual cortex (Sillito *et al.* 1990) and contrast sensitivity of visual cortex neurones in layers II and III are both AP5-sensitive (Daw *et al.* 1993). However, even though lesions of visual cortex generally block pattern discrimination tasks similar to that involved in the visual platform test, we do not yet have direct evidence that cortical ablations disrupt the exact task used by Morris *et al.* (1986*a*). One intriguing possibility is that non-NMDA forms of synaptic plasticity could be involved and, indeed, the claim of Johnston *et al.* (1992) that NMDA receptor-independent forms of synaptic plasticity may be quite widespread in the central nervous system raises the possibility that this form of plasticity may often mediate associative learning.

Is the apparent impairment in spatial learning caused by behavioural 'side effects' of the action of AP5 outside the hippocampus?

An almost diametrically opposite concern to Goddard's (1986) argument has been that chronic AP5 diffusion all over the brain would cause widespread NMDA receptor antagonism in many neural circuits whose functional consequences are bound to be complex. It follows that the apparent impairment in spatial learning could be due to the disruption of any number of psychological processes, such as attention, motivation, or even sensorimotor control (Mondadori and Weiskrantz 1991; Keith and Rudy 1990). We share the concerns of these and other critics, but are sceptical of the analytic utility of diffuse NMDA receptor blockade. In particular, we find it difficult to interpret effects of intraperitoneal injections of competitive or non-competitive NMDA antagonists. Such injections result in appreciable NMDA receptor blockade in the spinal cord, as well as all over the brain, and this leads, inexorably, to sensorimotor disturbances (such as disruption of supra-segmental reflexes). It has been claimed that these problems can be avoided by using low doses, but these then produce only the most subtle effects upon memory function (e.g. Wozniak et al. 1990). Indeed, with non-competitive antagonists, such as MK-801, matters may be yet more complicated because the time course with which a use-dependent block of the NMDA receptor develops may vary regionally as a function of the average level of neuronal excitability (see Morris 1990b). These problems can partly be obviated by chronic intraventricular infusion or, better still, by acute local intracerebral infusions, the two routes of administration we have chosen to include reference to in this chapter.

Three main sets of findings suggest that the spatial learning impairment in the water maze following chronic intraventricular (i.c.v.) infusion of AP5 is caused by blockade of NMDA receptors in the hippocampus. First, Morris et al. (1989) showed that acute intrahippocampal infusions of AP5 at a dose sufficient to block LTP caused a comparable behavioural impairment to that of chronic i.c.v. infusion. Autoradiographic visualization of labelled amino acid antagonists was used to establish that these small volumes (1 and 2 µl) were largely restricted to the hippocampus during the period of behavioural testing. Thus, AP5 diffusion outside the hippocampus is not necessary for the spatial learning impairment to occur (Fig. 15.2(A)).

Second, an extensive dose–response analysis in conjunction with in vivo microdialysis (S. Davis et al. 1992) established that the dose-related, AP5-induced impairment of spatial learning overlaps and parallels the disruption of dentate gyrus LTP in vivo (Fig. 15.2(B)), and that both these effects occur across a range of extracellular AP5 concentrations in hippocampus which exactly overlap those describing both the D-AP5 blockade of LTP in vitro (Harris et al. 1984) and D-AP5 displacement of [^{3}II]L-glutamate binding (Monaghan et al. 1988).

(A)

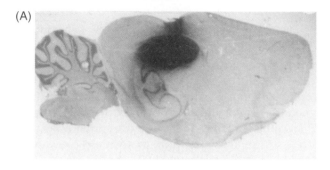

(B)

△ [³H]ʟ-Glut binding   (Monaghan *et al.* 1988)
□ LTP *in vitro*   (Harris *et al.* 1984)
▼ LTP *in vivo*
◆ Spatial learning

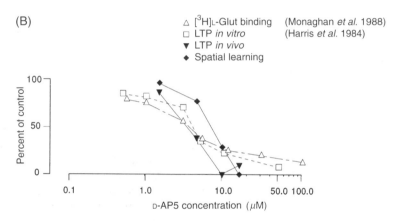

Fig. 15.2 Two lines of evidence that blockade of hippocampal NMDA receptors is sufficient to cause an impairment of spatial learning. (A) Local infusions of 1 or 2 µl of [³H]AP4 ([³H]AP5 was unavailable at the time this study was done) showed that the drug could be largely restricted to the dorsal hippocampus. Such infusions (of AP5) are sufficient to impair spatial learning (see Morris *et al.* 1989). (B) A comparison of the effects of AP5 upon [³H]-glutamate binding, LTP *in vitro*, LTP *in vivo*, and spatial learning. There is some indication that the dose–response relationship for spatial learning is to the right of the other functions, indicating some sparing of learning at concentrations sufficient to block hippocampal LTP, but the proximity of these functions is striking (see Morris *et al.* 1990*a*).

Third, several studies have established that other hippocampal-dependent tasks are also impaired by intraventricular infusion of NMDA antagonists (e.g. Tonkiss *et al.* 1988; Lyford *et al.* 1993; Rawlins *et al.* 1993). Tonkiss *et al.* (1988) found that AP5 impaired the operant schedule called DRL (differential reinforcement of low rates of response) in a similar manner to hippocampal lesions. In this schedule, rats are reinforced with food reward on each occasion they press a lever in an operant chamber if the response occurs a set minimum interval after the previous response (e.g. 18 s). Both AP5 and hippocampal lesions reduced the animals' efficiency in collecting reward and altered the function describing the relative frequency of inter-response times in a comparable manner. Using both AP5 and discrete hippocampal lesions, Rawlins and his colleagues have conducted a detailed follow up of two apparently conflicting lesion studies published by Aggleton *et al.* (1986) and Raffaele and Olton (1988). Aggleton *et al.* (1986) found no effect of hippocampal lesions in a task requiring recognition of numerous complex objects (goal boxes in a maze into which the animals could run). Raffaele and Olton (1988) found an impairment in recognizing which of two simple objects (one black and one white goal box) was seen most recently. This conflict of results has important implications for what role, if any, the hippocampus might play in recognition memory. There were several procedural differences between the studies that Rawlins and his colleagues considered of which the most important seem to be object complexity and frequency of repetition. Using a procedurally identical delayed matching to sample paradigm for all stimulus conditions, they have found that neither hippocampal lesions nor AP5 causes any impairment when multiple complex goal boxes are used (absolute recognition) but both cause a substantial impairment with two simple goal boxes (recognition of recency). Interestingly, the parallels between the effects of hippocampal lesions and AP5 extended to a third condition in which only two goal boxes were used (recognition of recency) but both goal boxes were complex. In this case, both treatments caused a substantial recognition impairment early in each testing session, which declined across the 20 trials of each day to near control levels. This result suggests that rats with hippocampal lesions can use other brain systems to recognize objects and, with difficulty and provided these objects differ in multiple ways, to recognize which of two objects was seen most recently. It is intriguing that intraventricular infusions of D-AP5 cause a comparable impairment. The parallels between the effects of hippocampal lesions and blocking hippocampal NMDA receptors are, however, not exact. There are certain learning tasks that are impaired by lesions but unaffected by AP5 (a point we shall pursue in the next section). Nonetheless, these three sets of studies collectively suggest that relatively selective blockade of hippocampal NMDA receptors, leaving fast synaptic transmission unaffected, is a sufficient condition for impairing several of the types of learning thought to involve hippocampal processing.

Does AP5 disrupt the dynamic system properties of the hippocampus and is this responsible for the learning impairment?

The argument presented in the preceding section points to blockade of hippocampal NMDA receptors as affecting certain kinds of learning, but this does not, of course, imply that blockade of hippocampal synaptic plasticity must be the cause of these impairments. AP5 may be having other effects within the hippocampus. Indeed, the striking similarity between the effects of AP5 and frank lesions raises the question of whether

AP5 infusion so disrupts the dynamic system properties of hippocampal circuitry that it is functionally equivalent to a temporary lesion. If this were the case, the fact that AP5 impairs LTP could be beside the point; the hippocampus would no longer be working properly and hippocampal-dependent learning would suffer for that fact.

There are several observations which lend support to this criticism. For example, Leung and Desborough (1988) reported that acute intraventricular infusion of AP5 disrupts hippocampal rhythmic slow activity (RSA or 'theta') which is known to impair spatial learning when disrupted in other ways (Winson 1978). However, Leung and Desborough's disruption of RSA only occurred in association with gross ataxia and this is not seen with chronic i.c.v. infusion. Abraham and Mason (1988) have shown that AP5 reduces the frequency of complex-spike bursting from presumed CA1 pyramidal cells and Herron *et al.* (1986) have discovered that NMDA receptors do participate in high-frequency synaptic transmission in the hippocampus. These observations also indicate that the hippocampus is, in some sense, not working properly under the influence of AP5; but the force of the critical implication can be turned on its head if one recognizes that short bursts of high-frequency firing in CA1 cells may be precisely the pattern that is normally associated with the induction of synaptic change, as suggested by the phenomenon of prime-burst potentiation (Larson and Lynch 1988; Otto *et al.* 1991). Finally, because hippocampal long-term depression (LTD) can sometimes be disrupted by AP5 (Abraham and Wickens 1991; Desmond *et al.* 1991; Dudek and Bear 1992; Mulkey and Malenka 1992), blocking NMDA receptors *in vivo* with AP5 may be blocking LTP, LTD, or both.

Notwithstanding the interpretive difficulties that these observations create, there are several findings which suggest that blocking hippocampal NMDA receptors has effects that can, at least, be dissociated from those of hippocampal lesions. For example, S. Davis (1990) trained rats in the water maze according to a protocol called 'delayed matching to spatial sample' in which the platform is hidden in a different position each day but there are four trials to that day's location. On the first trial (the nominal 'sample trial'), the animals have no way of knowing where the platform is located. However, on the second and succeeding trials, they should be able to escape faster by remembering the location of the platform on the first trial (the nominal 'choice trials'). Morris *et al.* (1990) had earlier used this protocol to establish that the task is severely impaired by selective ibotenate hippocampal lesions (although, interestingly, relatively unaffected by selective subiculum lesions). In normal rats, most of the savings occur between trials 1 and 2, with little improvement thereafter (Fig. 15.3(A)). Unexpectedly, S. Davis (1990) found this task to be unaffected by chronic i.c.v. infusions of AP5 when the interval between trials was 30 s (Fig. 15.3(b)). In a follow-up, she explored the effects of lengthening the inter-

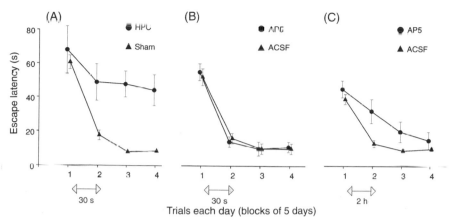

Fig. 15.3 Delayed matching to spatial sample. Rats were trained in a water maze with the platform moving location between days. It remained in the same place for each of four daily trials. Thus, memory of where the animal discovers the platform to be on Trial 1 of each day is indexed by savings in latency to escape on Trials 2–4. The interval between Trials 1 and 2 was either 30 s or 2 h, all remaining trials being conducted at a 30 s interval. (A) Impairment of spatial memory in rats given ibotenate hippocampal lesions. (B) No impairment in AP5-treated rats with a 30 s inter-trial interval. (C) Impairment on Trial 2 in AP5-treated rats with a 2 h inter-trial interval. (After S. Davis (1990).)

val between trials 1 and 2 to 2 h. Rats treated with artificial cerebrospinal-fluid (aCSF) continued to show substantial savings between trials 1 and 2, while AP5-treated rats did not (Fig. 15.3(C)). The interval between trials 2 and 3, and between trials 3 and 4, remained at 30 s. The performance of the AP5-treated rats improved on these trials to a point that was statistically indistinguishable from that of controls. These findings suggest that chronic intraventricular infusion of D-AP5 may leave short-term spatial memory intact while disrupting the formation of long-term spatial memory, whereas hippocampal lesions affect both short- and long-term spatial memory. A similar conclusion was reached by Tonkiss and Rawlins (1991).

Unfortunately, while S. Davis's (1990) results are suggestive, they are inconclusive for two reasons. First, the comparison between short-term and long-term spatial memory was conducted in different animals. To be confident of the dissociation, it is necessary to conduct a within-subjects comparison of time intervals. This has yet to be done. Second, the implication that leaving fast synaptic transmission and non-NMDA-dependent synaptic plasticity in hippocampus intact may be all that is necessary for short-term spatial memory should be tested directly by exploring the effects of temporarily blocking hippocampal AMPA receptors or using drugs which interfere with mossy-fibre potentiation. The former manipulation, which has recently been used in studies of fear conditioning (see below), should be functionally equivalent to a temporary lesion. There have been no investigations of mossy-fibre potentiation in memory and relatively few investigations of even mossy-fibre transmission in memory, other than the report by Frederickson *et al.* (1990) that temporarily chelating mossy-fibre bouton zinc by means of intrahippocampal infusions of DEDTC causes an impairment of short-term spatial memory in a formally similar paradigm to that used by S. Davis (1990).

Another approach to comparing the effects of AP5 and hippocampal lesions has been to compare retention and reversal learning of place-navigation in the water maze (Morris *et al.* 1990*a*; M. Good and R. G. M. Morris, unpublished). Rats were trained to find a hidden platform in one quadrant of the water-maze (e.g. north-east) and then (a) either implanted with minipumps containing AP5 or aCSF, or given ibotenate hippocampal lesions or sham surgery; and (b) either retrained to the same platform location (i.e. to north-east) or trained on a reversal (south-west). Our results indicate that hippocampal lesions disrupt both retention and new learning, while AP5 only impairs new learning and—even then—the deficit is statistically less severe than that of hippocampal lesions. This dissociation implies that the hippocampus is involved in the retrieval of spatial memory and that this retrieval process need not involve activation of NMDA receptors. Further, the dissociation implies that blocking NMDA receptors is not necessarily identical to making a frank lesion, although it clearly falls short of disproving that NMDA receptor blockade is leaving the dynamic system properties of the hippocampus unaffected other than blocking hippocampal synaptic plasticity (i.e. LTP or LTD).

Summary

A large body of work indicates that blockade of hippocampal NMDA receptors by AP5 causes impairments in the learning of a subset of tasks that are impaired by hippocampal lesions and that these behavioural impairments are associated with a disruption of associative NMDA-dependent LTP *in vivo*. However, both effects are dependent consequences of AP5 infusion and it is logically fallacious to assume that one dependent consequence of a treatment is the cause of the other. Thus, answering the third objection above, namely whether AP5 alters the systems properties of the hippocampus, may be exceedingly difficult.

Other ways to resolve the relationship between hippocampal LTP and learning include exploring the effects of blocking LTP downstream of the NMDA receptor, such as by interfering with certain protein kinases implicated in the expression of LTP such as Ca^{2+}/calmodulin-dependent protein kinase Type II, blocking enzymes responsible for synthesis of putative retrograde messengers, or interfering with proteolytic enzymes such as calpain. Such studies are under way, some using transgenic animals, and encouraging results have been reported (Grant *et al.* 1992; Silva *et al.*

1992). Another complementary strategy might be to explore the effect upon behaviour of drugs that improve LTP. No drugs that reliably improve LTP are yet available, but two candidates are a recently developed monoclonal antibody, B6B21, which enhances NMDA receptor channel activity in a glycine-like manner and the partial agonist at the same site, D-cycloserine (Thompson *et al.* 1992). These have recently been shown to cause enhancements in the rate with which a trace-conditioned eye-blink task is learned. Pseudoconditioning controls indicated that this enhancement of performance is most probably not due to sensitization effects. Moreover, examination of their effect during 'extinction' (i.e. when the conditioned response is no longer followed by the unconditional stimulus) indicated that they abolished the spontaneous recovery of behavioural performance that occurs between days. This is a fascinating observation because it points to a possible drug-induced enhancement of extinction—a form of long-term inhibitory learning—and an observation consistent with recent work showing that AP5 can disrupt the extinction of conditioned fear (see below). However, Thompson *et al.* (1992) are cautious about interpreting their results exclusively with respect to LTP in view of other findings indicating that eye-blink conditioning is associated with alterations in pyramidal cell excitability (Disterhoft *et al.* 1986).

NMDA receptor activity is necessary for certain forms of fear conditioning whose neural circuit properties are well delineated

Although it is clear that the hippocampus is critical for several different types of learning and plays an obligatory role in the transfer of short-term to long-term memory in humans, it is nonetheless difficult with our present understanding to envision how changes in the hippocampus translate directly into changes in behaviour. Because of this, it is difficult to see how NMDA receptors in the hippocampus could participate in memory. To make this translation, it is necessary to study the role of NMDA receptors in a brain area that is known to be directly involved in behaviour and then study the role of those receptors under conditions where that behaviour changes with experience. An attractive candidate system for such an analysis is the role of NMDA receptors in the amygdala in conditioned fear.

Conditioned fear is the psychological term used to describe the cluster of behavioural effects that are produced by a stimulus following its association with an aversive situation. In the animal laboratory, conditioned fear can be demonstrated by pairing an initially neutral stimulus, such as light, with an aversive stimulus, such as footshock. After a small number of such stimulus pairings, the light comes to elicit the constellation of behaviours that are typically used to define a state of fear in animals—immobility, changes in heart rate, vocalization, hyper-reactivity to other stimuli, etc. These changes in behaviour develop as a consequence of Pavlovian conditioning and one (or more) of them may be measured to obtain an index of conditioned fear.

Similarities between classical fear conditioning and associative long-term potentiation

There are several similarities between associative NMDA receptor-dependent LTP and Pavlovian fear conditioning. In fear conditioning, an initially weak or neutral stimulus (conditioned stimulus, or CS), which has little behavioural effect by itself, is consistently paired with a strong aversive stimulus (unconditioned stimulus, or US). Following a small number of pairings, sometimes only one, the CS comes to produce effects formerly produced only by the US. These effects are, typically, not seen when the CS and US are presented at random in an unpaired fashion. Similarly, in associative LTP, activation of a weak input to a given post-synaptic cell is paired with activation of a second strong input projecting to the same cell. Following a number of pairings, sometimes only one, the initially weak synaptic input is potentiated (McNaughton *et al.* 1978; Levy and Steward 1979; Barrionuevo and Brown 1983). This potentiation of the weak input is not seen when an equal number of the weak and strong inputs are presented in an unpaired fashion (Brown *et al.* 1988). Because LTP *in vivo* is expressed as a change in fast synaptic transmission that can be blocked by the AMPA antagonist CNQX, local administration of CNQX to the site of plasticity for conditioning might be expected to block the expression of conditioned fear while administration of the NMDA antagonist AP5 should not. Local administration of AP5, on the other hand, would be expected to block learning.

Advantages of Pavlovian fear conditioning for analysing the role of NMDA receptors in learning and memory

In Pavlovian conditioning, delivery of both the conditioned and unconditioned stimuli is under precise experimental control. This is unlike the situation in spatial learning (see above) where the stimuli and the relationship between them about which the animal learns are, in general, not under good experimental control (e.g. they cannot be turned on or off). Conditioned fear can be produced by a single or a small number of CS–US pairings given at precise times over a few minutes (e.g. Gleitman and Holmes 1967; Shurtleff and Ayres 1981; Campeau *et al.* 1990; Kim and Fanselow 1992). It is therefore possible to specify quite precisely when learning is initiated and drugs may be given shortly before, shortly after, or, indeed, long after this critical time point in order to evaluate their effects on learning and consolidation.

When evaluating the effects of drugs such as excitatory amino acid antagonists on learning or the expression of memory, it is important to be able to test their effects upon other behavioural and cognitive processes that could, potentially, alter the formation or measurement of memory independently of any direct effect upon associative process *per se*. For example, as also discussed above, learning might appear to be blocked because of nothing more than a disruption of sensory processing of the CS or, if shock is used as the US, because the drugs are analgesic. Inadequate measurement of memory can also occur if the drugs are administered during learning but not during the subsequent testing phase because the 'state' of the animal is very different during these two conditions. These and other complicating factors can be evaluated using appropriate control procedures. More complex 'Higher order' conditioning paradigms such as second order conditioning or sensory preconditioning (Mackintosh 1983) can also be used to measure the effects of drugs on other types of associative conditioning than fear conditioning.

NMDA receptor antagonists block the formation but not the expression of fear conditioning

Conditioned freezing measured 24 h after training

If rats are placed into a novel cage and, a few minutes later, given up to three shocks in rapid succession, they will first react by flinching or trying to escape but then, shortly thereafter, stop almost all movement. This immobility response (generally called 'freezing') is a species-typical reaction to footshock and usually lasts about 8–10 min. When returned to the same test cage 24 h later, the animals will again freeze. This response can be shown to be a conditioned reaction, where the CS is the stimulus of the testing cage and the US the shock, because rats tested in a different cage will not freeze very much, especially if the appearance or smell of the two cages are dissimilar. Kim *et al.* (1991) discovered that this conditioned freezing response is dependent on NMDA receptors. They infused rats (i.c.v.) with either AP5 (25 nmol/rat) or saline, placed them in a testing cage and, 3 min later, presented three footshocks spaced 20 s apart. The following day, half the rats previously infused with AP5 were infused again with AP5 (Group AP5/AP5) and half with saline (Group AP5/Sal). Similarly, half the rats previously infused with saline were infused again with saline (Group Sal/Sal) and half with AP5 (Group Sal/AP5). Their behaviour was video-taped throughout the testing session and analysed with respect to freezing every 8 s over an 8 min test session. Freezing was defined as 'the absence of any visible movement of the body and vibrissae except for movement necessitated by respiration' (p. 127). Figure 15.4 shows the results. Animals infused with saline on both days remained immobile for as much as 20% of the test session. This is indicative of conditioned fear because previous studies have shown that non-shocked

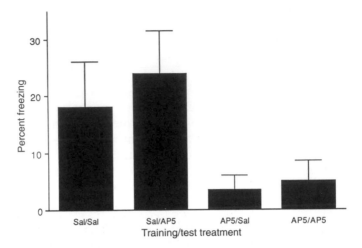

Fig. 15.4 AP5 blocks the acquisition but not the expression of conditioned freezing when given intraventricularly. The figure shows the mean percent (+SEM) freezing in groups given either saline before training and testing (Sal/Sal); saline before training but AP5 before testing (Sal/AP5); AP5 before training but saline before testing (AP5/Sal); or AP5 before both training and testing (AP5/AP5). Groups were tested 24 h after being given three shocks in training. Freezing is expressed as the percentage of total observations during the 8 min test. (Adapted from Kim *et al.* (1991) with permission from the American Psychological Association.)

rats show very low levels of immobility under comparable test conditions. The important finding was that animals given infusions of AP5 prior to training on day 1 showed very little immobility on day 2 (Groups AP5/Sal and AP5/AP5), whereas rats trained with saline but tested on day 2 with either saline or AP5 (Groups Sal/Sal and Sal/AP5) showed high levels of immobility. These findings indicate that AP5 impairs learning but does not block the expression of conditioned fear. Other related experiments indicated that the AP5-induced impairment of fear conditioning is stereo-specific (L-AP5 was without effect), and unlikely to be due to analgesia, because AP5 did not alter several measures of pain sensitivity.

A subsequent study (Kim *et al.* 1992) examined whether the impairment of conditioned fear learning was a complete blockade of learning or simply below the threshold of measurement. A sensitive 'reminder' procedure developed by Riccio and Richardson (1984) was used in which rats are given weak shocks on day 1 and then tested 24 h later. Normally, little or no freezing is then observed. However, if the animals are given a single 'reminder' shock on day 2 and then tested again on day 3, their level of conditioned immobility is significantly higher than that shown by animals which are not 'reminded' about shock. In this way, a level of fear conditioning that is sub-threshold on day 2 can be detected on the following day. Kim *et al.* (1992) trained rats with AP5 on day 1, tested them with saline on day 2, and gave a reminder shock. On day 3, the AP5-treated rats behaved as if they had never received any footshocks on day 1, despite the presentation of the reminder shock on day 2. The authors conclude that 'AP5 blocks fear conditioning exclusively at the encoding or storage level'.

Freezing measured immediately after training

During the day 1 training sessions in the study of Kim *et al.* (1992) described above, shock presentation elicited high levels of freezing that peaked in about 2 min and then dissipated gradually over the next 8 min. Like long-term freezing measured 24 h later, this immediate immobility response appears to be associative in nature. Surprisingly, it does not occur if shocks are delivered immediately after placing rats in the testing cage (Blanchard *et al.* 1976; Fanselow 1986), presumably because the animals fail to associate the cues of the cage with shock. The immediate or short-term conditioned immobility is not blocked by AP5 infused (i.c.v.) for either 3 min (Kim *et al.* 1991, 1992) or 20 min (DeCola *et al.* 1991) before shock. That is, AP5 appears to block long-term but not short-term memory, a result which echoes the water maze findings of S. Davis (1990) described above.

The role of NMDA receptors in the amygdala in fear-conditioning

A great deal of evidence from many different laboratories, using a variety of experimental techniques, indicates that the amygdala plays a crucial role in conditioned fear and probably anxiety (Gloor 1960; Gray 1982; Kapp *et al.* 1984, 1990; Sarter and Markowitsch 1985; Kapp and Pascoe 1986; LeDoux 1987; Davis 1992*a*). Many of the amygdaloid projection areas are critically involved in specific signs that are used to measure fear and anxiety (Fig. 15.5). Electrical stimulation of the amygdala elicits a pattern of behaviours that mimic natural or conditioned states of fear; lesions of the amygdala block innate or conditioned fear; and local infusion of drugs into the amygdala has anxiolytic effects in several behavioural tests. The amygdala may also be a critical site of plasticity that mediates both the acquisition and extinction of conditioned fear. Recent studies have shown that both NMDA-dependent (Gean *et al.* 1993) and NMDA-independent (Chapman and Bellavance 1992) LTP can occur in amygdala brain slices or *in vivo* following tetanic stimulation of that part of the medial geniculate nucleus which projects to the lateral nucleus of the amygdala (Clugnet and LeDoux 1990). Thus, if convergence between light and shock occurs at the amygdala, and if an NMDA-dependent process is involved in the acquisition of conditioned fear, then local infusion of NMDA antagonists into the amygdala should block the acquisition of conditioned fear. A key test of this prediction was conducted using a paradigm called fear-potentiated startle.

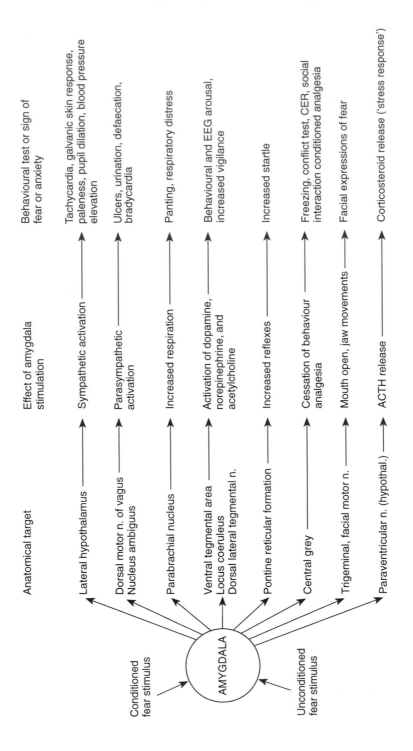

Fig. 15.5 Schematic diagram showing direct connections between the central nucleus of the amygdala and a variety of hypothalamic and brainstem target areas that may be involved in different animal tests of fear and anxiety. (From Davis (1992*a*) with permission from Wiley–Liss, Inc.)

Anatomical target | Effect of amygdala stimulation | Behavioural test or sign of fear or anxiety

Lateral hypothalamus → Sympathetic activation → Tachycardia, galvanic skin response, paleness, pupil dilation, blood pressure elevation

Dorsal motor n. of vagus Nucleus ambiguus → Parasympathetic activation → Ulcers, urination, defaecation, bradycardia

Parabrachial nucleus → Increased respiration → Panting, respiratory distress

Ventral tegmental area Locus coeruleus Dorsal lateral tegmental n. → Activation of dopamine, norepinephrine, and acetylcholine → Behavioural and EEG arousal, increased vigilance

Pontine reticular formation → Increased reflexes → Increased startle

Central grey → Cessation of behaviour analgesia → Freezing, conflict test, CER, social interaction conditioned analgesia

Trigeminal, facial motor n. → Mouth open, jaw movements → Facial expressions of fear

Paraventricular n. (hypothal.) → ACTH release → Corticosteroid release ('stress response')

AMYGDALA

Conditioned fear stimulus

Unconditioned fear stimulus

Fear-potentiated startle

Miserendino *et al.* (1990) examined fear-potentiated startle using a paradigm in which rats were first trained to be fearful of a light (by consistently pairing it with footshock) and then eliciting the startle reflex by a loud auditory stimulus either in the presence or absence of the light. The amplitude of the animal's behavioural response was measured in a specially designed box. Conditioned fear is indicated by a relatively higher startle amplitude in the presence of the light. This effect is associative (i.e. conditioned), because it does not occur following 'random' or unpaired presentations of lights and shocks (Davis and Astrachan 1978), and seems to be a good measure of fear because it is selectively blocked by lesions of the amygdala or drugs which reduce anxiety in people (Davis 1992*b*).

Rats were implanted with bilateral cannulas aimed at the basolateral nucleus of the amygdala, which is known to have high levels of NMDA receptors (Monaghan and Cotman 1985) and 1 week later infused with aCSF or various doses of AP5. Five minutes later they were presented with the first of 10 light-shock pairings presented at an average inter-trial interval of 4 min, creating a 45 min training session. The infusions and training procedures were repeated the following day. One week later, all animals were tested for fear-potentiated startle without any drug infusions. Figure 15.6 shows that AP5 caused a dose-related attenuation of fear-potentiated startle, with a total blockade at the higher doses.

Observation of the animals during training found no evidence of catalepsy or ataxia (cf. Leung and Desborough 1988). The effect did not seem to result from a decrease in sensitivity to footshock, because local infusion of AP5 into the amygdala did not alter either overall reactivity to footshock or the slope of reactivity as a function of different footshock intensities. In contrast to the blockade of acquisition, AP5 did not block the expression of fear-potentiated startle because its infusion immediately before testing did not block potentiated startle in animals previously trained in the absence of the drug. Potentiated startle was also blocked when the more potent NMDA antagonist, 3-(2-carboxypiperazin-4-yl)-propyl-1-phosphonic acid (CPP) was given before training. Other experiments reported by Miserendino *et al.* (1990) showed that 40 nmol/side of propranolol, which has local anaesthetic effects (Weiner 1985) and alters one-trial inhibitory avoidance conditioning (Liang *et al.* 1986), did not block or even attenuate fear-potentiated startle after local infusion into the amygdala prior to training. In addition, AP5 given after training but 1 week before testing did not block potentiated startle, ruling out any permanent damage to the amygdala or receptor blockade caused by residual drug during testing. Local infusion of AP5 did not affect visual prepulse inhibition, a sensitive measure of visual processing in rats (Wecker and Ison 1986), and, finally, infusion of AP5 into deep cerebellar nuclei did not block acquisition even at a dose

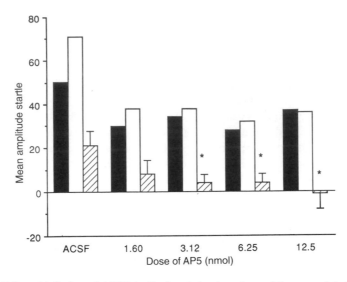

Fig. 15.6 Local infusion of AP5 into the basolateral nucleus of the amygdala blocks the acquisition of fear-potentiated startle. Figure shows the mean amplitude startle response during the test session on noise-alone trials (black bars) and light and noise trials (white bars), and the difference between these two trial types (+ SEM), following bilateral infusion of various doses of the NMDA antagonist AP5 into the amygdala during the training session which occurred 1 week before the test session. (From Miserendino *et al.* (1990) with permission from Macmillan Magazines Ltd.)

eight times that required to block acquisition after local infusion into the amygdala. These data indicate, therefore, that AP5's blockade of conditioning probably does not result from local anaesthetic effects, permanent damage to the amygdala, or blockade of visual transmission, and does not occur if infused into a different part of the brain. Similar results have also been found using an auditory rather than a visual conditioned stimulus (Campeau *et al.* 1992).

Freezing

Using very similar doses to those outlined above, Fanselow *et al.* (1991) have found that local infusion of AP5 into the basolateral nucleus of the amygdala before training blocks conditioned freezing measured 24 h later when the CS is the stimulus of the testing cage. This effect was highly localized, because infusion into the immediately adjacent central nucleus had no effect. Increasingly, infusion of AP5 in the hippocampus also was able to block conditioned freezing measured 24 h later (Young *et al.* 1992), consistent with recent work showing the dependence of contextual, compared with explicit cue, fear conditioning on both the amygdala and the hippocampus (Kim and Fanselow 1992; Phillips and LeDoux 1992).

Inhibitory avoidance

A more complex measure used to assess fear conditioning is inhibitory avoidance. In this paradigm, mice or rats are typically placed on the bright side of a two compartment box. A few seconds later they tend to move to the other, darker compartment, expressing a natural preference shown by many rodents to hide in dark places. However, when they do, they are confined, given a footshock, and then returned to their home cage. Between 24 and 48 h later, they are again placed on the bright side of the box and the length of time it takes them to cross over to the dark, previously shocked side is taken as a measure of the strength of fear of the dark compartment. A great deal of evidence now indicates that the amygdala is critically involved in the consolidation of memory measured with this inhibitory avoidance task (cf. McGaugh *et al.* 1992).

In an extensive series of experiments, Kim and McGaugh (1992) found that intra-amygdala infusion of DL-AP5 (5–50 nmol), D-AP5 (0.15–5 nmol), or CPP (0.5 or 1.5 nmol) prior to training caused a dose-dependent impairment of performance measured 48 h later using a multiple-trial step through avoidance paradigm (Fig. 15.7). The potency of the drugs was consistent with their relative affinities at the NMDA receptor. This effect was not seen when AP5 was infused into the striatum, immediately above the amygdala. Intra-amygdala infusion of 15 or 50 nmol of DL-AP5 did not affect footshock sensitivity or locomotor activity and the blockade of

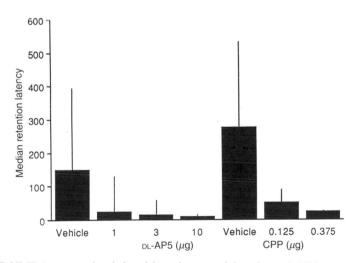

Fig. 15.7 NMDA antagonists infused into the amygdala prior to inhibitory avoidance training block retention measured 48 h later. The figure shows the median latency (+ interquartile range) to re-enter shock compartment following local infusion during training of various doses of either AP5 (A) or CPP (B). (Adapted from Kim and McGaugh (1992) with permission from Elsevier Science Publishers.)

memory formation could not be attributed to state-dependent effects. Although infusion of DL-AP5 prior to testing did affect performance, this effect was not shared by D-AP5 (5 nmol) or MK-801 (1.5 nmol), suggesting non-specific effects on neural transmission caused by the inactive L-isomer of AP5.

More recently, Izquierdo *et al.* (1992) found that immediate post-training infusion of AP5 (25 nmol) into either the amygdala, medial septum, or hippocampus blocked step-down inhibitory avoidance measured 18 h after training. In an important extension of this work, this same group showed that AP5 was amnesic when infused into either the hippocampus or amygdala immediately after training, but not thereafter (Jerusalinsky *et al.* 1992). However, the AMPA antagonist CNQX was amnesic if infused into the hippocampus or amygdala either immediately or 90 or 180 min after training, but not 360 min after training. In contrast, AP5 infused into the entorhinal cortex was amnesic when given either 90 or 180 min after training but not immediately or 360 min after training (Ferreira *et al.* 1992; Jerusalinsky *et al.* 1992). These data suggest, therefore, that a process sensitive first to AP5 and then to CNQX in the amygdala and hippocampus is critical for post-training memory processing of this step-down inhibitory task. Later on, an AP5-sensitive process in the entorhinal cortex may come into play. This exciting approach is beginning to point to a precise timing and sequence of brain structures involved in the formation of long-term memories and the role of excitatory amino acid receptors in these different structures during this process.

Inhibitory avoidance measured immediately after training

In the multiple-trial step-through avoidance procedure used by Kim and McGaugh (1992), rats are allowed to re-enter the shock compartment until they remain in the lighted compartment for 100 s or more before being returned to their home cage. This procedure allows a measure of acquisition of inhibitory avoidance where the number of trials (i.e. the number of times the animals goes into the dark compartment) is used as a measure of acquisition. Importantly, doses of DL-AP5 or CPP that blocked the formation of long-term inhibitory avoidance did not affect the rate of acquisition of short-term inhibitory avoidance. Once again, this is consistent with the freezing data above and the lack of effect of AP5 in the water maze using a multiple trial procedure with short inter-trial intervals.

Non-NMDA antagonists block the expression of conditioned fear

As mentioned earlier, once learning has occurred, local infusion of AP5 into the amygdala does not block the expression of either fear-potentiated startle or inhibitory avoidance. In contrast, Fig. 15.8 shows that local infusion of the AMPA antagonist CNQX into the amygdala dose-dependently blocks the expression of fear-potentiated startle using either a

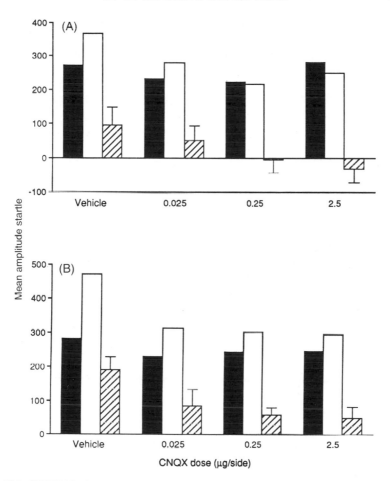

Fig. 15.8 CNQX blocks the expression of fear-potentiated startle when infused into the amygdala. Figure shows mean startle amplitudes in the presence and absence of the visual (A) or auditory (B) conditioned stimulus, and the difference scores (+ SEM) after pretest intra-amygdala infusion of various doses of CNQX or its vehicle, NaOH. (From Kim *et al.* (1993) with permission from Academic Press.)

visual (top panel) or auditory (bottom panel) conditioned stimulus (Kim *et al.* 1993). At the highest doses, the blockade is complete because the small residual effect seen using an auditory conditioned stimulus represents a slight unconditioned effect because it is of the same magnitude as one would find following unpaired noise-shock pairings (Campeau and Davis 1992). Importantly, CNQX blocked the expression of fear-potentiated startle but had no systematic effect on baseline startle after local infusion into the amygdala.

Using a step-down inhibitory avoidance paradigm, Izquierdo *et al.*

(1993) found that local infusion of CNQX at doses similar to those described above blocked the expression of inhibitory avoidance when infused directly into the amygdala or the dorsal hippocampus right before testing. Liang (1991) also reported that CNQX infused in the amygdala before testing blocked the expression of step-through inhibitory avoidance. This blockade occurred when testing was carried out 24 h after training but not 21 days after training. This suggests, at least for the inhibitory avoidance, that non-NMDA receptors in the amygdala are critical for the expression of recently formed memories but not older, well established ones, perhaps because brain areas other than the amygdala become the eventual sites of storage over time. In fact, more recent evidence shows that infusion of CNQX into both the amygdala and hippocampus blocks the expression of inhibitory avoidance when infused either 6, 13, or 20 days after training (Bianchin *et al.* 1993).

Effects of NMDA antagonists on second order conditioning and extinction

Effects of NMDA antagonists on second-order conditioning using fear-potentiated startle

As mentioned earlier, i.c.v. administration of AP5 or local infusion into the amygdala does not alter pain sensitivity as measured by the hot-plate test or the threshold for shock-induced activity or vocalization. While these measures would seem to rule out any gross effects of AP5 on peripheral pain sensitivity, it is not clear how these measures relate to the transmission of shock information in the amygdala, which is probably critical for the formation of conditioned fear. Without a careful analysis of changes in shock-induced, single-unit activity in the amygdala, it is difficult to rule out the possibility that AP5 impairs fear conditioning by reducing the ability of footshock to activate neurones in the amygdala. This ambiguity can partly be addressed using second order conditioning which consists of first pairing a neutral stimulus, such as light, with a shock (first order association) and then pairing a second neutral stimulus, such as a tone, with the light (second order association) in the absence of further shock presentations. Second order fear conditioning is said to have occurred if increased fear (i.e. increased startle) is observed in the presence of the tone relative to that shown by control groups that have the tone and light presented together in a non-paired fashion or which have the tone and light paired, but the light and shock presented in an unpaired fashion.

W. A. Falls and M. Davis (unpublished) now have preliminary evidence that local infusion of AP5 into the amygdala blocks the formation of second order conditioning. Because this procedure does not involve shock presentation during the second order conditioning phase, the blockade of this type of excitatory conditioning cannot be attributed to an interruption of shock information at the level of the amygdala. Furthermore, because these same doses of AP5 do not block the expression of fear-potentiated startle to the light (Miserendino *et al.* 1990), the blockade of second order conditioning cannot be ascribed to a blockade of activation of amygdala neurones by the light during the second order conditioning phase. Taken together, these data provide further evidence that AP5 in the amygdala blocks excitatory conditioning without affecting gross sensory transmission in the amygdala.

NMDA antagonists delay extinction of fear-potentiated startle

Clinically, the inability to eliminate fear and anxiety ranks as one of the major problems in psychiatry. Although a good deal is known about neural systems involved in the acquisition of fear, much less is known about the neural systems that might be involved in the extinction of conditioned fear (see LeDoux *et al.* 1989). To begin to approach this problem, we measured whether blockade of excitatory amino acid receptors at the level of the amygdala would alter the process of experimental extinction (Falls *et al.* 1992). Rats were implanted with bilateral cannulae aimed at the basolateral nucleus of the amygdala and trained for potentiated startle in the usual way. One week later, all animals were given an initial short test session and subsequently matched into four groups each having equivalent levels of fear-potentiated startle. The next day half the animals were presented with 30 light-alone 'extinction' trials at a 1 min inter-trial interval in which shocks were omitted. Five minutes before this extinction session, one group was infused with 50 nmol/side of AP5 and one group with the aCSF vehicle. The two remaining groups were treated identically, except that no lights were presented. They were placed into the test cages immediately after receiving either AP5 or aCSF. Twenty-four hours later, all rats were tested for fear-potentiated startle.

Figure 15.9 shows that animals infused with AP5 or aCSF but not given light-alone extinction trials had levels of potentiated startle equivalent to that observed in their initial test, i.e. no measurable extinction had occurred. Animals infused with aCSF immediately before the light-alone trials had very little potentiated startle on their second test, indicating that extinction had occurred. In contrast, animals infused with AP5 immediately before their light-alone trials displayed levels of potentiated startle that did not differ from their initial test or from the groups not given light-alone trials, and significantly higher levels than the group given aCSF and light-alone trials. These data indicate, therefore, that AP5 infused into the amygdala blocked extinction of fear-potentiated startle suggesting that an NMDA-dependent mechanism in the vicinity of the amygdala may be important for extinction of conditioned fear.

Summary

Four different laboratories, using three different measures of conditioned fear (fear-potentiated startle, freezing, and inhibitory avoidance) have now

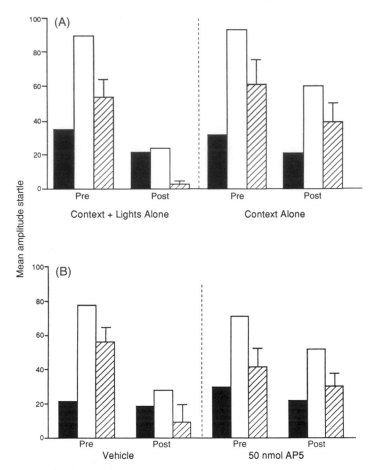

Fig. 15.9 (A) Lights presented in the absence of shock are required to produce extinction. The figure shows the mean amplitude startle response on noise-alone trials (black bars) and light and noise trials (white bars), and the difference between these two trial types (+ SEM, hatched bars) prior to (Pre) or following (Post) presentation of 60 lights (left panel) or an equivalent amount of exposure to the experimental context (right panel). (B) AP5 blocks extinction after local infusion into the balsolateral nucleus of the amygdala. Left panel: rats infused with the vehicle immediately before light-alone presentations showed a significant reduction in fear-potentiated startle (i.e. extinction). Right panel: rats infused with AP5 did not show extinction. (From Falls *et al.* (1992) with permission from the Society for Neuroscience.)

reported that local infusion of NMDA antagonists into the amygdala block the acquisition but not the expression of conditioned fear. In each case, the effective doses of AP5 are very similar. At first blush, this may seem inconsistent with the report of Chapman and Bellavance (1992) showing that LTP in the amygdala produced by electrical stimulation of the external capsule was only blocked by AP5 at doses that also decreased synaptic transmission. However, Gean *et al.* (1993) have now reported NMDA-dependent LTP in the basolateral amygdaloid nucleus when afferent stimulation was initiated in the endopyriform cortex. It would appear, therefore, that both NMDA-dependent and NMDA-independent forms of LTP occur in the amygdala, like they do in the hippocampus. The current literature is at least consistent with the hypothesis that NMDA-dependent LTP may be critical for the acquisition of conditioned fear. However, much more work needs to be done to evaluate whether other treatments, known to alter NMDA-dependent LTP, will also alter the acquisition of conditioned fear when applied directly in the amygdala.

Filial imprinting illustrates that certain forms of early learning depend upon and include changes in NMDA receptors

There has recently been considerable interest in the idea that the organization of the growing nervous system in young animals is dependent, at least partially, on patterns of activity in specific neural circuits (Constantine-Paton 1990). 'Activity-dependent self-organization' of the nervous system (Chapter 14) is an important idea for several reasons—the possibility of a link between the neurobiological mechanisms of neural development and those involved in learning being perhaps the most important. Other important insights that could emerge from its study include that of understanding how excitotoxicity ever evolved in the first place—the death of neurones ('cell death') and the pruning of their connections ('synapse elimination') being very important aspects of neural development. However, while parallels between the mechanisms of learning and those of development have been a frequent topic of comment, there are relatively few examples of research specifically addressing the issue of how learning occurs in young animals and whether there is any overlap between the mechanisms used and those guiding the architecture of the growing nervous system. A possible exception is recent work on filial imprinting.

If visually naive domestic chicks, about 1 day old, are exposed to a visually striking object, such as a rotating red box, they learn to approach that object and avoid others. This learning process is called 'filial imprinting' (Bateson 1976) and the object to which it is normally directed in nature is, of course, the mother hen. Distress calls emitted by the chick in the absence of the imprinted object show a striking reduction in its presence, presumably reflecting the comfort and security normally provided by the chick's mother. The nature of the learning process engaged in imprinting remains a matter of dispute (Bolhuis 1991), but it is clear that the chicks learn to recognize the imprinted object and to distinguish it from other similar ones. This learning takes place at a critical stage of postnatal development and may therefore engage neurobiological mechanisms similar to those involved in other aspects of development.

A large body of research implicates the intermediate extent of the hyperstriatum ventrale (IMHV) of the left brain as one key area involved in imprinting (see Horn 1991 for review). Briefly, incorporation of radio-active uracil into RNA has been found to be higher in IMHV than elsewhere; lesions in this area impair both acquisition and, if given shortly after training, retention also; and increases in the mean length and area of the post-synaptic density (PSD) of axospinous synapses associated with imprinting are restricted to the left IMHV. Of particular relevance to the present review, work from McCabe and Horn's laboratory has implicated NMDA receptors in the synaptic mechanisms that underly, or are altered by, imprinting.

The first indication of an involvement in NMDA receptors in imprinting arose from the discovery that imprinting training was associated with a change in post-synaptic densities and that this change was an increase in the number of glutamate receptors. McCabe and Horn (1988) investigated the effects of imprinting upon $[^3H]$L-glutamate binding to synaptic membranes prepared from the left and right IMHV. Training was associated with an increase in L-glutamate binding in the left but not the right IMHV. When the proportion of this increase due to alteration in NMDA or non-NMDA receptors was partialled out, it was found, somewhat surprisingly, that imprinting was associated with a significant increase in NMDA-sensitive L-glutamate binding. Moreover, when chicks which learned well were compared with chicks that failed to learn, a significantly higher level of NMDA-sensitive L-glutamate binding was found in the 'good learners' than in the 'bad learners'. While this latter correlation does not indicate the direction of causality (i.e. is it animals with higher NMDA-receptor binding that learn well, or is that learning causes an increase in NMDA-receptor binding?), there are two main reasons for thinking that it is the learning that induces the change in receptors. First, Horn (1991) have pointed out that the variance in the amount of NMDA receptor binding in good learners and that in bad learners is no smaller than that in untrained, dark-reared chicks. Second, a subsequent study has replicated the training associated increase in NMDA-sensitive L-glutamate binding and shown that it takes approximately 8 h to develop after an imprinting training schedule lasting approximately 3 h (McCabe and Horn 1991). Thus, it seems that learning in this very young animal can cause an increased expression of a specific subtype of excitatory amino acid receptors. As the electron microscopy work has revealed no change in the number of shaft or spine synapses, it seems likely that synapses in IMHV gain additional NMDA receptors as a result of imprinting.

Changes in NMDA-sensitive binding do not directly implicate NMDA receptors in the learning process of imprinting *per se*. Indeed, the delayed time course of the change suggests a role in retention rather than learning.

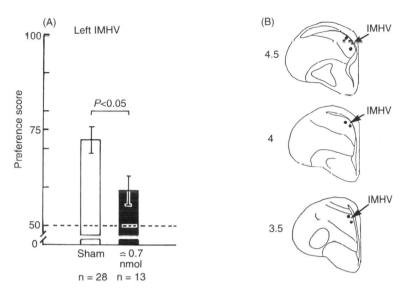

Fig. 15.10 AP5 impairs filial imprinting. (A) Infusion of 0.7 nmol of D-AP5 into the left IMHV impairs preference for an imprinting object. (B) Locations of the infusion cannulae in the chick brain. (After McCabe *et al.* (1992).)

However, direct evidence for a role in learning has been reported by McCabe *et al.* (1992) who have found that local intracerebral infusions of D-AP5 into the left IMHV prior to training cause a dose-related impairment of imprinting (Fig. 15.10).

What are the general implications of these findings? First, they imply that NMDA receptor-dependent learning is not some peculiarity of structures such as the hippocampus and amygdala in the rodent brain. NMDA receptors are also involved in other forms of learning, in a different species, and, importantly, at an early stage of life. The time-dependence of the increase in NMDA receptor number raises the intriguing possibility that imprinting could induce an alteration in the threshold for subsequent learning via an NMDA receptor mechanism. Second, given that NMDA receptor activity has been implicated in the activity-dependent refinement of neural circuits during so-called 'critical periods' of postnatal life, the involvement of NMDA receptors in early learning points to an overlap between the mechanisms of information storage and the organization of the nervous system.

Conclusion

Ten years have passed since the discovery that NMDA receptors played a key role in triggering a particular form of associative synaptic plasticity in the nervous system. Over this period, numerous behavioural studies have explored whether their activation is necessary for several kinds of learning. In this review, we hope we have explained the logic of this research enterprise and the key findings to have emerged so far. In our view, there is now extremely good evidence that *NMDA receptors are involved in the acquisition of new information but not in its subsequent retrieval or expression*. NMDA receptors participate in several different forms of learning, depending critically on the local circuits and neural systems of which they are a part. The types of learning which the hippocampus, amygdala, and IMHV carry out are quite different and, thus, it makes no sense to claim that NMDA receptors play a specific role in learning other than their physiological function of detecting conjunctions between presynaptic activity and sustained post-synaptic depolarization, and signalling them to the intracellular compartment of neurones by calcium. These brain areas receive different kinds of information and process them differently, but all make use of this physiological property of NMDA receptors in the service of the learning process in which they are engaged.

There are, however, numerous outstanding problems for future research. One that is relevant to each of the behavioural tests that have been reviewed is that no amount of research studying whether LTP is *necessary* for learning will ever be persuasive in the absence of studies definitively establishing that LTP occurs naturally during learning. Uncomfortable as it is, we have to face up to the complications of demonstrating that this synaptic mechanism is actually engaged during learning. In addition to using single-unit recording techniques (none of them easy), it would be intriguing to devise methods of visualizing NMDA receptors actually being activated during learning. A second issue involves specifying more precisely how synaptic changes in a given brain area can lead directly to a change in behaviour. In the hippocampus, a great deal is known about local synaptic circuitry yet little is known about how this relates directly to behaviour. In the amygdala, much more is known about how its outputs could directly modulate targets involved in specific signs of fear, yet much less is known about synaptic circuitry within this structure. Hence, a major challenge for future research will involve first measuring whether LTP actually occurs in a given brain structure during learning and, if so, how this change in synaptic strength translates neurally into a change in behaviour. Until that time, we can only surmise that an NMDA form of LTP underlies learning.

Acknowledgements

The work described in this chapter was supported by research grants from the Medical Research Council (RGMM) and NIMH grant MH-47840, Research Scientist Development Award MH-00004, and a grant from the Air Force Office of Scientific Research (MD).

References

Abraham, W. C. and Mason, S. E. (1988). Effects of the NMDA receptor/channel antagonists CPP and MK801 on hippocampal field potentials and long term potentiation in anaesthetised rats. *Brain Research*, **462**, 40–6.

Abraham, W. C. and Wickens, J. R. (1991). Heterosynaptic long-term depression is facilitated by blockade of inhibition in area CA1 of the hippocampus. *Brain Research*, **546**, 336–40.

Aggleton, J. P., Blindt, H. S., and Rawlins, J. N. P. (1986). The effects of combined amygdaloid-hippocampal lesions upon object recognition and spatial working memory. *Behavioural Neuroscience*, **103**, 962–74.

Barrionuevo, G. and Brown, T. H. (1983). Associative long-term potentiation in hippocampal slices. *Proceedings of the National Academy of Science, USA*, **80**, 7347–51.

Bateson, P. P. G. (1976). Specificity and the origins of behaviour. *Advances in the Study of Behaviour*, **6**, 1–20.

Bianchin, M., Walz, R., Ruschel, A. C., Zanatta, M. S., DaSilva, R. C., Bueno e Silva, M., Paczko, N., Medina, J. H., and Izquierdo, I. (1993). Memory expression is blocked by the infusion of CNQX into the hippocampus and/or the amygdala up to 20 days after training. *Behavioral and Neural Biology*, **59**, 83–6.

Blanchard, R. J., Fukunaga, K. K., and Blanchard, D. C. (1976). Environmental control of defensive reactions to footshock. *Bulletin of the Psychonomics Society*, **8**, 129–30.

Bliss, T. V. P. and Lømo, T. (1973). Long-lasting potentiation of synaptic transmission in the dentate area of the anaesthetised rabbit following stimulation of the perforant path. *Journal of Physiology* (London), **232**, 331–56.

Bolhuis, J. J. (1991). Mechanisms of avian imprinting: a review. *Biological Reviews*, **66**, 303–45.

Brennan, P. A. and Keverne, E. B. (1989). Impairment of olfactory memory by local infusions of non-selective excitatory amino acid receptor antagonists into the accessory olfactory bulb. *Neuroscience*, **33**, 463–8.

Brown, T. H., Chapman, P. F., Kairiss, E. W., and Keenan, C. L. (1988). Long-term synaptic potentiation. *Science*, **242**, 724–8.

Butcher, S. P., Hamberger, A., and Morris, R. G. M. (1991). Intracerebral distribution of D,L-2-amino-phosphonopentanoic acid (AP5) and the dissociation of different types of learning. *Experimental Brain Research*, **83**, 521–6.

Cajal, R. Y. (1911). *Histologie du systeme nerveux de l'homme et des vertebres*, Vol. II. Maluine, Paris.

Campeau, S. and Davis, M. (1992). Fear potentiation of the acoustic startle reflex using noises of various spectral frequencies as conditioned stimuli. *Animal Learning and Behavior*, **20**, 177–86.

Campeau, S., Liang, K. C., and Davis, M. (1990). Long-term retention of fear-potentiated startle following a short training session. *Animal Learning and Behavior*, **18**, 462–8.

Campeau, S., Miserendino, M. J. D., and Davis, M. (1992). Intra-amygdala infusion of the *N*-methyl-D-aspartate receptor antagonist AP5 blocks acquisition but not expression of fear-potentiated startle to an auditory conditioned stimulus. *Behavioural Neuroscience*, **106**, 569–74.

Chapman, P. F. and Bellavance, L. L. (1992). Induction of long-term potentiation in the basolateral amygdala does not depend on NMDA receptor activation. *Synapse*, **11**, 310–18.

Clugnet, M. C. and LeDoux, J. E. (1990). Synaptic plasticity in fear conditioning circuits: induction of LTP in the lateral nucleus of the amygdala by stimulation of the medial geniculate body. *Journal of Neuroscience*, **10**, 2818–24.

Collingridge, G. L., Kehl, S. J., and McLennan, H. (1983). Excitatory amino acids in synaptic transmission in the Schaffer collateral-commissural pathway of the rat hippocampus. *Journal of Physiology* (London), **334**, 33–46.

Constantine-Paton, M. (1990). NMDA receptor as a mediator of activity-dependent synaptogenesis in the developing brain. *Cold Spring Harbor Symposium on Quantitative Biology*, **55**, 431–44.

Davis, M. (1992a). The role of the amygdala in fear and anxiety. *Annual Review of Neuroscience*, **15**, 353–75.

Davis, M. (1992b). The role of the amygdala in conditioned fear. In *The amygdala: neurobiological aspects of emotion, memory, and mental dysfunction*, (ed. J. P. Aggleton), pp. 255–306. Wiley–Liss, New York.

Davis, M. and Astrachan, D. I. (1978). Conditioned fear and startle magnitude: effects of different footshock or backshock intensities used in training. *Journal of Experimental Psychology: Animal Behavioural Processes*, **4**, 95–103.

Davis, S. (1990). *The role of the NMDA receptor in the hippocampus in certain forms of learning*. Unpublished Ph.D. thesis, The University of Edinburgh.

Davis, S., Butcher, S. P., and Morris, R. G. M. (1992). The *N*-methyl-D-aspartate receptor antagonist 2-amino-5-phosphonopentanoate (AP5) impairs spatial learning and LTP *in vivo* at comparable intracerebral concentrations to those that block LTP *in vitro*. *Journal of Neuroscience*, **12**, 21–34.

Daw, N. W., Stein, P. S. G., and Fox, K. (1993). The role of NMDA receptors in information processing. *Annual Review of Neuroscience*, **16**, 207–22.

DeCola, J. P., Kim, J. J., and Fanselow, M. S. (1991). NMDA antagonist MK-801 blocks associative fear conditioning but not nonassociative sensitization of conditional fear. *Society of Neuroscience Abstracts*, **17**, 485.

Desmond, N. L., Colbert, C. M., Zhang, D. X., and Levy, W. B. (1991). NMDA receptor antagonists block the induction of long-term depression in the hippocampal dendate gyrus of the anesthetized rat. *Brain Research*, **552**, 93–8.

Disterhoft, J. F., Coulter, D. A., and Alkon, D. L. (1986). Conditioning specific changes of rabbit hippocampal neurons measured *in vitro*. *Proceedings of the National Academy of Science, USA*, **83**, 2733–7.

Dudek, S. and Bear, M. F. (1992). Homosynaptic long-term depression in area CA1 of hippocampus and the effects of NMDA receptor blockade. *Proceedings of the National Academy of Science, USA*, **89**, 4363–7.

Falls, W. A., Miserendino, M. J. D., and Davis, M. (1992). Extinction of fear-potentiated startle: blockade by infusion of an NMDA antagonist into the amygdala. *Journal of Neuroscience*, **12**, 854–63.

Fanselow, M. S. (1986). Associative vs. topographical accounts of the immediate shock freezing deficit in rats: Implications for the response selection rules governing species-specific defensive reactions. *Learning and Motivation*, **17**, 16–39.

Fanselow, M. S., Kim, J. J., and Landeira-Fernandez, J. (1991). Anatomically selective blockade of pavlovian fear conditioning by application of an NMDA antagonist to the amygdala and periaqueductal gray. *Society of Neuroscience Abstracts*, **17**, 659.

Ferreira, M. B. C., DaSilva, R. C., Median, J. H., and Izquierdo, I. (1992). Late posttraining memory processing by entorhinal cortex: involvement of NMDA and GABAergic receptors. *Pharmacology, Biochemistry and Behaviour*, **41**, 767–71.

Frederickson, R. E., Frederickson, C. J., and Danscher, G. (1990). *In situ* binding of bouton zinc reversibly disrupts performance on a spatial memory task. *Behavioural Brain Research*, **38**, 25–33.

Gean, P. W., Chang, F. C., Huang, C. C., Lin, J. H., and Way, L. J. (1993). Long-term enhancement of EPSP and NMDA receptor-mediated synaptic transmission in the amygdala. *Brain Research Bulletin*, **31**, 7–11.

Gleitman, H. and Holmes, P. A. (1967). Retention of incompletely learned CER in rats. *Psychonomic Science*, **7**, 19–20.

Gloor, P. (1960). Amygdala. In *Handbook of Physiology, Section I, Neurophysiology*, (ed. J. Field), pp. 1395–420. American Physiology Society, Washington, DC.

Goddard, G. V. (1986). A step nearer the neural substrate. *Nature*, **319**, 721–2.

Good, M. and Honey, R. C. (1991). Conditioning and contextual retrieval. *Behavioural Neuroscience*, **105**, 499–509.

Grant, S. G. N., O'Dell, T. J., Karl, K. A., Stein, P. L., Soriano, P., and Kandel, E. R. (1992). Impaired long-term potentiation, spatial learning and hippocampal development in *fyn* mutant mice. *Science*, **258**, 1903–9.

Gray, J. A. (1982). *The neuropsychology of anxiety*.

Harris, E. W., Ganong, A. H., and Cotman, C. W. (1984). Long-term potentiation in the hippocampus involves activation of N-methyl-D-aspartate receptors. *Brain Research*, **323**, 132–7.

Hebb, D. O. (1949). *The organisation of behaviour: a neuropsychological theory*. Wiley, New York.

Herron, C. E., Lester, R. J., Coan, E. J., and Collingridge, G. L. (1986). Frequency-dependent involvement of NMDA receptors in the hippocampus: A novel synaptic mechanism. *Nature*, **322**, 265–8.

Hirsh, R. (1974). The hippocampus and contextual retrieval of information from memory: a theory. *Behavioural Biology*, **12**, 421–44.

Horn, G. (1985). *Memory, imprinting and the brain*. Clarendon Press, Oxford.

Horn, G. (1991). Imprinting and recognition memory: a review of neural mechanisms. In *Neural and behavioural plasticity: the use of the domestic chick as a model*, (ed. R. J. Andrew), pp. 219–61. Oxford University Press, Oxford.

Izquierdo, I., Da Cunha, C., Rosat, R., Jerusalinsky, D., Beatriz, M., Ferreira, C., and Medina, J. H. (1992). Neurotransmitter receptors involved in post-training memory processing by the amygdala, medial septum, and hippocampus of the rat. *Behavioral and Neural Biology*, **58**, 16–26.

Izquierdo, I., Bianchin, M., Bueno e Silva, M., Zanatta, M. S., Walz, R., Ruschel, A. C., Da Silva, R. C., Paczko, N., and Medina, J. H. (1993). CNQX infused into rat hippocampus or amygdala disrupts the expression of memory of two different tasks. *Behavioral and Neural Biology*, **59**, 1–4.

Jerusalinsky, D., Ferreira, M. B. C., Walz, R., DaSilva, R. C., Bianchin, M., Ruschel, A. C., Zanatta, M. S., Medina, J. H. and Izquierdo, I. (1992). Amnesia by post-training infusion of glutamate receptor antagonists into the amygdala, hippocampus, and entorhinal cortex. *Behavioral and Neural Biology*, **58**, 76–80.

Johnston, D., Williams, S. H., Jaffe, D., and Gray, R. (1992). NMDA-receptor independent long-term potentiation. *Annual Review of Physiology*, **54**, 489–505.

Kandel, E. R. and Schwartz, J. H. (1982). Molecular biology of learning: modulation of transmitter release. *Science*, **218**, 433–43.

Kapp, B. S. and Pascoe, J. P. (1986). Correlation aspects of learning and memory: vertebrate model systems. In *Learning and memory: a biological view* (ed. J. L. Martinez and R. P. Kesner), pp. 399–440. Academic Press, New York.

Kapp, B. S., Pascoe, J. P., and Bixler, M. A. (1984). The amygdala: a neuroanatomical systems approach to its contribution to aversive conditioning. In *The neuropsychology of memory*, (ed. N. Butters and L. S. Squire), pp. 473–88. The Guilford Press, New York.

Kapp, B. S., Wilson, A., Pascoe, J. P., Supple, W. F., and Whalen, P. J. (1990). A neuroanatomical systems analysis of conditioned bradycardia in the rabbit. In *Neurocomputation and learning: foundations of adaptive networks*, (ed. M. Gabriel and J. Moore). Bradford Books, New York.

Keith, J. R. and Rudy, J. W. (1990). Why NMDA-receptor-dependent long-term potentiation may not be a mechanism of learning and memory: reappraisal of the NMDA-receptor blockade strategy. *Psychobiology*, **18**, 251–7.

Khanna, J. M., Wu, P. H., Wiener, B., and Kalaut, H. NMDA antagonists inhibit rapid tolerance to ethanol. *Brain Research Bulletin*, 1991, **26**, 643–5.

Kim, J. J. and Fanselow, M. S. (1992). Modality-specific retrograde amnesia of fear. *Science*, **256**, 675–7.

Kim, M. and McGaugh, J. L. (1992). Effects of intra-amygdala injections of NMDA receptor antagonists on acquisition and retention of inhibitory avoidance. *Brain Research*, **585**, 35–48.

Kim, J. J., DeCola, J. P., Landeira-Fernandez, J., and Fanselow, M. S. (1991). *N*-methyl-D-aspartate receptor antagonist APV blocks acquisition but not expression of fear conditioning. *Behavioural Neuroscience*, **105**, 160–7.

Kim, J. J., Fanselow, M. S., DeCola, J. P., and Landeira-Fernandez, J. (1992). Selective impairment of long-term but not short term conditional fear by the *N*-methyl-D-aspartate antagonist APV. *Behavioural Neuroscience*, **106**, 591–6.

Kim, M., Campeau, S., Falls, W. A., and Davis, M. (1993). Infusion of the non-NMDA receptor antagonist CNQX into the amygdala blocks the expression of fear-potentiated startle. *Behavioral and Neural Biology*, **59**, 5–8.

Larson, J. and Lynch, G. (1988). Role of *N*-methyl-D-aspartate receptors in the induction of synaptic potentiation by burst stimulation patterned after the hippocampal theta-rhythm. *Brain Research*, **441**, 111–18.

LeDoux, J. E. (1987). Emotion. In *Handbook of Physiology*, (ed. F. Plum), Section 1, Vol. 5, *Higher functions of the brain*, pp.416–59. American Psychological Society, Bethesda, MD.

LeDoux, J. E., Romanski, L., and Xagoraris, A. (1989). Indelibility of subcortical memories. *Journal of Cognitive Neuroscience*, **1**, 238–43.

Leung, L.-W.S. and Desborough, K. A. (1988). APV, an *N*-methyl-D-aspartate receptor antagonist, blocks the hippocampal theta rhythm in behaving animals. *Brain Research*, **463**, 148–52.

Levy, W. B., Jr and Steward, O. (1979). Synapses as associative memory elements in the hippocampal formation. *Brain Research*, **175**, 233–45.

Liang, K. C. (1991). Pretest intra-amygdala injection of lidocaine or glutamate antagonists impairs retention performance in an inhibitory avoidance task. *Society of Neuroscience Abstracts*, **17**, 486.

Liang, K. C., Juler, R. G., and McGaugh, J. L. (1986). Modulating effects of post-training epinephrine on memory: involvement of the amygdala noradrenergic systems. *Brain Research*, **368**, 125 33.

Lincoln, J., Coopersmith, R., Harris, E. W., Cotman, C. W., and Leon, M. (1988). NMDA receptor activation and early olfactory learning. *Brain Research*, **467**, 309–12.

Lyford, G. L., Gutnikov, S. A., Clark, A. M., and Rawlins, J. N. P. (1993). Determinants of non-spatial working-memory deficits in rats given intraventricular infusions of the NMDA antagonist AP5. *Neuropsychologia*, **31**, 1079–98.

McCabe, B. J. and Horn, G. (1988). Learning and memory: regional changes in *N*-methyl-D-aspartate receptors in the chick brain after imprinting. *Proceedings of the National Academy of Science, USA*, **85**, 2849–53.

McCabe, B. J. and Horn, G. (1991). Synaptic transmission and recognition memory: Time course of changes in *N*-methyl-D-aspartate receptors after imprinting. *Behavioural Neuroscience*, **105**, 289–94.

McCabe, B. J., Davey, J. E., and Horn, G. (1992). Impairment of learning by localised injection of an *N*-methyl-D-aspartate receptor antagonist into the hyperstriatum ventrale of the domestic chick. *Behavioural Neuroscience*, **106**, 947–53.

McGaugh, J. L., Introini-Collison, I. B., Cahill, L., Kim, M., and Liang, K. C. (1992). Involvement of the amygdala in neuromodulatory influences on memory storage. In *The amygdala: neurobiological aspects of emotion, memory, and mental dysfunction*, (ed. J. P. Aggleton), pp. 431–51. Wiley–Liss, New York.

Mackintosh, N. J. (1983). *Conditioning and associative learning*. Oxford University Press, Oxford.

McNaughton, B. L., Douglas, R. M., and Goddard, G. V. (1978). Synaptic enhancement in fascia dentata: cooperativity among co-active efferents. *Brain Research*, **157**, 277 93.

Miserendino, M. J. D., Sananes, C. B., Melia, K. R., and Davis, M. (1990). Blocking of acquisition but not expression of conditioned fear-potentiated startle by NMDS antagonists in the amygdala. *Nature*, **345**, 716–18.

Monaghan, D. T. and Cotman, C. W. (1985). Distribution of *N*-methyl-D-aspartate-sensitive L-[^{3}H]glutamate binding sites in rat brain. *Journal of Neuroscience*, **5**, 2909–19.

Monaghan, D. T., Olverman, H. J., Nguyen, L., Watkins, J. C., and Cotman, C. W. (1988). Two classes of *N*-methyl-D-aspartate recognition sites: differential distribution and differential regulation by glycine. *Proceedings of the National Academy of Science, USA*, **85**, 9836–40.

Mondadori, C. and Weiskrantz, L. (1991). Memory facilitation induced by *N*-methyl-D-aspartate blockade. In *Long term potentiation: a debate of current issues*, (ed. M. Baudry and J. L. Davis), pp. 259–66. MIT Press, Cambridge, MA.

Morris, R. G. M. (1981). Spatial localisation does not require the presence of local cues. *Learning and Motivation*, **12**, 239–60.

Morris, R. G. M. (1984). Developments of a watermaze procedure for studying spatial learning in the rat. *Journal of Neuroscience Methods*, **11**, 47–60.

Morris, R. G. M. (1989). Synaptic plasticity and learning: selective impairment of learning and blockade of long-term potentiation *in vivo* by the *N*-methyl-D-aspartate receptor antagonist, AP5. *Journal of Neuroscience*, **9**, 3040–57.

Morris, R. G. M. (1990*a*). Towards a representational hypothesis of the role of hippocampal synaptic plasticity in spatial and other forms of learning. *Cold Spring Harbor Symposium on Quantitative Biology*, **55**, 161–74.

Morris, R. G. M. (1990*b*). It's heads they win, tails I lose! *Psychobiology*, **18**, 261–6.

Morris, R. G. M., Garrud, P., Rawlins, J. N. P., and O'Keefe, J. (1982). Place navigation impaired in rats with hippocampal lesions. *Nature*, **297**, 681–3.

Morris, R. G. M., Anderson, E., Lynch, G. S., and Baudry, M. (1986*a*). Selective impairment of learning and blockade of long-term potentiation by an *N*-methyl-D-aspartate receptor antagonist, AP5. *Nature*, **319**, 774–6.

Morris, R. G. M., Hagan, J. J., and Rawlins, J. N. P. (1986*b*). Allocentric spatial learning by hippocampectomised rats: a further test of the spatial-mapping and working-memory theories of hippocampal function. *Quarterly Journal of Experimental Psychology*, **38B**, 365–95.

Morris, R. G. M., Halliwell, R. F., and Bowery, N. (1989). Synaptic plasticity and learning. II: Do different kinds of plasticity underly different kinds of learning? *Neuropsychologia*, **27**, 41–59.

Morris, R. G. M., Davis, S., and Butcher, S. P. (1990*a*). Hippocampal synaptic plasticity and NMDA receptors: a role in information storage? *Philosophical Transactions of the Royal Society of London*, Series B, **329**, 187–204.

Morris, R. G. M., Schenk, F., Tweedie, F., and Jarrard, L. E. (1990*b*). Ibotenate lesions of hippocampus and/or subiculum: dissociating components of allocentric spatial learning. *European Journal of Neuroscience*, **2**, 1016–28.

Morrisett, R. A., Martin, D., Wilson, W. A., Savage, D. D., and Schwartzwelder, H. S. (1989). Prenatal exposure to ethanol decreases the sensitivity of the adult rate hippocampus to *N*-methyl-D-aspartate. *Alcohol*, **6**, 415–20.

Mulkey, R. M. and Malenka, R. C. (1992). Mechanisms underlying induction of homosynaptic long-term depression in area CA1 of the hippocampus. *Neuron*, **9**, 967–75.

O'Keefe, J. and Nadel, L. (1978). *The hippocampus as a cognitive map*. Oxford University Press, Oxford.

Otto, T., Eichenbaum, H., Wiener, S. I., and Wible, C. G. (1991). Learning-related patterns of CA1 spike trains parallel stimulation parameters optimal for inducing hippocampal long-term potentiation. *Hippocampus*, **1**, 181–92.

Phillips, R. G. and LeDoux, J. E. (1992). Differential contribution of amygdala and hippocampus to cued and contextual fear conditioning. *Behavioural Neuroscience*, **106**, 274–85.

Raffaele, K. C. and Olton, D. S. (1988). Hippocampal and amygdaloid involvement in working memory for nonspatial stimuli. *Behavioural Neuroscience*, **102**, 355–69.

Rawlins, J. N. P., Lyford, G. L., Seferiades, A., Deacon, R. M. J., and Cassaday, H. J. (1993). Critical determinants of non-spatial working memory deficits in rats with conventional lesions of hippocampus or fornix. *Behavioural Neuroscience*, **107**, 420–33.

Riccio, D. C. and Richardson, R. (1984). The status of memory following experimentally induced amnesias: gone, but not forgotten. *Physiological Psychology*, **12**, 59–72.

Sarter, M. and Markowitsch, H. J. (1985). Involvement of the amygdala in learning and memory: A critical review, with emphasis on anatomical relations. *Behavioural Neuroscience*, **99**, 342–80.

Shurtleff, D. and Ayres, J. J. B. (1981). One-trial backward excitatory fear conditioning in rats: Acquisition, retention, extinction, and spontaneous recovery. *Animal Learning and Behavior*, **9**, 65–74.

Sillito, A., Murphy, P. C., Salt, T. E., and Moddy, C. I. (1990). The dependence of retino geniculate transmission in the cat on NMDA receptors. *Journal of Neurophysiology*, **63**, 347–55.

Silva, A. J., Paylor, R., Wehner, J. M., and Tonegawa, S. (1992). Impaired spatial learning in a calcium-calmodulin kinase II mutant mice. *Science*, **257**, 206–11.

Staubli, U., Thibault, O., DiLorenzo, M., and Lynch, G. (1989). Antagonism of NMDA receptors impairs acquisition but not retention of olfactory memory. *Behavioural Neuroscience*, **103**, 54–60.

Sutherland, R. J., Whishaw, I. Q., and Kolb, B. (1983). A behavioural analysis of spatial localisation following electrolytic, kainate, or colchicine induced damage to the hippocampal formation. *Behavioural Brain Research*, **7**, 133–53.

Thompson, L. T., Moskal, J. R., and Disterhoft, J. F. (1992). Hippocampus-dependent learning facilitated by a monoclonal antibody or D cycloserine. *Nature*, **359**, 638–41.

Tonkiss, J. and Rawlins, J. N. P. (1991). The competitive NMDA antagonist AP5, but not the non-competitive antagonist MK-801, induces a delay-related impairment in spatial working memory in rats. *Experimental Brain Research*, **85**, 349–58.

Tonkiss, J., Morris, R. G. M., and Rawlins, J. N. P. (1988). Intra-ventricular infusion of the NMDA antagonist AP5 impairs performance on a non-spatial operant DRL task in the rat. *Experimental Brain Research*, **73**, 181–8.

Trujillo, K. A. and Akil, H. (1991). Inhibition of morphine tolerance and dependence by the NMDA receptor antagonist MK-801. *Science*, **251**, 85–7.

Wecker, J. R. and Ison, J. R. (1986). Visual function measured by reflex modification in rats with inherited retinal dystrophy. *Behavioural Neuroscience*, **100**, 679–84.

Weiner, N. (1985). Drugs that inhibit adrenergic nerves and block adrenergic receptors. In *The pharmacological basis of therapeutics*, (ed. A. Gilman, L. S. Goodman, T. W. Rall, and F. Murad), pp. 181–214. Macmillan, New York.

Willetts, J., Balster, R. L., and Leander, J. D. (1990). The behavioural pharmacology of NMDA receptor antagonists. *Trends in Pharmacological Science*, **11**, 423–8.

Winson, J. (1978). Loss of hippocampal theta rhythm results in a spatial memory deficit in the rat. *Science*, **201**, 160–3.

Wozniak, D. F., Olney, J. W., Kettinger, L., Bice, M., and Miller, J. P. (1990). Behavioural effects of MK-801 in the rat. *Psychopharmacology*, **101**, 47–56.

Young, S. L., Fanselow, M. S., and Bohenek, D. L. (1992). The dorsal hippocampus and contextual fear conditioning. *Society of Neuroscience Abstracts*, **18**, 1564.

Zilles, K. (1985). *The cortex of the rat*. Springer-Verlag, Berlin.

16 Clinical implications of NMDA receptors

PAUL L. HERRLING

Introduction

In the past the major clinical applications of chemical therapeutic agents were frequently first discovered in the clinic following their introduction in another area and before their mechanism of action was known in any detail, e.g. chlorpromazine was first used as a sedative to potentiate anaesthesia (Laborit *et al.* 1952) before its antipsychotic potential was discovered (Delay *et al.* 1952).

In the field of excitatory amino acids a different trend seems to prevail. The discovery of such agents about thirty years ago led, after alternating periods of scepticism and enthusiasm (Watkins 1988) concerning their role as major excitatory transmitters in the mammalian central nervous system, to the recent explosion of publications, particularly on *N*-methyl-D-aspartate (NMDA; Anonymous 1989). These studies on the physiology and pharmacology of excitatory amino acids led to a new understanding of the high degree of complexity of excitatory transmission in the brain, far removed from the early concept that post-synaptic depolarization caused excitation and hyperpolarization inhibition. As a consequence of this recent knowledge, workers in the field have proposed therapeutic applications for drugs modulating excitatory amino acid systems, ranging across the entire field of psychiatry and neurology, although only a very limited number of such compounds have reached the stage of clinical evaluation.

This review will attempt a summary of the proposed therapeutic applications for drugs modulating excitatory amino acids and a short description of the rationale which led to these proposals. The emphasis will be on NMDA-modulating compounds, but mention will also be made of possible clinical applications for compounds acting at non-NMDA receptors.

Therapeutic applications for drugs modulating excitatory amino acid systems

Anticonvulsive therapy

One of the earliest observations relating to application of glutamate and aspartate to the mammalian brain was their ability to cause convulsions

(Hayashi 1954). More recently the view that excessive activity of excitatory amino acid transmission might be the cause of epileptic episodes was further strengthened by the observation that NMDA receptor agonists can induce cells to fire in rhythmic bursts in several brain regions including the cortex, hippocampus, and caudate nucleus as reviewed by Meldrum (1985). It was therefore proposed that anticonvulsant therapy in man might be achieved by the use of antagonists of the NMDA receptor complex. This approach was predominantly pursued by Meldrum and colleagues using a wide range of animal models, including primates (Meldrum 1985; Meldrum and Kerwin 1987).

Interestingly, antagonists of the NMDA receptor, both of the competitive type, such as 2-amino-7-phosphonoheptanoate (AP7) (Meldrum 1986) and 3-((±)-2-carboxypiperazin-4-yl)-propyl-1-phosphonate (CPP) (Davies *et al.* 1986), as well as NMDA channel blockers like dizocilpine (MK-801) (Meldrum 1988) all display anticonvulsant properties in animal models of epilepsy. MK-801 also reduces the frequency of convulsive episodes in man (Troupin *et al.* 1986). Non-NMDA antagonists such as 6-cyano-7-nitroquinoxaline-2,3-dione (CNQX: FG9065) do not seem to be as effective in some models of epilepsy (Jensen and Sheardown 1988). The potential treatment of high pressure neurological syndrome (HPNS) by NMDA antagonists has also been investigated. A relatively selective and competitive NMDA antagonist, AP7, is able to more than double the atmospheric pressure at which tremor occurs in HPNS and also protects against pressure-induced myoclonus and convulsions (Meldrum *et al.* 1983). Drugs with such properties might be useful whenever work at high pressure is required, such as in the deep-sea environment.

Neuroprotection

Selective destruction of neuronal cell bodies in the CNS with sparing of passing axons and glial cells can be achieved by local or in some cases also systemic application of excitatory amino acid agonists (Lucas and Newhouse 1957; Rothman and Olney 1987). This property of excitatory amino acids led to the widespread experimental use of agents like kainate, ibotenate, quinolinate, etc. as tools in neurobiology whenever selective neuronal destruction was required (Fuxe *et al.* 1983). Such excitotoxic properties which are shared by excitatory amino acids endogenous to the mammalian brain were also the basis of several hypotheses relating to the causation of certain neurodegenerative diseases (Albers *et al.* 1989; Choi 1990). Thus, clinical syndromes in which selective premature neuronal death occurs might at least in some cases be due to excessive activation of excitatory amino acid systems, resulting from pathologically increased release and/or decrease of uptake. Alternatively, exogenous excitotoxins occurring in the environment might be responsible for such symptoms.

Hypoxic/ischaemic damage to the central nervous system

Exposure of mammalian brain tissue in cultures to hypoxic episodes results in progressive neuronal deterioration and death. Rothman (1984) demonstrated that this neuronal death could be partly prevented *in vitro* by applying the broad-spectrum excitatory amino acid antagonist γ-D-glutamylglycine to cultures during hypoxic episodes. Intrahippocampal injections of the competitive NMDA antagonist, AP7, in rats reduced hippocampal neuronal damage following experimental forebrain ischaemia (Simon *et al.* 1984). NMDA channel blockers such as MK-801 have also been shown to reduce the volume of neuronal damage due to middle cerebral artery occlusion in cats (Ozyurt *et al.* 1988). Similar findings were obtained in rats with a non-competitive NMDA antagonist of unknown mechanism, ifenprodil (Gotti *et al.* 1988) and in cats with competitive NMDA antagonists such as D-CPP-ene (SDZ EAA 494) (Bullock *et al.* 1990). Recently, additional evidence has accumulated suggesting an excitotoxic role of NMDA receptors in spinal cord injury (Faden *et al.* 1990; Liu *et al.* 1991), in perinatal hypoxic conditions (Kjellmer 1991; Young *et al.* 1990), and in concussive brain injury (Katayama *et al.* 1990).

It was therefore proposed that excitatory amino acids interacting with the NMDA system might be responsible for neuronal death following hypoxic/ischaemic conditions, possibly also in man, due to their selective neurotoxic properties (Choi 1990). Clinical studies might be planned to evaluate the effects of drugs inhibiting the NMDA system in **stroke, head injury**, and **post-cardiac arrest**. An important feature of these studies will be to determine if a beneficial effect of such drugs can be demonstrated even when applied several hours after the occurrence of the injury, as in normal clinical practice some time usually elapses before patients are diagnosed and treatment can begin. Preliminary animal studies indicate that post-injury treatment with NMDA antagonists might still have protective effects (Woodruff *et al.* 1988).

Endogenous neurotoxins

Some compounds endogenous to the human brain such as the tryptophan metabolite quinolinic acid, a selective NMDA agonist in some parts of the brain, have been shown to be neurotoxic (Stone *et al.* 1987). Schwarcz and co-workers have performed a series of elegant studies aimed at elucidating the metabolism and distribution of quinolinic acid in the mammalian brain, including man (Schwarcz *et al.* 1983). As it appears that quinolinic acid is not released upon depolarization of neurones and does not have a specific uptake system, it is unlikely to be a neurotransmitter in the mammalian brain. However, Schwarcz and colleagues have hypothesized that it might be released under pathological conditions (Schwarcz *et al.* 1988*a,b*; Freese *et al.* 1990). Furthermore, they showed that there is only an intracellular metabolic mechanism for this agent; there is no extracellular inactivation mechanism for quinolinic acid except for diffusion. Upon its release it might therefore cause neurotoxic damage (Whetsell *et al.* 1988) in such conditions as **Huntington's disease** or in **hepatic encephalopathy**, as suggested by Moroni and colleagues (1986). **Amyotrophic lateral sclerosis** is another degenerative disease with selective neuronal death where an abnormality of endogenous excitatory amino acids has been implicated (Allaoua *et al.* 1992; Perry *et al.* 1990; Plaitakis 1990; Rothstein *et al.* 1990), in addition to the possible involvement of exogenous excitotoxins (see below). Because NMDA antagonists provoke release of dopamine in basal ganglia (Imperato *et al.* 1990) and because they cause monoamine-like locomotor stimulation in monoamine-depleted rodents, it has been proposed (Carlsson and Carlsson 1990; Greenamyre and O'Brien 1991; Svensson *et al.* 1991) that NMDA antagonists could be useful agents in **Parkinson's** disease. Furthermore, these agents protect substantia nigra neurones from MPP$^+$ toxicity in animals (Turski *et al.* 1991; Turski and Stephens 1992) and potentiate the effects of L-DOPA in monoamine-depleted rats (Klockgether and Turski 1990).

Exogenous excitotoxins

Amyotrophic lateral sclerosis, **Alzheimer-type dementia**, and **Parkinsonism** are all syndromes where post-mortem investigations reveal neuronal death in discrete areas, namely neurones in cortex and the spinal cord (Rothstein *et al.* 1992), cholinergic cells of the basal forebrain, and dopamine cells of the substantia nigra, respectively. These findings are similar to those obtained by injecting excitotoxins into the same regions in animal models and therefore the involvement of environmental excitotoxins in their aetiology has been investigated by several groups.

In the 1950s the Chamorro population of Guam and Rota in the western Pacific exhibited an incidence of symptoms usually associated with the diseases described above that was 50–100 times higher than in the continental US. Since then, the incidence has declined, inducing researchers to look for an environmental change to account for this phenomenon (Spencer *et al.* 1987*a*). Suspicion focused on compounds found in the seed of *Cycas circinalis* (false sago palm) which was used on these islands as a food source until after the Second World War. Spencer and his colleagues (1987*b*) isolated amongst others β-*N*-methylamino-L-alanine (BMAA) and characterized it as a possible excitotoxic agent, responsible for the neurodegenerative symptoms. However, the hypothesis is still controversial and other toxins have been proposed (Duncan *et al.* 1992). A similar investigation into the causes of another motoneurone disease, **lathyrism**, showed that it might result from the ingestion of β-*N*-oxalylamino-L-alanine (BOAA) found in the seeds of *Lathyrus sativus* (chickling or grass pea). The excitotoxic action of BOAA is antagonized in animal models by non-NMDA excitatory amino acid antagonists, and that of BMAA by specific NMDA antagonists (Spencer *et al.* 1987*b*).

Some forms of **shellfish poisoning** are characterized not by paralysis but by central nervous system symptoms including convulsions. An agent possibly responsible for these symptoms might be domoic acid found in a seaweed (*Chondria armata*) and used as food by some edible mussels as proposed by Glavin and collaborators (1989). Preliminary animal data show that broad-spectrum excitatory amino acid antagonists such as kynurenic acid could be effective as antidotes for domoic acid poisoning (Glavin *et al.* 1990).

In the above cases it would suffice to eliminate these plants from the diet to achieve prevention. However, these examples demonstrate that environmental agents exogenous to the human body might cause neuronal degeneration mediated by excitatory amino acid receptors. It would therefore be important to test excitatory amino acid antagonists in neurodegenerative diseases of as yet unknown origin, such as amyotrophic lateral sclerosis which occurs in regions where *Cycas* is not part of the diet. They could prevent further neurological deterioration after the beginning of treatment.

Indirect excitotoxicity following viral infection

The **acquired immunodeficiency syndrome (AIDS)** is often accompanied by neurological symptoms including dementia. Histological observations have led some authors to suggest that endogenous excitatory amino acids might be caused by the virus to reach excitotoxic levels. There are two lines of evidence supporting this hypothesis: firstly, quinolinic acid levels (see above) are elevated in the spinal cord fluid of HIV-1 infected patients (Heyes *et al.* 1991) and secondly, mononuclear phagocytes infected with HIV-1 secrete a neurotoxin whose effect can be blocked by NMDA antagonists (Giulian *et al.* 1990).

In some cases the **measles** virus also causes neurodegeneration which resembles excitotoxic lesions. Andersson and his colleagues (1991) therefore applied the non-competitive NMDA antagonist MK-801 to mice treated with a neurotropic measles virus and achieved neuroprotection relative to untreated animals.

Neuronal protection in the ageing brain

Neurodegenerative diseases of the ageing brain such as Alzheimer's and Parkinson's diseases, as mentioned above, are characterized by selective premature neuronal loss, but with the exception of the cases described above, no causative agents of an environmental nature such as poisons or viruses have yet been identified. Some investigators have therefore explored the possibility that endogenous or exogenous neurotoxins acting via excitatory amino acid receptors might be involved (Maragos *et al.*

1987). There is circumstantial evidence for such an involvement in Alzheimer's disease, as these authors have found a prominent loss of NMDA binding sites in the cortex and hippocampus of *post mortem* brains (Greenamyre 1986), at least in patients who died in an advanced state of disease. In the same regions muscarinic cholinergic, benzodiazepine, and GABA binding sites were not decreased relative to controls. Furthermore, β-amyloid was seen to increase the vulnerability of cortical neurones to excitotoxins (Koh *et al.* 1990). These results are consistent with the excitotoxic hypothesis as it could be imagined that precisely those neurones are affected that have a high density of NMDA receptors. A further observation possibly relevant to this hypothesis is that D-aspartate seems to accumulate in the brain with increasing age (Man *et al.* 1983); however, the site of accumulation is white matter not grey. The excitotoxic hypothesis is only one of many advanced with respect to the causes of Alzheimer's disease, but it has the advantage that it will be testable as soon as NMDA antagonists are clinically available (Palmer and Gershon 1990). However, here again, one can only hope for cessation of the progressing deterioration after beginning treatment.

Psychiatric disturbances

This area is as speculative as the above-mentioned ones. Attention has focused on schizophrenia and anxiety, mainly based on theoretical considerations. This is due, at least for schizophrenia, to the fact that there are no 'schizophrenic' animals that can be used as models and that the current drugs are developed according to the dopamine hypothesis of schizophrenia for which there are many animal models, though none well-suited for testing the excitatory amino acid hypothesis.

Schizophrenia

Freed (1988) has put forward a number of arguments for the involvement of excitatory amino acids in schizophrenia which centre around the corticostriatal pathway. He proposes that the antipsychotic effect of dopamine antagonists is due to a secondarily induced subsensitivity of the corticostriatal excitatory amino acid synapse. His arguments are that antidopaminergic agents produce an acute, non-specific sedation but that the anti-psychotic effects develop more slowly over days and weeks, at a time when tolerance has developed to the sedative effects. Dopaminergic supersensitivity, also known to develop only after repeated administration of strong dopamine receptor antagonists, might be responsible for the tolerance to sedation. Because the corticostriatal excitatory synapse is located on the same dendritic spines of medium spiny neurones as nigro-striatal dopaminergic synapses, the former synapse may become secondarily subsensitive. In support of this hypothesis are the observations that dopamine inhibits cortically evoked excitatory post-synaptic potentials (EPSPs) in striatal cells (Herrling and Hull 1980) and repeated neuroleptic administration to mice reduces their sensitivity to quisqualate (Freed 1988). Non-NMDA receptors might be the receptors predominantly involved in the cortico-striatal EPSP (Herrling *et al.* 1983; Herrling 1985); however, NMDA receptors may also play a role in this synapse (Cherubini *et al.* 1988). It will be of interest to learn whether non-NMDA antagonists such as CNQX (Honoré 1989) cause a catalepsy like that induced by haloperidol. If not, such agents might turn out to be anti-psychotics with lower incidence of extrapyramidal side effects in clinical use (Meldrum and Kerwin 1987). Further evidence linking excitatory amino acid receptors and schizophrenia are the finding that a glutamate receptor gene is expressed in lower quantity in schizophrenics than in normals (Harrison *et al.* 1991) and that NMDA receptor-mediated glutamate release is deficient in synaptosomes from schizophrenics (Sherman *et al.* 1991).

Anxiety

The idea that competitive NMDA antagonists might be anxiolytic in man comes from observations in animal tests indicating that they were active in conflict situations but were different in many respects from benzodiazepines (Liebman and Bennett 1988; Stephens and Andrews 1988; Serrano *et al.* 1989; Trullas *et al.* 1989; Bennett *et al.* 1990; Dunn *et al.* 1990; Kehne *et al.* 1991).

Drugs of abuse

Several lines of evidence indicate an interaction of NMDA receptors with tolerance phenomena:

1. NMDA antagonists inhibit tolerance to ethanol (Khanna *et al.* 1991) and ethanol withdrawal-induced seizures (Liljequist 1991).

2. There are differences in NMDA receptor densities in mice prone or resistant to ethanol withdrawal seizures (Valverius *et al.* 1990).

3. Trujillo and Akil (1991) report that MK-801 inhibits morphine tolerance and dependence in mice.

Hormonal disturbances

Several groups have described effects of excitatory amino acid modulating drugs on hormonal parameters (Van den Pol *et al.* 1990). *N*-Methyl-D-aspartate increased serum levels of luteinizing hormone (LH) and growth hormone (GH) while kainic acid increased only GH levels (Mason *et al.* 1983; Estienne *et al.* 1990*a,b*; Lopez *et al.* 1990; Urbanski and Ojeda 1990; Brann and Mahesh 1991; Farah *et al.* 1991). Kynurenic acid, a broad-spectrum excitatory amino acid antagonist, reduces synaptic excitation in slices of the supraoptic nucleus of rats, a nucleus known to regulate endocrine functions (Gribkoff and Dudek 1988). The competitive NMDA antagonist, 2-amino-5 phosphonopentanoate (AP5), suppresses pulsatile LH release in rats (Arslan *et al.* 1988). These observations open the possibility that excitatory amino acid modulating drugs might be of use in some forms of **endocrine disturbances**.

Other neurological indications

Muscle relaxation

NMDA antagonists have been shown to block synaptic responses involved in spinal reflexes (Davies 1988) and to be strong muscle relaxants in animal models of spasticity (Turski *et al.* 1987, 1988). It is therefore possible that they could be used in some forms of **clinical spasticity**.

Disturbances of the auditory system

Broad-spectrum antagonists of excitatory amino acids such as kynurenic acid (Bobbin and Caesar 1987) and α-D-glutamylamino-methylsulphonic acid (GAMS) affect the excitability of the auditory nerve after perfusion into the cochlea, indicating that the hair cell transmitter might act at non-NMDA excitatory amino acid receptors (Ehrenberger and Brix 1983). In one clinical study (Ehrenberger and Brix 1983) both glutamate and glutamate diethylester were described to alleviate **tinnitus** (ear ringing) after intravenous injection.

Anaesthesia and analgesia

Many dissociative anaesthetics have been found to be NMDA channel blockers (see Chapter 3 and Lodge *et al.* 1988). The clinical use of these drugs, however, has been limited by psychotomimetic effects. The possibility must be explored that competitive NMDA antagonists at high doses might be anaesthetics (see below for discussion of side effects). Some animal data suggest that NMDA receptors are involved in nociceptive pathways (Davies and Lodge 1987; Eaton and Salt 1987; Aanonson 1990; Haley *et al.* 1990; Klepstad *et al.* 1990; Salt 1992; in humans: Kristensen *et al.* 1992).

Migraine

Some researchers have proposed that cortical spreading depression is the trigger for **migraine** attacks (Lauritzen 1990) and there is evidence linking NMDA receptors to this phenomenon (Marranes *et al.* 1988) leading to the suggestion that NMDA antagonists might be useful in treating migraine attacks (Hansen *et al.* 1988). Recently it was reported that excitatory amino acid levels are elevated in migraine (Ferrari *et al.* 1990).

Cognition enhancers

NMDA antagonists have been shown to impair some forms of memory formation (see below). This has led to the hypothesis that a moderate up-regulation of NMDA receptor function could lead to an improved cognitive function without excitotoxic or pro-convulsive effects. A site of choice for such an up-regulation is the strychnine-insensitive modulatory glycine site (SIGS) on the NMDA receptor (Johnson and Ascher 1987; Thomson 1990). A D-serine analogue (D-cycloserine) has been found to have partial agonistic properties at the SIGS (Hood *et al*. 1989; Henderson *et al*. 1990; Emmett *et al*. 1991), and indeed displays cognition enhancing properties in animals (Monahan *et al*. 1989; Herberg and Rose 1990; Thompson *et al*. 1992).

Side effects

It can be predicted that peripheral side effects of excitatory amino acid modulating drugs resulting from interactions with peripheral excitable tissue will be relatively few since in contrast to other transmitter systems such as the acetylcholine, noradrenaline, dopamine, and serotonin systems, excitatory amino acid receptors seem, with very few exceptions (Moroni *et al*. 1986; Erdoe 1991; Wiley *et al*. 1991; Bertrand *et al*. 1992), to be confined to the central nervous system.

Nevertheless, as with most other therapeutically effective chemical agents, it is to be expected that the clinical use of drugs modulating excitatory amino acid systems will be limited by their side effects. The nature of limiting side effects will probably depend on the potential therapeutic indication. In the following, some side effects that can be inferred from the neurobiology of excitatory amino acids are discussed. Toxicological, organ-specific side effects which are independent of the interaction with excitatory amino acid receptors are not discussed as they might vary with the chemical nature of the agents used.

Muscle relaxation and sedation

These properties of excitatory amino antagonists (see above) might be a limiting factor in their use in epilepsy. The therapeutic margin needs to be distinctly better than that of existing anti-epileptic drugs to allow widespread use of excitatory amino acid antagonists in this indication.

Psychotomimetic effects

As mentioned above, some NMDA channel blockers used as anaesthetics in man, such as ketamine, display psychotomimetic effects. There is growing evidence that these effects are associated with the inhibition of the NMDA system and not with properties of dissociative anaesthetics unrelated to excitatory amino acid systems (Lodge *et al*. 1988; Øye *et al*. 1992). Nevertheless, there are also data (France and co-workers 1989) indicating that the competitive NMDA antagonist *cis*-4-(phosphonomethyl)-2-piperidine carboxylic acid (CGS 19755) does not produce

ketamine like discriminative stimuli in rhesus monkeys. Should psychotomimetic effects be associated with NMDA receptor blockade this would
mean that such agents might have to be restricted to acute indications
where such side effects are not too disturbing in view of the clinical benefit,
e.g. in head trauma. Furthermore, the psychotomimetic effects might be
dose-dependent and could possibly be dissociated from the beneficial effect
of NMDA antagonists. Meanwhile clear psychotomimetic effects have
been observed with competitive NMDA antagonists at high doses
(Kristensen *et al*, 1992).

Effects on learning performance and neuronal plasticity

NMDA antagonists inhibit some forms of learning performance in rats (see
Chapter 15 and Morris *et al.* (1986) and Parada-Turska and Turski (1990)).
If this also applies to human learning performance it would limit the use of
such agents, e.g. in epilepsy where the onset of treatment is often before
adult age. However, here again extrapolation to the clinical situation is
difficult as it seems that the effect of NMDA antagonists is task-dependent
and associated with high doses (Mondadori *et al.* 1988). At lower doses
performance in some paradigms of learning such as step-down shock avoidance are even improved by NMDA antagonists (Mondadori *et al.* 1988).
This aspect requires special attention in the clinic.

Neuronal plasticity during development has also been shown to be
influenced by modulators of the NMDA receptor system (see Chapter 14
and Kleinschmidt *et al.* (1987)). As plasticity probably also occurs in the
human adult NMDA antagonists might interfere with this function.

Effects on sensory systems

In addition to the effects on auditory and nociceptive systems described
above, there is considerable evidence that excitatory amino acid receptors
are involved in all levels of sensory transmission, e.g. in the visual (Kemp
and Sillito 1983; Miller and Slaughter 1986; Tang and Ho 1988) and
somatosensory systems (Salt 1987; Salt and Eaton 1990; Mansbach 1991).
These processes involve both NMDA and non-NMDA receptors, but it is
still unclear what contributions these different receptor systems make to sensory perception. There is evidence, however, that NMDA antagonists affect
brightness discrimination in rats (Tang and Ho 1988). It will be important
to determine if effects of amino acid receptor modulating drugs on sensory
processes in man are of such magnitude as to limit their clinical use.

Conclusion

Research into the neurobiology of excitatory amino acid systems has
yielded a wealth of information on many physiological functions of the
mammalian central nervous system. This was mainly due to the dis-

covery of specific pharmacological tools in which J. C. Watkins played a predominant role ever since the discovery of excitatory amino acids. One consequence of this new knowledge was the proposal of many potential therapeutic indications for drugs interacting with these systems. If agents which modulate excitatory amino acids prove to be useful in any of these therapeutic areas then the neurobiological investigation of excitatory amino acids will not only have been scientifically fascinating but will also have contributed to improved clinical treatment of patients, thereby reaching the ultimate goal of the biomedical researcher.

Acknowledgements

Thanks to Dr T. Bucher for commenting on the manuscript and Ms H. Peis for secretarial assistance.

References

Aanonsen, L. M., Lei, S., and Wilcox, G. L. (1990). Excitatory amino acid receptors and nociceptive neurotransmission in rat spinal cord. *Pain*, **41**, 309–21.

Albers, G. W., Goldberg, M. P., and Choi, D. W. (1989). N-methyl-D-aspartate antagonists: ready for clinical trial in brain ischemia? *Annals of Neurology*, **25**, 398–403.

Allaoua, H., Chaudieu, I., Krieger, C., Boksa, P., Privat, A., and Quirion, R. (1992). Alterations in spinal cord excitatory amino acid receptors in amyotrophic lateral sclerosis patients. *Brain Research*, **579**, 169–72.

Andersson, T., Schultzberg, M., Schwarcz, R., Löve, A., Wickman, C., and Kristensson, K. (1991). *European Journal of Neuroscience*, **3**, 66–71.

Anonymous (1989). *The Scientist*, February 20, p. 14.

Arslan, M., Pohl, C. R., and Plant, T. M. (1988). DL-2-amino-5-phosphono-pentanoic acid, a specific N-methyl-D-aspartic acid receptor antagonist, suppresses pulsatile LH release in the rat. *Neuroendocrinology*, **47**, 465–8.

Bennett, D. A., Lehmann, J., Bernard, P. S., Liebman, J. M., Williams, M., Wood, P. L., Boast, C. A., and Hutchison, A. J. (1990). CGS 19755: a novel competitive N-methyl-D-aspartate (NMDA) receptor antagonist with anticonvulsant, anxiolytic and anti-ischemic properties. In *Current and Future trends in anticonvulsant, anxiety, and stroke therapy*, pp. 519–24.

Bertrand, G., Gross, R., Puech, R., Loubatières-Mariani, M. M., and Bockaert, J. (1992). Evidence for a glutamate receptor of the AMPA subtype which mediates insulin release from rat perfused pancreas. *British Journal of Pharmacology*, **106**, 354–9.

Bobbin, R. P. and Ceasar, G. (1987). Kynurenic acid and γ-D-glutamylamino-methylsulfonic acid suppress the compound action potential of the auditory nerve. *Hearing Research*, **25**, 77–81.

Brann, D. W. and Mahesh, V. B. (1991). Endogenous excitatory amino acid regulation of the progesterone-induced LH and FSH surge in estrogen-primed ovariectomized rats. *Neuroendocrinology*, **53**, 107–10.

Bullock, R., Graham, D. I., Chen, M.-H., Lowe, D., and McCulloch, J. (1990).

Focal cerebral ischemia in the cat: pretreatment with a competitive NMDA receptor antagonist, D-CPP-ene. *Journal of Cerebral Blood Flow and Metabolism*, **10**, 668–74.

Carlsson, M. and Carlsson, A. (1990). Interactions between glutamatergic and monoaminergic systems within the basal ganglia—implications for schizophrenia and Parkinson's disease. *Trends in Neurosciences*, **13**, 272–6.

Cherubini, E., Herrling, P. L., Lanfumey, L., and Stanzione, P. (1988). Excitatory amino acids in synaptic excitation of rat striatal neurones *in vitro*. *Journal of Physiology*, **400**, 677–90.

Choi, D. W. (1990). The role of glutamate neurotoxicity in hypoxic-ischemic neuronal death. *Annual Review of Neuroscience*, **13**, 171–82.

Davies, J. (1988). A reappraisal of the role of NMDA and non-NMDA receptors in neurotransmission in the cat dorsal horn. In *Frontiers in excitatory amino acid research*, (ed. E. Cavalheiro, J. Lehmann, and L. Turski), pp. 355–62. Liss, New York.

Davies, J., Evans, R. H., Herrling, P. L., Jones, A. W., Olverman, H. J., Pook, P., and Watkins, J. C. (1986). CPP, a new potent and selective NMDA antagonist. Depression of central neuron responses, affinity for [^{3}H]D-AP5 binding sites on brain membranes and anticonvulsant activity. *Brain Research*, **382**, 169–73.

Davies, S. N. and Lodge, D. (1987). Evidence for involvement of N-methyl-aspartate receptors in 'wind-up' of class 2 neurones in the dorsal horn of the rat. *Brain Research*, **424**, 402–6.

Delay, J., Deniker, P., and Havl, J. M. (1952). Utilisation thérapeutique psychiatrique d'une phénothiazine d'action centrale sélective. *Annales Médicales Psychologiques*, **110**, 112–17.

Duncan, M. W., Marini, A. M., Watters, R., Kopin, I. J., and Markey, S. P. (1992). Zinc, a neurotroxin to cultured neurons, contaminates cycad flour prepared by traditional guamanian methods. *Journal of Neuroscience*, 1523–37.

Dunn, R. W., Corbett, R., Martin, L. L., Payack, J. F., Laws-Ricker, R., Wilmot, C. A., Rush, D. K., Cornfeldt, M. L., and Fielding, S. (1990). Preclinical anxiolytic profiles of 7189 and 8319, novel non-competitive NMDA antagonists. In *Current and future trends in anticonvulsant, anxiety, and stroke therapy*, pp. 495–512.

Eaton, S. A. and Salt, T. E. (1987). N-Methyl-D-aspartate antagonists reduce the responses of rat thalamic neurones to noxious stimulation. *Journal of Physiology* (London), **394**, 114P.

Ehrenberger, K. and Brix, R. (1983). Glutamic acid and glutamic acid diethylester in tinnitus treatment. *Acta Otolaryngologia*, **95**, 599–605.

Emmett, M. R., Mick, S. J., Cler, J. A., Rao, T. S., Iyengar, S., and Wood, P. L. (1991). Actions of D-cycloserine at the N-methyl-D-aspartate-associated glycine receptor site *in vivo*. *Neuropharmacology*, **30**, 1167–71.

Erdoe, S. L. (1991). Excitatory amino acid receptors in the mammalian periphery. *Trends in Pharmacological Sciences*, **12**, 426–9.

Estienne, M. J., Schillo, K. K., Hileman, S. M., Green, M. A., and Hayes, S. H. (1990*a*). Effect of N-methyl-D,L-aspartate on luteinizing hormone secretion in ovariectomized ewes in the absence and presence of estradiol. *Biology of Reproduction*, **42**, 126–30.

Estienne, M. J., Schillo, K. K., Green, M. A., and Hileman, S. M. (1990*b*). Growth hormone release after N-methyl-D,L-aspartate in sheep: dose response and effect of an opioid antagonist. *Journal of Animal Sciences*, **68**, 3198–203.

Faden, A. I., Ellison, J. A., and Noble, L. J. (1990). Effects of competitive and non-competitive NMDA receptor antagonists in spinal cord injury. *European Journal of Pharmacology*, **175**, 165–74.

Farah, J. M., Rao, T. S., Mick, S. J., Coyne, K. E., and Iyengar, S. (1991). *N*-methyl-D-aspartate treatment increases circulating adrenocorticotropin and luteinizing hormone in the rat. *Endocrinology*, **128**, 1875–80.

Ferrari, M. D., Odink, J., Bos, K. D., Malessy, M. J. A., and Bruyn, G. W. (1990). Neuroexcitatory plasma amino acids are elevated in migraine. *Neurology*, **40**, 1582–6.

France, C. P., Wood, J. H., and Ornstein, P. (1989). The competitive *N*-methyl-D-aspartate (NMDA) antagonist CGS 19755 attenuates the rat-decreasing effects of NMDA in rhesus monkeys without producing ketamine-like discriminative stimulus effects. *European Journal of Pharmacology*, **159**, 133–9.

Freed, W. J. (1988). The therapeutic latency of neuroleptic drugs and nonspecific postjunctional supersensitivity. *Schizophrenia Bulletin*, **14**, 269–77.

Freese, A., Swartz, K. J., During, M. J., and Martin, J. B. (1990). Kynurenine metabolites of tryptophan: implications for neurologic diseases. *Neurology*, **40**, 691–5.

Fuxe, K., Roberts, P., and Schwarcz, R. (1983). *Excitotoxins*. Macmillan Press, London.

Giulian, D., Vaca, K., and Noonan, C. A. (1990). Secretion of neurotoxins by mononuclear phagocytes infected with HIV-1. *Science*, **250**, 1593–6.

Glavin, G. B., Pinsky, C., and Bose, R. (1989). Mussel poisoning and excitatory amino acid receptors. *Trends in Pharmaceutical Sciences*, **10**, 15–16.

Glavin, G. B., Pinsky, C., and Bose, R. (1990). Domoic acid-induced neurovisceral toxic syndrome: characterization of an animal model and putative antidotes. *Brain Research Bulletin*, **24**, 701–3.

Gotti, B., Duverger, D., Bertin, J., Carter, C., Dupont, R., Frost, J., Gaudilliere, B., MacKenzie, E., Rousseau, J., Scatton, B., and Wick, A. (1988). Ifendopril and SL 82.0715 as cerebral anti-ischemic agents. I. Evidence for efficacy in models of focal cerebral ischemia. *Journal of Pharmacology and Experimental Therapeutics*, **247**, 1211–21.

Greenamyre, J. T. (1986). The role of glutamate in neurotransmission and in neurologic disease. *Archives of Neurology*, **43**, 1058–63.

Greenamyre, J. T. and O'Brien, C. F. (1991). *N*-methyl-D-aspartate antagonists in the treatment of Parkinson's disease. *Archives of Neurology*, **48**, 977–81.

Gribkoff, V. K. and Dudek, F. E. (1988). The effects of the excitatory amino acid antagonist kynurenic acid on synaptic transmission to supraoptic neuroendocrine cells. *Brain Research*, **442**, 152–6.

Haley, J. E., Sullivan, A. F., and Dickenson, A. H. (1990). Evidence for spinal *N*-methyl-D-aspartate receptor involvement in prolonged chemical nociception in the rat. *Brain Research*, **518**, 218–26.

Hansen, A. J., Lauritzen, M., and Wieloch, T. (1988). NMDA antagonists inhibit cortical spreading depression, but not anoxic depolarization. In *Frontiers in excitatory amino acid research*, (ed. E. A. Cavalheiro, J. Lehmann, and L. Turski), pp. 661–6. Liss, New York.

Harrison, P. J., McLaughlin, D., and Kerwin, R. W. (1991). Decreased hippocampal expression of a glutamate receptor gene in schizophrenia. *Lancet*, **337**, 450–2.

Hayashi, T. A. (1954). Effects of sodium glutamate on the nervous system. *Keio Journal of Medicine*, **3**, 183–92.

Henderson, G., Johnson, J. W., and Ascher, P. (1990). Competitive antagonists and partial agonists at the glycine modulatory site of the mouse N-methyl-D-aspartate receptor. *Journal of Physiology*, **430**, 189–212.

Herberg, L. J. and Rose, J. C. (1990). Effects of D-cycloserine and cycloleucine, ligands for the NMDA-associated strychnine-insensitive glycine site, on brain-stimulation reward and spontaneous locomotion. *Pharmacology, Biochemistry and Behavior*, **36**, 735–8.

Herrling, P. L. (1985). Pharmacology of the corticocaudate excitatory postsynaptic potential in the cat: evidence for its mediation by quisqualate- or kainate-receptors. *Neuroscience*, **14**, 417–26.

Herrling, P. L. and Hull, C. D. (1980). Iontophoretically applied dopamine depolarizes and hyperpolarizes the membrane of cat caudate neurons. *Brain Research*, **192**, 441–62.

Herrling, P. L., Morris, R., and Salt, T. E. (1983). Effects of excitatory amino acids and their antagonists on membrane and action potentials of cat caudate neurones. *Journal of Physiology*, **339**, 207–22.

Heyes, M. P., Brew, B. J., Martin, A., Price, R. W., Salazar, A. M., Sidtis, J. J., Yergey, J. J., Mouradian, M. M., Sadler, A. E., Keilp, J., Rubinow, D., and Markey, S. P. (1991). Quinolinic acid in cerebrospinal fluid and serum in HIV-1 infection: relationship to clinical and neurological status. *Annals of Neurology*, **29**, 202–9.

Honoré, T. (1989). Excitatory amino acid receptor subtypes and specific antagonists. *Medicinal Research Reviews*, **9**, 1–23.

Hood, W. F., Compton, R. P., and Monahan, J. B. (1989). D-Cycloserine: a ligand for the N-methyl-D-aspartate coupled glycine receptor has partial agonist characteristics. *Neuroscience Letters*, **98**, 91–5.

Imperato, A., Scrocco, M. G., Bacchi, S., and Angelucci, L. (1990). NMDA receptors and *in vivo* dopamine release in the nucleus accumbens and caudatus. *European Journal of Pharmacology*, **187**, 555–6.

Jensen, L. H. and Sheardown, M. (1988). Lack of potent antiepileptic effect of specific non-NMDA EAA receptor antagonist. In *Frontiers in excitatory amino acid research*, (ed. E. A. Cavalheiro, J. Lehmann, and L. Turski), pp. 219–26. Liss, New York.

Johnson, J. and Ascher, P. (1987). Glycine potentiates the NMDA response in cultured mouse brain neurons. *Nature*, **325**, 529–31.

Katayama, Y., Becker, D. P., Tamura, T., and Hovda, D. A. (1990). Massive increase in extracellular potassium and the indiscriminate release of glutamate following concussive brain injury. *Journal of Neurosurgery*, **73**, 889–900.

Kehne, J. H., McCloskey, T. C., Baron, B. M., Chi, E. M., Harrison, B. L., Whitten, J. P., and Palfreyman, M. G. (1991). NMDA receptor complex antagonists have potential anxiolytic effects as measured with separation-induced ultrasonic vocalizations. *European Journal of Pharmacology*, **193**, 283–92.

Kemp, J. A. and Sillito, A. M. (1983). The nature of the excitatory transmitter mediating X and Y cell inputs to the cat dorsal lateral geniculate nucleus. *Journal of Physiology*, **323**, 377–91.

Khanna, J. M., Wu, P. H., Weiner, J., and Kalant, H. (1991). NMDA antagonists inhibit rapid tolerance to ethanol. *Brain Research Bulletin*, **26**, 643–5.

Kjellmer, I. (1991). Mechanisms of perinatal brain damage. *Annals of Medicine*, **23**, 675–9.

Klepstad, P., Maurset, A., Moberg, E. R., and Oye, I. (1990). Evidence of a role for NMDA receptors in pain perception. *European Journal of Pharmacology*, **187**, 513–18.

Kleinschmidt, A., Bear, M. F., and Singer, W. (1987). Blockade of 'NMDA' receptors disrupts experience-dependent plasticity of kitten striate cortex. *Science*, **238**, 355–8.

Klockgether, T. and Turski, L. (1990). NMDA antagonists potentiate antiparkinsonian actions of L-Dopa in monoamine-depleted rats. *Annals of Neurology*, **25**, 539–46.

Koh, J., Yang, L. L., and Cotman, C. W. (1990). β-Amyloid protein increases the vulnerability of cultured cortical neurons to excitotoxic damage. *Brain Research*, **533**, 315–20.

Kristensen, J. D., Svensson, B., and Cordly, I. St. The NMDA-receptor antagonist CPP abolishes neurogenic 'wind-up pain' after intratheral administration in humans. *Pain*, **5A**: 749–753 (PS2).

Laborit, H., Huguenard, P., and Alluaume, R. (1952). Un nouveau stabilisateur végétatif (le 4560 RP). *La Presse Médicale*, **60**, 206–8.

Lauritzen, M. (1988). Cortical spreading depression: a putative migraine mechanism. *Trends in Neurosciences*, **10**, 8–12.

Liebman, J. M. and Bennett, D. A. (1988). Anxiolytic actions of competitive N-methyl-D-aspartate receptor antagonists: a comparison with benzodiazepine modulators and dissociative anesthetics. In *Frontiers in excitatory amino acid research*, (ed. E. A. Cavalheiro, J. Lehmann, and L. Turski), pp. 301–8. Liss, New York.

Liljequist, S. (1991). The competitive NMDA receptor antagonist, CGP 39551, inhibits ethanol withdrawal seizures. *European Journal of Pharmacology*, **192**, 197–8.

Liu, D., Thangnipon, W., and McAdoo, D. J. (1991). Excitatory amino acids rise to toxic levels upon impact injury to the rat spinal cord. *Brain Research*, **547**, 344–8.

Lodge, D., Aram, J. A., Church, J., Davies, S. N., Martin, D., Millar, J., and Zeman, S. (1988). Sigma opiates and excitatory amino acids. In *Excitatory amino acids in health and disease*, (ed. D. Lodge), pp. 237–59. Wiley and Sons, New York.

Lopez, F. J., Donoso, A. O., and Negro-Vilar, A. (1990). Endogenous excitatory amino acid neurotransmission regulates the estradiol-induced LH surge in ovarie ectomized rats. *Endocrinology*, **126**, 1771–3.

Lucas, D. R. and Newhouse, J. P. (1957). The toxic effect of sodium-L-glutamate on the inner layers of the retina. *Archives of Ophthalmology*, **58**, 193–204.

Man, E. H., Sandhouse, M. E., Burg, J., and Fisher, G. H. (1983). Accumulation of D-aspartic acid with age in the human brain. *Science*, **220**, 1407–8.

Mansbach, R. S. (1991). Effects of NMDA receptor ligands on sensorimotor gating in the rat. *European Journal of Pharmacology*, **202**, 61–6.

Maragos, W. F., Greenamyre, J. T., Penney, J. B., and Young, A. B. (1987). Glutamate dysfunction in Alzheimer's disease: an hypothesis. *Trends in Neurosciences*, **10**, 65–8.

Marranes, R., Willems, R., De Prins, E., and Wauquier, A. (1988). Evidence for a role of the N-methyl-D-aspartate (NMDA) receptor in cortical spreading depression in the rat. *Brain Research*, **457**, 226–40.

Mason, G. A., Bissette, G., and Nemeroff, C. B. (1983). Effects of excitotoxic amino acids on pituitary hormone secretion in the rat. *Brain Research*, **289**, 366–9.

Meldrum, B. (1985). Possible therapeutic applications of antagonists of excitatory amino acid neurotransmitters. *Clinical Science*, **68**, 113 22.

Meldrum, B. (1986). Drugs acting on amino acid neurotransmitters. *Advances in Neurology*, **43**, 687–706.

Meldrum, B. S. (1988). What are the future prospects for agents decreasing excitatory neurotransmission as anti-epileptic agents? In *Frontiers in excitatory acid research*, (ed. E. A. Calvalheiro, J. Lehmann, and L. Turski), pp. 195–202. Liss, New York.

Meldrum, B. S. and Kerwin, R. W. (1987). Glutamate receptors and schizophrenia. *Journal of Psychopharmacology*, **1**, 217–21.

Meldrum, B., Wardley-Smit, B., Halsey, M., and Rostain, J. C. (1983). 2-Amino-phosphonoheptanoic acid protects against the high pressure neurological syndrome. *European Journal of Pharmacology*, **87**, 501–2.

Miller, R. F. and Slaughter, M. M. (1986). Excitatory amino acid receptors of the retina: diversity of subtypes and conductance mechanisms. *Trends in Neurosciences*, **9**, 211–18.

Monahan, J. B., Handelmann, G. E., Hood, W. F., and Cordi, A. A. (1989). D-cycloserine, a positive modulator of the N-methyl-D-aspartate receptor, enhances performance of learning tasks in rats. *Pharmacology, Biochemistry and Behavior*, **34**, 649–53.

Mondadori, C., Ortmann, R., Petschke, F., Buerki, H., D'Amato, F., Meisburger, J. G., and Fagg, G. E. (1988). In *Frontiers in excitatory acid research*, (ed. E. A. Cavalheiro, J. Lehmann, and L. Turski), pp. 419–26. Liss, New York.

Moroni, F., Lombardi, G., Carla, V., Pellegrini, D., Carassale, G. L., and Cortesini, C. (1986). Content of quinolinic acid and of other tryptophan metabolites increases in brain region of rats used as experimental models of hepatic encephalopathy. *Journal of Neurochemistry*, **46**, 869–74.

Moroni, F., Luzzi, S., Franchi-Micheli, S., and Zilletti, L. (1986). The presence of NMDA-type receptors for glutamic acid in the guinea pig myenteric plexus. *Neuroscience Letters*, **68**, 57–62.

Morris, R. G. M., Anderson, E., Lynch, G. S., and Baudry, M. (1986). Selective impairment of learning and blockade of long-term potentiation by an N-methyl-D-aspartate receptor antagonist, AP5. *Nature*, **319**, 774–6.

Øye, V., Paulsen, O., and Maurset, A. (1992). Effects of ketamine on sensory perception: evidence for a role of N-methyl-D-aspartate receptors. *Journal of Pharmacology and Experimental Therapeutics*, **260**, 1209–13.

Ozyurt, E., Graham, D. I., Woodruff, G. N., and McCulloch, J. (1988). Protective effect of the glutamate antagonist, MK-801 in focal cerebral ischemia in the cat. *Journal of Cerebral Blood Flow and Metabolism*, **8**, 138 43.

Palmer, A. M. and Gershon, S. (1990). Is the neuronal basis of Alzheimer's disease cholinergic or glutamatergic? *FASEB Journal*, **4**, 2745–52.

Parada-Turska, J. and Turski, W. A. (1990). Excitatory amino acid antagonists and memory: effect of drugs acting at N-methyl-D-aspartate receptors in learning and memory tasks. *Neuropharmacology*, **29**, 1111–16.

Perry, T. L., Krieger, C., Hansen, S., and Eisen, A. (1990). Amyotrophic lateral sclerosis: amino acid levels in plasma and cerebrospinal fluid. *Annals of Neurology*, **28**, 12–17.

Plaitakis, A. (1990). Glutamate dysfunction and selective motor neuron degeneration in amyotrophic lateral sclerosis: a hypothesis. *Annals of Neurology*, **28**, 3–8.

Rothman, S. M. (1984). Synaptic release of excitatory amino acid neurotransmitter mediates anoxic neuronal death. *Journal of Neuroscience*, **4**, 1884–91.

Rothman, S. M. and Olney, J. W. (1987). Excitotoxicity and the NMDA receptor. *Trends in Neurosciences*, **10**, 299–301.

Rothstein, J. D., Tsai, G., Kuncl, R. W., Clawson, L., Cornblath, D. R., Drachman, D. B., Pestronk, A., Stauch, B. L., and Coyle, J. T. (1990). Abnormal excitatory amino acid metabolism in amyotrophic lateral sclerosis. *Annals of Neurology*, **28**, 18–25.

Rothstein, J. D., Martin, L. J., and Kuncl, R. W. (1992). Decreased glutamate transport by the brain and spinal cord in amyotrophic lateral sclerosis. *New England Journal of Medicine*, **326**, 1464–8.

Salt, T. E. (1987). Excitatory amino acid receptors and synaptic transmission in the rat ventrobasal thalamus. *Journal of Physiology*, **391**, 499–510.

Salt, T. E. (1992). The possible involvement of excitatory amino acids and NMDA receptors in thalamic pain mechanisms and central pain syndromes. *APS Journal*, **1**, 52–4.

Salt, T. E. and Eaton, S. A. (1990). Postsynaptic potentials evoked in ventrobasal thalamus neurones by natural sensory stimuli. *Neuroscience Letters*, **114**, 295–9.

Schwarcz, R., Whetsell, W. O., and Mangano, R. M. (1983). Quinolinic acid: an endogenous metabolite that produces axon-sparing lesions in rat brain. *Science*, **219**, 316–18.

Schwarcz, R., Speciale, C., Gramsbergen, J. B. P., and Turski, W. (1988*a*). Kynurenines in the mammalian brain. In *Frontiers in excitatory amino acid research*, (ed. E. A. Cavalheiro, J. Lehmann, and L. Turski), pp. 613–20. Liss, New York.

Schwarcz, R., Whetsell, W. O., and Turski, W. A. (1988*b*). Kynurenines and nerve cell death. *Neurodegenerative Disorders*, 7–19.

Serrano, A., D'Angio, M., and Scatton, B. (1989). NMDA antagonists block restraint-induced increase in extracellular DOPAC in rat nucleus accumbens. *European Journal of Pharmacology*, **162**, 157–66.

Sherman, A. D., Hegwood, T. S., Baruah, S., and Waziri, R. (1991). Deficient NMDA-mediated glutamate release from synaptosomes of schizophrenics. *Biological Psychiatry*, **30**, 1191–8.

Simon, R. P., Swan, J. H., Griffith, T., and Meldrum, B. S. (1984). Blockade of *N*-methyl-D-aspartate receptors may protect against ischemic damage in the brain. *Science*, **226**, 850–2.

Spencer, P. S., Hugon, J., Ludolph, A., Nunn, P. B., Ross, S. M., Roy, D. N., and Schaumburg, H. H. (1987*a*). Discovery and partial characterization of primate motor-system toxins. In *Selective neuronal death*, (Ciba Foundation symposium 126), pp. 221–38. Wiley, New York.

Spencer, P. S., Nunn, P. B., Hugon, J., Ludolph, A. C., Ross, S. M., Roy, D. N., and Robertson, R. C. (1987*b*). Guam amyotrophic lateral sclerosis-parkinsonism-dementia linked to a plant excitant neurotoxin. *Science*, **237**, 517–22.

Stephens, D. N. and Andrews, J. S. (1988). *N*-methyl-D-aspartate antagonists in animal models of anxiety. In *Frontiers in excitatory amino acid research*, (ed. E. A. Cavalheiro, J. Lehmann, and L. Turski), pp. 309–16. Liss, New York.

Stone, T. W., Connick, J. H., Winn, P., Hastings, M. H., and English, M. (1987). Endogenous excitotoxic agents. In *Selective neuronal death* (Ciba Foundation symposium 126), pp. 204–20. Wiley, New York.

Svensson, A., Pilehlad, E., and Carlsson, M. (1991). A comparison between the non-competitive NMDA antagonist dizocilpine (MK-801) and the competitive NMDA antagonist D-CPP-ene with regard to dopamine turnover and locomotor-stimulatory properties in mice. *Journal of Neural Transmission*, **85**, 117–29.

Tang, A. H. and Ho, P. M. (1988). Both competitive and non-competitive antagonists of N-methyl-D-aspartic acid disrupt brightness discrimination in rats. *European Journal of Pharmacology*, **151**, 143–6.

Thomson, A. M. (1990). Glycine is a coagonist at the NMDA receptor/channel complex. *Progress in Neurobiology*, **35**, 53–74.

Thompson, L. T., Moskai, J. R., and Disterhoft, J. F. (1992). Hippocampus-dependent learning facilitated by a monoclonal antibody or D-cycloscrine. *Nature*, **359**, 638–41.

Troupin, A. S., Mendius, J. R., Cheng, F., and Risinger, M. W. (1986). MK-801. In *New anticonvulsant drugs*, (ed. B. S. Meldrum and R. J. Porter), pp. 191–201. J. Libbey, London.

Trujillo, K. A. and Akil, H. (1991). Inhibition of morphine tolerance and dependence by the NMDA receptor antagonist MK-801. *Science*, **251**, 85–7.

Trullas, R., Jackson, B., and Skolnick, P. (1989). Anxiolytic properties of 1-aminocyclo-propane-carboxylic acid, a ligand at strychnine-insensitive glycine receptors. *Pharmacology, Biochemistry and Behavior*, **34**, 313–16.

Turski, L. and Stephens, D. N. (1992). Excitatory amino acid antagonists protect mice against MPP$^+$ seizures. *Synapse*, **10**, 120–5.

Turski, L., Klockgether, T., Sontag, K. H., Herrling, P. L., and Watkins, J. C. (1987). Muscle relaxant and anticonvulsant activity of 3-($\pm$)-2-carboxy-piper-azine-4-yl)propyl-1-phosphonic acid, a novel N-methyl-D-aspartate antagonist, in rodent. *Neuroscience Letters*, **73**, 143–8.

Turski, L., Klockgether, T., Turski, W. A., Ikonomidou, C., Schwarz, M., and Sontag, K. H. (1988). Muscle relaxant action of excitatory amino acid antagonists: sites of action. In *Frontiers in excitatory amino acid research*, (ed. E. A. Cavalheiro, J. Lehmann, and L. Turski), pp. 343–50. Liss, New York.

Turski, L., Bressler, K. Rettig, K.-J., Loeschmann, P.-A., and Wachtel, H. (1991). Protection of substantia nigra from MPP$^+$ neurotoxicity by N-methyl-D-aspartate antagonists. *Nature*, **349**, 414–18.

Urbanski, H. F. and Ojeda, S. R. (1990). A role for N-methyl-D-aspartate (NMDA) receptors in the control of LH secretion and initiation of female puberty. *Endocrinology*, **126**, 1774–6.

Valverius, P., Crabbe, J. C., Hoffmann, P. L., and Tabakoff, B. (1990). NMDA receptors in mice bred to be prone or resistant to ethanol withdrawal seizures. *European Journal of Pharmacology*, **184**, 185–9.

Van den Pol, A. N., Wuarin, J.-P., and Dudek, F. E. (1990). Glutamate, the dominant excitatory transmitter in neuroendocrine regulation. *Science*, **250**, 1276–8.

Watkins, J. C. (1988). Thirty years of excitatory amino acid research. In *Frontiers in excitatory amino acid research*, (ed. E. A. Cavalheiro, J. Lehmann, and L. Turski), pp. 3–10. Liss, New York.

Whetsell, W. O., Koehler, C., and Schwarcz, R. (1988). Quinolinic acid: a glia-derived excitotoxin in the mammalian central nervous system. In *The biochemical pathology of astrocytes*, pp. 191–202. Liss, New York.

Wiley, J. W., Lu, Y., and Owyang, C. (1991). Evidence for a glutamatergic neural pathway in the myenteric plexus. *American Journal of Physiology and Gastro-enterology*, **261**, G693–G700.

Woodruff, G. N., Foster, A. C., Wong, E. H. F., Gill, R., Kemp, J. A., and Iversen, L. L. (1988). Excitatory amino acids and neurodegenerative disorders: possible therapeutic indications. In *Excitatory amino acids in health and disease*, (ed. D. Lodge), pp. 379–89. Wiley, London.

Young, R. S. K., Petroff, O. A. C., Novotny, E. J., and Wong, M. (1990). Neonatal excitotoxic brain research. *Developmental Neuroscience*, **12**, 210–20.

17 The NMDA receptor in epilepsy

SUZANNE CLARK, STEVEN STASHEFF,
DARRELL V. LEWIS, DAVID MARTIN, AND
WILKIE A. WILSON

Introduction

Few things have generated more excitement in the field of epilepsy than studies suggesting that N-methyl-D-aspartate (NMDA) receptors may play a role in the development and expression of seizures. It is possible that antagonists of the NMDA receptor channel complex[1] may become a new class of anti-epileptic drugs which not only suppress seizures, but in some cases may be able to prevent the development of the epileptic condition altogether. Given the significance of the latter possibility, it is not surprising that the NMDA receptor has become the focus of intense study.

Since the first edition of this book, the field of NMDA-related epilepsy research has expanded dramatically. In this brief period of time a wealth of new pharmacologic agents has been developed that has facilitated a wide range of *in vivo* and *in vitro* studies. In this chapter we will briefly review some of the earlier studies covered in the previous edition and then focus on the large number of recent advances.

Background

Early investigations of the glutamatergic system suggested that this excitatory amino acid system might play a role in epilepsy. Glutamate and aspartate were found to cause convulsions (Hayashi 1952), glutamate levels were found to be elevated in human epileptic foci (Perry and Hansen 1981), and anatomical studies revealed that NMDA receptors were located in brain regions involved in epilepsy (see Chapter 6). Furthermore, the voltage-sensitive block of NMDA receptors by magnesium was recognized to be important for epilepsy, since the strong neuronal depolarizations seen during epileptic activity could remove the block and increase NMDA receptor-mediated currents (Coan and Collingridge 1985).

The most striking finding about the NMDA receptor was its role in neuroplasticity (Collingridge *et al.* 1983). This was pertinent to epilepsy because neuroplasticity appeared to be involved in certain aspects of the clinical condition. The NMDA antagonists were the tools needed to

---

[1] From this point onward we will refer to 'the NMDA receptor channel complex' as simply the NMDA receptor. However, if a study focuses on the receptor, channel, or modulatory sites, this will be specified.

investigate epileptic neuroplasticity and have helped to distinguish between the processes of **epileptogenesis** and **expression**.

Epileptogenesis is a process that occurs when normal neural tissue is transformed to a relatively permanent epileptic state. The term *expression* refers simply to the *occurrence* of epileptiform activity, but does not imply that there is an underlying epileptic condition in the tissue. For example, healthy animals (or brain slices taken from them) normally do not express epileptiform activity in response to mild stimuli. However, they can be forced to do so if administered a powerful stimulus or convulsant drugs. In contrast, after epileptogenesis, epileptiform activity may occur spontaneously or in response to previously mild stimuli.

Epileptogenesis and expression have different pharmacologic profiles in respect to NMDA receptor antagonists. Both *in vivo* and *in vitro* studies have found that epileptogenesis can be blocked by NMDA receptor antagonists. In contrast, these same studies have found that *expression* may not be blocked, or may be blocked only by higher concentrations of NMDA antagonists.

One of the major challenges in epilepsy is to identify the damage caused by epileptogenesis that is responsible for the chronic epileptic condition. Spontaneous seizures may result from defects in excitatory or inhibitory synaptic or cellular processes. It is possible that there is a range of aetiologies, rather than a single defect. Therefore, it is in the context of multiple aetiologies that this review proceeds and, although we will focus primarily on the possible role of the NMDA receptor, it is not possible to rule out the involvement of other neural excitatory and inhibitory systems in epilepsy.

The nature of epileptiform activity: epileptiform bursts and seizures

The two most commonly studied types of epileptiform activity are interictal spikes and seizures; the NMDA receptor may play a role in each. However, the importance of that role can vary, depending on the experimental conditions, the brain region under evaluation, and whether the tissue has previously undergone epileptogenesis.

Interictal spikes differ from seizures in that they do not normally disrupt behaviour and therefore are not usually the target of anticonvulsant therapy (Niedermeyer 1990). However, interictal spikes are considered to be markers of an abnormal area of the brain and may be used to help localize an epileptic seizure focus. Epileptiform bursts (interictal spikes recorded *in vitro*) are brief discharges (50–200 ms) that involve the synchronous firing of many neurones and appear to be triggered synaptically (Johnston and Brown 1984).

On a cellular level, each neurone undergoes a large depolarization (the paroxysmal depolarizing shift, or PDS) which can trigger multiple action potentials (Matsumoto and Ajmone Marsan 1964). The PDS is thought to be generated and sustained by synaptic and/or intrinsic cellular mechanisms (for review see Speckmann and Elger 1991). The synaptic component of the PDS may involve both NMDA and non-NMDA receptor activation, for the PDS can be reduced by antagonists of NMDA (Lee and Hablitz 1990) or non-NMDA (Lee and Hablitz 1989) receptors. A combination of both antagonists may completely block the PDS when either agent alone cannot (Lee and Hablitz 1989).

On the network level, NMDA- and non-NMDA-mediated potentials may contribute to burst triggering and duration. NMDA receptor antagonists can slow the frequency of spontaneous bursts (for review see Dingledine *et al.* 1990) and can shorten the duration of each burst (Herron *et al.* 1985; Anderson *et al.* 1987). However, NMDA receptor activity is not always necessary for burst generation: electrically triggered bursts are not blocked by NMDA antagonist (Anderson *et al.* 1987), nor are spontaneous bursts which occur with convulsants such as kainic acid (Neuman *et al.* 1988) or 4-aminopyridine (Psarropoulou and Avoli 1992). In the high potassium model, spontaneous epileptiform burst frequency was not reduced by D-APV, but was reduced by the non-NMDA receptor antagonist 6-cyano-7-nitro-quinoxaline-2,3-dione (CNQX) (Chamberlin *et al.* 1990).

How do these properties of epileptiform bursts relate to the treatment of seizures? It is thought that epileptiform bursts may help trigger seizures or may set up conditions favourable to seizure activity. Thus, drugs that reduce epileptiform bursts may consequently suppress seizure activity.

Compared with epileptiform bursts, seizures are longer, more complex events of synchronous cellular firing. Seizures can often severely disrupt behaviour and thus are often the target of anticonvulsant medication. Seizures are probably generated by both synaptic and non-synaptic processes. Synaptic processes may contribute to the triggering and spread of a seizure, whereas non-synaptic processes (possibly mediated by changes in ionic concentrations, ephaptic interactions, or gap junctions) may help to support seizure activity during conditions in which synaptic transmission is reduced. For example, synaptic activity is reduced or blocked when extracellular calcium concentrations ($[Ca^{2+}]_o$) decrease; such conditions have been recorded during seizures *in vivo* (Pumain *et al.* 1985). Evidence that this drop in $[Ca^{2+}]_o$ may contribute to seizure activity comes from *in vitro* studies using hippocampal slices. If slices are exposed to artificial cerebral spinal fluid (ACSF) with abnormally low concentrations of calcium, spontaneous seizure-like events occur (Taylor and Dudek 1982). The seizures are not blocked by APV, suggesting that NMDA receptor activation is not necessary for non-synaptic, seizure-like activity (Heinemann *et al.* 1985).

This complex nature of seizure activity may explain the results obtained with NMDA antagonists. In certain experimental models NMDA antagonists suppress seizures, in others they do not (for reviews see Dingledine *et al.* (1990) and Clark and Wilson (1992)). It is possible that seizures generated in some models have a stronger non-synaptic drive, and thus would be less sensitive to agents like the NMDA receptor antagonists. Alternatively, the seizures could be driven by other excitatory mechanisms which, although synaptically mediated, do not depend on NMDA receptor activation.

Another variable affecting the role of NMDA receptor activity in seizures is the brain region under evaluation. For example, NMDA receptors do not play a major role in low-frequency synaptic transmission in the hippocampus (Collingridge *et al.* 1983), in contrast to cerebral cortex (Thomson 1985). Consequently, NMDA antagonists may have a stronger anticonvulsant effect against epileptic activity arising in cortical regions with a prominent NMDA-mediated component to synaptic activity.

The NMDA receptor and the ontogeny of seizure susceptibility

Development plays an important role in epilepsy, manifest as an increased seizure susceptibility in immature humans and animals. This may be partially due to developmentally regulated changes in the number or distribution of NMDA receptors, as well as to the active role NMDA receptors play in neuronal development (for reviews see McDonald and Johnston (1990) and Constantine-Paton *et al.* (1990)).

A number of studies have identified developmentally regulated changes in NMDA receptor activity that could contribute to seizure susceptibility. When measured with the grease-gap method, the magnesium block of the NMDA receptor channel is less potent and less efficacious in hippocampal slices from 10–15 day old rats than in slices from adults (Nadler *et al.* 1990). Similarly, in area CA1 of hippocampal slices, synaptically evoked extracellular NMDA excitatory post-synaptic potentials (EPSPs) from young (<35 day old) rats were larger and less sensitive to magnesium than were adult (>75 day old) rats (Morrisett *et al.* 1990*a*). In area CA3, NMDA-evoked responses were less voltage-sensitive in hippocampal slices from immature rats than in adults (Ben-Ari *et al.* 1988).

Enhanced NMDA receptor-mediated activity could also be due to transient periods of increased excitatory input. In the hippocampus of immature rats there is a period of increased excitatory amino acid input of the infrapyramidal zone of area CA3 during a period of enhanced seizure susceptibility (Swann *et al.* 1991). Similarly, transient periods of increased NMDA receptor binding have been measured during phases of high seizure susceptibility in rats (Tremblay *et al.* 1988; McDonald *et al.* 1990) and humans (Piggott *et al.* 1993).

NMDA receptors also have a developmentally regulated sensitivity to calcium. Lowering $[Ca^{2+}]_o$ to 1 mM enhanced NMDA-induced potentials in immature but not mature rats (Brady *et al.* 1991). This finding is significant in the light of the drop in $[Ca^{2+}]_o$ that has been measured *in vivo* during seizures (Pumain *et al.* 1985).

Receptor kinetics are also changed in young animals in a direction that could enhance epileptic activity. The decay time of the NMDA excitatory post-synaptic current (EPSC) is significantly prolonged in slices of the superior colliculus from 10–15 day old rats when compared with 23–33 day old rats (Hestrin 1992).

These results provide evidence that the NMDA receptor may play a role in the enhanced expression of seizure activity early in development, since the changes in NMDA receptor activity are in the direction that could result in enhanced excitatory activity.

Experimental evidence for an NMDA receptor-mediated role in epilepsy

Acute *in vivo* animal models of epilepsy

There is considerable evidence from *in vivo* studies that NMDA antagonists can suppress epileptiform activity. Early investigations found these antagonists had anticonvulsant action in several chemical models of epilepsy (Croucher *et al.* 1982; Meldrum *et al.* 1983*a*), maximal electroshock seizures (Czuczwar *et al.* 1984), and high pressure neurological syndrome (Meldrum *et al.* 1983*c*). The results from these early studies were promising and, as the selectivity of each agent was characterized, there appeared to be a correlation between anticonvulsant action *in vivo* and NMDA receptor or channel binding affinity (for review see Chapman 1991).

Many new antagonists were soon developed and tested in models of epilepsy. (This subject will be covered in more depth elsewhere (see Chapters 19 and 20); we will discuss only a few of the many studies here.) Although behavioural side effects limited the effectiveness of some agents, others had favourable therapeutic profiles. However, the results depended somewhat on the experimental model used in each study. For example, the competitive antagonist D-(−)4-(3-phosphonopropyl)piperazine-2-carboxylic acid (D-CPP) and its unsaturated derivative D-(−)(E)-4-(3-phosphonoprop-2-enyl)piperazine-2-carboxylic acid (D-CPP-ene) suppressed seizures in two acute animal models: the DBA/2 mouse and the photosensitive baboon (Patel *et al.* 1990). Both of these agents had favourable therapeutic ratios against seizures and had a duration of action of up to 48 h in baboons. In contrast, in four rodent models of epilepsy, CPP caused motor toxicities at (or near) effective anticonvulsant doses (Löscher *et al.* 1988). The discrepancy between models may predict a potential variation in human response or they may simply reflect differences between species or experimental models.

In general, the competitive antagonists of the receptor are associated with fewer side effects than non-competitive antagonists of the channel. For example, in mice, NMDA-induced seizures were blocked by both competitive and non-competitive NMDA antagonists, but the competitive antagonists were associated with fewer side effects than the non-competitive antagonists (Koek and Colpaert 1990).

The correlation between NMDA receptor affinity (or potency) and anti-convulsant effectiveness may not always hold. In the maximal electroshock seizure (MES) model, the therapeutic index (toxic dose$_{50}$/MES-effective dose$_{50}$) of two non-competitive, open-channel antagonists did not correlate with their potency against NMDA-induced depolarization. When ($\pm$)-5-aminocarbonyl-10,11-dihydro-5H-dibenzo[a,d]cyclohepten-5,10-imine (ADCI) was compared with (+)-5-methyl-10,11-dihydro-5H-dibenzo (a,d)cyclohepten-5,10-imine maleate (dizocilpine, also known as MK-801), ADCI had a more favourable therapeutic index than dizocilpine (5.5 and 0.27, respectively) (Rogawski *et al.* 1991). This was true despite the fact that ADCI was a less potent antagonist than dizocilpine against NMDA-mediated depolarization (IC$_{50}$ verses NMDA of 15.2 and 0.60, respectively) (Rogawski *et al.* 1991; Yamaguchi and Rogawski 1992). These results suggest that behavioural side effects may limit the usefulness of non-competitive antagonists with high potency, but perhaps not those of lower potency.

Furthermore, in some models the NMDA antagonists do not block seizures, even when the same species of experimental animal is used. For example, in the strain of mice used in the MES study discussed above, the NMDA antagonists APV or phencyclidine (PCP) had only a weak effect against seizures evoked with the non-NMDA agonists kainate or quisqualate (Koek and Colpaert 1990). Similarly, seizures produced by the convulsant 4-aminopyridine (4-AP) were not inhibited by the NMDA antagonists (+)-MK-801 or ($\pm$)-CPP (Yamaguchi and Rogawski 1992) although they were inhibited by ADCI (Rogawski *et al.* 1991). Therefore, although NMDA receptor activity can contribute to seizure generation *in vivo*, it may not be necessary if seizures can be triggered by other means.

Other sites on the NMDA receptor may also serve as targets for anti-convulsant drug development. Some of the most promising agents are those targeted at the strychnine-insensitive glycine site on the NMDA receptor (the 'glycine site'). The antagonists of this glycine site (7-chloro-kynurenic acid and HA 966) were effective against seizures evoked in mice by intracerebroventricular (i.c.v.) NMDA (Koek and Colpaert 1990). This study also compared the glycine site antagonists with competitive and non-competitive NMDA antagonists. Once again, non-competitive antagonists were associated with the highest level of side effects whereas glycine site antagonists did not have behavioural toxicities. (Similar positive results with 7-chlorokynurenic acid were seen against kindled seizures (Croucher and Bradford 1990), as discussed in the next section.)

Chronic *in vivo* models of epilepsy

Many of the acute *in vivo* models discussed above use healthy, non-epileptic animals. However, the neuronal processes in healthy animals may differ significantly from those in epileptic animals. Therefore, it is important to develop animal models which may more closely resemble the human epileptic condition. For that reason, a number of investigators have turned to chronic models of epilepsy to attempt to reproduce the pathology seen in human epilepsy. In several chronic *in vivo* models, changes have been found in NMDA receptors that may cause (or contribute to) the epileptic condition.

Kindling

One of the most widely studied chronic models is kindling. Kindling is a model of both epileptogenesis and seizure expression (McNamara *et al.* 1985). In kindling, epileptogenesis is usually induced by delivering an initially subconvulsive train of electrical stimuli at periodic intervals to a specific site in the brain. The trains evoke a progressively more intense response that eventually develops into a behavioural seizure. After a number of trains, seizure intensity reaches a plateau, at which point the animal is considered 'fully kindled'. Fully kindled animals can be used to study seizure expression and to test anticonvulsants, whereas the early phases of kindling can be used to study epileptogenesis.

In the kindling model, the NMDA channel blocker dizocilpine has dose-dependent effects against epileptogenesis and seizure expression. Kindling epileptogenesis is suppressed by low doses of dizocilpine, whereas fully kindled seizures are not suppressed unless higher doses are used (De Sarro *et al.* 1985; McNamara 1988). Although dizocilpine suppressed fully kindled seizures in several other studies (Gilbert 1988; Sato *et al.* 1988) it did so at doses that have been previously reported to cause profound behavioural depression (McNamara *et al.* 1988).

What can explain this kindling-induced decrease in dizocilpine effectiveness? Although there are a number of possibilities, one possibility is that NMDA receptor activity is enhanced. NMDA receptor activity could be directly enhanced by an increase in effectiveness or number of receptors, or by an increase in neurotransmitter release. It could be indirectly enhanced by changes in inhibitory processes. In either case, a higher concentration of the antagonist might be required to offset an increase in activity (McNamara *et al.* 1992).

Several kindling studies have measured a change in NMDA receptor-mediated activity. Kindling caused an increase in NMDA-mediated synaptic activity in the dentate gyrus. In slices from unkindled rats, perforant path stimulation of dentate granule cells evokes EPSPs that lacked an NMDA-mediated component. In contrast, after kindling there was a component of the EPSP that appeared to be NMDA-mediated, for it was voltage-sensitive, blocked by DL-APV, and enhanced by lowering magnesium concentrations (Mody and Heinemann 1987).

The kindling process can also alter agonist-induced calcium influx. NMDA agonists cause an influx of calcium through NMDA receptors which can be measured as a drop in $[Ca^{2+}]_o$. In normal, non-epileptic tissue this drop is limited to superficial cortical layers. This is thought to reflect the location of NMDA receptors, because the influx is blocked by APV, but not by antagonists of voltage-sensitive calcium channels (Pumain *et al.* 1987). In hippocampal slices from kindled rats, exogenously applied agonists (aspartate or homocysteic acid) caused a drop in $[Ca^{2+}]_o$ that was more widely distributed across cell layers than in slices from control rats (Wadman *et al.* 1985). Similar results have been seen in the chronic cobalt animal model (Pumain *et al.* 1986) and in slices from surgical sections removed from humans for seizure control (Louvel *et al.* 1992). An expanded NMDA receptor-mediated calcium influx could be relevant to epilepsy for several reasons: the decrease in extracellular calcium concentrations could reduce charge screening, rendering the neuronal membrane more excitable (Frankenhaeuser and Hodgkin 1957). Furthermore, as calcium flows into cells it can affect cellular processes and second messenger systems that may also contribute to epileptic activity (Perlin and De Lorenzo 1992).

Kindling also changes other responses to NMDA agonists. Martin *et al.* (1992) used the grease-gap method to compare agonist-induced depolarizations in hippocampal slices from kindled and control rats. Kindling significantly increased the sensitivity to NMDA: in area CA3 of hippocampal slices from kindled and control rats, the EC_{50} of NMDA was 35 and 151 μM, respectively. This effect was measured 1–2 months after the last kindled seizure; a smaller, but still significant, effect could be measured one day after the last kindled seizure.

Kindling can also alter several NMDA-mediated second messenger processes. A kindling-induced change was measured in phosphoinositide (PI) hydrolysis mediated by several receptor-mediated systems. In hippocampal slices from kindled rats, NMDA more potently suppressed carbachol-induced phosphatidyl inositol turnover than did slices from control rats (Morrisett *et al.* 1989).

Kindling has also been found to change the binding properties of the NMDA receptor channel complex, although the direction of the change varies across studies. Binding to different sites on the NMDA receptor channel complex has been found to increase (Yeh *et al.* 1989), decrease (Okazaki *et al.* 1989), or remain unchanged (Jones and Johnson 1989; Akiyama *et al.* 1992). Some of these differences in NMDA receptor channel binding may be due to the different ligands used, the anatomical areas studied, or the time points measured.

In summary, the kindling model has helped to ascertain that epileptogenesis depends on NMDA receptor activation. Although kindling development is also suppressed by other classes of drugs such as γ-aminobutyric acid (GABA) agonists (for reviews see McNamara *et al.* (1985) and Sato *et al.* (1990)) and commonly used anticonvulsants (Silver *et al.* 1991), it is not clear if these agents act directly to inhibit epileptogenesis or indirectly by suppressing net NMDA receptor activity.

Furthermore, several kindling studies found that NMDA receptor activity was enhanced by kindling. This enhancement could be a direct result of the kindling stimulus trains, for strong stimuli have been shown to potentiate NMDA receptor-mediated synaptic transmission (Bashir *et al.* 1991). Although kindling appears to enhance several NMDA receptor-mediated processes, it is important to determine if these changes in NMDA activity are a *cause* of kindled seizures or are a kindling-induced change that is unrelated to seizure expression.

Kainic acid

Another chronic model in which changes in the NMDA receptor-mediated responses have been measured is the kainic acid model. Kainic acid can cause chronic seizures and damage to the hippocampal formation reminiscent of temporal lobe sclerosis (Tauck and Nadler 1985), a pathologic finding in certain types of human epilepsy. Turner and Wheal (1991) administered kainic acid at a dose titrated to cause loss of hippocampal neurones in area CA3 but not area CA1. One week after treatment, the CA1 pyramidal cells from kainic acid-treated rats had changes in several properties that could potentially contribute to epileptiform activity. The neurones could fire graded bursts of action potentials, a characteristic previously reported to occur in slices from humans with epilepsy (Schwartzkroin *et al.* 1983; Avoli and Olivier 1987). EPSPs evoked in area CA1 appeared to have an NMDA-mediated component, for they were voltage-sensitive, suppressed by D-APV, and had a prolonged duration (see Fig. 17.1). It is not clear whether this increase in NMDA-mediated activity is due to a direct increase in NMDA receptors or a decrease in inhibition. Inhibition appears to be compromised in the kainic acid model (Wheal *et al.* 1984), perhaps due to loss of excitatory drive to inhibitory GABAergic interneurones, rather than a loss of inhibitory inputs on to the excitatory cells (Williams *et al.* 1993).

Pilocarpine

The cholinergic agonist pilocarpine can also cause neuronal damage and chronic limbic seizure. In hippocampal slices from pilocarpine-treated rats, the EPSPs in the dentate granule cells appeared to have an enhanced NMDA-mediated component compared with controls (Isokawa and Mello 1991). This enhancement could result from a loss of inhibition, since inhibitory post-synaptic potentials (IPSPs) could not be synaptically evoked.

In summary, the results from the studies using chronic *in vivo* models suggest that the NMDA receptor is involved in epileptogenesis and that chronic epileptic conditions may be associated with long-term enhancement of NMDA receptor-mediated activity. However, these results do not rule out the importance of concomitant changes in other synaptic and

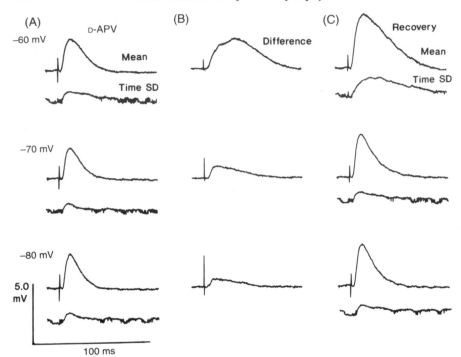

(A) D-APV
−60 mV
Mean
Time SD

−70 mV

−80 mV

5.0 mV

100 ms

(B) Difference

(C) Recovery
Mean
Time SD

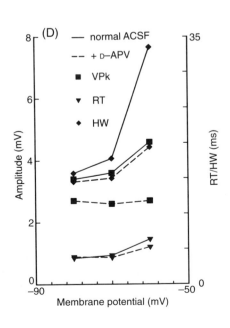

(D)
— normal ACSF
--- + D−APV
■ VPk
▼ RT
◆ HW

Amplitude (mV)

RT/HW (ms)

Membrane potential (mV)

Fig. 17.1 Voltage- and D-APV-sensitive components of EPSPs in area CA1 in a slice from a kainic acid treated rat. Shown in (A) and (B) are intracellular recordings of EPSPs evoked by stimuli in stratum radiatum at three different resting membrane potentials in D-APV (20 μM) or control ACSF (recovery). The mean potential (upper trace) and time standard deviation (SD) (lower trace) are shown in (A) and (C). (A) EPSPs evoked in D-APV at membrane potentials of −60, −70, and −80 mV. (B) Difference between EPSPs evoked in D-APV or after recovery in control ACSF. (C) Recovery from D-APV. In this example D-APV caused only a small change in the actual peak voltage. However, there was a range of D-APV sensitivity in these slices; EPSPs in some slices were almost completely suppressed by D-APV (see Figure 6 of Turner and Wheal 1991). In lesioned slices, D-APV decreased the EPSPs to an average of 17 per cent of their control values, an effect markedly different from control slices. (D) Summary of changes in the peak magnitude and waveform parameters of the EPSP in (A) and (C) as functions of both D-APV exposure and resting membrane potential. The EPSP peak and half-width were decreased in an additive manner by D-APV and hyperpolarization. (VPk: peak voltage, RT: rise time, HW: half-width.) (Reproduced with permission from Turner and Wheal (1991).)

---

cellular processes; further study is needed to determine which changes are actually necessary for seizure activity in these models.

Genetic models of epilepsy

Early studies using genetic models of epilepsy found that NMDA receptor antagonists suppressed seizures in the photosensitive baboon *Papio papio* (Meldrum *et al.* 1983*b*) and the audiogenic seizure-prone mouse (DBA/2) (Croucher *et al.* 1982; Meldrum *et al.* 1983*a*). More recent studies have confirmed these results and have sought to identify the mechanism underlying this involvement.

Genetic audiogenic seizures, in which seizures are evoked in susceptible mice or rats by loud noise, were one of the early models in which NMDA antagonists were found to have anticonvulsant activity (Croucher *et al.* 1982; Jones *et al.* 1984). These seizures may arise in NMDA receptor-mediated auditory pathways. Faingold *et al.* (1992) found evidence for this in the genetically epilepsy-prone rat (GEPR). Audiogenic seizures were suppressed by local injection of the NMDA antagonists 2-amino-7-phosphonoheptanoate (AP7) or CPP into the inferior colliculus, the area where these seizures are thought to be generated. Local injections of L-canaline, a glutamate synthesis inhibitor, also decreased or blocked audiogenic seizures.

The epileptic mouse is a genetic model of temporal lobe epilepsy in which seizures can be induced by handling (tossing). Flavin *et al.* (1991) compared potassium-evoked aspartate release from hippocampal slices taken from epileptic mice that had previously had seizures and normal (C57BL/6J) control mice. Although there was no difference in basal levels, there was an increase in the potassium-evoked release of aspartate in slices from epileptic mice. Glutamate release was not changed, nor was GABA release. These results suggest that previous seizures may cause persistent changes in the release of selected excitatory amino acids.

Several genetic animal models resemble human absence seizures. Absence seizures are marked by behavioural arrest during which time brief bursts of spike-wave discharges are recorded. These bursts are thought to be mediated by inhibitory and excitatory synaptic connections between the cortex and thalamus (Gloor and Fariello 1988). Absence seizures may arise from defects in a number of different neurotransmitter systems and intrinsic cellular processes, including changes in noradrenergic innervation (Noebels 1984), T-type calcium channels (Coulter *et al.* 1989), $GABA_A$ and $GABA_B$ receptors (Crunelli and Lereshe 1991; Hosford *et al.* 1992; Marescaux *et al.* 1992; Snead 1992), γ-hydroxybutyric acid receptors (Snead 1992) as well as in NMDA receptors (Peeters *et al.* 1990).

Several *in vivo* studies have examined the role of NMDA receptors in genetic models of absence. In the WAG/Rij rat, an i.c.v. dose of agonist (NMDA) increased absence seizures, whereas the seizures were decreased by the NMDA antagonist 2-amino-7-phosphonoheptanoic acid (Peeters *et al.* 1990). Although dizocilpine had a similar effects in this model, it also caused agitation in these animals. This behavioural side effect could have reduced spike-wave discharges, since absence seizures are suppressed by an increase in alertness (Peeters *et al.* 1989). The 'genetic absence epilepsy rat' from Strasbourg (GAERS) responded somewhat differently: both NMDA agonists and antagonists decreased spike wave discharges (Marescaux *et al.* 1992).

Although absence seizures differ from convulsive seizures in their behavioural presentation and mechanism of generation, both types of seizures are associated with changes in calcium influx. In the GAERS model, Pumain *et al.* (1992) measured the decrease in $[Ca^{2+}]_o$ in response to iontophoretic application of NMDA in the sensorimotor cortex, an area of the brain with prominent spike-wave discharges. The GAERS rat had an expanded distribution of NMDA-mediated calcium responses, including both superficial and deep cortical layers, when compared with control rats. As discussed above, a similar change in calcium responses has been found in models of convulsive seizures. Since absence seizures and convulsive seizures differ in many ways, it is interesting to see that this NMDA receptor-mediated change is common to both.

Acute *in vitro* models of epilepsy and the NMDA receptor

One of the most common *in vitro* models in which to study epileptiform activity is the brain slice preparation. Brain slices are often used to study acute epileptogenesis and expression, although some aspects of chronic epileptogenesis can be studied with cultured cells or slices.

Epileptiform activity has been recorded in slices from the hippocampus

(Taylor and Dudek 1982; Herron *et al.* 1985), entorhinal cortex (Wilson *et al.* 1988; Jones and Lambert 1990), neocortex (Aram and Lodge 1988), amygdala (Gean and Shinnick-Gallagher 1988), and inferior colliculus (Pierson *et al.* 1989). All of these areas have NMDA receptors (see Chapter 6), so it is not surprising that NMDA receptor antagonists can modify either epileptogenesis or the expression of epileptiform activity in slices from these areas.

Each type of slice often has a characteristic firing pattern, depending on anatomy, ontogeny, and experimental conditions (for review see Clark and Wilson (1992)). Although epileptiform bursts are often easier to evoke in the commonly used models, electrographic seizures can also occur under certain conditions or if slices from young animals are used.

Epileptogenesis of electrographic seizures (EGSs) in slices

To develop an *in vitro* model of the epileptogenesis of seizures, we capital-ized on the ontological differences in EGS expression. Using hippocampal slices from adult rats, we had previously developed a model of epilepto-genesis of epileptiform bursts by giving repeated stimulus trains (see be-low) (Stasheff *et al.* 1985). We found that repeated stimulus trains could also evoke electrographic seizures if hippocampal slices were from younger rats (21–35 days old) (Anderson *et al.* 1988). To produce epileptogenesis of electrographic seizures, stimulus trains were repeated every 10 min until the trains gradually evoked longer and more intense after-discharges. After three to six stimulus trains, the after-discharges reached a plateau with respect to duration and firing pattern (see Fig. 17.2.) After-discharges that developed a characteristic 'tonic–clonic' firing pattern were classified as EGSs. This *in vitro* epileptogenesis is reminiscent of the development of seizures in the kindling model.

In our studies, the most striking effect of NMDA antagonists was on epileptogenesis (Stasheff *et al.* 1989). Figure 17.3 illustrates this effect. First, D-APV (50 μM) was bath-applied for 15 min, then the slice was stimulated every 10 min for a total of 10 trains. There was no significant increase in the number of after-discharges over the course of the trains (Fig. 17.3(A)). After the tenth train, the D-APV was washed off with control ACSF while stimulations were continued. There was a progressive development of the after-discharge until tonic–clonic EGSs were evoked (Fig. 17.3(B)).

These results suggested that antagonists of the NMDA receptors blocked epileptogenesis *in vitro*, similar to the effects seen in the *in vivo* kindling model. However, we wanted to confirm that we were not merely seeing a gradual wash-out of an anticonvulsant effect of D-APV. To that end, we modified the experiment so that epileptogenesis was first induced in the absence of D-APV. The first 10 trains were delivered to a new slice in control ACSF. After the tenth train, D-APV was applied. In Fig. 17.3(C),

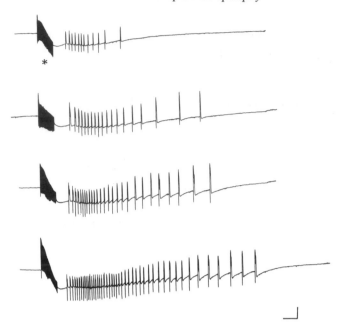

Fig. 17.2 Induction of electrographic seizures. Extracellular field recordings from area CA3 of the hippocampal slice showing the progressive enhancement of after-discharges evoked by successive stimulus trains (asterisk). The first stimulus train elicited an after-discharge with a short duration. Each successive train evoked an after-discharge of a longer duration and more complex firing pattern. By the fourth stimulus train, there was a rapidly firing (tonic) phase in the early part of the after-discharge followed by a phase of complex bursts resembling those during the clonic phase of a seizure. When after-discharges develop this pattern characterized by 'tonic–clonic' phases and a constant duration, they are given the designation electrographic seizures (EGSs).

Fig. 17.3 D-APV prevents epileptogenesis of electrographic seizures (EGSs), but does not block established EGS expression in area CA3 of hippocampal slices. (A) Extracellular recording of stimulus train-evoked after-discharges in the presence of D-APV (50 μM). Stimulus trains (arrows) were repeated at 10 min intervals. From the first to the eighth train there was no significant enhancement of the after-discharges while D-APV was present. (B) Next, D-APV was washed off with control ACSF. During this period stimulus trains evoked progressively longer after-discharges, typical of normal epileptogenesis in hippocampal slices. (C) In a different slice, 10 stimulus trains were given in control ACSF to allow complete epileptogenesis (ACSF control). Then increasing concentrations of D-APV (25, 50, and 100 μM) were applied. Stimulus trains were continued at 10 min intervals. There was no significant effect of D-APV on EGS expression even at the highest concentration used. (Reproduced with permission from Stasheff *et al.* (1989), copyright 1989 by the AAAS.)

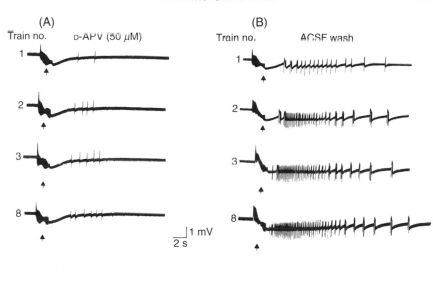

(A) Train no.   D-APV (50 μM)

1

2

3

8

⌐|1 mV
2 s

(B) Train no.   ACSF wash

1

2

3

8

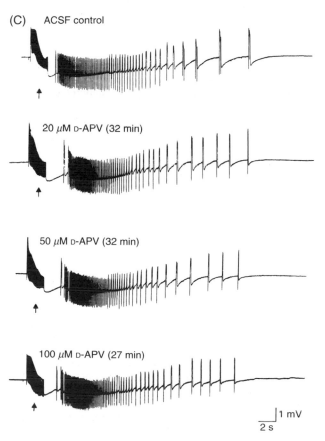

(C)   ACSF control

20 μM D-APV (32 min)

50 μM D-APV (32 min)

100 μM D-APV (27 min)

⌐|1 mV
2 s

EGSs are shown before and after D-APV was applied. The EGS firing pattern was not significantly altered by any concentration of the antagonist. Overall, D-APV did not significantly depress the number of bursts within an EGS, nor the EGS duration or tonic–clonic firing pattern. D-APV did occasionally reduce the duration of the individual bursts within the later clonic portion of the EGSs. The non-competitive antagonist dizocilpine also blocked epileptogenesis without blocking seizure expression (Stasheff *et al*. 1989). APV also suppressed epileptogenesis in a model using sine-wave stimulus trains to induce epileptogenesis in hippocampal slices (Bawin *et al*. 1991).

Although NMDA antagonists did not block EGS expression, the antagonists could raise the seizure threshold. Normally, EGSs have a distinct threshold (Anderson *et al*. 1988). NMDA antagonists could raise this threshold, but if the intensity of a stimulus train was increased, the train set off an EGS with a complete stereotypical tonic–clonic pattern (Cohen *et al*. 1992). Thus, NMDA antagonists appeared to suppress EGS triggering, but did not appear to modify the regenerative mechanisms driving the EGS firing pattern.

One of the goals in the study of epilepsy is to identify how epileptogenesis changes the cells and/or networks to render them permanently epileptic. As discussed above in the kainate model, there is evidence that neuronal inhibition may be reduced. In the *in vitro* brain slice models there is evidence both for (Stelzer *et al*. 1987) and against (Higashima 1988; Bawin *et al*. 1991) a loss of inhibition after epileptogenesis. In our own studies, we did not detect a decrease in inhibition after epileptogenesis, except at very low stimulus intensities (unpublished observations). However, over the course of epileptogenesis there was an increase in spontaneous antidromic action potentials recorded in area CA3 of hippocampal slices (Stasheff and Wilson 1990). As was seen for EGSs, the epileptogenesis-associated increase in antidromic action potentials was prevented by NMDA antagonists (Stasheff and Wilson 1993). In contrast, after epileptogenesis the antidromic action potentials were not blocked by NMDA antagonists. They were blocked by bicuculline or picrotoxin, suggesting that these antidromic action potentials were triggered by a $GABA_A$-mediated process.

There are many other models that evoke EGSs in slices and, as seen with the *in vivo* studies, there is a range of effects seen with NMDA antagonists (for reviews see Clark and Wilson (1992) and Dingledine *et al*. (1990)). For example, in the low magnesium model, EGSs were blocked by NMDA antagonists (Avoli *et al*. 1987; Sagratella *et al*. 1987; Jones and Heinemann). In contrast, in the low calcium model, spontaneous EGS were not blocked by APV (Heinemann *et al*. 1985).

Epileptiform bursts in slices

Although epileptiform bursts differ from seizures in duration and firing pattern, there are several similarities between these two types of activity.

As with the epileptogenesis of seizures, the epileptogenesis of burst activity is blocked by NMDA receptor antagonists (Anderson *et al.* 1987). Furthermore, burst epileptogenesis is blocked by NMDA antagonists regardless of the experimental method used to induce epileptogenesis. For example, NMDA antagonists block burst epileptogenesis induced by stimulus trains, kainic acid, NMDA, or high potassium (Anderson *et al.* 1987; Ben-Ari and Gho 1988). As discussed previously, epileptiform burst expression is blocked by NMDA antagonists in some slice models, but not all, as was seen with models of electrographic seizure expression.

The NMDA receptor in epileptic human tissue

Human epileptic tissue has often been examined to search for clues about chronic epilepsy. Human tissue provides unique challenges, for it can be difficult to secure adequate control tissue. Nevertheless, if done properly, these studies can provide important information about the human epileptic condition.

Several studies have documented the presence of NMDA-mediated potentials in human brain slices from surgical sections removed during surgery for intractable seizures. Avoli and Olivier (1987) characterized the responses evoked in layer III–V neurones in neocortical slices. A single strong stimulus could evoke bursts of action potentials that occurred during a late, slow depolarizing potential. This late potential appeared to be NMDA receptor-mediated, for it was voltage-sensitive and reduced by APV. Similarly, Urban *et al.* (1990) found that 70 per cent of human hippocampal slices studied appeared to have NMDA receptor-mediated synaptic potentials in the dentate, for they were enhanced by low magnesium and reduced by D-APV or CPP. NMDA receptor-mediated potentials have also been recorded in slices from children. Wuarin *et al.* (1992) measured responses in neocortical slices from paediatric surgical sections in a solution containing bicuculline and CNQX (a combination chosen to enhance and isolate NMDA potentials). As in adult tissue, synaptic potentials in these slices appeared to have NMDA receptor-mediated components, for EPSPs were voltage-sensitive and reduced by APV.

Brain slices from humans have also been exposed to convulsants. Neocortical slices exposed to bicuculline generated spontaneous bursts and after-discharges that were suppressed by APV; magnesium-free solutions caused spontaneous electrographic seizures that were suppressed by either competitive (CPP) or non-competitive (dizocilpine) antagonists (Avoli 1991).

There are several studies in which human control tissue was available. Louvel *et al.* (1992) measured the laminar profile of agonist-induced changes in $[Ca^{2+}]_o$ in slices from control and epileptic tissue (frontal cortex removed during surgery for tumours and human temporal or frontal cortex removed during surgery for epilepsy, respectively). Human epileptic tissue had an expanded laminar profile of NMDA-mediated $[Ca^{2+}]_o$ responses, as seen in the cobalt, kindling, and genetic absence animal models discussed previously. A similar change was seen in response to the application of glutamate, but not quisqualate or kainic acid, suggesting that the change may be specific to NMDA receptor-mediated processes.

A biochemical study of human tissue measured the amount of several amino acids in temporal neocortex that had been classified pre-operatively as either spiking or non-spiking (Sherwin *et al.* 1988). When surgical samples of the two types were compared, the spiking samples had higher concentrations of glutamate, aspartate, and glycine. No changes were detected in GABA or taurine.

Several studies have explored the changes in glutamatergic receptor binding in human epileptic tissue. NMDA and non-NMDA receptor binding has been increased, decreased or unchanged, depending on the receptor subtype or the area of the brain under study (Hosford *et al.* 1991; McDonald *et al.* 1989; and Ben-Ari *et al.* 1992).

These studies using human tissue demonstrate that NMDA-mediated potentials *can* be evoked in slices from human tissue. They also suggest that NMDA receptor-mediated responses may be changed in human epileptic tissue. Further experiments comparing epileptic and control human tissue may help to characterize properties unique to epileptic tissue as well as to determine which of these unique properties are responsible for seizure expression in humans.

Alcohol withdrawal seizures

Ethanol can affect NMDA receptor activation by several mechanisms. It can antagonize NMDA-mediated responses within concentration ranges (5–50 mM) that cause intoxication in humans (Lovinger *et al.* 1989). It can also decrease the release of glutamate and aspartate at concentrations of ≥ 25 mM and ≥ 50 mM, respectively (Martin and Swartzwelder 1992). Ethanol also decreases GABA release in this study, but only at higher concentrations (100 mM).

There is growing evidence that NMDA receptors may be involved in seizures associated with alcohol withdrawal. This may be due to the effect of chronic ethanol exposure on the NMDA receptor. Chronic ethanol exposure has been associated with up-regulation of NMDA receptor-linked channels (Grant *et al.* 1990). During abrupt withdrawal of ethanol, this receptor up-regulation may be responsible for a transient period of increased seizure susceptibility. In mice undergoing ethanol withdrawal, seizure susceptibility parallels changes in NMDA receptor binding (Gulya *et al.* 1991).

Other *in vivo* experiments support the hypothesis that ethanol withdrawal seizures may be mediated by NMDA receptors. Ethanol withdrawal seizures were blocked by dizocilpine in rats (Morrisett *et al.* 1990*b*).

Dizocilpine and ADCI were effective against ethanol withdrawal seizures in mice (Grand *et al.* 1992). ADCI had lower motor toxicities than dizocil pine and was also active against whole body tremors during withdrawal, an effect that dizocilpine lacked (Grant *et al.* 1992).

Although withdrawal from chronic ethanol exposure can *cause* seizures, acute application of ethanol can decrease seizure activity. Ethanol may exert this effect by blocking NMDA receptor activation or by suppressing excitatory amino acid release. Ethanol (60–300 mM) has an anticonvulsant effect on stimulus-train evoked EGSs in hippocampal slices (Cohen *et al.* 1992). Similarly, in slices of the amygdala exposed to low levels of magnesium, ethanol (100 mM) reduces stimulus-evoked after-discharges (Gean 1992). This effect occurred at concentrations similar to those that suppressed evoked NMDA synaptic potentials in this preparation.

Anticonvulsants and the NMDA receptor

Several studies have investigated the effect of common anticonvulsants on NMDA receptor activity. In some of the studies the drug effect occurred at (or near) the concentrations that exist in human CSF during treatment for seizure control (e.g. approximately 4–13 μM for carbamazepine (Loiseau and Duche 1989) and 4–8 μM for phenytoin (Woodbury 1989). In cultured neurones from the spinal cord, carbamazepine (20–50 μM) reduced NMDA-induced currents, whereas phenytoin (1–50 μM) did not (Lampe and Bigalke 1990). In cortical wedges from the DBA/2 mouse, carbamaze pine (1.25–10 μM) reduced NMDA-evoked depolarization (Lancaster and Davies 1992).

Other studies have found no effect of carbamazepine on NMDA receptor activity. In whole cell recordings of cultured hippocampal neurones, carbamazepine did not block NMDA-induced currents at 30 μM and caused only a slight suppression at 300 μM (Rogawski *et al.* 1991). In hemisected rat spinal cord, carbamazepine (40 μM) did not appreciably block responses evoked by NMDA, quisqualate, or kainate (Olpe *et al.* 1991). Similarly, carbamazepine (30 mg/kg i.p.) could not block the effect of these agonists *in vivo* when they were administered iontophoretically (Olpe *et al.* 1991).

Anticonvulsant barbiturates reduce glutamatergic activity, but have a stronger effect on non-NMDA than NMDA receptors (for review see Rogawski and Porter 1990). In slices of rat striatum, phenobarbital an tagonized $^{22}Na^+$ efflux evoked by kainic and quisqualic acid, but did not block NMDA-induced $^{22}Na^+$ efflux (Teichberg *et al.* 1984).

Several anticonvulsants suppress excitatory amino acid release. Pheny toin, carbamazepine, phenobarbital, and valproate decreased aspartate release from rat cortical slices, although in some cases at concentrations above therapeutic levels (Crowder and Bradford 1987). In rat cortical slices, potassium-evoked release of D-aspartate was inhibited by phenytoin, phenobarbitone, and mephobarbital, but also at concentrations above the therapeutic levels (Skerritt and Johnston 1983). Phenytoin was the only drug that depressed spontaneous release in normal potassium solutions (Skerritt and Johnston 1983). The investigational anticonvulsant lamotrigine suppressed release of both glutamate and aspartate from cortical slices exposed to veratrine; it had less of an effect against GABA release (Leach *et al.* 1986). In contrast, lamotrigine did not suppress release of these neurotransmitters evoked by potassium, suggesting that lamotrigine may decrease release through its effect on sodium channels by suppressing neuronal firing (Leach *et al.* 1986). This may be the mechanism by which phenytoin and carbamazepine reduce release, for they can also suppress sodium channel activity (for review see MacDonald (1989)). Carbamazepine also can increase potassium conductance (Zona *et al.* 1990) and block calcium channels (F. Brugger, personal communication) at (or near) therapeutic concentrations; it may exert its anticonvulsant effect through one or more of these mechanisms.

Although these anticonvulsants may directly or indirectly alter the activity of glutamatergic receptor systems, this is not thought to be their primary anticonvulsant mechanism, for these drugs act on many other neurotransmitter systems and neuronal processes at therapeutic concentrations (for reviews see MacDonald (1989) and Rogowski and Porter (1990)). Nevertheless, if a drug reduces NMDA receptor activity, it is possible that this property might facilitate the primary anticonvulsant mechanism of action.

Potential limitations of NMDA receptor antagonists in epilepsy treatment

In addition to general concerns about reversible behavioural toxicity, there are several concerns about the use of NMDA antagonists that relate specifically to the treatment of epilepsy. These effects are:

(1) behavioural changes due to indirect neurotoxicity;

(2) suppression of certain types of learning and memory;

(3) disruptions of normal synaptic development;

(4) enhanced susceptibility to NMDA antagonist-induced side effects in chronic epilepsy.

NMDA antagonist-induced neurotoxicity has been seen in the cingulate and retrosplenial cerebral cortex. Although this toxicity can be attenuated pharmacologically with anticholinergic or GABAergic drugs (Olney *et al.* 1991), there are obvious risks associated with the use of potentially neurotoxic drugs in a patient population that may already have some degree of neuronal cell loss.

The effects on learning are also important to consider in the epileptic population, many of whom are stricken during critical periods for learning. Although it can be argued that several of the commonly used anticonvulsants also disrupt learning, comparative studies will need to be done to select the least disruptive drugs.

NMDA antagonists may be associated with a unique, developmentally associated risk for epilepsy. This risk may be due to the role NMDA receptors play in normal neuronal development (McDonald and Johnston 1990). Experimental evidence for this risk was obtained in a study using a noise-induced animal model of epilepsy. Using this model, Pierson and Swann (1991) set out to test the ability of NMDA antagonists to protect rats from noise-induced seizure susceptibility. In this models, when immature rats are exposed to a loud noise, that exposure results in subsequent long-term susceptibility to noise induced-seizures. This susceptibility becomes manifest several days after the initial exposure and persists into adulthood. Normally, if the initial noise exposure is given during the peak age for this phenomenon (postnatal day (PND) 14), 22 per cent of the rats become predisposed to noise-induced seizures.

Based on the studies in kindling and slices, NMDA antagonists were expected to block noise-induced epileptogenesis and thus prevent the subsequent development of seizure susceptibility. Surprisingly, the antagonists had the opposite effect. In rats pre-treated with dizocilpine (MK801) or PCP before the noise exposure, the drug pretreatment *increased* long-term seizure susceptibility to 100 per cent (see Fig. 17.4(A)). However, neither dizocilpine nor PCP affected susceptibility when administered in the absence of noise exposure. MK-801 pretreatment enhanced long-term susceptibility (see Fig. 17.4(B)). In addition to increasing susceptibility, dizocilpine lengthened the window of time during which rats were vulnerable to the initial noise exposure. In contrast, after epileptogenesis has occurred, the noise-evoked seizures can be suppressed with dizocilpine.

These results suggest that there may be a specific window of susceptibility for the seizure-enhancing effects of NMDA antagonists. One possible scenario for the mechanism underlying this window is based on the role of the NMDA receptor in normal synaptic development (McDonald and Johnston 1990). During normal development, there is a brief period of exuberant axonal connectivity (for review see Swann *et al.* (1993)). Later in development these extra synaptic connections are eliminated through a process of pruning. The pruning process can be pharmacologically disrupted by NMDA antagonists. For example, DL-APV can disrupt normal synapse elimination in the cerebellum (Rabacchi *et al.* 1992). If NMDA receptor antagonists disrupt pruning in areas of the brain susceptible to seizures, then the unpruned exuberant connections could predispose the network to seizures (Swann *et al.* 1993).

NMDA antagonists do not enhance seizure susceptibility under all conditions; in certain situations they can be protective. Stafstrom *et al.* (1993) studied this property in kainic acid-induced status epilepticus. In young

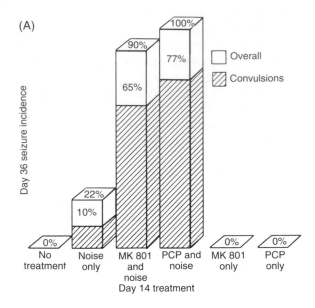

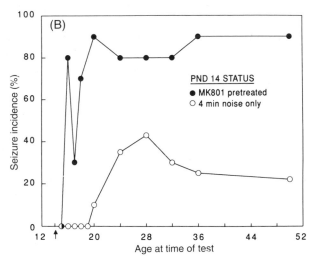

Fig. 17.4 Effect of NMDA antagonist pretreatment on the ontogeny and enhancement of subsequent seizure susceptibility. (A) The effect of single neonatal dizocilpine or PCP pre-treatments on the level of adult susceptibility induced by 4 min noise exposure. The term 'overall' refers to the sum of all non-convulsive (wild running-only) and all convulsive seizures. Rats (PND 14) were administered either dizocilpine or PCP 30 min before a 4 min noise exposure. They were subsequently tested for noise-evoked seizures on PND 36. The drug pretreatment/noise exposure combination significantly increased the incidence of seizures ($P < 0.005$). Note that neither antagonists alone caused an increase in seizure incidence, but that the combination of noise and antagonists exposure

rats, an episode of status epilepticus is associated with an increased susceptibility to seizures later in development. Pretreatment with dizocilpine reduced this delayed susceptibility. It is possible that dizocilpine treatment may prevent epileptogenesis as long as it is not administered during critical periods of synaptic development.

In addition to the role NMDA receptors play in synapse elimination, they also appear to be involved in neural migration. NMDA receptor antagonists decrease normal granule cell migration in the cerebellum (Komuro and Rakic 1993). In humans, areas of abnormal neural migration have been associated with seizure foci (Palmini *et al.* 1991). It is possible that NMDA receptor antagonists may disrupt neural migration in humans if given during periods of neural migration. This could be especially important in treating epilepsy during pregnancy. However, it is important to note that this period is sensitive to many insults; even commonly used anticonvulsants have been associated with postnatal developmental defects, although the effect of the drugs cannot always be separated out from the effect of a severe maternal seizure disorder, which may also be disruptive to development (Ransom and Elmore 1991).

Another potential problem with the use of NMDA antagonists for epilepsy is that they may be administered chronically to control seizures. As is the case with many chronically administered drugs, symptoms of withdrawal may occur if they are abruptly discontinued. Based on the results from an *in vitro* study, withdrawal of NMDA antagonists could result in seizures. When cultured hippocampal neurones were chronically exposed to the antagonist kynurenate (10 μm), the abrupt withdrawal of the antagonist precipitated seizure-like epileptiform activity and cell death (Furshpan and Potter 1989). The seizure-like activity appeared to be mediated by NMDA receptors, for it was attenuated by APV.

The neurologic side effects of the NMDA antagonists may also be more pronounced in patients with epilepsy. When compared with normal rats, kindled rats had more PCP-like stereotypies in response to two competitive NMDA antagonists, CGP37849 and CGP39551, and the non-competitive antagonist dizocilpine (Löscher and Hönack 1991). Even when tested at low doses to enhance the effect of the anticonvulsant valproate, dizocilpine (0.05 mg/kg) caused behavioural side effects and reduced the therapeutic index of the valproate in kindled rats (Dziki *et al.* 1992). Thus, in screening

---

greatly enhanced susceptibility. (B) Effect of dizocilpine pretreatment on the ontogeny of seizure susceptibility. At the optimal age for seizure susceptibility (PND 14), dizocilpine was administered 30 min before a 4 min noise exposure (arrow). Control rats were exposed to the noise, but were not given dizocilpine. Between PND 15 and 52, each rat was tested once for noise-evoked seizure susceptibility. In rats pre-treated with dizocilpine, the seizures occurred earlier, had a higher incidence ($P < 0.01$, except on PND 15), and did not decrease with age compared with control rats. (Modified and reproduced, with permission, from Pierson and Swann (1991).)

for side effects, it may be important to test NMDA antagonists in an animal model in which epileptogenesis has already occurred, such as the kindling or kainic acid models.

Promise for NMDA receptor antagonists

Based on the animal models of epilepsy, it may be possible to predict situations in which the NMDA receptor antagonists may be most effective for treating epilepsy in humans. For example, in the case of seizure expression, seizures that occur in the non-epileptic brain (e.g. during alcohol withdrawal) may respond well to treatment to NMDA antagonists. Similarly, seizures that arise within circuits which have a large NMDA synaptic component may also be more sensitive to the antagonists.

Another situation in which the NMDA antagonists may hold promise is in epileptogenesis. In many cases it is not possible to pinpoint the exact time or cause of epileptogenesis. However, there are certain medical conditions that are associated with an increased risk of epilepsy. For example, there may be an increased risk of developing epilepsy after an episode of status epilepticus (Lothman and Bertram 1993). Status epilepticus may be associated with excessive activation of excitatory amino acid receptors; this may mediate epileptogenesis, causing the development of a chronic epileptic condition (Wasterlain *et al.* 1993). Epileptogenesis associated with severe head injury may also be due the NMDA-mediated processes, although is also thought to involve neural damage secondary to haemorrhage and subsequent iron-induced free-radical production (Willmore 1992). There is also speculation that chronic seizures may cause a previously healthy areas of the brain to develop into a new focus (Andermann and Oguni 1990, but see also Blume 1990). In these potentially epileptogenic conditions, NMDA antagonists may prevent the epileptogenic process.

Summary

Many *in vivo* and *in vitro* studies support the hypothesis that NMDA receptors contribute to the development and expression of epilepsy. Although further investigations will be needed to define the risks and to determine the optimal conditions for the use of NMDA antagonists, there clearly is promise for these new agents. Based on the evidence above, the NMDA antagonists may have a unique place in the treatment of epilepsy by preventing the development of this disruptive and potentially debilitating condition.

Acknowledgements

We thank Dr David A. Hosford and Deborah Barr for helpful and insightful comments. Supported by the Veterans' Administration and by NINCDS 17771.

References

Akiyama, K., Yoneda, Y., Ogita, K., Itoh, T., Daigen, A., Sora, I., Kohira, I., Ujike, H., and Otsuki, S. (1992). Ionotropic excitatory amino acid receptors in discrete brain regions of kindled rats. *Brain Research*, **587**, 73–82.

Andermann, F. and Oguni, H. (1990). Do epileptic foci in children migrate? The pros. *Electroencephalography and Clinical Neurophysiology*, **76**, 96–9.

Anderson, W. W., Swartzwelder, H. S., and Wilson, W. A. (1987). The NMDA receptor antagonist 2-amino-5-phosphonovalerate blocks stimulus train-induced epileptogenesis but not epileptiform bursting in the rat hippocampal slice. *Journal of Neurophysiology*, **57**, 1–21.

Anderson, W. W., Swartzwelder, H. S., and Wilson, W. A. (1988). Regenerative, all-or-none, electrographic seizures in the rat hippocampal slice in physiological magnesium medium. In *Synaptic plasticity in the hippocampus*, (ed. H. L. Haas and G. Buzaki), pp. 180–5. Springer-Verlag, Berlin.

Aram, J. A. and Lodge, D. (1988). Validation of a neocortical slice preparation for the study of epileptiform activity. *Journal of Neuroscience Methods*, **23**, 211–44.

Avoli, M. (1991). Excitatory amino acid receptors in the human epileptogenic neocortex. *Epilepsy Research*, **10**, 33–40.

Avoli, M. and Olivier, A. (1987). Bursting in human epileptogenic neocortex is depressed by an *N*-methyl-D-aspartate antagonist. *Neuroscience Letters*, **76**, 249–54.

Avoli, M., Louvel, J., Pumain, R., and Olivier, A. (1987). Seizure-like discharges induced by lowering $[Mg^{2+}]_o$ in the human epileptogenic neocortex maintained *in vitro*. *Brain Research*, **417**, 199–203.

Bashir, Z. I., Alford, S., Davies, S. N., Randall, A. D., and Collingridge, G. L. (1991). Long-term potentiation of NMDA receptor-mediated synaptic transmission in the hippocampus. *Nature*, **349**, 156–8.

Bawin, S. M., Satmary, W. M., Mahoney, M. D., and Adey, W. R. (1991). Transition from normal to epileptiform activity in kindled rat hippocampal slices. *Epilepsy Research*, **8**, 107–16.

Ben-Ari, Y. and Gho, M. (1988). Long-lasting modification of the synaptic properties of rat CA3 hippocampal neurones induced by kainic acid. *Journal of Physiology*, **404**, 365–84.

Ben-Ari, Y., Cherubini, E., and Krnjevic, K. (1988). Changes in voltage dependence of NMDA currents during development. *Neuroscience Letters*, **94**, 88–92.

Ben-Ari, Y., Represa, A., Tremblay, E., Robain, O., LeGal LaSalle, G., Rovira, C., Gho, M., and Cherubini, E. (1992). Epileptogenesis and neuronal plasticity: studies on kainate receptor in the human and rat hippocampus. *Epilepsy Research*, **S8**, 369–73.

Blume, W. T. (1990). Do epileptic foci in children migrate? The cons. *Electroencephalography and Clinical Neurophysiology*, **76**, 96–9.

Brady, R. J., Smith, K. L., and Swann, J. W. (1991). Calcium modulation of the *N*-methyl-D-aspartate (NMDA) response and electrographic seizures in immature hippocampus. *Neuroscience Letters*, **124**, 92–6.

Chamberlin, N. L., Traub, R. D., and Dingledine, R. (1990). Role of EPSPs in initiation of spontaneous synchronized burst firing in rat hippocampal neurons bathed in high potassium. *Journal of Neurophysiology*, **64**, 1000–8.

Chapman, A. G. (1991). Excitatory amino acid antagonists and therapy of epilepsy.

In *Excitatory amino acid antagonists*, (ed. B. Meldrum), pp. 265–86. Blackwell Scientific Publications, Oxford, UK.

Clark, S. and Wilson, W. A. (1992). Brain slice models of epilepsy: neuronal networks and actions of antiepileptic drugs. In *Drugs for control of epilepsy: neuronal networks and actions of antiepileptic drugs* (ed. C. L. Faingold and G. H. Fromm), pp. 89–123. CRC Press, Boca Raton, FL.

Coan, E. J. and Collingridge, G. L. (1985). Magnesium ions block an N-methyl-D-aspartate receptor-mediated component of synaptic transmission in rat hippocampus. *Neuroscience Letters*, **53**, 21–6.

Cohen, S. M., Martin, D., Morrisett, R. A., Wilson, W. A., and Swartzwelder, H. S. (1992). Proconvulsant and anticonvulsant properties of ethanol: studies of electrographic seizures *in vitro*. *Brain Research*, **601**, 80–7.

Collingridge, G. L., Kehl, S. S., and McLennan, H. (1983). Excitatory amino acids in synaptic transmission in the schaffer collateral-commissural pathway of the rat hippocampus. *Journal of Physiology* (London), **344**, 33–46.

Constantine-Paton, M., Cline, H. T., and Debski, E. (1990). Patterned activity, synaptic convergence, and the NMDA receptor in developing visual pathways. *Annual Review of Neuroscience*, **13**, 129–54.

Coulter, D. A., Huguenard, J. R., and Prince, D. A. (1989). Characterisation of ethosuximide reduction of low-threshold calcium current in thalamic neurons. *Annals of Neurology*, **25**, 582–93.

Croucher, M. J. and Bradford, H. F. (1990). 7-Chlorokynurenic acid, a strychnine-insensitive glycine receptor antagonist, inhibits limbic seizure kindling. *Neuroscience Letters*, **118**, 29–32.

Croucher, M. J., Collins, J. F., and Meldrum, B. J. (1982). Anticonvulsant action of excitatory amino acid antagonists. *Science*, **216**, 899–901.

Crowder, J. M. and Bradford, H. F. (1987). Common anticonvulsants inhibit Ca^{2+} uptake and amino acid neurotransmitter release *in vitro*. *Epilepsia*, **28**, 378–82.

Crunelli, V. and Leresche, N. (1991). A role of $GABA_B$ receptors in excitation and inhibition of thalamocortical cells. *Trends in Neuroscience*, **14**, 16–21.

Czuczwar, S. J., Turski, L., Schwartz, M., Turski, W. A., and Kleinrok, Z. (1984). Effects of excitatory amino-acid antagonists on the anticonvulsant action of phenobarbital or diphenylhydantoin in mice. *European Journal of Pharmacology*, **100**, 357–62.

De Sarro, G., Meldrum, B. S., and Reavill, C. (1985). Anticonvulsant action of 2-amino-7-phosphonoheptanoic acid in the substantia nigra. *European Journal of Pharmacology*, **106**, 175–9.

Dingledine, R., McBain, C. J., and McNamara, J. D. (1990). Excitatory amino acid receptors in epilepsy. *Trends Pharmacological Science*, **11**, 334–8.

Dziki, M., Löscher, W., and Hönack, D. (1992). Kindled rats are more sensitive than non-kindled rats to the behavioural effects of combined treatment with MK-801 and valproate. *European Journal of Pharmacology*, **222**, 273–8.

Faingold, C. L., Naritoku, D. K., Copley, C. A., Randall, M. E., Riaz, A., Boersma Anderson, C. A., and Arnerić, S. P. (1992). Glutamate in the inferior colliculus plays a critical role in audiogenic seizure initiation. *Epilepsy Research*, **13**, 95–105.

Flavin, H. J., Wieraszko, A., and Seyfried, T. N. (1991). Enhanced aspartate release from hippocampal slices of epileptic (El) mice. *Journal of Neurochemistry*, **56**, 1007–11.

Frankenhaeuser, B. and Hodgkin, A. L. (1957). The action of calcium on the electrical properties of squid axons. *Journal of Physiology*, **137**, 218–44.

Furshpan, E. J. and Potter, D. D. (1989). Seizure-like activity and cellular damage in rat hippocampal neurons in cell culture. *Neuron*, **3**, 199–207.

Gean, P.-W. (1992). Ethanol inhibits epileptiform activity and NMDA receptor-mediated synaptic transmission in rat amygdaloid slices. *Brain Research Bulletin*, **28**, 417–21.

Gean, P.-W. and Shinnick-Gallagher, P. (1988). Characterization of the epileptiform activity induced by magnesium-free solution in rat amygdala slices: an intracellular study. *Experimental Neurology*, **101**, 248–55.

Gilbert, M. E. (1988). The NMDA-receptor antagonist, MK-801, suppresses limbic kindling and kindled seizures. *Brain Research*, **463**, 90–9.

Gloor, P. and Fariello, R. G. (1988). Generalized epilepsy: some of its cellular mechanisms differ from those of focal epilepsy. *Trends in Neuroscience*, **11**, 63–8.

Grant, K. A., Valverius, P., Hudspith, M., and Tabakoff, B. (1990). Ethanol withdrawal seizures and the NMDA receptor complex. *European Journal of Pharmacology*, **176**, 289–96.

Grant, K. A., Snell, L. D., Rogawski, M. A., Thurkauf, A., and Tabakoff, B. (1992). Comparison of the effects of the uncompetitive N-methyl-D-aspartate antagonist (±)-5-aminocarbonyl-10,11-dihydro-5H-benzo[a,d]cyclohepten-5,10-imine (ADCL) with its structural analogs dizocilpine (MK-801) and carbamazepine on ethanol withdrawal seizures. *Journal of Pharmacology and Experimental Therapeutics*, **260** 1017–22.

Gulya, K., Grant, K. A., Valverius, P., Hoffman, P. L., and Tabakoff, B. (1991). Brain regional specificity and time-course of changes in the NMDA receptor-ionophore complex during ethanol withdrawal. *Brain Research*, **547**, 129–34.

Hayashi, T. A. (1952). A physiological study of epileptic seizures following cortical stimulation in animals and its application to human clinics. *Japanese Journal of Physiology*, **3**, 46–64.

Heinemann, U., Franceschetti, S., Hamon, B., Konnerth, A., and Yaari, Y. (1985). Effects of anticonvulsants on spontaneous epileptiform activity which develops in the absence of chemical synaptic transmission in hippocampal slices. *Brain Research*, **325**, 349–52.

Herron, C. E., Williamson, R., and Collingridge, G. L. (1985). A selective N-methyl-D-aspartate antagonist depresses epileptiform activity in rat hippocampal slices. *Neuroscience Letters*, **61**, 255–60.

Hestrin, S. (1992). Developmental regulation of NMDA receptor-mediated synaptic currents at a central synapse. *Nature*, **357**, 686–9.

Higashima, M. (1988). Inhibitory processes in development of seizure activity in hippocampal slices. *Experimental Brain Research*, **72**, 37–44.

Hosford, D. A., Crain, B. J., Cao, Z., Bonhaus, D. W., Friedman, A. H., Okazaki, M. M., Nadler, J. V., and McNamara, J. O. (1991). Increased AMPA-sensitive quisqualate receptor binding and reduced NMDA receptor binding in epileptic human hippocampus. *Journal of Neuroscience*, **11**, 428–34.

Hosford, D., Clark, S., Cao, Z., Wilson, W. A., Lin, F.-H., Morrisett, R. A., and Huin, A. (1992). The role of $GABA_B$ receptor activation in absence seizures of lethargic (lh/lh) mice. *Science*, **257**, 398–401.

Isokawa, M. and Mello, L. E. (1991). NMDA receptor-mediated excitability in dendritically deformed dentate granule cells in pilocarpine-treated rats. *Neuroscience Letters*, **129**, 69–73.

Johnston, D. and Brown, T. H. (1984). The synaptic nature of the paroxysmal depolarizing shift in hippocampal neurons. *Annals of Neurology*, **16** (suppl.), S65–71.

Jones, A. W., Croucher, M. J., Meldrum, B. S., and Watkins, J. C. (1984). Suppression of audiogenic seizures in DBA/2 mice by two new dipeptide NMDA receptor antagonists. *Neuroscience Letters*, **45**, 157–61.

Jones, R. S. G. and Heinemann, U. (1988). Synaptic and intrinsic responses of medial entorhinal cortical cells in normal and magnesium-free medium *in vitro*. *Journal of Neurophysiology*, **57**, 1476–96.

Jones, R. S. G. and Lambert, J. D. C. (1990). Synchronous discharges in the rat entorhinal cortex *in vitro*: site of initiation and the role of excitatory amino acid receptors. *Neuroscience*, **34**, 657–70.

Jones, S. M. and Johnson, K. M. (1989). Effects of amygdaloid kindling on NMDA receptor function and regulation. *Experimental Neurology*, **106**, 52–60.

Koek, W. and Colpaert, F. C. (1990). Selective blockade of N-methyl-D-aspartate (NMDA)-induced convulsions by NMDA antagonists and putative glycine antagonists: relationship with phencyclidine-like behavioral effects. *Journal of Pharmacology and Experimental Therapeutics*, **252**, 349–57.

Komuro, H. and Rakic, P. (1993). Modulation of neuronal migration by NMDA receptors. *Science*, **260**, 95–7.

Lampe, H. and Bigalke, H. (1990). Carbamazepine blocks NMDA-activated currents in cultured spinal cord neurons. *NeuroReport*, **1**, 26–8.

Lancaster, J. M. and Davies, J. A. (1992). Carbamazepine inhibits NMDA-induced depolarizations in cortical wedges prepared from DBA/2 mice. *Experientia*, **48**, 751–3.

Leach, M. J., Marden, C. M., and Miller. A. A. (1986). Pharmacological studies on lamotrigine, a novel potential antiepileptic drug: II. Neurochemical studies on the mechanism of action. *Epilepsia*, **27**, 490–7.

Lee, W.-L. and Hablitz, J. J. (1989). Involvement of non-NMDA receptors in picrotoxin-induced epileptiform activity in the hippocampus. *Neuroscience Letters*, **107**, 129–34.

Lee, W.-L. and Hablitz, J. J. (1990). Effect of APV and ketamine on epileptiform activity in the CA1 and CA3 regions of the hippocampus. *Epilepsy Research*, **61**, 87–94.

Loiseau, P. and Duche, B. (1989). Carbamazepine: clinical use. In *Antiepileptic drugs* (3rd edn), (ed. F. E. Dreifuss, R. H. Mattson, B. S. Meldrum, and J. K. Penry) , pp. 533–54. Raven Press Ltd, New York.

Löscher, W. and Hönack, D. (1991). The novel competitive N-methyl-D-aspartate (NMDA) antagonist CGP 37849 preferentially induces phencyclidine-like behavioral effects in kindled rats: attenuation by manipulation of dopamine, alpha-1 and serotonin$_{1A}$ receptors. *Journal of Pharmacology and Experimental Therapeutics*, **257**, 1146–53.

Löscher, W., Nolting, B., and Hönack, D. (1988). Evaluation of CPP, a selective NMDA antagonist, in various rodent models of epilepsy. Comparison with other NMDA antagonists, and with diazepam and phenobarbital. *European Journal of Pharmacology*, **152**, 9–17.

Lothman, E. W. and Bertram, E. H., III (1993). Epileptogenic effects of status epilepticus. *Epilepsia*, **34** (Suppl. 1), S59–S70.

Louvel, J., Pumain, R., Roux, R. X., and Chodkievicz, J. P. (1992). Recent advances in understanding epileptogenesis in animal models and in humans. *Advances in Neurology*, **57**, 517–24.

Lovinger, D. L., White, G., and Weight, F. F. (1989). Ethanol inhibits NMDA-activated ion current in hippocampal neurons. *Science*, **243**, 1721–4.

McDonald, J. W. and Johnston, M. V. (1990). Physiological and pathophysiological roles of excitatory amino acids during central nervous system development. *Brain Research Reviews*, **15**, 41–70.

McDonald, J. W., Garofalo, E. A., Hood, T., Sackellares, J. C., Gilman, S., McKeever, P. E., Troncoso, J. C., and Johnston, M. V. (1989). Altered excitatory and inhibitory amino acid receptor binding in hippocampus of patients with temporal lobe epilepsy. *Annals of Neurology*, **29**, 529–41.

McDonald, J. W., Johnston, M. V., and Young, A. B. (1990). Differential ontogenic development of three receptors comprising the NMDA receptor/channel complex in the rat hippocampus. *Experimental Neurology*, **110**, 237–47.

MacDonald, R. L. (1989). Antiepileptic drug actions. *Epilepsia*, **30** (Suppl. 1), S19–28.

McNamara, J. O., Bonhaus, D. W., Shin, C., Crain, B. J., Gellman, R. L., and Giacchino, J. L. (1985). The kindling model of epilepsy: a critical review. *Critical Reviews in Clinical Neurobiology*, **1**, 341–91.

McNamara, J. O., Russell, R. D., Rigsbee, L., and Bonhaus, D. W. (1988). Anticonvulsant and antiepileptogenic actions of MK-801 in the kindling and electroshock models. *Neuropharmacology*, **27**, 563–8.

McNamara, J. O., Morrisett, R., and Nadler, J. V. (1992). Recent advances in understanding mechanisms of the kindling model. *Advances in Neurology*, **57**, 555–60.

Marescaux, C., Vergnes, M., and Depaulis, A. (1992). Genetic absence epilepsy in rats from Strasbourg—A review. *Journal of Neural Transmission* (Suppl.) **35**, 37–69.

Martin, D. and Swartzwelder, H. S. (1992). Ethanol inhibits release of excitatory amino acids from slices of hippocampal area CA1. *European Journal of Pharmacology*, **219**, 469–72.

Martin, D., McNamara, J. O., and Nadler, J. V. (1992). Kindling enhances sensitivity of CA3 hippocampal pyramidal cells to NMDA. *Journal of Neuroscience*, **12**, 1928–35.

Matsumoto, H. and Ajmone Marsan, C. (1964). Cortical cellular phenomena in experimental epilepsy: interictal manifestations. *Experimental Neurology*, **9**, 286–304.

Meldrum, B. S., Croucher, M. J., Czuczwar, S. J., Collins, F. J., Curry, K., Joseph, M., and Stone, T. W. (1983a). A comparison of the anticonvulsant potency of ($\pm$) 2-amino-5-phosphono-pentanoic acid and ($\pm$) 2-amino-7-phosphonoheptanoic acid. *Neuroscience*, **9**, 925–30.

Meldrum, B. S., Croucher, M. J., Badman, G., and Collins, J. F. (1983b). Antiepileptic action of excitatory amino acid antagonists in the photosensitive baboon, *Papio papio. Neuroscience Letters*, **39**, 101–4.

Meldrum, B. S., Wardley-Smit, B., Halsey, M., and Rostain, J.-C. (1983c). 2-Amino-phosphonoheptanoic acid protects against the high pressure neurological syndrome. *European Journal of Pharmacology*, **87**, 501–2.

Mody, I. and Heinemann, U. (1987). NMDA receptors of dentate gyrus granule cells participate in synaptic transmission following kindling. *Nature*, **326**, 701–4.

Morrisett, R. A., Chow, C., Nadler, J. V., and McNamara, J. O. (1989). Biochemical evidence for enhanced sensitivity to N-methyl-D-aspartate in the hippocampal formation of kindled rats. *Brain Research*, **469**, 25–8.

Morrisett, R. A., Mott, D. D., Lewis, D. V., Wilson, W. A., and Swartzwelder, H. S. (1990*a*). Reduced sensitivity of the N-methyl-D-aspartate component of synaptic transmission to magnesium in hippocampal slices from immature rats. *Developmental Brain Research*, **56**, 257–62.

Morrisett, R. A., Rezvani, A. H., Overstreet, D., Janowsky, D. S., Wilson, W. A., and Swartzwelder, H. S. (1990*b*). MK-801 potently inhibits alcohol withdrawal seizures in rats. *European Journal of Pharmacology*, **176**, 103–5.

Nadler, J. V., Martin, D., Bowe, M. A., Morrisett, R. A., and McNamara, J. O. (1990). Kindling, prenatal exposure to ethanol and postnatal development selectively alter responses of hippocampal pyramidal cells to NMDA. In *Excitatory amino acids and neuronal plasticity*, (ed. Y. Ben-Ari), pp. 407–18. Plenum Press, New York.

Neuman, R., Cherubini, E., and Ben-Ari, Y. (1988). Epileptiform bursts elicited in CA$_3$ hippocampal neurons by a variety of convulsants are not blocked by N-methyl-D-aspartate antagonists. *Brain Research*, **459**, 265–74.

Niedermeyer, E. (1990). Introduction to electroencephalography. In *The epilepsies: diagnosis and management*, pp. 42 and 264. Urban & Schwarzenberg, Baltimore, MD.

Noebels, J. L. (1984). A single gene error of noradrenergic axon growth synchronizes central neurones. *Nature*, **310**, 409–11.

Okazaki, M. M., McNamara, J. O., and Nadler, J. V. (1989). N-methyl-D-aspartate receptor autoradiography in rat brain after angular bundle kindling. *Brain Research*, **482**, 358–64.

Olney, J. W., Labruyere, J., Wang, G., Wozniak, D. F., Price, M. T., and Sesma, M. A. (1991). NMDA antagonist neurotoxicity: mechanism and prevention. *Science*, **254**, 1515–18.

Olpe, H.-R., Schmutz, M., Brugger, F., Wicki, U., Ferrat, T., Pozza, M. and Steinmann, M. (1991). Mechanism of action of antiepileptic drugs with special reference to carbamazepine and valproate. *Biological Psychiatry*, **2**, 252–4.

Palmini, A., Andermann, F., Olivier, A., Tampierei, D., and Robitaille, Y. (1991). Focal neuronal migration disorders and intractable partial epilepsy: results of surgical treatment. *Annals of Neurology*, **30**, 750–7.

Patel, S., Chapman, A. G., Graham, J. L., Meldrum, B. S., and Frey, P. (1990). Anticonvulsant activity of the NMDA antagonists, D(−)4-(3-phosphonopropyl) piperazine-2-carboxylic acid (d-CPP) and D(−)(E)-4-(phosphonoprop-2-enyl) piperazine-2-carboxylic acid (D-CPPene) in a rodent and a primate model of reflex epilepsy. *Epilepsy Research*, **7**, 3–10.

Peeters, B. W. M. M., Van Rijn, C. M., Luijtelaar, E. L. J. M., and Coenen, A. M. L. (1989). Antiepileptic and behavioural actions of MK-801 in an animal model of spontaneous absence epilepsy. *Epilepsy Research*, **3**, 178–81.

Peeters, B. W. M. M., Van Rijn, C. M., Vossen, J. M. H., and Coenen, A. M. L. (1990). Involvement of NMDA receptors in non-convulsive epilepsy in WAG/Rij rats. *Life Science*, **47**, 523–9.

Perlin, J. B. and DeLorenzo, R. J. (1992). Calcium and epilepsy. In *Recent advances in epilepsy*, No. 5, (ed. T. A. Pedley and B. S. Meldrum), pp. 15–36. Churchill Livingstone, Edinburgh.

Perry, T. L. and Hansen, S. (1981). Amino acid abnormalities in epileptogenic foci. *Neurology* (New York), **31**, 872–6.

Pierson, M. and Swann, J. (1991). Sensitization to noise-mediated induction of seizure susceptibility by MK 801 and phencyclidine. *Brain Research*, **560**, 229–36.

Pierson, M. G., Smith, K. L., and Swann, J. W. (1989). A slow NMDA-mediated synaptic potential underlies seizures originating from midbrain. *Brain Research*, **486**, 381–6.

Piggot, M. A., Perry, E. K., Perry, R. H., and Scott, D. (1993). *N*-methyl-D-aspartate (NMDA) and non-NMDA binding sites in developing human frontal cortex. *Neuroscience Research Communications*, **12**, 9–16.

Psarropoulou, C. and Avoli, M. (1992). CPP, an NMDA-receptor antagonist, blocks 4-aminopyridine-induced spreading depression episodes but not epileptiform activity in immature rat hippocampal slices. *Neuroscience Letters*, **135**, 139–43.

Pumain, R., Menini, C., Heinemann, U., Louvel, J., and Silva-Barrat, C. (1985). Chemical synaptic transmission is not necessary for epileptic seizures to persist in the baboon *Papio papio*. *Experimental Neurology*, **89**, 250–8.

Pumain, R., Louvel, J., and Kurcewicz, I. (1986). Long-term alterations in amino acid-induced ionic conductances in chronic epilepsy. *Advances in Experimental Medicine and Biology*, **203**, 439–47.

Pumain, R., Kurcewicz, I., and Louvel, J. (1987). Ionic changes induced by excitatory amino acids in the rat cerebral cortex. *Canadian Journal of Physiology and Pharmacology*, **65**, 1067–77.

Pumain, R., Louvel, J., Gastard, M., Kurcewicz, I., and Vergnes, M. (1992). Responses to *N*-methyl-D-aspartate are enhanced in rats with petit mal-like seizures. *Journal of Neural Transmission*, **35** (Suppl.), 97–108.

Rabacchi, S., Bailly, Y., Delhaye-Bouchaud, N., and Mariani, J. (1992). Involvement of the *N*-methyl-D-aspartate (NMDA) receptor in synapse elimination during cerebellar development. *Science*, **256**, 1823–5.

Ransom, B. R. and Elmore, J. G. (1991). Effects of antiepileptic drugs on the developing central nervous system. *Advances in Neurology*, **55**, 225–37.

Rogawski, M. A. and Porter, R. J. (1990). Antiepileptic drugs: pharmacological mechanisms and clinical efficacy with consideration of promising developmental stage compounds. *Pharmacological Reviews*, **42**, 223–86.

Rogawski, M. A., Yamaguchi, S.-I., Jones, S. M., Rice, K. C., Thurkauf, A., and Monn, J. A. (1991). Anticonvulsant activity of the low-affinity uncompetitive *N*-methyl-D-aspartate antagonist (±)-5-aminocarbonyl-10,11-dihydro-5H-dibenzo[*a,b*]dyclohepten-5,10-imine (ADC1): comparison with the structural analogs dizocilpine (MK-801) and carbamazepine. *Journal of Pharmacology and Experimental Therapeutics*, **259**, 30–7.

Sagratella, S., Frank, C., and Scotti de Carolis, A. (1987). Effects of ketamine and (+)cyclazocine on 4-aminopyridine and "magnesium free" epileptogenic activity in hippocampal slices of rats. *Neurophamacology*, **261**, 1181–4.

Sato, K., Morimoto, K., and Okamoto, M. (1988). Anticonvulsant action of a non-competitive antagonist of NMDA receptors (MK-801) in the kindling model of epilepsy. *Brain Research*, **463**, 12–20.

Sato, M., Racine, R. J., and McIntyre, D. C. (1990). Kindling: basic mechanisms and clinical validity. *Electroencephalography and Clinical Neurophysiology*, **76**, 459–72.

Schwartzkroin, P. A., Turner, D. A., Knowles, W. D., and Wyler, A. R. (1983). Studies of human and monkey "epileptic" neocortex in the *in vitro* slice preparation. *Annals of Neurology*, **13**, 249–57.

Sherwin, A., Robitaille, Y., Quesney, F., Olivier, A., Villemure, J., Leblanc, R., Feindel, W., Andermann, E., Gotman, J., Andermann, F., Ethier, R., and Kish, S. (1988). Excitatory amino acids are elevated in human epileptic cerebral cortex. *Neurology*, **38**, 920–3.

Silver, J. M., Shin, C., and McNamara, J. O. (1991). Antiepileptogenic effects of conventional anticonvulsants in the kindling model of epilepsy. *Annals of Neurology*, **29**, 356–63.

Skerrit, J. H. and Johnston, G. A. R. (1983). Inhibition of amino acid transmitter release from rat brain slices by phenytoin and related anticonvulsants. *Clinical and Experimental Pharmacology and Physiology*, **10**, 527–33.

Snead, O. C. (1992). Evidence for GABA$_B$-mediated mechanisms in experimental generalized absence seizures. *European Journal of Pharmacology*, **213**, 343–9.

Speckmann, E.-J. and Elger, C. E. (1991). The neurophysiological basis of epileptic activity: a condensed overview. *Epilepsy Research*, Suppl. **2**, 1–7.

Stafstrom, C. E., Homes, G. L., and Thompson, J. L. (1993). MK801 pretreatment reduces kainic acid-induced spontaneous seizures in prepubescent rats. *Epilepsy Research*, **14**, 41–8.

Stasheff, S. F. and Wilson, W. A. (1990). Increased ectopic action potential generation accompanies epileptogenesis *in vitro*. *Neuroscience Letters*, **111**, 144–50.

Stasheff, S. F., Mott, D. D., and Wilson, W. A. (1993). Axon terminal hyperexcitability associated with epileptogenesis *in vitro*: II. Pharmacological regulation by NMDA and GABA$_A$ receptors. *Journal of Neurophysiology*, **70**, 976–84.

Stasheff, S. F., Bragdon, A. C., and Wilson, W. A. (1985). Induction of epileptiform activity in hippocampal slices by trains of electrical stimuli. *Brain Research*, **344**, 296–302.

Stasheff, S. F., Anderson, W. W., Clark, S., and Wilson, W. A. (1989). NMDA antagonists differentiate epileptogenesis from seizure expression in an *in vitro* seizure model. *Science*, **245**, 648–51.

Stelzer, A., Slater, N. T., and ten Bruggencate, G. (1987). Activation of NMDA receptors blocks GABAergic inhibition in an *in vitro* model of epilepsy. *Nature*, **326**, 698–701.

Swann, J. W., Gomez, C. M., Rice, F. L., Smith, K. L., and Turner, J. N. (1991). Anatomical studies of CA3 hippocampal neurons and networks during postnatal development. *Society of Neuroscience Abstracts*, **17**, 1131.

Swann, J. W., Smith, K. L., Brady, R. J., and Pierson, M. G. (1993). Neurophysiological studies of alterations of seizure susceptibility during brain development. In *Concepts and models in epilepsy research*, (ed. P. Schwartzkroin), pp. 209–43. Cambridge University Press, Cambridge, UK.

Tauck, D. L. and Nadler, J. V. (1985). Evidence of functional mossy fiber sprouting in hippocampal formation of kainic acid-treated rats. *Journal of Neuroscience*, **5**, 1016–22.

Taylor, C. P. and Dudek, R. E. (1982). Synchronous neural afterdischarges in rat hippocampal slices without active chemical synapses. *Science*, **218**, 810–12.

Teichberg, V. I., Tal, N., Goldberg, O., and Luini, A. (1984). Barbiturates, alcohols and the CNS excitatory neurotransmission: specific effects on the kainate and quisqualate receptors. *Brain Research* **291**, 285–92.

Thomson, A. M. (1986). A magnesium-sensitive post-synaptic potential in rat cerebral cortex resembles neuronal responses to *N*-methylaspartate. *Journal of Physiology*, **370**, 531–49.

Tremblay, E., Roisin, M. P., Represa, A., Charriaut-Marlangue, C., and Ben-Ari, Y. (1988). Transient increased density of NMDA binding sites in the developing rat hippocampus. *Brain Research*, **461**, 393–6.

Turner, D. A. and Wheal, H. V. (1991). Excitatory synaptic potentials in kainic acid-denervated rat CA1 pyramidal neurons. *Journal of Neuroscience*, **11**, 2786–94.

Urban, L., Aitken, P. G., and Somjen, G. G. (1990). An NMDA-mediated component of excitatory synaptic input to dentate granule cells in 'epileptic' human hippocampus studied *in vitro*. *Brain Research*, **515**, 319–22.

Wadman, W. J., Heinemann, U., Konnerth, A., and Newhaus, S. (1985). Hippocampal slices of kindled rats reveal calcium involvement of epileptogenesis. *Experimental Brain Research*, **57**, 404–7.

Wasterlain, C. G., Fujikawa, D. G., Penix, L., and Sankar, R. (1993). Pathophysiological mechanisms of brain damage from status epilepticus. *Epilepsia*, **34** (Suppl. 1) S37–S53.

Wheal, H. V., Ashwood, T. J., and Lancaster, B. (1984). A comparative *in vitro* study of the kainic acid lesioned and bicuculline treated hippocampus: chronic and acute models of focal epilepsy. In *Electrophysiology of epilepsy*, (ed. P. Schwartzkroin and H. V. Wheal), pp. 173–200. Academic Press, New York.

Williams, S., Vachon, P., and Lacaille, J.-C. (1993). Monosynaptic GABA-mediated inhibitory postsynaptic potentials in CA1 pyramidal cells of hyperexcitable hippocampal slices from kainic acid-treated rats. *Neuroscience*, **52**, 541–54.

Willmore, L. F. (1992). Post-traumatic epilepsy-mechanisms and prevention. In *Recent advances in epilepsy*, (ed. T. A. Pedley and B. S. Meldrum), pp. 107–17. Churchill Livingstone, Edinburgh.

Wilson, W. A., Swartzwelder, H. S., Anderson, W. W., and Lewis, D. V. (1988). Seizure activity *in vitro*: a dual focus model. *Epilepsy Research*, **2**, 289–93.

Woodbury, D. M. (1989). Phenytoin; absorption, distribution, and excretion. In *Antiepileptic drugs* (3rd edn), (ed. F. E. Dreifuss, R. H. Mattson, B. S. Meldrum, and J. K. Penry), pp. 177–95. Raven Press, New York.

Wuarin, J. P., Peacock, W. J., and Dudeck, F. E. (1992). Single-electrode voltage-clamp analysis of the *N*-methyl-D-aspartate component of synaptic responses in neocortical slices from children with intractable epilepsy. *Journal of Neurophysiology*, **67**, 84–93.

Yamaguchi, S. and Rogawski, M. A. (1992). Effects of anticonvulsant drugs on 4-aminopyridine-induced seizures in mice. *Epilepsy Research*, **11**, 9–16.

Yeh, G. C., Bonhaus, D. W., Nadler, J. V., and McNamara, J. O. (1989). *N*-methyl-D-aspartate receptor plasticity in kindling: quantitative and qualitative alterations in the *N*-methyl-D-aspartate receptor-channel complex. *Proceedings of the National Academy of Sciences, USA*, **86**, 8157–60.

Zona, C., Tancredi, V., Palma, E., Pirrone, G. C., and Avoli, M. (1990). Potassium currents in rat cortical neurons in culture are enhanced by the antiepileptic drug carbamazepine. *Canadian Journal of Physiology and Pharmacology*, **68**, 545–7.

18 NMDA receptors, neuronal development, and neurodegeneration

JOHN GARTHWAITE

Introduction

In several brain regions, N-methyl-D-aspartate (NMDA) receptors are specially effective during the developmental period, where they appear to play important roles in the formation and stabilization of developing synapses. The early activation of NMDA receptors could also provide signals which promote neuronal survival, growth, and differentiation. In the first part of this article an attempt is made to review this area of NMDA receptor research and to place the information into a chronological framework.

As neurones mature, they can then become vulnerable to a more established phenomenon, that of irreversible damage inflicted by excessive or prolonged activation of glutamate receptors. This phenomenon has achieved potential clinical significance following evidence from animal models that glutamate receptor blockade can prevent cell death taking place in a number of neurodegenerative disorders of the types that affect humans. A major question concerns the mechanism of this destructive action. Following detailed descriptions of the neurotoxicity of glutamate receptor agonists in several brain areas *in vivo*, the use of *in vitro* preparations (brain slices and cultures) has, in recent years, been extended to try to understand the link between receptor activation and neuronal death and is starting to highlight some of the instrumental events, both at the level of the cell membrane and beyond. These will be discussed in the second part.

NMDA receptors and neuronal development

Neurones in numerous areas of the brain (hippocampus, cortex, cerebellum, and striatum) exhibit heightened responses of various sorts to NMDA receptor agonists during development (Dupont *et al*. 1987; Garthwaite *et al*. 1987; Tsumoto *et al*. 1987; Hamon and Heinemann 1988; McDonald *et al*. 1988; Tremblay *et al*. 1988; Bode-Greuel and Singer 1989; Represa *et al*. 1989). Binding studies have also indicated that there is a transient expression of NMDA receptors in the developing spinal cord ventral horn (Kalb *et al*. 1992). Functionally, the increased sensitivity to NMDA that occurs in the developing hippocampus (Hamon and Heinemann 1988) coincides with an increase in the magnitude of long-term potentiation that can be produced by brief high frequency stimulation (Harris and Teyler 1984), a phenomenon that depends on NMDA receptor activation. Likewise, in the developing visual cortex, where NMDA receptors are believed to play a role in the establishment of use-dependent modifications in ocular dominance and orientation selectivity (Collingridge and Singer 1990; Constantine-Paton *et al.* 1990), neurones are more susceptible to long-term potentiation than in the adult (Kato *et al.* 1991).

Synaptic plasticity in the hippocampus and visual cortex are discussed elsewhere in this volume and so, here, the focus will be on the trophic and morphogenic consequences of NMDA receptor activation and on the way that these receptors participate in synaptic and non-synaptic transmission during neuronal differentiation. Many of the pertinent findings have come from studies of the cerebellum. This brain region has long been a favourite one for developmental neurobiologists because it contains only a small number of neuronal types which are formed in a known sequence and which can readily be identified from their morphology and their position in the strikingly uniform and geometrically simple laminated structure. The principal synaptic interrelationships (shown schematically in Fig. 18.1)

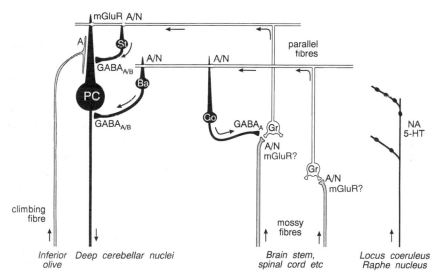

Fig. 18.1 Schematic wiring diagram of the cerebellar cortex indicating the subclasses of glutamate and GABA receptors that have been shown to be synaptically relevant. A question mark indicates that the neurone possesses the respective receptor, but that its role in synaptic transmission has not been established. Neurones whose function is inhibitory are shown in black; excitatory fibres and neurones are stippled or unfilled. Abbreviations: A, AMPA receptors; N, NMDA receptors; mGluR, metabotropic glutamate receptors; Ba, basket cell; Go, Golgi cell; Gr, granule cell; PC, Purkinje cell; St, stellate cell; NA, noradrenaline; 5-HT, 5-hydroxytryptamine.

have been established for many years and glutamate is the likely transmitter at each of the main excitatory synapses, that is, between mossy
fibres and granule cells, between granule cell axons (parallel fibres) and
their targets—Purkinje cells and inhibitory interneurones (basket, stellate,
and Golgi cells)—and between climbing fibres and Purkinje cells.

When do neurones first acquire glutamate receptors?

Woodward *et al.* (1971) were the first to examine in detail the developmental appearance of chemosensitivity to putative transmitters in central
neurones. Using iontophoretic methods, they showed that rat Purkinje
cells *in vivo* were sensitive to glutamate as early as on the day of birth,
which predates by about 3 days the appearance of synapses and which
corresponds to a time when Purkinje cells have no dendrites. (These
neurones originate some 4–7 days before birth.) More recent studies *in
vitro* have shown that Purkinje cells in the newborn are also sensitive to
aspartate and quisqualate but they fail to respond to N-methyl-DL-aspartate
(NMDLA), suggesting that only non-NMDA receptors are present early
on (Dupont *et al.* 1987). However, by the end of the first postnatal week
(when synaptogenesis has begun), Purkinje cells also respond to N-methyl-
DL-aspartate (NMA) (Dupont *et al.* 1987) or NMDA itself (Garthwaite *et
al.* 1987; Rosenmund *et al.* 1992).

In situ hybridization autoradiography has indicated that there may be a
developmental switch in AMPA receptor subunits expressed by Purkinje
cells and other neurones. Thus, at postnatal day 4, the predominant
mRNAs seen in Purkinje cells were of the GluR1 and GluR3 subunits,
whereas the GluR2 subunit appeared later, to reach its peak at postnatal
day 14 (Pellegrini-Giampietro *et al.* 1992). As the absence of GluR2
implies a Ca^{2+} permeable receptor channel, this result suggests that activation of early AMPA receptors on Purkinje cells could directly elicit a Ca^{2+}
influx through the membrane of these cells. A similar situation may also
exist for neurones in the cortex and striatum (Pellegrini-Giampietro *et al.*
1992).

The developmental appearance of NMDA receptors on the other major
type of neurone in the cerebellar cortex, the granule cell, is somewhat
different. In the rat, cerebellar granule cells are formed mainly during the
second and third weeks after birth from dividing cells in the external
granule cell layer (see Fig. 18.4 for a histological illustration of the immature cerebellar cortex). Shortly after their final division, they emit fibres
horizontally (these will become the parallel fibres) and then the cell bodies
migrate down through the molecular layer to reach the granule cell layer
several days later. It is here that granule cells normally first meet and form
synapses with mossy fibres. The first functional synapses with mossy fibres
form around postnatal days 5–7 (Crepel 1974; Puro and Woodward 1977).

Granule cells seem to be equipped with NMDA receptors from very early on in their differentiation. In cerebellar slices, morphological changes (reversible swelling) produced by NMDA can be detected under appropriate conditions in granule cells even before they have begun to migrate (G. Garthwaite *et al*. 1986), a finding supported by recent patch electrode recordings (Rossi and Slater 1993). Analogous responses of premigratory granule cells to kainate have also been found using the same method (unpublished observation) suggesting that non-NMDA receptors are also present, a conclusion consistent with *in situ* hybridization histochemistry showing that premigratory granule cells express mRNA for the GluR4c subunit of AMPA receptors (Gallo *et al*. 1992).

Neurones in the cerebral cortex appear similar to cerebellar granule cells. Thus, in the rat, functional NMDA receptors are expressed on neurones within the cortical plate, but not on cells in the ventricular zone (the germinal zone), indicating that they attain sensitivity at some time between cessation of mitosis and the end of migration, but before the appearance of synapses (LoTurco *et al*. 1991). Analogous results have been found in the turtle cerebral cortex (Blanton *et al*. 1990; Blanton and Kriegstein 1992) where the developmental sequence of receptor acquisition appears to be: $GABA_A$ and NMDA receptors, followed by $GABA_B$ and non-NMDA receptors.

NMDA receptor activation may promote early differentiation

The question arises as to whether any significance can be attached to the expression of NMDA receptors on neurones so long before they receive any synaptic contact. Are these receptors ever activated? Recent evidence from both cerebral cortex and cerebellum, at least *in vitro*, suggests that NMDA receptors may be under tonic activation by an endogenous agonist, presumably glutamate, prior to synapse formation (Blanton *et al*. 1990; Blanton and Kriegstein 1992; Rossi and Slater 1993). In cerebellar granule cells, the degree of tonic receptor activation increased as the cells progressed from their premigratory phase to their migratory phase and on to when they entered the internal granule cell layer and ceased migration (Rossi and Slater 1993).

Assuming that NMDA receptors are activated prior to synapse formation, what functions might they perform? Pearce *et al*. (1987) have studied the very early outgrowth of neurites from granule cells in culture. This normally occurs during the first few hours after plating. If NMDA receptors are blocked with kynurenic acid or 2-amino-5-phosphonovalerate (APV), however, neurite outgrowth is inhibited in a manner that can be overcome by adding glutamate or NMDA to the culture fluid. Addition of a glutamate-metabolizing enzyme, on the other hand, inhibits outgrowth to the same extent as did APV. These results suggest that endogenous glutamate released into the culture medium (giving a concentration of 7–10 μM in serum-free conditions (R. D. Burgoyne, personal communication)) was promoting neurite outgrowth through its action on NMDA receptors; this effect has further been suggested to involve protein kinase C (Cambray-Deakin *et al.* 1990). When examined more precisely, NMDA receptor activation increased by 9-fold the growth rate of cultured granule cell neurites and enhanced by 28 per cent the proportion of processes equipped with a growth cone; NMDA antagonists, on the other hand, induced a retraction of pre-existing processes (Rashid and Cambray-Deakin 1992).

The activity of the enzyme, glutaminase, in cultured granule cells is also greatly enhanced by NMDA receptor activation (Moran and Patel 1989). Glutaminase is involved in the synthesis of the neurotransmitter pool of glutamate and thus has been considered a useful marker for the bio-chemical differentiation of glutamatergic neurones. In these experiments, NMDA was added to the neurones after they had been cultured for 2 days; this led to concentration-dependent, progressive increase in enzyme activity per cell which could be inhibited by APV or the NMDA channel blocker, MK-801. Cycloheximide and actinomycin D also inhibited this effect, suggesting that it is brought about by *de novo* synthesis of both RNA and protein.

An interesting new finding indicates that NMDA receptors may also participate in neuronal migration itself (Komuro and Rakic 1993). The study was conducted on mouse cerebellar slices in which living cells were labelled with a fluorescent marker, allowing long-term monitoring of their movement by confocal microscopy. Whilst blockade of AMPA/kainate receptors and $GABA_{A/B}$ receptors had no effect, NMDA antagonists significantly de-creased (by up to 50%) the rate of cell movement. Removal of Mg^{2+}, or of glycine, had the reverse effect and lowering Ca^{2+} was markedly inhibitory.

All these findings are consistent with the idea that NMDA receptor stimulation by glutamate could participate in the differentiation and migration of neurones before they receive any synaptic contact. Whether glutamate has such a paracrine role *in vivo* or not remains to be examined, but, as the *in vitro* studies suggest (see above), it is conceivable that, while still in the external layer or during their migration through the molecular layer, granule cells become exposed to concentrations of glutamate sufficient to have these effects, as a result of the release of the amino acid from nearby axons of the earlier-formed granule cells, or possibly from the radial glial cells (Bergmann glia) down whose processes they migrate.

Changes in chemosensitivity with maturation

The excitatory action of NMDA on Purkinje cells appears to be main-tained during the main developmental period but thereafter becomes greatly reduced, unlike that of non-NMDA receptor agonists or of gluta-mate (Dupont *et al.* 1987; Garthwaite *et al.* 1987). In the adult, NMDA often produces an inhibition of Purkinje cell firing due to activation of nearby inhibitory interneurones, which remain sensitive to NMDA (Crepel *et al*, 1982; Quinlan and Davies 1985; Garthwaite and Garthwaite 1984, 1986*a*). The decline in the sensitivity of Purkinje cells may be brought about by the progressive investment of their dendrites by parallel fibres because in a mutant mouse (the staggerer) where parallel fibres synapses do not form, Purkinje cells reputedly stay sensitive to NMDA (Dupont *et al*. 1984). Alternatively, it may be related to the climbing fibre innervation. During postnatal days 5–14, Purkinje cells are multiply innervated by climbing fibres, the transmitter of which may activate NMDA receptors (Kimura *et al*. 1985; Sekiguchi *et al*. 1987), before the adult one-to-one relationship is established (Crepel *et al*. 1976). The staggerer mutant, however, retains the immature, multiple, climbing fibre innervation (Crepel *et al*. 1980). It is possible, therefore, that the normal loss of responsiveness to NMDA is due to a delayed loss of NMDA receptors following the regression, by 14 days, of supernumerary climbing fibres.

Granule cells, too, display pronounced and selective changes in sensitivity to exogenous NMDA. Soon after their arrival in the internal granule cell layer, granule cells express enough receptors to be vulnerable to the neurotoxic effect of NMDA (Garthwaite and Garthwaite 1986*a*) and high-amplitude Mg^{2+}-sensitive depolarizing responses to NMDA can be recorded from them over 8–14 days after birth (Garthwaite *et al*. 1987). During the following week, the size of the responses to NMDA, relative to those to either kainate or quisqualate, becomes much smaller. The capacity of NMDA to kill granule cells is reduced in parallel (Garthwaite and Garthwaite 1986*a*), indicating that this does not simply represent a gradual increase in relative chemosensitivity to non-NMDA agonists. Near adult values of both measures of NMDA sensitivity are reached at 21 days when the basic wiring of the cerebellar circuitry is complete.

Role in synaptic transmission

The participation of NMDA receptors in the early synaptic activation of granule cells by mossy fibres has been studied in cerebellar slices (Garthwaite and Brodbelt 1989). In the 14 day old, a sizeable component of the population response could be inhibited by APV even during low frequency stimulation with millimolar concentrations of Mg^{2+} in the perfusing solution and after the non-NMDA receptor-mediated components had been blocked by 6-cyano-2,3-dihydroxy-7-nitro-quinoxaline, CNQX (Fig. 18.2(a)). The APV-sensitive component could, however, be greatly enhanced in size by removal of Mg^{2+} (Fig. 18.2(b)) and it could be observed in relative isolation (in the absence or presence of Mg^{2+}) at low stimulation voltages. In support of these findings, patch electrode recording from cerebellar slices suggests that NMDA receptors make up a much larger proportion of the evoked excitatory post-synaptic current in developing granule cells than when these cells are more mature (D'Angelo *et al*. 1990, 1993).

The NMDA system on developing granule cells can thus be activated

(a) 1.2 mM Mg²⁺   **(b) Mg²⁺– free**

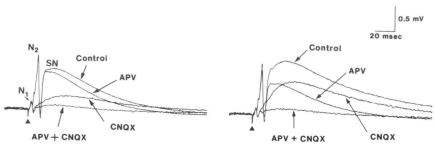

Fig. 18.2 Role of NMDA and non-NMDA receptors in the mossy fibre-granule cell pathway in developing (14 day old) rat cerebellum (Garthwaite and Brodbelt 1989). Population responses to low frequency stimulation of mossy fibres (stimulus applied at arrowheads) were recorded in slices using a gap technique. The main potentials are designated N_1 (probably the presynaptic action potential), N_2 (population granule cell spike and underlying synaptic currents) and SN (slow negative wave thought to be elicited by different mossy fibres from those producing N_2). The NMDA antagonist, APV (30 μM) inhibits a component of the SN wave even in the presence of Mg^{2+} (a). This NMDA receptor-mediated component can be seen in relative isolation after non-NMDA receptors are blocked with CNQX (10 μM) and its size is selectively increased by removal of Mg^{2+} (b).

unusually easily by the mossy fibre transmitter. With maturation, this is lost: in the adult for example, removal of Mg^{2+} (Fig. 18.3) or high frequency stimulation (Garthwaite and Brodbelt 1990) is needed to reveal a NMDA receptor-mediated component of the synaptic response, much as in other areas of adult brain.

A comparable situation to that of the early mossy fibre–granule cell synapses exists in the cerebral cortex, including the visual cortex, where NMDA receptors participate in synaptic responses in the developing tissue more prominently than in the adult (Tsumoto *et al.* 1987; Kato *et al.* 1991; Carmignoto and Vicini 1992; Fox *et al.* 1992; Burgard and Hablitz 1993).

The question of whether the NMDA receptors present on developing Purkinje cells are synaptically relevant remains uncertain. In the parallel fibre pathway, NMDA receptors only appeared to operate in synapses with inhibitory interneurones (Garthwaite and Beaumont 1989) and at climbing fibre–Purkinje cell synapses, in 11–17 day old rats, the climbing fibre response seemed to be wholly mediated by non-NMDA receptors (Konnerth *et al.* 1990). The possibility that NMDA receptors are involved in either pathway at earlier ages has still not been examined.

Mechanisms underlying enhanced NMDA sensitivity

One explanation may be that there is a higher density of NMDA receptors at certain states of development, so that even though the individual cur-

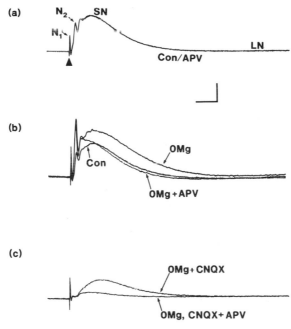

Fig. 18.3 NMDA and non-NMDA receptors in mossy fibre-granule cell pathway in slices of adult rat cerebellum. Details as in Fig. 2. Note that, unlike in the immature tissue, removal of Mg^{2+} is needed to reveal an APV-sensitive wave. Calibration, 0.1 mV, 20 msec.

rents going through NMDA channels are small at normal resting potential and in the presence of Mg^{2+}, the summation of large numbers of these currents is sufficient to elicit marked excitatory post-synaptic potentials (EPSPs). In some brain regions, this explanation has been supported by binding experiments (Tremblay *et al.* 1988; Bode-Greuel and Singer 1989; Represa *et al.* 1989).

Another possibility is that the receptors or channels are different from those in the adult. An analogy here would be the acetylcholine receptor in skeletal muscle which is known to have distinct adult and immature molecular forms, reflecting different subunit compositions (Mishina *et al.* 1986). The functional significance of the immature form in developing muscle is that it produces long duration miniature endplate currents in response to spontaneous transmitter release and these cause the spontaneous muscle contractions that are necessary for normal neuromuscular development (Jaramillo *et al.* 1988). The currents associated with the adult form of the receptor are not long-lasting enough to do this.

Recent work indicates that this analogy may indeed be appropriate. Hestrin (1992) recorded excitatory currents produced either by synaptic release of transmitter, or by fast NMDA application to membrane patches, in neurones of the superior colliculus and found that their duration was several times longer at early developmental stages compared with older animals. Complementary results have been obtained in the frontal and visual subdivisions of the cerebral cortex (Carmignoto and Vicini 1992; Burgard and Hablitz 1993).

Other results suggest that there may be lesser voltage-dependence of NMDA currents in immature neurones. Ben Ari *et al.* (1988) have described unusual NMDA currents in rat hippocampal CA3 neurones during the postnatal period. Whereas the currents in adult neurones had their characteristic J-shaped current–voltage relationship, those in many of the immature cells did not show the region of negative slope conductance between -60 and -30 mV. Some showed only a positive slope throughout. A reduced voltage-dependence would mean that activation of NMDA receptors will evoke larger currents at more hyperpolarized membrane potentials than those on adult cells. Others have reported that immature CA1 pyramidal neurones in the hippocampus are less sensitive to Mg^{2+} than their adult counterparts, again implying a reduced voltage-sensitivity (Bowe and Nadler 1990). However, this was not evident in cortical (LoTurco *et al.* 1991), superior collicular (Hestrin 1992), or cerebellar granular (D'Angelo *et al.* 1993) neurones studied with patch electrodes.

One explanation may be that the second messenger modulation of NMDA receptor currents changes with development: protein kinase C, for example has been suggested to enhance currents by reducing the Mg^{2+} block of the receptor channel (Chen and Huang 1992). Another possibility is that the subunit composition of NMDA receptor subunits varies during development. Coexpression of the ubiquitous NMDAR1 (NR1) subunit with the NR2C subunit gives rise to currents that are both longer-lasting and less Mg^{2+}-sensitive than with the NR2A or NR2B subunits (Kutsuwada *et al.* 1992; Monyer *et al.* 1992; Ishii *et al.* 1993). The NR2C subunit is mainly located in cerebellar granule cells. However, developmental studies, so far only done in the mouse (Watanabe *et al.* 1992), indicate that NR2C mRNA becomes evident at about 7 days after birth and continues on into adulthood, arguing against a transient developmental expression. Two other subunits, on the other hand, are transiently expressed: the NR2D shows a widespread distribution in immature animals but virtually disappears by 21 days after birth, and the NR2B is strongly evident in many areas at 7 days but thereafter, in the cerebellum and brain stem (midbrain, pons, and medulla) but not in the forebrain, the signals became markedly less. The properties conferred by the NR2D subunit have not yet been reported, but the findings support the expectation that there exist immature forms of the NMDA receptor. Moreover, there is evidence that the changes in NMDA receptor function that occur during maturation are not simply governed by a developmental clock, but are dependent on neuronal activity (Carmignoto and Vicini 1992; Fox *et al.* 1992).

Functional significance of NMDA currents in developing synapses

Since the NMDA system appears to be so readily activated by the neuro-transmitter in at least some developing synapses, it is tempting to assume that it plays a role there other than, or in addition to, one of simply mediating excitation. In particular it is to be expected that post-synaptic influx of Ca^{2+} through the NMDA channels and the subsequent activation or intracellular enzymes and second messenger systems, as well as the production of diffusible messengers such as nitric oxide (Garthwaite *et al.* 1988), would take place much as they do in the adult, but under milder conditions. In a sense, this is appropriate because one feature of immature pathways is that they tend to be easily fatigued (e.g. Puro and Woodward 1977) and so are unable to sustain the high frequency transmission that is normally needed to activate the NMDA system. The question is, how do the cells use the information?

NMDA receptor activation may prevent cell death

During synapse formation, initial 'low-level' contacts between synaptic partners are subject to a series of refinements which require their mutual interactions. These events are often regressive. First, there is a matching of the presynaptic neurone population to the numbers of target cells by the process of cell death. This is believed to work both ways: the presynaptic cells compete for trophic factors which are released from the target cells and if a presynaptic neurone fails to receive adequate amounts of trophic factor, perhaps because it fails to induce enough activity in its target cells, then it dies (Oppenheim 1985). At the same time, survival of the target cells may be dependent on the afferent neurones (Parks 1979; Okado and Oppenheim 1984; Clarke 1985; Linden and Pinon 1987).

Balazs *et al.* (1988) have suggested that NMDA receptor activation may be an important factor which promotes neuronal survival. They used almost pure cultures of cerebellar granule cells which, by being mostly deprived of their natural targets and having no mossy fibre input, would be expected to be doubly disadvantaged. Sure enough, after a few days, the majority of the granule cells died. However, if NMDA was included in the medium, this widespread loss of neurones was prevented. APV not only inhibited the effects of NMDA but also caused an additional loss of neurones grown without NMDA, indicating that these were sustained by the low levels of glutamate present in the medium. NMDA antagonism also induces neuronal death in developing spinal cord cultures (Brenne-man *et al.* 1990).

Addition of NMDA to the granule cell cultures, therefore, may either fool the neurones into thinking that they have been innervated or elicit the release of a trophic factor which would normally be provided by the target cells. Either explanation would be consistent with the *in vivo* observations:

in the weaver mutant, most granule cells fail to migrate (and so do not become innervated) and die soon after being produced, while those that survive are the few which become innervated by aberrant mossy fibres (Rakic and Sidman 1973); however, granule cell survival can also depend on the availability of their targets, the Purkinje cells (Chen and Hillman 1989).

Fine tuning of synaptic connections

In a later stage of synapse maturation, there is an activity-dependent fine tuning of synaptic connections in which some are stabilized and others— presumably the less effective or 'erroneous' ones—are eliminated (Changeux and Danchin 1976; Changeux and Mikishibi 1978). The potential function of NMDA receptors in one aspect of this process is exemplified most strikingly by studies of use-dependent changes in the visual system as discussed by Artola and Singer (Chapter 14). In the cerebellum, connections between climbing fibres and Purkinje cells and between mossy fibres and granule cells are subject to considerable pruning: in the former, withdrawal of supernumerary fibres takes place without substantial death of the parent neurones in the inferior olive (Crepel 1982) whereas the latter involves a large withdrawal of granule cell dendrites (Hamori and Somogyi 1983). The possibility that NMDA receptors participate in climbing fibre plasticity has now been studied (Rabacchi *et al.* 1992) and it was found that chronic *in vivo* application of NMDA antagonist prevented climbing fibre regression in about 50 per cent of the recorded Purkinje cells, suggesting that NMDA receptor activation is normally involved in the pruning mechanism.

NMDA receptors may promote morphogenesis

A striking feature of many developing neurones is the progressive matching of dendritic growth and arborization to the numbers of afferent fibres. This is thought to arise because new synapses are first made on the fine processes (filopodia) of dendritic growth cones and these synapses induce the transformation of the filopodia into growth cones and of the original growth cones into dendrites. NMDA receptors have recently been implicated in this mechanism (Brewer and Cotman 1989). The experiments used granule cells from the dentate gyrus grown in culture. Addition of glutamate or NMDA did not affect the numbers of processes arising from the soma but both agonists dramatically increased the degree of their secondary branching. This effect could be inhibited by the NMDA channel blocker, MK-801, and could not be duplicated by depolarizing the neurones with elevated K^+. It is therefore conceivable that activation of NMDA receptors in the early synapses leads to an influx of Ca^{2+} into dendritic growth cones and filopodia and this provides the necessary trigger for their transformation into dendritic branches and, in turn, for the genesis of new growth cones. Glutamate has also been reported to increase the size of neurones cultured from whole brain (Aruffo *et al.* 1987). In addition, nuclei were larger, the rough endoplasmic reticulum was more developed and mitochondria more abundant.

Conclusions

NMDA receptors may first be expressed at a very early stage of neuronal differentiation, even before migration and/or well before any synapses are formed. Should they encounter glutamate in sufficient concentration, the amino acid could, through these receptors, encourage early differentiation, such as axonal growth and the synthesis of transmitter enzymes, and assist in migration. In a later stage, a ready activation of NMDA currents by the transmitter appears to be a prominent feature of many developing synapses. The consequences of this may include, not only a more plastic synapse, but the provision of trophic support to prevent cell death, the triggering of dendritic branching and the fine tuning of synaptic connections. Near the end of the developmental period, the sensitivity of at least some neurones to NMDA declines apparently in an activity-dependent manner.

In this relatively new area of NMDA receptor research, the information available at present is still rather limited. Nevertheless, it is hoped that, in the near future, NMDA receptors can be fitted more formally into conceptual frameworks for the development and stabilization of synaptic connections (Changeux and Danchin 1976; Changeux and Mikoshiba 1978); it is anticipated that this will lead to the incorporation of new and more precise elements into these frameworks as they apply specifically to central synapses.

Glutamate receptors and neuronal degeneration

With each major advance in glutamate pharmacology that occurred over the years (see Chapter 1) there came, soon afterwards, correspondingly large steps in understanding that glutamate neurotoxicity and excitation were linked and that the linkage was at the level of the receptor (Olney 1984). Although NMDA was first recognized to be a potent neurotoxin in 1971 (Olney *et al.* 1971) much of the research in the subsequent decade and more was occupied with the mechanism triggered by kainate (McGeer *et al.* 1978). This mechanism, or at least its complex manifestations *in vivo*, is still poorly understood. With the development of good NMDA antagonists and their application to animal models of acute pathologies (see Chapters 19 and 20) the balance soon shifted in favour of the NMDA receptor. More recently, and for similar reasons, the AMPA receptor has also attracted increasing interest.

The main issues to be considered here are the events associated with glutamate receptor activation that culminate in neuronal degeneration. As with questions about glutamate receptor pharmacology and physiology, *in vitro* preparations, though not without potential artefact, have been invaluable in addressing this question experimentally and, accordingly, much of the following will refer to results obtained with these preparations.

Differential vulnerability

Different neuronal populations can show striking differences in their sensitivity to the toxic actions of glutamate receptor agonists. This emerged clearly from earlier *in vivo* studies and is well illustrated by the behaviour of cells in young rat cerebellar slices (Fig. 18.4). Here, dividing, premigratory and migrating granule cells are insensitive to the toxic effects of all agonists tested; differentiating granule cells in the internal layer are vulnerable to NMDA but not to kainate; Golgi cells are vulnerable to kainate but not to NMDA; neurones in the intracerebellar nuclei are vulnerable to

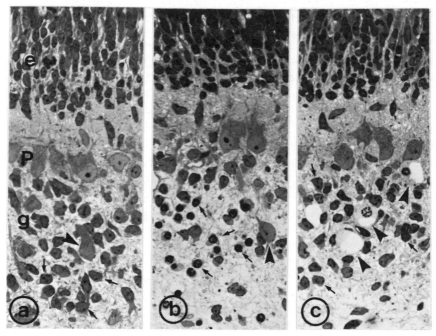

Fig. 18.4 NMDA and kainate neurotoxicity in young (8 day old) rat cerebellar slices. (a), Control slice (3 h incubation); e, P and g indicate the external granule cell, Purkinje cell, and internal granule cell layers respectively; arrowheads, Golgi cells; arrows, granule cells. (b), Slice exposed to 100 μM NMDA for 30 min followed by 90 min recovery in agonist-free medium. Granule cells in the internal layer are necrotic, Golgi cells are spared. (c), Slice exposed to 100 μM kainate in the same way shows sparing of granule cells and necrosis of Golgi cells.

both agonists whereas Purkinje cells at this age are not permanently damaged by either of these agonists (Garthwaite and Garthwaite 1986*a*; Hajos *et al.* 1986) but are selectively vulnerable to the toxic effects of AMPA (Garthwaite and Garthwaite 1991*a*).

There are also major differences in the toxic profiles of different agonists in young hippocampal slices. For example, NMDA kills all differentiating neurone types, whereas quisqualate is more selective for CA3 neurones and kainate is toxic only to a scattered population, possibly of inhibitory interneurones (Garthwaite and Garthwaite 1989). In addition, the toxicities of different agonists can have quite distinct pathological manifestations even in the same neurones, AMPA and quisqualate causing progressive shrinkage of neuronal somata and dendrites coupled with microvacuolation (dark cell degeneration) whereas NMDA elicits a classical necrotic profile consisting of pyknotic nuclei and swollen cytoplasm and mitochondria (e.g. Garthwaite and Garthwaite 1989, 1991*a*).

Dispersed cultures have also been used as models but, in these, it is much more difficult to identify the vulnerable neurones. Populations in cerebral cortical cultures that are relatively more sensitive to either NMDA or kainate have, nevertheless, been detected using NADPH diaphorase histochemistry (Koh and Choi 1988).

Developmental changes

Neurones have to reach a certain degree of maturation before they become vulnerable. As noted above, cerebellar granule cells, though they may express NMDA receptors early on, are resistant to NMDA toxicity until they have stopped migrating. Relatively undifferentiated neurones in the dentate gyrus of hippocampal slices (Garthwaite and Garthwaite 1989) and in cultures of fetal cerebral cortical neurones are also resistant (Choi *et al.* 1987). With maturation, a variety of changes can occur. Some neurones, such as cerebellar granule cells, are only transiently vulnerable to NMDA (Garthwaite and Garthwaite 1986*a*); others remain vulnerable into adulthood, e.g. hippocampal pyramidal cells and striatal neurones, although these too may be particularly susceptible during development (McDonald *et al.* 1988); others develop sensitivity relatively slowly, e.g. cerebellar Golgi cells; some never become vulnerable, e.g. Purkinje cells (Garthwaite and Garthwaite 1986*a*). Kainate, in general, becomes a more efficacious toxin as development proceeds, a phenomenon that, in part, may reflect the importance of the afferent innervation in the toxic mechanism (McGeer *et al.* 1978). AMPA, on the other hand, is a potent neurotoxin in immature brain (McDonald *et al.* 1990; Garthwaite and Garthwaite 1991*a*).

Possible reasons for selective vulnerability

In some cases, it seems most likely that the relative density of receptor subtypes is a major determining factor. For example, in the adult cerebellum, electrophysiological studies have indicated that non-NMDA agonists are powerful excitants for Purkinje cells whereas NMDA, at best, is only weak (Crepel and Audinat 1991). Accordingly, these neurones can be killed by kainate, quisqualate, and AMPA but not by NMDA. The developmental decline in the toxicity of NMDA towards cerebellar granule cells is also paralleled by a fall in the ability of NMDA to depolarize these neurones (Garthwaite *et al.* 1987).

Chemosensitivity, however, is almost certainly not the only factor involved. One example is the granule cell in young rat cerebellum; kainate and NMDA are both very effective depolarizers of these neurones but only NMDA is toxic (J. Garthwaite *et al.* 1986). When the morphological changes occurring during the first few minutes of exposure to the agonists were investigated, granule cells initially exhibited obvious swelling in response to kainate, consistent with a powerful depolarizing effect, but after 5 min they began to shrink and eventually regained close to their original size despite the continued presence of the agonist (Hajos *et al.* 1986). Exposure of the slices to kainate in the absence of Ca^{2+} appeared to prevent this apparent desensitization because the swelling then increased dramatically and persisted, though it was reversible on washout of agonist. The same procedure applied to slices incubated with NMDA also induced huge swelling of several neuronal populations, including some that are resistant to NMDA toxicity (G. Garthwaite *et al.* 1986), implying that these, too, are normally protected by a similar Ca^{2+}-dependent type of desensitization. A comparable mechanism may protect certain neurones from excessive AMPA receptor activation, as inhibitors of the desensitization of this receptor have been found to augment quisqualate, glutamate, and AMPA neurotoxicity in hippocampal cultures (Zorumski *et al.* 1990).

Exposure periods needed to produce irreversible damage

These depend on the applied concentration. In young rat cerebellar slices, for example, a 5 min exposure to 1 mM NMDA kills about 50 per cent of vulnerable granule cells; the corresponding times with concentrations of 300 μM, 100 μM, and 50 mM are 10 min, near 20 min, and 30 min respectively (Fig. 18.5). In cortical cultures, exposures of between 5 min and 24 h—depending on the agonist and its concentration—are required to produce widespread cell death (Koh and Choi 1988). Thus, glutamate toxicity can range from being very acute to being slow to develop, depending on the degree of receptor activation.

Ca^{2+} and glutamate neurotoxicity

It is now generally accepted that Ca^{2+} is the all-important ion in mediating the transition to neuronal death in the case of NMDA neurotoxicity (Meldrum and Garthwaite 1990). This is based partly on results showing that irreversible damage is prevented by reducing extracellular Ca^{2+} or by

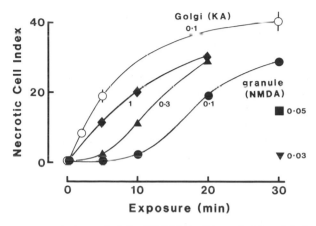

Fig. 18.5 Exposure periods needed for NMDA (solid symbols) and kainate (unfilled symbols) to inflict irreversible damage to granule cells and Golgi cells, respectively. In all cases, the slices were given a 90 min recovery period following the exposures. The different symbols refer to different agonist concentrations (in mM as indicated). Values represent mean numbers of necrotic cells in the granule cell layer per 10^4 (with NMDA) or 10^5 (kainate) μm^2.

increasing intracellular Ca^{2+} buffering and partly because of the correlation that exists between intracellular Ca^{2+} loading and cell death (Garthwaite and Garthwaite 1986*b*; Hartley *et al.* 1993). The evidence also strongly suggests that non-NMDA receptor-mediated degeneration is also Ca^{2+}-dependent, though there are differences from the NMDA-mediated mechanism (G. Garthwaite *et al.* 1986; Garthwaite and Garthwaite 1991*b*).

Do neurones become overloaded with Ca^{2+}?

This was studied in cerebellar slices exposed to NMDA, using an electron microscopic technique that allows visualization of the subcellular sites of Ca^{2+} accumulation (Garthwaite and Garthwaite 1986*b*). During the first 5 min of exposure of the neurones to 100 μM NMDA, substantial Ca^{2+} accumulation occurred but this was localized to the Golgi apparatus and nucleus, leaving the cytoplasm relatively clear; accordingly, the neurones were able to recover on removal of the agonist. With a longer exposure, however, Ca^{2+} deposits additionally appeared in a population of swollen mitochondria and could also be seen apparently free throughout the cytoplasm. The precise levels reached are not known but, given the relatively low sensitivity of the technique, cytoplasmic Ca^{2+} may even have risen as high as 100 μM, i.e. an increase of more than 1000-fold above normal resting values. When the agonist is removed at this point, the neurones became necrotic during a subsequent recovery period. These results suggest that the transition from reversible to irreversible neuronal damage is

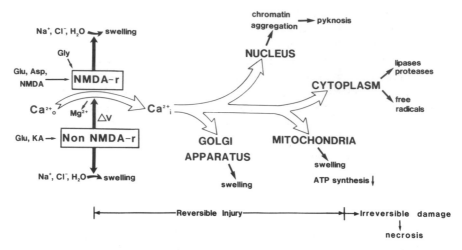

Fig. 18.6 Progress to the stage of irreversible neuronal damage as a result of a sustained influx of Ca^{2+} following activation of NMDA receptors (NMDA-r) and its potentiation by simultaneous depolarization through non-NMDA receptors (non NMDA-r).

associated with an overloading of the mechanisms which serve to keep cytoplasmic Ca^{2+} at low levels.

Sources of the lethal Ca^{2+} load

Since the above technique detected minimal intracellular Ca^{2+} in neurones not exposed to agonists and since extracellular Ca^{2+} was needed to produce degeneration, it can be concluded that the overload in these neurones is due mainly to entry of Ca^{2+} from the outside rather than to release from intracellular stores. The NMDA-gated channels with their effective high Ca^{2+} permeability are likely to represent the major route. Activation of voltage sensitive Ca^{2+} channels alone (by depolarizing the neurones with high K^+) is insufficient to cause cell death under identical conditions (J. Garthwaite *et al.* 1986). Because of the voltage-dependent properties of NMDA receptor channels, however, depolarization enhances Ca^{2+} influx and so potentiates NMDA toxicity. Thus, in the presence of 1.2 mM Mg^{2+}, non-NMDA receptor activation (with kainate) or depolarization with K^+ can convert a non-toxic concentration of NMDA into a toxic one (Garthwaite and Garthwaite 1987).

Whilst receptor-mediated Ca^{2+} entry is probably a necessary primary event in at least some cells, the ensuing rise in intracellular Ca^{2+} may be supplemented by a release of Ca^{2+} from internal stores. The relative contribution of the latter, moreover, may vary with the receptor being activated (see Lei *et al.* 1992; Frandsen and Schousboe, 1993). If it is assumed that a requirement for cell death is that Ca^{2+} rises above a certain threshold for a certain duration, quantitatively minor sources could be enough to tip the balance.

Other routes of Ca^{2+} entry may be more critical under different conditions or in different cells. To take two examples, in cultured retinal ganglion cells, L-type Ca^{2+} channel antagonists, at concentrations likely to act relatively specifically (0.5–1 μM), were found to have marked neuroprotective effects against glutamate and NMDA toxicities, although the extracellular Ca^{2+} was abnormally high (10 mM) in these experiments (Sucher *et al.* 1991); and, in rat optic nerve (in which glutamate is non-toxic), the major route of lethal Ca^{2+} entry under anoxic conditions appears to be through reversal of the Na^+-Ca^{2+} exchanger as a result of intracellular Na^+ loading (Stys *et al.* 1992).

How does excess Ca^{2+} cause cell death?

In cerebellar slices, there is a close association between many of the prominent cytopathological changes leading up to the stage of irreversible neuronal damage and the sites of intracellular Ca^{2+} accumulation (Garthwaite and Garthwaite 1986*b*). Thus, one of the earliest changes is a swelling of the cisternae of the Golgi apparatus. These also are the early sites of Ca^{2+} uptake (presumably with anions and water). Chromatin in the nuclei starts to aggregate and, coincidentally, Ca^{2+} accumulation in the nucleus can be detected. As Ca^{2+} in the nucleus increases, so the chromatin becomes progressively more clumped. A population of mitochondria also undergo swelling, seemingly in proportion to the amount of Ca^{2+} inside them (Fig. 18.6).

None of these pathological changes occurs when the neurones are exposed to NMDA in Ca^{2+}-free conditions, when other changes linked to NMDA-induced depolarization (such as swelling and Na^+ influx) continue, so it is likely that they are caused specifically by Ca^{2+}. In the case of mitochondria, accumulation of Ca^{2+} plus phosphate is thought to be responsible for the swelling and it is associated with impairment of oxidative phosphorylation. The clumping of chromatin is presumably associated with loss of nuclear function; it can progress rapidly to frank pyknosis, a characteristic feature of dead cells.

As well as causing pathological changes in organelles, sustained increases in Ca^{2+} could also influence several other processes which could contribute directly or indirectly to cell death. These include ionic channels or pumps as well as a variety of Ca^{2+} sensitive enzymes. Evidence exists that some of these mechanisms are important in the destructive cascade:

1. Elevated Ca^{2+} is able to inhibit K^+ currents (Chen and Wong 1991; Marrion *et al.* 1991), depress responses to GABA mediated through $GABA_A$ receptors (Inoue *et al.* 1986; Stelzer *et al.* 1988), augment responses to NMDA (Markram and Segal 1991), and inhibit the activity of the Na^+-K^+ pump (Fukuda and Prince 1992). All these would be expected

to contribute a feed-forward effect, further increasing intracellular Ca^{2+} as well as promoting other ionic disturbances. In cultured hippocampal neurones, a persistent depolarization of 20 mV or more occurred after washout of glutamate (0.5 mM; 10 min application); moreover, although the neurones remained viable during the initial stages, the appearance of the depolarization was predictive of a subsequent degeneration (Coulter *et al.* 1992). Several other studies have shown that in the aftermath of a glutamate exposure, and sometimes after a recovery of cytosolic Ca^{2+} to near pre-exposure levels, there occurred a persistent rise in cytosolic Ca^{2+} that was dependent on Ca^{2+} influx and which was also predictive of degeneration (e.g. Randall and Thayer 1992; Wadman and Connor 1992; Tymianski *et al.* 1993). Both the extended depolarization and the secondary Ca^{2+} elevations were dependent on an initial glutamate-induced Ca^{2+} influx.

These and other events set in motion in response to one insult may also render the neurones hypersensitive to later NMDA receptor activation. This can be seen in cerebellar slices: under normal conditions, neurones of the intracerebellar nuclei survive a 5 min exposure to 100 μM NMDA, but degenerate after a 10 min exposure (Hajos *et al.* 1986). If they are exposed for 5 min, left to recover for 1 h in the presence of APV, and then exposed for another 5 min after washout of APV, the neurones do not recover but instead go on to degenerate much as if they had been given a single 10 min exposure (Fig. 18.7).

2. Phospholipase A2 activation leads to the production of arachidonic acid. Arachidonic acid itself is potentially dangerous as it can increase NMDA receptor currents, induce a lasting inhibition of glutamate uptake, and activate protein kinase C (PKC) (Attwell *et al.* 1993). Moreover, during its metabolism, arachidonic acid can give rise to free radicals and these highly reactive species can damage proteins, membranes, and DNA. In cultured cerebellar granule cells, NMDA (but not kainate) receptor activation has been shown to lead to the Ca^{2+}-dependent production of superoxide ions, an effect that could not be reproduced by activation of voltage-sensitive Ca^{2+} channels; NMDA toxicity towards these cells was also inhibited by trappers of superoxide ions, which were assumed to penetrate cells, but not by superoxide dismutase which is likely to remain extracellular (Lafon-Cazal *et al.* 1993). The antioxidant, ubiquinone, has also been shown to protect the same neurones against glutamate-induced neuronal death (Favit *et al.* 1992).

3. The activation of proteases such as calpain has often been invoked as part of Ca^{2+}-mediated cell death because, in theory, these enzymes could cause cytoskeletal breakdown due to degradation of spectrin (Seubert *et al.* 1988; Siman *et al.* 1989), microtubules (Sandoval and Weber 1978), and neurofilaments (Schlaepfer and Hasler 1979) and to blebbing of the cell surface (Nicotera *et al.* 1986). Two forms of calpain have been identified,

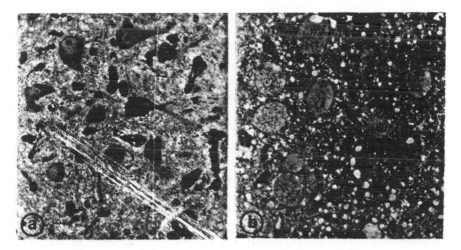

Fig. 18.7 Intracerebellar nucleus neurones given a non-lethal exposure to NMDA are hypervulnerable to a second exposure. In (a), the neurones were exposed to 100 μM NMDA for 5 min (+ 2 h recovery in the presence of 100 μM D,L-APV) and appear unharmed. In (b), they were exposed to NMDA for 5 min, recovered for 1 h in the presence of APV and, after a 10 min washout of the APV, they were exposed to NMDA again for 5 min and recovered for 1 h with APV, This second challenge with NMDA caused the neurones to degenerate.

calpain I and II, the former requiring less Ca^{2+} (about 50 μM for half-maximal activity) than the latter (about 0.5 mM), but the substrate specificity for the two types is similar. NMDA, in neurotoxic concentrations, induced calpain I-mediated spectrin degradation (Siman *et al.* 1989) and calpain inhibitors have been found to reduce ischaemic damage in hippocampal neurones (Lee *et al.* 1991) and, in immature cerebellar slices, to reduce by 70 per cent AMPA-mediated degeneration of Purkinje cells (Caner *et al.* 1993).

4. An involvement of PKC is suggested by the results of Mattson (1991) showing that artificial activation of this enzyme leads to the death of cultured human cortical neurones and by results on rat cultured cerebellar granule cells demonstrating that down-regulation of PKC (Favaron *et al.* 1990) or inhibitors of the enzyme such as calphostin C (Felipo *et al.* 1993) protect against glutamate toxicity. PKC activation and its translocation into membranes may be linked to activation of a sustained Ca^{2+} entry pathway leading to cell death (see above; Favaron *et al.* 1990; Wadman and Connor 1992).

5. Nitric oxide (NO) is a diffusible, free radical species that is synthesized by the enzyme NO synthase. Whilst performing many important physiological functions, NO is also potentially toxic through its ability to inactivate key iron/sulphur-containing enzymes and react with superoxide ions

to generate peroxynitrite, a precursor of more toxic free radicals, such as the hydroxyl radical. Some cells, notably macrophages, exploit the toxic properties of NO to aid in their cytostatic and cytotoxic effects on invading micro-organisms and parasites (Moncada *et al.* 1991). In the brain, a major stimulus for NO synthase activation is in cytosolic Ca^{2+} that follows NMDA receptor activation (Garthwaite *et al.* 1988; Garthwaite 1991) and NO, a powerful stimulator of soluble guanylate cyclase, serves to couple NMDA receptors to increased cyclic GMP levels. Some experiments on cultured cortical neurones have suggested that NO also mediates NMDA neurotoxicity as the cell death could be reduced by NO synthase inhibitors and duplicated by NO-donating compounds (Dawson *et al.* 1993). This result has been partially supported by some other laboratories (Reif 1993; Vige *et al.* 1993) but not by others using similar cultures of cortex (Regan *et al.* 1993) or cultures of other brain areas (e.g. Demerle-Pallardy *et al.* 1991; Pauwels and Leysen 1992; Lafon-Cazal *et al.* 1993). Likewise, *in vivo*, NO synthase inhibitors have been found to partially protect hippocampal neurones from NMDA neurotoxicity in one study (Moncada *et al.* 1992) but to have no effect, or worsen the damage, in others (Haberny *et al.* 1992; Lerner-Natoli *et al.* 1992).

Conclusions

The neuronal cell death which follows excessive activation of glutamate receptors on vulnerable neurones probably arises mainly from the activation of NMDA and AMPA receptors. In both cases, the damage is Ca^{2+}-dependent and is likely to be caused by a failure of homeostatic mechanisms serving to maintain intracellular Ca^{2+} at low levels. Loss of organelle function and cell membrane integrity represents the final stage but before this happens, there may be several intervening steps. There is currently no consensus on what these steps are, and different mechanisms may operate in different cells. Moreover, many of the results have been obtained from cultured cells and their relevance to neurones *in vivo* must remain in question. Nevertheless, this area of research is ultimately likely to lead both to a much fuller understanding of the biology of neurodegeneration and to the identification of key mechanisms around which new neuroprotective agents can be designed.

References

Aruffo, C., Ferszt, R., Hildebrandt, A. G., and Cervos-Navarro, J. (1987). Low doses of L-monosodium glutamate promote neuronal growth and differentiation *in vitro*. *Developmental Neuroscience*, **9**, 228–39.

Attwell, D., Miller, B., and Sarantis, M. (1993). Arachidonic acid as a messenger in the central nervous system. *Seminars in the Neurosciences*, **5**, 159–69.

Balazs, R., Hack, N., and Jorgensen, O. S. (1988). Stimulation of the *N*-methyl-D-aspartate receptor has a trophic effect on differentiating cerebellar granule cells. *Neuroscience Letters*, **87**, 80–6.

Ben-Ari, Y., Cherubini, E., and Krnjevic, K. (1988). Changes in voltage dependence of NMDA currents during development. *Neuroscience Letters*, **94**, 88–92.

Blanton, M. G. and Kriegstein, A. R. (1992). Properties of amino acid transmitter receptors of embryonic cortical neurons when activated by exogenous and endogenous agonists. *Journal of Neurophysiology*, **67**, 1185–200.

Blanton, M. G., LoTurco, J. J., and Kriegstein, A. R. (1990). Endogenous neurotransmitter activates N-methyl-D-aspartate receptors on differentiating neurons in embryonic cortex. *Proceedings of the National Academy of Science, USA*, **87**, 8027–30.

Bode-Greuel, K. M. and Singer, W. (1989). The development of N-methyl-D-aspartate receptors in cat visual cortex. *Developmental Brain Research*, **46**, 197–204.

Bowe, M. A. and Nadler, J. V. (1990). Developmental increase in the sensitivity to magnesium of NMDA receptors on CA1 hippocampal pyramidal cells. *Developmental Brain Research*, **56**, 55–61.

Brenneman, D. E., Forsythe, I. D., Nicol, T., and Nelson, P. G. (1990). N-Methyl-D-aspartate receptors influence neuronal survival in developing spinal cord cultures. *Developmental Brain Research*, **51**, 63–8.

Brewer, G. J. and Cotman, C. W. (1989). NMDA receptor regulation of neuronal morphology in cultured hippocampal neurons. *Neuroscience Letters*, **99**, 268–73.

Burgard, E. C. and Hablitz, J. J. (1993). Developmental changes in NMDA and non-NMDA receptor-mediated synaptic potentials in rat neocortex. *Journal of Neurophysiology*, **69**, 230–40.

Cambray-Deakin, M. A., Adu, J., and Burgoyne, R. D. (1990). Neuritogenesis in cerebellar granule cells *in vitro*: a role for protein kinase C. *Developmental Brain Research*, **53**, 40–6.

Caner, H., Collins, J. L., Harris, S. M., Kassell, N. F., and Lee, K. S. (1993). Attenuation of MPA-induced neurotoxicity by a calpain inhibitor. *Brain Research*, **607**, 354–6.

Carmignoto, G. and Vicini, S. (1992). Activity-dependent decrease in NMDA receptor responses during development of the visual cortex. *Science*, **258**, 1007–11.

Changeux, J.-P. and Danchin, A. (1976). Selective stabilization of developing synapses as a mechanism for the specification of neuronal networks. *Nature*, **264**, 705–12

Changeux, J.-P. and Mikoshiba, K. (1978). Genetic and 'epigenetic' factors regulating synapse formation in vertebrate cerebellum and neuromuscular junction. *Progress in Brain Research*, **48**, 44–66.

Chen, S. and Hillman, D. E. (1989). Regulation of granule cell number by a predetermined number of Purkinje cells in development. *Developmental Brain Research*, **45**, 137–47.

Chen, L. and Huang, L.-Y. M. (1992). Protein kinase C reduces Mg^{2+} block of NMDA-receptor channels as a mechanism of modulation. *Nature*, **356**, 521–3.

Chen, Q. X. and Wong, R. K. S. (1991). Intracellular Ca^{2+} suppressed a transient potassium current in hippocampal neurons. *Journal of Neuroscience*, **11**, 337–43.

Choi, D. W., Maulucci-Gedde, M., and Kriegstein, A. R. (1987). Glutamate neurotoxicity in cortical cell culture. *Journal of Neuroscience*, **7**, 357–68.

Clarke, P. G. H. (1985). Neuronal death during development in the isthmo-optic nucleus of the chick: sustaining role of afferents from the tectum. *Journal of Comparative Neurology*, **234**, 365–79.

Collingridge, G. L. and Singer, W. (1990). Excitatory amino acid receptors and synaptic plasticity. *Trends in Pharmacological Sciences*, **11**, 290–6.

Constantine-Paton, M., Cline, H. T., and Debski, E. (1990). Patterned activity, synaptic convergence, and the NMDA receptor in developing visual pathways. *Annual Review of Neuroscience*, **13**, 129–54.

Coulter, D. A., Sombadi, S., and DeLorenzo, R. J. (1992). Electrophysiology of glutamate neurotoxicity *in vitro*: induction of a calcium-dependent extended neuronal depolarization. *Journal of Neurophysiology*, **68**, 362–73.

Crepel, F. (1974). Excitatory and inhibitory processes acting upon cerebellar Purkinje cells during maturation in the rat: Influence of hypothyroidism. *Experimental Brain Research*, **20**, 403–20.

Crepel, F. (1982). Regression of functional synapses in the immature mammalian cerebellum. *Trends in Neuroscience*, **5**, 266–9.

Crepel, F. and Audinat, E. (1991). Excitatory amino acid receptors of cerebellar Purkinje cells: Development and plasticity. *Progress in Biophysics and Molecular Biology*, **55**, 31–46.

Crepel, F., Mariani, J., and Delhaye-Bouchaud, N. (1976). Evidence for a multiple innervation of Purkinje cells by climbing fibres in the immature rat cerebellum. *Journal of Neurobiology*, **7**, 567–78.

Crepel, F., Delhaye-Bouchaud, N., Guastavino, J. M., and Sampaio, I. (1980). Multiple innervation of cerebellar Purkinje cells by climbing fibres in staggerer mutant mouse. *Nature*, **283**, 483–4.

Crepel, F., Dhanjal, S. S., and Sears, T. A. (1982). Effect of glutamate, aspartate and related derivatives on cerebellar Purkinje cell dendrites in the rat: an *in vitro* study. *Journal of Physiology*, **329**, 297–317.

D-Angelo, E., Rossi, P., and Garthwaite, J. (1990). Dual-component NMDA receptor currents at a single central synapse. *Nature*, **346**, 467–70.

D-Angelo, E., Rossi, P., and Taglietti, V. (1993). Different proportions of *N*-methyl-D-aspartate and non-*N*-methyl-D-aspartate receptor currents at the mossy fibre-granule cell synapse of developing rat cerebellum. *Neuroscience*, **53**, 121–30.

Dawson, V. L., Dawson, T. M., Uhl, G. R., and Snyder, S. H. (1993). Mechanisms of nitric oxide-mediated neurotoxicity in primary brain cultures. *Journal of Neuroscience*, **13**, 2651–61.

Demerle-Pallardy, C., Lonchampt, M.-O., Chabrier, P.-E., and Braquet, P. (1991). Absence of implication of L-arginine/nitric oxide pathway on neuronal cell injury induced by L-glutamate or hypoxia. *Biochemical and Biophysical Research Communications*, **181**, 456–64.

Dupont, J.-L., Fournier, E., Gardette, R., and Crepel, F. (1984). Effect of excitatory amino acids on Purkinje cell dendrites in cerebellar slices from normal and staggerer mice. *Neuroscience*, **12**, 613–19.

Dupont, J.-L., Gardette, R., and Crepel, F. (1987). Postnatal development of the chemosensitivity of rat cerebellar Purkinje cells to excitatory amino acids: an in vitro study. *Developmental Brain Research*, **34**, 59–68.

Favaron, M., Manev, H., Siman, R., Bertolino, M., Szekely, A. M., Costa, E., DeErausquin, G., and Guidotti, A. (1990). Down-regulation of protein kinase C protects cerebellar granule neurons in primary culture from glutamate-induced neuronal death. *Proceedings of the National Academy of Science, USA*, **87**, 1983–7.

Favit, A., Nicoletti, F., Scapagnini, U., and Canonico, P. L. (1992). Ubiquinone protects cultured neurons against spontaneous and excitotoxin-induced degeneration. *Journal of Cerebral Blood Flow and Metabolism*, **12**, 638–45.

Felipo, V., Minana, M.-D., and Grisolia, S. (1993). Inhibitors of protein kinase C prevent the toxicity of glutamate in primary neuronal cultures. *Brain Research*, **604**, 192–6.

Fox, K., Daw, N., Sato, H., and Czepita, D. (1992). The effect of visual experience on development of NMDA receptor synaptic transmission in kitten visual cortex. *Journal of Neuroscience*, **12**, 2672–84.

Frandsen, A. and Schousboe, A. (1993). Excitatory amino acid-mediated cytotoxicity and calcium homeostasis in cultured neurons. *Journal of Neurochemistry*, **60**, 1202–11.

Fukuda, A. and Prince, D. A. (1992). Excessive intracellular Ca^{2+} inhibits glutamate-induced Na^+-K^+ pump activation in rat hippocampal neurons. *Journal of Neurophysiology*, **68**, 28–35.

Gallo, V., Upson, L. M., Hayes, W. P., Vyklicky, L., Jr, Winters, C. A., and Buonanno, A. (1992). Molecular cloning and developmental analysis of a new glutamate receptor subunit isoform in cerebellum. *Journal of Neuroscience*, **12**, 1010–23.

Garthwaite, G. and Garthwaite, J. (1984). Differential sensitivity of rat cerebellar cells *in vitro* to the neurotoxic effects of excitatory amino acid analogues. *Neuroscience Letters*, **48**, 361–7.

Garthwaite, G. and Garthwaite, J. (1986a). *In vitro* neurotoxicity of excitatory amino acid analogues during cerebellar development. *Neuroscience*, **17**, 755–67.

Garthwaite, G. and Garthwaite, J. (1986b). Amino acid neurotoxicity: intracellular sites of calcium accumulation associated with the onset of irreversible damage to rat cerebellar neurones *in vitro*. *Neuroscience Letters*, **71**, 53–8.

Garthwaite, G. and Garthwaite, J. (1987). Receptor-linked ionic channels mediate *N*-methyl-D-aspartate neurotoxicity in rat cerebellar slices. *Neuroscience Letters*, **83**, 241–6.

Garthwaite, G. and Garthwaite, J. (1989). Neurotoxicity of excitatory amino acid receptor agonists in young rat hippocampal slices. *Journal of Neuroscience Methods*, **29**, 33–42.

Garthwaite, G. and Garthwaite, J. (1991a). AMPA neurotoxicity in cerebellar and hippocampal slices: histological evidence for three mechanisms. *European Journal of Neuroscience*, **3**, 715–28.

Garthwaite, G and Garthwaite, J. (1991b). Mechanisms of AMPA neurotoxicity in cerebellar and hippocampal slices. *European Journal of Neuroscience*, **3**, 729–36.

Garthwaite, G., Hajos, F., and Garthwaite, J. (1986). Ionic requirements for neurotoxic effects of excitatory amino acid analogues in rat cerebellar slices. *Neuroscience*, **18**, 437–47.

Garthwaite, G., Yamini, B., Jr, and Garthwaite, J. (1987). Selective loss of Purkinje and granule cell responsiveness to *N*-methyl-D-aspartate in rat cerebellum during development. *Developmental Brain Research*, **36**, 288–92.

Garthwaite, J. (1991). Glutamate, nitric oxide and cell-cell signalling in the nervous system. *Trends in Neuroscience*, **14**, 60–7.

Garthwaite, J. and Beaumont, P. S. (1989). Excitatory amino acid receptors in the parallel fibre pathway in rat cerebellar slices. *Neuroscience Letters*, **107**, 151 6.

Garthwaite, J. and Brodbelt, A. R. (1989). Synaptic activation of *N*-methyl-D-aspartate and non-*N*-methyl-D-aspartate receptors in the mossy fibre pathway in adult and immature rat cerebellar slices. *Neuroscience*, **29**, 401–12.

Garthwaite, J. and Brodbelt, A. R. (1990). Glutamate as the principal mossy fibre transmitter in rat cerebellum: pharmacological evidence. *European Journal of Neuroscience*, **2**, 177–80.

Garthwaite, J., Garthwaite, G., and Hajos, F. (1986). Amino acid neurotoxicity: relationship to neuronal depolarization in rat cerebellar slices. *Neuroscience*, **18**, 449–60.

Garthwaite, J., Charles, S. L., and Chess-Williams, R. (1988). Endothelium-derived relaxing factor release on activation of NMDA receptors suggests role as intercellular messenger in the brain. *Nature*, **336**, 385–8.

Haberny, K. A., Pou, S., and Eccles, C. U. (1992). Potentiation of quinolinate-induced hippocampal lesions by inhibition of NO synthesis. *Neuroscience Letters*, **146**, 187–90.

Hajos, F., Garthwaite, G., and Garthwaite, J. (1986). Reversible and irreversible neuronal damage caused by excitatory amino acid analogues in rat cerebellar slices. *Neuroscience*, **18**, 417–36.

Hamon, B. and Heinemann, U. (1988). Developmental changes in neuronal sensitivity to excitatory amino acids in area CA1 of the rat hippocampus. *Developmental Brain Research*, **38**, 286–90.

Hamori, J. and Somogyi, J. (1983). Differentiation of cerebellar mossy fiber synapses in the rat: a quantitative electron microscope study. *Journal of Comparative Neurology*, **220**, 365–77.

Harris, K. M. and Teyler, T. J. (1984). Developmental onset of long-term potentiation in area CA1 of the rat hippocampus. *Journal of Physiology*, **346**, 27–48.

Hartley, D. M., Kurth, M. C., Bjerkness, L., Weiss, J. H., and Choi, D. W. (1993). Glutamate receptor-induced $^{45}Ca^{2+}$ accumulation in cortical cell culture correlates with subsequent neuronal degeneration. *Journal of Neuroscience*, **13**, 1993–2000.

Hestrin, S. (1992). Developmental regulation of NMDA receptor-mediated synaptic currents at a central synapse. *Nature*, **357**, 686–9.

Inoue, M., Oomura, Y., Yakushiji, T., and Akaike, N. (1986). Intracellular calcium ions decrease the affinity of the GABA receptor. *Nature*, **324**, 156–8.

Ishii, T., Moriyoshi, K., Sugihara, H., Sakurada, K., Kadotani, H., Yokoi, M., Akazawa, C., Shigemoto, R., Mizuno, N., Masu, M., and Nakanishi, S. (1993). Molecular characterization of the family of the *N*-methyl-D-aspartate receptor subunits. *Journal of Biological Chemistry*, **268**, 2836–43.

Jaramillo, F., Vicini, S., and Schuetze, S. M. (1988). Embryonic acetylcholine receptors guarantee spontaneous contractions in rat developing muscle. *Nature*, **335**, 66–8.

Kalb, R. G., Lidow, M. S., Halsted, M. J., and Hockfield, S. (1992). *N*-methyl-D-aspartate receptors are transiently expressed in the developing spinal cord ventral horn. *Proceedings of the National Academy of Science, USA*, **89**, 8502–6.

Kato, N., Artola, A., and Singer, W. (1991). Developmental changes in the susceptibility to long-term potentiation of neurones in rat visual cortex slices. *Developmental Brain Research*, **60**, 43–50.

Kimura, H., Okamoto, K., and Sakai, Y. (1985). Pharmacological evidence for L-aspartate as the neurotransmitter of cerebellar climbing fibres in the guinea-pig. *Journal of Physiology*, **365**, 103–19.

Koh, J.-Y. and Choi, D. W. (1988). Vulnerability of cultured cortical neurons to damage by excitotoxins: differential susceptibility of neurons containing NADPH-diaphorase. *Journal of Neuroscience*, **8**, 2153–63.

Komuro, H. and Rakic, P. (1993). Modulation of neuronal migration by NMDA receptors. *Science*, **260**, 95–7.

Konnerth, A., Llano, I., and Armstrong, C. M. (1990). Synaptic currents in cerebellar Purkinje cells. *Proceedings of the National Academy of Science, USA*, **87**, 2662–5.

Kutsuwada, T., Kashiwabuchi, N., Mori, H., Sakimura, K., Kushiya, E., Araki, K., Meguro, H., Masaki, H., Kumanishi, T., Arakawa, M., and Mishina, M. (1992). Molecular diversity of the NMDA receptor channel. *Nature*, **358**, 36–41.

Lafon-Cazal, M., Pietri, S., Culcasi, M., and Bockaert, J. (1993). NMDA-dependent superoxide production and neurotoxicity. *Nature*, **364**, 535–7.

Lee, K. S., Frank, S., Vanderklish, P., Arai, A., and Lynch, G. (1991). Inhibition of proteolysis protects hippocampal neurons from ischemia. *Proceedings of the National Academy of Science, USA*, **88**, 7233–7.

Lei, S. Z., Zhang, D., Abele, A. E., and Lipton, S. A. (1992). Blockade of NMDA receptor-mediated mobilization of intracellular Ca^{2+} prevents neurotoxicity. *Brain Research*, **598**, 196–202.

Lerner-Natoli, M., Rondouin, G., de Bock, F., and Bockaert, J. (1992). Chronic NO synthase inhibition fails to protect hippocampal neurones against NMDA toxicity. *Neuroreport*, **3**, 1109–12.

Linden, R. and Pinon, L. P. (1987). Dual control by targets and afferents of developmental neuronal death in the mammalian central nervous system: a study in the parabigeminal nucleus of the rat. *Journal of Comparative Neurology*, **266**, 141–9.

LoTurco, J. J., Blanton, M. G., and Kriegstein, A. R. (1991). Initial expression and endogenous activation of NMDA channels in early neocortical development. *Journal of Neuroscience*, **11**, 792–9.

McDonald, J. W., Silverstein, F. S., and Johnston, M. V. (1988). Neurotoxicity of N-methyl-D-aspartate is markedly enhanced in developing rat central nervous system. *Brain Research*, **459**, 200–3.

McDonald, J. W., Trescher, W. H., and Johnston, M. V. (1990). The selective ionotropic-type quisqualate receptor agonist AMPA is a potent neurotoxin in immature rat brain. *Brain Research*, **526**, 165–8.

McGeer, E. G., Olney, J. W., and McGeer, P. L. (ed.) (1978). *Kainic acid as a tool in neurobiology*. Raven Press, New York.

Markram, H. and Segal, M. (1991). Calcimycin potentiates responses of rat hippocampal neurons to N-methyl-D-aspartate. *Brain Research*, **540**, 322–4.

Marrion, N. V., Zucker, R. S., Marsh, S. J., and Adams, P. R. (1991). Modulation of M-current by intracellular Ca^{2+}. *Neuron*, **6**, 533–45.

Mattson, M. (1991). Evidence for the involvement of protein kinase C in neurodegenerative changes in cultured human cortical neurons. *Experimental Neurology*, **112**, 95–103.

Meldrum, B. S. and Garthwaite, J. (1990). Excitatory amino acid neurotoxicity and neurodegenerative disease. *Trends in Pharmacological Sciences*, **11**, 379–87.

Mishina, M., Takai, T., Imoto, K., Noda, M., Takahashi, T., Numa, S., Methfessel, C., and Sakmann, B. (1986). Molecular distinction between fetal and adult forms of muscle acetylcholine receptor. *Nature*, **321**, 406–11.

Moncada, S., Palmer, R. M. J., and Higgs, E. A. (1991). Nitric oxide: physiology, pathophysiology, and pharmacology. *Pharmacological Reviews*, **43**, 109–42.

Moncada, C., Lekieffre, D., Arvin, B., and Meldrum, B. (1992). Effect of NO synthase inhibition on NMDA- and ischaemia-induced hippocampal lesions. *Neuroreport*, **3**, 530–2.

Monyer, H., Sprengel, R., Schoepfer, R., Herb, A., Higuchi, M., Lomeli, H., Burnashev, N., Sakmann, B., and Seeburg, P. H. (1992). Heteromeric NMDA receptors: molecular and functional distinction of subtypes. *Science*, **256**, 1217–21.

Moran, J. and Patel, A. J. (1989). Stimulation of the *N*-methyl-D-aspartate receptor promotes the biochemical differentiation of cerebellar granule neurons and not astrocytes. *Brain Research*, **486**, 15–25.

Nicotera, P., Hartzell, P., Davis, G., and Orrenius, S. (1986). The formation of plasma membrane blebs in hepatocytes exposed to agents that increase cytosolic Ca^{2+} is mediated by the activation of a non-lysosomal proteolytic system. *FEBS Letters*, **209**, 139–44.

Okado, N. and Oppenheim, R. W. (1984). Cell death of motoneurones in the chick embryo spinal cord. IX. The loss of motoneurons following removal of afferent input. *Journal of Neuroscience*, **4**, 1639–52.

Olney, J. W. (1984). Excitotoxins: an overview. In *Excitotoxins*, (ed. K. Fuxe, P. J. Roberts, and R. Schwarcz), pp. 82–96. Macmillan, London.

Olney, J. W., Ho, O. L., and Rhee, V. (1971). Cytotoxic effects of acidic and sulphur containing amino acids on the infant mouse central nervous system. *Experimental Brain Research*, **14**, 61–76.

Oppenheim, R. W. (1985). Naturally occurring cell death during neural development. *Trends in Neuroscience*, **8**, 487–93.

Parks, T. N. (1979). Afferent influences on the development of the brain stem auditory nuclei of the chicken: otocyst ablation. *Journal of Comparative Neurology*, **83**, 665–78.

Pauwels, P. J. and Leysen, J. E. (1992). Blockade of nitric oxide formation does not prevent glutamate-induced neurotoxicity in neuronal cultures from rat hippocampus. *Neuroscience Letters*, **143**, 27–30.

Pellegrini-Giampietro, D. E., Bennett, M. V. L., and Zukin, R. S. (1992). Are Ca^{2+}-permeable kainate/AMPA receptors more abundant in immature brain? *Neuroscience Letters*, **144**, 65–9.

Pearce, I. A., Cambray-Deakin, M. A., and Burgoyne, R. D. (1987). Glutamate acting on NMDA receptors stimulates neurite outgrowth from cerebellar granule cells. *FEBS Letters*, **223**, 143–7.

Puro, D. G. and Woodward, D. J. (1977). Maturation of evoked mossy fiber input to rat cerebellar Purkinje cells (II). *Experimental Brain Research*, **28**, 427–41.

Quinlan, J. E. and Davies, J. (1985). Excitatory and inhibitory responses of Purkinje cells, in the rat cerebellum *in vivo*, induced by excitatory amino acids. *Neuroscience Letters*, **60**, 39–46.

Rabacchi, S., Bailly, Y., Delhaye-Bouchaud, N., and Mariani, J. (1992). Involvement of the *N*-methyl-D-aspartate (NMDA) receptor in synapse elimination during cerebellar development. *Science*, **256**, 1823–5.

Rakic, P. and Sidman, R. L. (1973). Organization of the cerebellar cortex secondary to deficit of granule cells in weaver mutant mice. *Journal of Comparative Neurology*, **152**, 133–62.

Randall, R. D. and Thayer, S. A. (1992). Glutamate-induced calcium transient triggers delayed calcium overload and neurotoxicity in rat hippocampal neurons. *Journal of Neuroscience*, **12**, 1882–95.

Rashin, N. A. and Cambray-Deakin, M. A. (1992). *N*-methyl-D-aspartate effects on the growth, morphology and cytoskeleton of individual neurons *in vitro*, *Developmental Brain Research*, **67**, 301–8.

Regan, R. R., Renn, K. E., and Panter, S. S. (1993). NMDA neurotoxicity in murine cortical cell cultures is not attenuated by hemoglobin or inhibition of nitric oxide synthesis. *Neuroscience Letters*, **153**, 53–6.

Reif, D. W. (1993). Delayed production of nitric oxide contributes to NMDA-mediated neuronal damage. *Neuroreport*, **4**, 566–8.

Represa, A., Tremblay, E., and Ben-Ari, Y. (1989). Transient increase of NMDA-binding sites in human hippocampus during development. *Neuroscience Letters*, **99**, 61 6.

Rosenmund, C., Legendre, P., and Westbrook, G. L. (1992). Expression of NMDA channels on cerebellar Purkinje cells acutely dissociated from newborn rats. *Journal of Neurophysiology*, **68**, 1901–5.

Rossi, D. J. and Slater, N. T. (1993). The developmental onset of NMDA receptor-channel activity during neuronal migration. *Neuropharmacology*, **32**, 1239–48.

Sandoval, I. V. and Weber, K. (1978). Calcium-induced inactivation of microtubule formation in brain extracts. *European Journal of Biochemistry*, **92**, 463–70.

Schlaepfer, W. W. and Hasler, M. B. (1979). Characterization of the calcium-induced disruption of neurofilaments in rat peripheral nerve. *Brain Research*, **168**, 299–309.

Sekiguchi, M., Okamoto, K., and Sakai, Y. (1987). NMDA-receptors on Purkinje cell dendrites in guinea pig cerebellar slices. *Brain Research*, **437**, 402–6.

Seubert, P., Larson, J., Oliver, M., Jung, M. W., Baudry, M., and Lynch, G. (1988). Stimulation of NMDA receptors induces proteolysis of spectrin in hippocampus. *Brain Research*, **460**, 189–94.

Siman, R., Nosek, J. C., and Kegerise, C. (1989). Calpain I activation is specifically related to excitatory amino acid induction of hippocampal damage. *Journal of Neuroscience*, **9**, 1579–90.

Stelzer, A., Kay, A. R., and Wong, R. K. S. (1988). $GABA_A$-receptor function in hippocampal cells is maintained by phosphorylation factors. *Science*, **241**, 339–41.

Stys, P. K., Waxman, S. G., and Ransom, B. R. (1992). Ionic mechanisms of anoxic injury in mammalian CNS white matter: role of Na^+ channels and Na^+-Ca^{2+} exchanger. *Journal of Neuroscience*, **12**, 430–9.

Sucher, N. J., Lei, S. Z., and Lipton, S. A. (1991). Calcium channel antagonists attenuate NMDA receptor-mediated neurotoxicity of retinal ganglion cells in culture. *Brain Research*, **297**, 297–302.

Tremblay, E., Roisin, M. P., Represa, A., Charriaut-Marlangue, C., and Ben-Ari, Y. (1988). Transient increased density of NMDA binding sites in the developing rat hippocampus. *Brain Research*, **461**, 393–6.

Tsumoto, T., Hagihara, K., Sato, H., and Hata, Y. (1987). NMDA receptors in the visual cortex of young kittens are more effective than those of adult cats. *Nature*, **327**, 513–14.

Tymianski, M., Charlton, M. P., Carlen, P. L., and Tator, C. H. (1993). Secondary Ca^{2+} overload indicates early neuronal injury which precedes staining with viability indicators. *Brain Research*, **607**, 319–23.

Vige, X., Carreau, A., Scatton, B., and Nowicki, J. P. (1993). Antagonism by NG-nitro-L-arginine of L-glutamate-induced neurotoxicity in cultured neonatal rat cortical neurons. Prolonged application enhances neuroprotective efficacy. *Neuroscience*, **55**, 893–901.

Wadman, W. J. and Connor, J. A. (1992). Persisting modification of dendritic calcium influx by excitatory amino acid stimulation in isolated CA1 neurons. *Neuroscience*, **48**, 293–305.

Watanabe, M., Inoue, Y., Sakimura, K., and Mishina, M. (1992). Developmental changes in distribution of NMDA receptor channel subunit mRNAs. *Neuroreport*, **3**, 1138–40.

Woodward, D. J., Hoffer, B. J., Siggins, G. R., and Bloom, F. E. (1971). The ontogenetic development of synaptic junctions, synaptic activation, and responsiveness to neurotransmitter substances in rat cerebellar Purkinje cells. *Brain Research*, **34**, 73–97.

Zorumski, C. F., Thio, L. L., Clark, G. D., and Clifford, D. B. (1990). Blockade of desensitization augments quisqualate excitotoxicity in hippocampal neurons. *Neuron*, **5**, 61–6.

19   Competitive NMDA antagonists as drugs

B. S. MELDRUM AND A. G. CHAPMAN

The potential clinical applications of *N*-methyl-D-aspartate (NMDA) antagonists were initially defined on the basis of animal models. Epilepsy was the first target syndrome identified (Croucher *et al.* 1982) and remains an important potential therapeutic area. By 1985 (Meldrum 1985) other proposed targets included ischaemic brain damage, tremor and spasticity, and anxiety. Today stroke and traumatic injury of the spinal cord and brain are the most important clinical targets. Phase II clinical trials are now in progress. Parkinson's disease may also be a target. The possibility of using NMDA antagonists as long-term therapies in chronic neurodegenerative disorders seems relatively remote, largely because of the problem of side effects. Table 19.1 lists potential therapeutic targets for NMDA antagonists. Before reviewing preclinical and clinical data relating to the therapeutic prospects of NMDA antagonists we shall briefly review currently available compounds.

Drugs currently available

The competitive NMDA antagonists currently under evaluation are all structural analogues of 2-amino-5-phosphonopentanoate (AP5) and 2-amino-7-phosphonoheptanoate (AP7). The molecular formulae of some potent antagonists are given in Fig. 19.1. Antagonist activity resides in the D(−) isomer. The phosphono group can be replaced by a tetrazole, with similar bulk.

Table 19.1   Therapeutic targets for NMDA antagonists

1. Epilepsy, myoclonus, status epilepticus, and epileptogenesis (head injury)
2. Spasticity, tremor, and Parkinson's disease
3. Anxiety
4. Pain and hyperalgesia
5. Emesis
6. Ischaemic brain damage, cardiac arrest, open heart surgery, stroke, and perinatal asphyxia
7. Traumatic injury of brain and spinal cord
8. Chronic neurodegenerative disorders, amyotrophic lateral sclerosis, and Huntington's disease

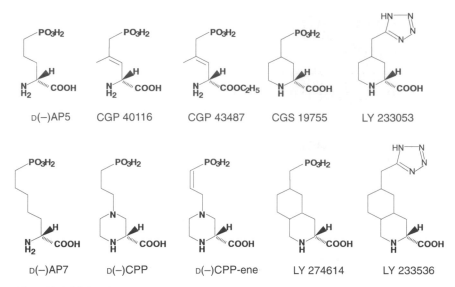

Fig. 19.1 Molecular formulae of D(−)AP5, 2-amino-5-phosphonopentanoic acid; D(−)AP7, 2-amino-7-phosphonoheptanoic acid; CGP 40116 (the active isomer of CGP 37849, 2-amino-4-methyl-5-phosphono-3-pentenoic acid); D(−)CPP, D(−)3-(2-carboxypiperazin-4-yl)-propyl-1-phosphonic acid; CGP 43487 (the active isomer of CGP 39551, 2-amino-4-methyl-5-phosphono-3-pentenoate-1-ethyl ester; D(−)CPP-ene, D(−)3-(2-carboxypiperazin-4-yl)-propenyl-1-phosphonic acid; CGS 19755, 1-(cis-2-carboxypiperidine-4-yl)-propyl-1-phosphonic acid; LY 274614, 6-phosphono-decahydroiso-quinoline-3-carboxylic acid; LY 233053, (cis-(+)4-((2H-tetrazol-5-yl)methylpiperidine-2-carboxylic acid); LY 233536, 6-tetrazole-decahydroisoquinoline-3-carboxylic acid.

Their relative potencies as NMDA antagonists *in vitro* match their relative potencies *in vivo* as anticonvulsants when they are given by the intracerebroventricular (i.c.v.) or intravenous (i.v.) route. All compounds are also active by the oral route but with a slower onset of activity. CGP 39551, the ethyl ester of CGP 37849, has greater relative potency with oral administration.

Epilepsy

Clinical epilepsy takes many forms and has several different underlying biochemical and pathological causes. Some acquired forms may be related to an excessive sensitivity of NMDA receptor-mediated responses (Meldrum 1991). Thus in kindled rats there is evidence for enhanced NMDA receptor-mediated responses in the hippocampus (Martin *et al.* 1992).

Rodent models

Competitive NMDA antagonists have been assessed in a wide range of rodent models of epilepsy (Fig. 19.2). In DBA/2 mice they are more

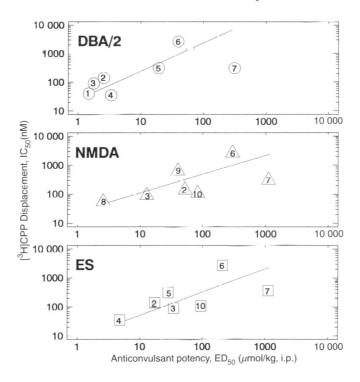

Fig. 19.2 Correlation between NMDA receptor affinities (as estimated by displacement from brain membrane preparations of [³H]CPP (compounds 1–7) or [³H]CGS 19755 (compounds 8–10)) and anticonvulsant activities in three rodent seizure models for the 10 competitive NMDA antagonists whose structures are given in Fig. 19.1. Compounds: 1, CPP-ene; 2, CPP; 3, CGS 19755; 4, CGP 37849; 5, CGP 39551; 6, AP7; 7, AP5; 8, LY 274614; 9, LY 233536; 10, LY 233053. Anticonvulsant ED_{50}s were determined against sound-induced clonic seizures in DBA/2 mice, against clonic NMDA-induced seizures in mice and maximal electroshock seizures. Sources given by Chapman (1991) from which this figure is reproduced.

potent than conventional anti-epileptic drugs when given by the i.c.v. route but of comparable potency when given intraperitoneally (i.p.) or orally (Chapman *et al.* 1987, 1990, 1991; Lehmann *et al.* 1988; Patel *et al.* 1990). Similar high potency and favourable therapeutic index is found against sound-induced seizures in genetically epilepsy-prone rats, particularly for CGP 39551 and CGP 37849 (Smith *et al.* 1993; De Sarro and De Sarro 1993). Protection is seen in a variety of chemically induced seizures, including seizures induced by NMDA, pentylenetetrazol, and DMCM (methyl-6,7-dimethoxy-4-ethyl-β-carboline-3-carboxylate) (Croucher *et al.* 1982; Czuczwar and Meldrum 1982; Chapman 1991). Protection is also seen in maximal electroshock seizures in rodents (Czuczwar *et al.* 1985).

Kindled seizures and the kindling process

Limbic seizures induced by electrical kindling of the amygdala have been proposed as a model of complex partial seizures in man. The fully kindled seizure can be suppressed by high doses of NMDA antagonists (Löscher and Hönack 1991). Competitive NMDA antagonists are active only at doses producing significant motor side effects. They do not reduce the duration of the after-discharge. (In contrast, non-NMDA antagonists both suppress the clinical seizure and shorten the after-discharge duration (Dürmüller *et al.*, 1994.)

The kindling process is regarded as a model for epileptogenesis (following traumatic brain injury or hippocampal lesions induced by prolonged convulsions). Administration of NMDA antagonists prior to each kindling stimulation blocks the kindling process (Morimoto *et al.* 1991). Activation of NMDA receptors seems to be essential for the kindling process very much as it is for the induction of long-term potentiation (LTP) in the hippocampus.

Photosensitive baboons

The suppression of light-induced myoclonic responses in the baboon, *Papio papio*, was first observed with AP5 and AP7 (Meldrum *et al.* 1983*b*). Subsequently, D-CPP-ene (Patel *et al.* 1990) and CGP 39551 and CGP 37849 (Chapman *et al.* 1991) were shown to provide potent and long-lasting suppression of myoclonic responses when given by the i.v. or oral route (see Figs 19.3 and 19.4). Oral administration was not associated with sedative or other side effects.

Clinical trials

Initial clinical trials in epilepsy usually involve the test compound being given in an add-on trial in drug-refractory adult patients with complex partial seizures. A preliminary trial of this kind has been conducted with D-CPP-ene (Sveinbjornsdottir *et al.* 1993). In eight patients with intractable complex partial seizures, D-CPP-ene (250 mg twice daily) was added to their existing therapy and increased to 500 mg twice daily after 2 weeks. No improvement in seizure control was observed and all patients were withdrawn because of side effects (impaired concentration, sedation, and ataxia). (Higher doses of D-CPP-ene were well tolerated in volunteers.) These preliminary data suggest that the poor efficacy of competitive NMDA antagonists in kindled seizures in rodents may be matched by poor efficacy in complex partial seizures in man. Clinical observations in generalized seizures would be of great interest.

Cerebroprotection in ischaemia

Activation of glutamate receptors during and after an episode of focal or global ischaemia appears to contribute importantly to the pathological

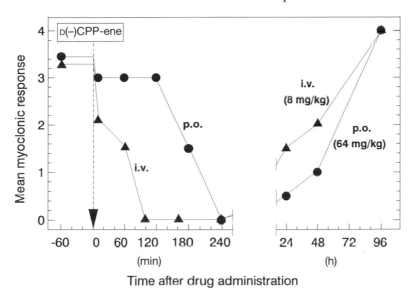

Fig. 19.3 Effect of D(−)CPP-ene on light-induced myoclonic responses in the Senegalese baboon, *Papio papio*. Myoclonic responses to stroboscopic stimulation graded as follows: 1, myoclonus of eyelids; 2, myoclonus of face; 3, myoclonus of trunk and limbs; 4, myoclonus persisting beyond the end of photic stimulation. Points represent the mean responses in four highly photosensitive baboons. At time zero baboons received D(+)CPP-ene, either 8 mg/kg intravenously or 64 mg/kg orally.

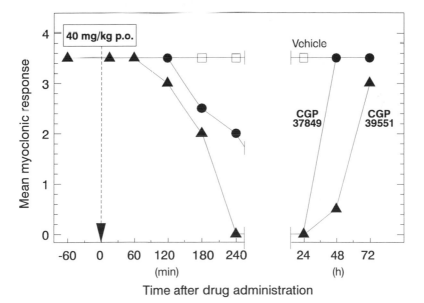

Fig. 19.4 Effect of CGP 37849 (40 mg/kg) or CGP 39551 (40 mg/kg) orally on light-induced myoclonic responses in *Papio papio*. Scoring of responses and presentation are as in Fig. 19.3.

outcome (Meldrum 1990). The role of increases in the extracellular concentration of glutamate and aspartate in determining this damage is not yet clear. Nevertheless, many experiments show that NMDA or non-NMDA antagonists can protect potently against brain damage occurring following focal or global ischaemia. Global ischaemia is observed clinically in cardiac arrest and similar circumstances where cerebral blood flow is transiently severely reduced. It is modelled in rodents by cardiac arrest or by transient occlusion of the carotid arteries in the neck combined either with reduction of mean arterial blood pressure to 50 mm Hg (two-vessel occlusion) or with prior cauterization of the vertebral arteries in the neck (four-vessel occlusion). NMDA antagonists confer little or no cerebroprotection in severe global ischaemia (four-vessel occlusion) but they do give some protection in the less severe two-vessel occlusion model, particularly if it is brief and repeated (Rod and Auer 1989; Swan and Meldrum 1990; Lin *et al.* 1992).

Focal ischaemia presents clinically as stroke and is commonly modelled by reversible or irreversible occlusion of one middle cerebral artery (MCA). Competitive NMDA receptor antagonists have a potent cerebroprotective action in MCA occlusion in the mouse, rat and cat (see Table 19.2). Reduction of the volume of cortex showing infarction is consistently observed with antagonist administration before or at the time of the occlusion. Delayed administration often requires a higher dose to provide protection and the therapeutic time window ends between 1 and 2 h after the occlusion. The therapeutic time window seems somewhat shorter for competitive NMDA antagonists than for MK-801 (see next chapter) probably as a result of the slower penetration of the competitive antagonists into the brain.

In animal models of focal ischaemia, NMDA receptor antagonists provide more dramatic and consistent cerebroprotection than any other class

Table 19.2 Competitive NMDA antagonists in MCA occlusion

Species	Compound	Dose (mg/kg)	Time start (min)	Cortical protection (%)	Reference
Cat	D-CPP-ene	15	−15	75	Chen *et al.* (1991)
			+60	30 *ns*	
Rat	2-AP7	100	+15	80	Roman *et al.* (1989)
	CGS 19755	10	−5	82	Simon and Shiraishi (1990)
			+5	72	
			+60	0	
Mouse	CGS 19755	10			Goyyi *et al.* (1990)

ns: nonsignificant; time start: initiation of drug administration in relation to onset of MCA occlusion.

of drug. This has led to the initiation of clinical trials of NMDA receptor antagonists in stroke (CGS 19755 has entered phase II trial in a five centre study in the US.)

Spinal trauma and head trauma

Spinal trauma is modelled in rats and rabbits by a percussion injury to the exposed spinal cord. Head trauma can be modelled in the rat by fluid percussion delivered to the cerebral cortex via a trephine hole. Outcome is assessed by neurological testing and by histopathology. Such procedures have shown a protective action of CPP in the spinal cord and brain (Faden *et al.* 1989, 1990).

There are many possible mechanisms by which NMDA receptor activation following cerebral trauma can contribute to the final pathological outcome. One concerns the production of toxins by microglia or macrophages that act via NMDA receptors (Giulian 1992). It is clear that many of these factors act substantially later than the time of injury. It is likely that the therapeutic time window in head injury is very much greater than in cerebral ischaemia. This factor, combined with the greater rapidity of transport to emergency care facilities and the greater tolerance of cognitive or behavioural side effects (in a comatose patient in intensive care), makes traumatic injury probably the best target for the cerebroprotective effect of NMDA antagonists.

A dose-escalation tolerability trial is in progress in Glasgow and shows that fairly high doses of CGS 19755 are well tolerated in comatose patients (Stewart *et al.* 1993).

Parkinsonism

An action of NMDA antagonists against spasticity was originally described in genetically spastic Wistar rats (Turski *et al.* 1985). An action against tremor has been reported in the high pressure neurological syndrome in rats and baboons (Meldrum *et al.* 1983a; Pearce *et al.* 1991). There is also strong evidence from rodent models of Parkinsonism and from MPTP-(n-methyl-4-phenyl-1,2,3,6-tetrahydropyridine) treated monkeys that the motor improvement induced by L-DOPA can be greatly enhanced by the co-administration of NMDA antagonists or non-NMDA antagonists (Klockgether and Turski 1990; Greenamyre and O'Brien 1991).

Analgesia

Analgesic effects of NMDA antagonists have been shown in animal models (France *et al.* 1990). NMDA receptors appear to play a crucial role in neuropathic pain and hyperalgesia. NMDA receptor antagonists prevent autotomy in rodents (induced by injury discharge) (Seltzer *et al.* 1991). The increase in spinal cord neuronal excitability induced by repetitive stimulation of afferents is blocked by competitive and non-competitive NMDA antagonists (Woolf and Thompson 1991).

Anxiolytic activity

An anxiolytic action of a competitive NMDA antagonist was first demonstrated in the four plate test (Stephens *et al.* 1986). Such an action has been confirmed in other rodent models (Kehne *et al.* 1991). Compared with other available anxiolytic agents, NMDA antagonists are not thought likely to offer significant improvement.

Chronic neurodegenerative disorders

There has been extensive speculation that NMDA receptor antagonists might be useful in chronic neurodegenerative disorders. There is strong circumstantial evidence that the selective pattern of cell loss in the striatum is determined by activation of NMDA receptors, probably in neurones compromised by impaired energy metabolism (Beal *et al.* 1991; Beal 1992). There is also evidence that activation of NMDA receptors may be important in AIDS dementia. For example, cerebrospinal fluid (CSF) quinolinic acid concentrations are markedly increased (Heyes *et al.* 1991).

The therapeutic application of NMDA antagonists in these conditions will, however, require the development of compounds with better side effect profiles than currently available compounds.

Adverse effects

The most obvious side effects of the acute administration of NMDA receptor antagonists in animals are sedation, muscular weakness, and ataxia. In rodents, splaying of the hind limbs is prominent and the 'chimney escape test' provides a sensitive quantitative test of motor impairment (Löscher and Schmidt 1988). The non-competitive antagonists of the phencyclidine/dizocilpine type differ in that they prominently induce enhanced motor activity and motor stereotypies such as head-weaving. Very high doses of competitive antagonists may also induce stereotypies (Compton *et al.* 1987). In discrimination studies with systemic administration in rodents and primates there is no cross-over between phencyclidine or ketamine and competitive NMDA antagonists (France *et al.* 1989; Koek *et al.* 1990).

Adverse effects of competitive NMDA antagonists on spatial learning have been shown in the Morris water maze in the rat (Morris *et al.* 1986). The motor side effects of competitive NMDA antagonists appeared more severe in kindled rats than in controls (Löscher and Honack 1991), suggesting that kindling or repeated seizures may alter the sensitivity of NMDA receptors to antagonists as well as to agonists.

Acute neurological side effects have not been prominent in trials in volunteers but preliminary data in patients with complex partial seizures and in stroke suggest that sedation, confusion, ataxia, and possibly tinnitus may be limiting side effects.

There is also substantial experimental evidence for the involvement of NMDA receptors in those processes of synaptogenesis that are under functional control. This includes for example the connections of the visual pathway that evolve *in utero*, under the control of spontaneous activity and postnatally under the control of image-evoked activity (Kleinschmidt *et al.* 1987; Bear *et al.* 1990). There is thus concern that sustained blockade of NMDA receptors could interfere not only with critical developmental processes, *in utero* or in early childhood, but also with restorative processes occurring following brain injury (i.e. post-ischaemia or trauma).

Future prospects

The future prospects for competitive NMDA antagonists as therapeutic agents are not yet clear. In epilepsy the best prospects may be in status epilepticus and in primary generalized seizures, but trials in these areas are not yet in evidence. Data for stroke are beginning to accumulate; we do not yet know which type of NMDA antagonist will be most appropriate. Data from head injury appear promising; here also it may take some time before the optimal agent acting on glutamatergic transmission is identified.

The cloning and expression of the genes for the NMDA receptor proteins, and the evidence that the subunit composition may vary in different parts of the brain, open up a large new field for pharmacological research. It may be possible to identify competitive antagonists that are specific for particular heteromeric forms of the receptor that are responsible for specific normal or abnormal functions. In this way it may prove possible to optimize anti-epileptic or other actions of the drugs.

References

Beal, M. F. (1992). Does impairment of energy metabolism result in excitotoxic neuronal death in neurodegenerative illnesses? *Annals of Neurology* **31**, 119–30.

Bear, M. F., Kleinschmidt, A., Gu, Q., and Singer, W. (1990). Disruption of experience-dependent synaptic modifications in striate cortex by infusion of an NMDA receptor antagonist. *Journal of Neuroscience*, **10**, 909–25.

Beal, M. F., Ferrante, R. J., Swartz, K. J., and Kowall, N. W. (1991). Chronic quinolinic acid lesions in rats closely resemble Huntington's disease. *Journal of Neuroscience*, **11**, 1649–59.

Chapman, A. G. (1991). Excitatory amino acid antagonists and therapy of epilepsy.

In *Excitatory amino acid antagonists*, (ed. B. S. Meldrum), pp. 265–86. Blackwell Scientific Publications Ltd, Oxford.

Chapman, A. G., Meldrum, B. S., Nanji, N., and Watkins, J. C. (1987). Anticonvulsant action and biochemical effects in DBA/2 mice of CPP (3-((+)-2-carboxypiperazine-4-yl)-propyl-1-phosphonate), a novel *N*-methyl-D-aspartate antagonist. *European Journal of Pharmacology*, **139**, 91–6.

Chapman, A. G., Graham, J., and Meldrum, B. S. (1990). Potent oral anticonvulsant action of CPP and CPPene in DBA/2 mice. *European Journal of Pharmacology*, **178**, 97–9.

Chapman, A. G., Graham, J. L., Patel, S., and Meldrum, B. S. (1991). Anticonvulsant activity of two orally active competitive NMDA-antagonists, CGP 37849 and CGP 39551 against sound-induced seizures in DBA/2 mice and photically-induced myoclonus in *Papio papio*. *Epilepsia*, **32**, 578–87.

Chen, M., Bullock, R., Graham, D. I., Frey, P., Lowe, D., and McCulloch, J. (1991). Evaluation of a competitive NMDA antagonist (D-CPPene) in feline focal cerebral ischemia. *Annals of Neurology*, **30**, 62–70.

Compton, R. P., Contreras, P. C., O'Donohue, T. L., and Monahan, J. B. (1987). The *N*-methyl-D-aspartate antagonist, 2-amino-7-phosphonoheptanoate, produces phencyclidine-like behavioral effects in rats. *European Journal of Pharmacology*, **136**, 133–4.

Croucher, M. J., Collins, J. F., and Meldrum, B. S. (1982). Anticonvulsant action of excitatory amino acid antagonists. *Science*, **216**, 899–901.

Czuczwar, S. J. and Meldrum, B. (1982). Protection against chemically induced seizures by 2-amino-7-phosphonoheptanoic acid. *European Journal of Pharmacology*, **83**, 335–8.

Czuczwar, S. J., Cavalheiro, E. A., Turski, L., Turski, W. A., and Kleinrok, Z. (1985). Phosphonic analogues of excitatory amino acids raise the threshold for maximal electroconvulsions in mice. *Neuroscience Research*, **3**, 86–90.

De Sarro, G. B. and De Sarro, A. (1993). Anticonvulsant properties of non-competitive antagonists of the *N*-methyl-D-aspartate receptor in genetically epilepsy-prone rats: Comparison with CPPene. *Neuropharmacology*, **32**, 51–8.

Dürmüller, N., Craggs, M., and Meldrum, B. (1994). The effect of the non-NMDA antagonists GYKI 52466 and NBQX and the competitive NMDA receptor antagonist D-CPPene on the development of amygdala kindling and on amygdala-kindled seizures. *Epilepsy Research*, **17**, 167–74.

Faden, A. I., Demediuk, P., Panter, S. S., and Vink, R. (1989). The role of excitatory amino acids and NMDA receptors in traumatic brain injury. *Science*, **244**, 798–800.

Faden, A. I., Ellison, J. A., and Noble, L. J. (1990). Effects of competitive and non-competitive NMDA receptor antagonists in spinal cord injury. *European Journal of Pharmacology*, **175**, 165–74.

France, C. P., Woods, J. H., and Ornstein, P. (1989). The competitive *N*-methyl-D-aspartate (NMDA) antagonist CGS 19755 attenuates the rate-decreasing effects of NMDA in rhesus monkeys without producing ketamine-like discriminative stimulus effects. *European Journal of Pharmacology*, **159**, 133–9.

France, C. P., Winger, G. D., and Woods, J. H. (1990). Analgesic, anesthetic, and respiratory effects of the competitive *N*-methyl-D-aspartate (NMDA) antagonist CGS 19755 in rhesus monkeys. *Brain Research*, **526**, 355–8.

Giulian, D. (1992). Brain inflammatory cells, neurotoxins, and acquired immunodeficiency syndrome. In *Excitatory amino acids*, (ed. R. P. Simon), pp. 229–34. Thieme Medical Publishers, Inc., New York.

Gotti, B., Benavides, J., MacKenzie, E. T., and Scatton, B. (1990). The pharmacotherapy of focal cortical ischaemia in the mouse. *Brain Research*, **522**, 290–307.

Greenamyre, J. T. and O'Brien, C. F. (1991). *N*-methyl-D-aspartate antagonists in the treatment of Parkinson's disease. *Archives of Neurology*, **48**, 977–81.

Heyes, M. P., Brew, B. J., Martin, A., Price, R. W., Salazar, A. M., Sidtis, J. J., Yergey, J. A., Mouradian, M. M., Sadler, A. E., Keilp, J., Rubinow, D., and Markey, S. P. (1991). Quinolinic acid in cerebrospinal fluid and serum in HIV-1 infection: relationship to clinical and neurological status. *Annals of Neurology*, **29**, 202–9.

Kehne, J. H., McCloskey, T. C., Baron, B. M., Chi, E. M., Harrison, B. L., Whitten, J. P., and Palfreyman, M. G. (1991). NMDA receptor complex antagonists have potential anxiolytic effects as measured with separation-induced ultrasonic vocalizations. *European Journal of Pharmacology*, **193**, 283–92.

Kleinschmidt, A., Bear, M. F., and Singer, W. (1987). Blockade of 'NMDA' receptors disrupts experience-dependent plasticity of kitten striate cortex. *Science*, **238**, 355–8.

Klockgether, T. and Turski, L. (1990). NMDA antagonists potentiate antiparkinsonian actions of L-dopa in monoamine-depleted rats. *Annals of Neurology*, **28**, 539–46.

Koek, W., Woods, J. H., and Colpaert, F. C. (1990). *N*-methyl-D-aspartate antagonism and phencyclidine-like activity: a drug discrimination analysis. *Journal of Pharmacology and Experimental Therapeutics*, **253**, 1017–25.

Lehmann, J., Chapman, A. G., Meldrum, B. S., Hutchison, A., Tsai, C., and Wood, P. L. (1988). CGS 19755 is a potent and competitive antagonist at NMDA-type receptors *in vitro* and *in vivo*. *European Journal of Pharmacology*, **154**, 89–93.

Lin, B., Dietrich, W. D., Kraydieh, S., Busto, R., Globus, M.Y.T., and Ginsberg, M. D. (1992). MK-801 protects in a model of repeated episodes of brief normothermic forebrain ischemia in rats. *Society of Neuroscience Abstracts*, **18**, 1256.

Löscher, W. and Hönack, D. (1991). Anticonvulsant and behavioral effects of two novel competitive *N*-methyl-D-aspartate acid receptor antagonists, CGP 37849 and CGP 39551, in the kindling model of epilepsy. Comparison with MK-801 and carbamazepine. *Journal of Pharmacology and Experimental Therapeutics*, **256**, 432–40.

Löscher, W. and Schmidt, D. (1988). Which animal models should be used in the search for new antiepileptic drugs? A proposal based on experimental and clinical considerations. *Epilepsy Research*, **2**, 145–81.

Martin, D., McNamara, J. O., and Nadler, J. V. (1992). Kindling enhances sensitivity of CA3 hippocampal pyramidal cells to NMDA. *Journal of Neuroscience*, **12**, 1928–35.

Meldrum, B. S. (1985). Possible therapeutic applications of antagonists of excitatory amino acid neurotransmitters. *Clinical Science*, **68**, 113–22.

Meldrum, B. S. (1990). Protection against ischaemic neuronal damage by drugs acting on excitatory neurotransmission. *Cerebrovascular Brain Metabolism Reviews*, **2**, 27–57.

Meldrum, B. S. (1991). Excitatory amino acid neurotransmission in epilepsy and anticonvulsant therapy. In *Excitatory amino acids* (ed. B. S. Meldrum, F. Moroni, R. P. Simon, and J. H. Woods), pp. 655–70. Raven Press, New York.

Meldrum, B., Wardley-Smith, B., Halsey, M. J., and Rostain, J.-C. (1983). 2-amino-phosphonoheptanoic acid protects against the high pressure neurological syndrome. *European Journal of Pharmacology*, **87**, 501–2.

Meldrum, B. S., Croucher, M. J., Badman, G., and Collins, J. F. (1983). Antiepileptic action of excitatory amino acid antagonists in the photosensitive baboon, *Papio papio*. *Neuroscience Letters*, **39**, 101–4.

Morimoto, K., Katayama, K., Inoue, K., and Sato, K. (1991). Effects of competitive and noncompetitive NMDA receptor antagonists on kindling and LTP. *Pharmacology, Biochemistry and Behaviour*, **40**, 893–9.

Morris, R. G. M., Anderson, E., Lynch, G. S., and Baudry, M. (1986). Selective impairment of learning and blockade of long-term potentiation by an *N*-methyl-D-aspartate receptor antagonist, AP5. *Nature*, **319**, 774–6.

Patel, S., Chapman, A. G., Graham, J. L., Meldrum, B. S., and Frey, P. (1990). Anticonvulsant activity of the NMDA antagonists, D(−)4-(3-phosphonopropyl) piperazine-2-carboxylic acid (D-CPP) and D(−) (E)-4-(3-phosphonoprop-2-enyl)piperazine-2-carboxylic acid (D-CPPene) in a rodent and a primate model of reflex epilepsy. *Epilepsy Research*, **7**, 3–10.

Pearce, P. C., Halsey, M. J., Maclean, C. J., Ward, E. M., Webster, M.-T., Luff, N. P., Pearson, J., Charlett, A., and Meldrum, B. S. (1991). The effects of the competitive NMDA receptor antagonist CPP on the high pressure neurological syndrome in a primate model. *Neuropharmacology*, **30**, 787–96.

Rod, M. R. and Auer, R. N. (1989). Pre- and post-ischemic administration of dizocilpine (MK-801) reduces cerebral necrosis in the rat. *Canadian Journal of Neurological Science*, **16**, 340–4.

Roman, R., Bartkowski, H., and Simon, R. P. (1989). The specific NMDA receptor antagonist AP-7 attenuates focal ischemic brain injury. *Neuroscience Letters*, **104**, 19–24.

Seltzer, Z., Cohn, S., Ginzburg, R., and Beilin, B. (1991). Modulation of neuropathic pain behavior in rats by spinal disinhibition and NMDA receptor blockade of injury discharge. *Pain*, **45**, 69–75.

Simon, R. P. and Shiraishi, K. (1990). *N*-methyl-D-aspartate antagonist reduces stroke size and regional glucose metabolism. *Annals of Neurology*, **27**, 606–11.

Smith, S. E., Al-Zubaidy, Z. A., Chapman, A. G., and Meldrum, B. S. (1993). Excitatory amino acid antagonists, lamotrigine and BW 1003C87 as anticonvulsants in the genetically epilepsy-prone rat. *Epilepsy Research*, **15**, 101–15.

Stephens, D. N., Meldrum, B. S., Weidmann, R., Schneider, C., and Grutzner, M. (1986). Does the excitatory amino acid receptor antagonist 2-APH exhibit anxiolytic activity? *Psychopharmacology*, **90**, 166–9.

Stewart, L., Bullock, R., Jones, M., Kotake, A., and Teasdale, G. M. (1993). The cerebral haemodynamic and metabolic effects of the competitive NMDA antagonist CGS 19755 in humans with severe head injury. 2nd *International Neurotrauma Symposium*, Glasgow, 4–9 July (Abstract).

Sveinbjornsdottir, S., Sander, J. W. A. S., Upton, D., Thompson, P. J., Patsalos, P. N., Hirt, D., Emre, M., Lowe, D., and Duncan, J. S. (1993). The excitatory amino acid antagonist D-CPP-ene (SDZ EAA-494) in patients with epilepsy. *Epilepsy Research*, **16**, 165–74.

Swan, J. H. and Meldrum, B. S. (1990). Protection by NMDA antagonists against selective cell loss following transient ischaemia. *Journal of Cerebral Blood Flow and Metabolism*, **10**, 343–51.

Turski, L., Schwarz, M., Turski, W. A., Klockgether, T., Sontag, K.-H., and Collins, J. F. (1985). Muscle relaxant action of excitatory amino acid antagonists. *Neuroscience Letters*, **53**, 321–6.

Woolfe, C. J. and Thompson, S. W. N. (1991). The induction and maintenance of central sensitization is dependent on *N*-methyl-D-aspartate receptor activation; implications for the treatment of post-injury pain hypersensitivity states. *Pain*, **44**, 293–9.

20 Non-competitive NMDA antagonists as drugs

L. L. IVERSEN AND J. A. KEMP

Introduction

The 'excitotoxic theory', suggesting that the neuronal damage which results from ischaemic, hypoxic, hypoglycaemic, and traumatic insults is caused, at least in part, by excessive release of glutamate and a subsequent overactivation of post-synaptic receptors, is no longer dogma but firmly supported by experimental evidence (Choi 1991; McCulloch *et al.* 1992). The N-methyl-D-aspartate (NMDA) receptor plays a key role in mediating this toxicity, probably due to its high permeability to calcium (MacDermott *et al.* 1986), a known mediator of cell damage (Schanne *et al.* 1979). Much of the evidence supporting a role for NMDA receptors has come from studies with selective antagonists. Initially, these were performed with competitive antagonists of the glutamate recognition site, such as D-2-amino-5-phosphonopentanoate (D-AP5) and D-2-amino-5-phosphono-heptanoate (D-AP7), which were shown to be neuroprotective in animal studies (Schwarcz and Meldrum 1985). More recently, however, much work has concentrated on antagonists acting in a non-competitive manner with glutamate at the NMDA receptor complex.

The first of these described were compounds which acted at the level of the ion channel and include potent antagonists, such as phencyclidine and dizocilpine (MK-801), which penetrate readily into the central nervous system (CNS) following systemic administration. This feature made them more attractive candidates as drugs than the highly polar competitive antagonists but, unfortunately, they also possessed undesirable side effects, including behavioural stimulant (Tricklebank *et al.* 1989) and cardiovascular (Lewis *et al.* 1989) effects. Although these side effects may limit the therapeutic usefulness of channel blockers, these compounds, because of their non-competitive nature and pharmacokinetic profile, have dramatic neuroprotective effects in certain animal models of neurodegeneration (see later) and have played a major part in establishing the excitotoxic theory. However, due to the possible limitations of the channel blockers, more recent work has concentrated on substances which act at different sites on the NMDA receptor complex and much of this effort, including our own, has targeted the glycine co-agonist site.

Pharmacology of non-competitive NMDA antagonists

Dizocilpine (MK-801) and related compounds

Dizocilpine was originally described as a potent anticonvulsant agent with anxiolytic and central sympathomimetic properties and an unknown mechanism of action (Clineschmidt *et al.* 1982*a,b*). We discovered that it was a potent NMDA receptor antagonist (Wong *et al.* 1986) and several findings suggested it acted as an open channel blocker. The specific binding of [^{3}H]dizocilpine was completely inhibited by dissociative anaesthetics, such as phencyclidine (PCP) and ketamine (Wong *et al.* 1986), which had previously been shown to produce a use- and voltage-dependent block of NMDA receptors (Honey *et al.* 1985). Furthermore, functional studies showed that the blocking effect of dizocilpine itself was markedly agonist-dependent (Wong *et al.* 1986; Huettner and Bean 1988), even more so than PCP and ketamine (Kemp *et al.* 1991). This agonist-dependency could also be demonstrated in radioligand binding experiments. Thus, in well-washed membranes, [^{3}H]dizocilpine binding was enhanced by glutamate and glycine site agonists and inhibited by antagonists of these sites (Foster and Wong 1987), suggesting that [^{3}H]dizocilpine bound preferentially to the activated form of the NMDA receptor. A clear correlation was also shown between the regional distribution of sites in the CNS labelled by [^{3}H]dizocilpine, NMDA-sensitive [^{3}H]L-glutamate binding and strychnine-insensitive [^{3}H]glycine binding (Bowery *et al.* 1988).

A number of other channel blockers of the NMDA receptor have been synthesized with the aim of developing neuroprotective agents (Fig. 20.1)

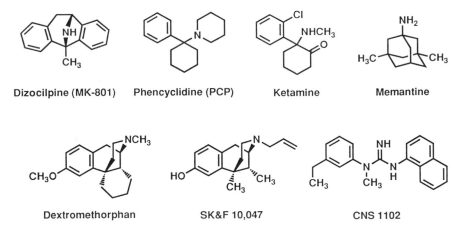

Fig. 20.1 Non-competitive NMDA receptor antagonists-channel blockers.

and amongst these are a series of substituted guanidines (Keana *et al.* 1989).One of the most potent and selective of this series, CNS 1102 (*N*-(1-naphthyl)-*N'*-(*m*-ethylphenyl)-*N'*-methylguanidine), has been shown to be neuroprotective both *in vitro* and *in vivo* (McBurney *et al.* 1991; Park *et al.* 1991).

Other types of non-competitive NMDA antagonists

Following the discovery of the glycine-site on the NMDA receptor complex (Johnson and Ascher 1987) it was rapidly shown that HA-966 (Fletcher and Lodge 1988; Foster and Kemp 1989) and kynurenic acid (Watson *et al.* 1988) antagonized NMDA responses by an action at this site (Fig. 20.2). It was also recognized that there were differences in the antagonist properties of these two compounds due to the fact that HA-966 was a low-efficacy partial agonist (Foster and Kemp 1989) whilst kynurenic acid, and the higher affinity 7-chloro analogue, were full antagonists (Kemp *et al.* 1988). The affinity and selectivity of kynurenic acids for the glycine site were enhanced further by combined 5- and 7-substituents (Foster *et al.* 1992). Modification of the heterocyclic ring led to the 4-substituted tetrahydro-quinolines and the most potent glycine-site antagonist to date, the 4-*trans*-phenylurea, L-689,560 (Foster *et al.* 1992). Unfortunately, whilst being highly active *in vitro*, the antagonists derived from the kynurenic series to date have poor CNS bioavailability and are only weakly active when given systemically.

In contrast, HA-966 has several marked CNS effects when administered

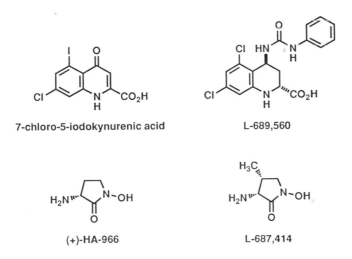

7-chloro-5-iodokynurenic acid   L-689,560

(+)-HA-966   L-687,414

Fig. 20.2 Non-competitive NMDA receptor antagonists-glycine site compounds.

systemically and some of these actions reside in the different enantiomers of HA-966 (Singh *et al*. 1990). Thus, the glycine site activity is conferred by the (R)-(+) enantiomer of racemic HA-966 whilst the (S)-(−) enantiomer is responsible for its γ-butyrolactone-like sedative effects (Singh *et al*. 1990). Substitution with methyl at the 4-position results in an increase in activity in (R)-(+) *cis*-β-methyl-HA-966 (L-687,414), which has a 10 times higher affinity than (+)HA-966 but a slightly lower level of efficacy (Kemp *et al*. 1991). Although of much lower affinity than the full antagonists, such as L-689,560, L-687,414 has better CNS bioavailability and is more potent *in vivo* following systemic administration. Thus, at present L-687,414 is the most useful compound with which to study the *in vivo* properties of glycine-site antagonists/low efficacy partial agonists. Such studies have revealed that, like other NMDA antagonists, L-687,414 is anticonvulsant (Saywell *et al*. 1991) and neuroprotective (see later) but appears to have a better separation than ion channel blockers, between the doses required for these effects and those which produce the undesirable sedative/ataxic effects.

Other non-competitive NMDA receptor antagonists with different and, as yet, unclear mechanism of action are ifenprodil and eliprodil. Binding studies with [³H]ifenprodil (Shoemaker *et al*. 1990) and its effects on [³H]TCP binding (Carter *et al*. 1989) have suggested an interaction with the polyamine site, although there is some doubt whether this is a simple competitive interaction. An electrophysiological study (Legendre and West-brook 1991) has indicated two components to its NMDA receptor blocking action, neither of which appears to involve directly the polyamine site.

Neuroprotective effects of dizocilpine and other NMDA antagonists

Neurotoxins

Dizocilpine has been found to protect against NMDA-related excitotoxic damage in a variety of *in vitro* models. Using chick embryo retina *in vitro*, dizocilpine was found to be the most potent compound in protecting against NMDA-induced damage (Olney *et al*. 1987). A similar conclusion was reached in studies demonstrating the ability of dizocilpine and other non-competitive NMDA antagonists to protect mouse cortical neurones in primary culture from damage following exposure to NMDA (Goldberg *et al*. 1988). These authors also found that the same drugs could prevent neuronal damage caused by transient exposure of tissue cultures to hypoxia (Table 20.1), a finding we have been able to confirm in our own laboratory (Priestley *et al*. 1990). Dizocilpine was also found to protect cultures of rat hippocampal neurones against NMDA-induced cell death (Peterson *et al*. 1989) and retinal ganglion cell cultures against L-glutamate (Hahn *et al*. 1988). In the latter model dizocilpine remained effective even when added

Table 20.1 NMDA antagonists in primary cultures of mouse cortical neurones

	EC$_{50}$ for neuroprotective actions of non-competitive antagonists (μM)	
Antagonist	Versus NMDA	Versus hypoxia
MK-801 (dizocilpine)	0.3	0.1
PCP (phencyclidine)	1	1
(+)-Cyclazocine	10	3
(+)-SKF 10,047	10	3
Pentazocine	30	30

EC$_{50}$ for each antagonist is defined as the concentration required to reduce lactate dehydrogenase efflux from damaged neurones to 50 per cent of the untreated control level (data from Goldberg et al. (1988)).

1 or 4 h after the initial exposure to glutamate (Levy and Lipton 1990). Excitotoxin or hypoxia-induced cell death in primary neuronal cultures has proved to be a valuable model to demonstrate the neuroprotective effects of other non-competitive NMDA antagonists, including dextrorphan and levorphanol (Choi et al. 1987), thiokynurenates (Moroni et al. 1992), HA-966, 7-chlorokynurenate (Priestley et al. 1990), and memantine (Erdö and Schäfer 1991).

Systemically administered dizocilpine also protects against neuronal degeneration in rat brain after intracerebral injections of NMDA and related agonists (Foster et al. 1987, 1988; Beal et al. 1988). A quantitative assessment of the neuroprotective effects of dizocilpine in the rat striatum was made by measuring the activity of marker enzymes for intrinsic neurones, using choline acetyltransferase (CAT) as a marker for cholinergic neurones and glutamic acid decarboxylase (GAD) as a marker for GABAergic neurones (Foster et al. 1987). Dizocilpine given 1 h before injections of NMDA or the NMDA agonist, quinolinic acid, into rat striatum afforded a complete protection against the loss of GAD and CAT normally produced by excitotoxin injections and remained partially effective even when administered up to 5 h after the excitotoxin injection (Foster et al. 1988). The specificity of dizocilpine was indicated by the observation that kainic acid- or α-amino-3-hydroxy-5-methyl-isoxazolepropionate (AMPA)-induced decrements in striatal CAT and GAD were not protected by dizocilpine at doses up to 10 mg/kg. The damage to rat arcuate nucleus caused by systemic administration of NMDA was completely prevented by pretreatment with dizocilpine (1 mg/kg) (Fuller et al. 1987) or L-glutamate (Lehmann and Jönsson 1992). McDonald et al. developed a perinatal rat model to study the protective effects of systemically administered NMDA antagonists against damage caused by intrastriatal injection of NMDA in 7 day old rat pups and demonstrated the efficacy of dizocilpine and PCP (McDonald *et al.* 1989*a,b*).

Global ischaemia

Dizocilpine is effective in a number of animal models of global ischaemia (Table 20.2). In the first studies performed with the compound we found that peripherally administered dizocilpine protected against the hippocampal damage produced by complete forebrain ischaemia in gerbils (Gill *et al.* 1987). Cerebral ischaemia was induced by occlusion of the common carotid arteries for 5 min. This brief period of global ischaemia led to no obvious neurological abnormalities or mortality. However, consistent neuronal damage and cell loss were observed histologically 4 days later, particularly in the population of large hippocampal pyramidal cells in the CA1 region. Measurements of neuronal damage in this region were made from both hippocampi in cresyl violet stained coronal sections. Pretreatment of gerbils with dizocilpine 1 h prior to ischaemia produced a dose-dependent decrease in the area of CA1 neuronal degeneration, with an ED_{50} of 0.3 mg/kg (i.p.). After pretreatment with higher doses (1–10 mg/kg) the majority of animals were completely protected. Surprisingly, dizocilpine remained fully effective in protecting hippocampal neurones when administered 30 min after the ischaemic insult, and partial neuroprotection was observed even when a single dose of dizocilpine was given 15 or 24 h after the artery occlusion (Gill *et al.* 1988).

The neuroprotective effects of dizocilpine in the gerbil were confirmed by Lawrence *et al.* (1987), who found an ED_{50} of approximately 1 mg/kg (i.p. 15 min before) for protection of CA1 hippocampal neurones following a more severe (10 min) bilateral artery occlusion, and by Kato *et al.* (1990) who found that a single dose of 3 mg/kg (i.p.) 30 min before repeated 2 min periods of artery occlusion protected hippocampal and thalamic neurones. Buchan and Pulsinelli (1990) and Corbett *et al.* (1990) claimed that the neuroprotective effects of dizocilpine in the gerbil model could be attributed to the hypothermia induced by the drug and were no longer seen in normothermic animals. Nevertheless, we continued to observe the neuroprotective effects of dizocilpine when the experiments were repeated with control of body temperature (Gill and Woodruff 1990). While hypothermia may contribute to the neuroprotective effects of dizocilpine under some conditions, it cannot explain the efficacy seen in the many models in which body temperature is monitored and controlled (Hattori and Wasterlain 1991).

Dizocilpine has also been tested in global forebrain ischaemia studies in the rat. In a model involving bilateral occlusion of the carotid arteries following reduction of blood pressure to less than 50 mm Hg, dizocilpine has generally been found to be effective in reducing cortical and hippo-

Table 20.2 Dizocilpine (MK-801): summary of neuroprotective studies in global ischaemia

Species	Procedure	Dizocilpine treatment	Neurological outcome	Neurohistological outcome	Reference
Gerbil	bilateral occlusion carotid (5–20 min)	(ED$_{50}$ = 0.3 mg/kg) 0.1–10.0 mg/kg i.p. 1 h before to 24 h after	Improved survival	reduced cell loss (hippocampus) at 4 days	Gill et al. (1987a, 1988)
Gerbil	bilateral occlusion carotid (10 min)	ED$_{50}$ = 1.0 mg/kg (15 min before)	–	reduced cell loss (hippocampus) at 4 days	Lawrence et al. (1987)
Rat	10 min bilateral occlusion carotid + temporary lowering blood pressure	0.2–3.0 mg/kg i.p. 1 h before; ED$_{50}$ = 0.5 mg/kg	–	reduced cell loss (cortex and hippocampus) at 7 days	Gill et al. (1987b)
		0.25 + 0.5 mg/kg i.v. 15 min before	–	reduced cell loss (hippocampus) at 7 days	Church et al. (1988)
		1.0 mg/kg i.v. 20 min before or 20 min after	–	reduced cell loss, (cortex striatum and hippocampus) at 7 days	Rod and Auer (1989)
		0.3–3.0 mg/kg i.p. 15 min and 5 h after	–	reduced cell loss (hippocampus) at 7 days	Swan and Meldrum (1990)
		0.1–5.0 mg/kg before and after	–	no reduction in cell loss (hippocampus)	Nellgård et al. (1991)
Rat	4-vessel occlusion (15 min)	various	–	no reduction in cell loss (hippocampus)	Buchan et al. (1991)
Rat	occlusion carotid + 2–3 h hypoxia in 7 day-old pups	1.0 mg/kg s.c. 1–1.25 h after	–	greatly reduced loss of cortical tissue at 5 days	McDonald et al. (1987)
		10 mg/kg i.p. 30 min before or 60 min after	–	large reduction in cortical, striatal, and hippocampal damage	Hattori et al. (1989)
		0.5–1.0 mg/kg during hypoxia	–	prevention of cell loss (hippocampus)	Ford et al. (1989)
Rat	carotid ligation + 75 min hypobaric	1.0 mg/kg i.p. 15 min before	–	greatly reduced brain damage	Olney et al. (1989)
Cat	17 min cardiac arrest	0.33 mg/kg i.v. at 5 min, then 0.075 mg/kg/h for 10 h	no improvement at 2, 4, and 7 days	–	Fleischer et al. (1988)
Dog	11 min aortic occlusion	0.15 mg/kg i.v. 5 min, then 0.075 mg/kg/h for 8 h	no improvement at 1, 2, or 3 days	no reduction in hippocampal damage	Michenfelder et al. (1989)
Dog	17 min cardiac arrest	0.3 mg/kg i.v. 5 min, then 0.075 mg/kg/h for 12 h	no improvement at up to 4 days	–	Sterz et al. (1989)
Pigtail monkey	complete cerebral ischaemia	0.3 mg/kg i.v. 5 min, then 0.15 mg/kg/h for 10 h	no improvement at 4 days	no reduction in hippocampal damage	Lanier et al. (1990)

campal damage, provided the drug was administered prior to the ischaemia or not more than 20 min after (Gill *et al.* 1987; Church *et al.* 1988; Rod and Auer 1989; Swan and Meldrum 1990) (Table 20.2). In the more severe 'four-vessel' occlusion model—which yields a complete cerebral ischaemia—it is clear that dizocilpine was ineffective (Buchan *et al.* 1991) and this was also the conclusion in large animal studies of complete cerebral ischaemia which seek to mimic the effects of cardiac arrest in man (Fleischer *et al.* 1988; Michenfelder *et al.* 1989; Sterz *et al.* 1989; Lanier *et al.* 1990). This may in part reflect the severity of these models and the variable outcome observed in the control groups.

Dramatic protective effects of dizocilpine have been reported in neonatal rat brain (McDonald *et al.* 1987; Ford *et al.* 1989; Hattori *et al.* 1989). Seven day old rats subjected to unilateral or bilateral carotid artery occlusion and subsequent hypoxia exhibited severe brain damage, which could be completely prevented by dizocilpine (1 mg/kg i.p.) given up to 1.25 h after the start of hypoxia. Protective effects have also been reported with dextromethorphan in a similar model (Prince and Feeser 1988), although much higher doses (20–35 mg/kg i.p.) were required. Olney *et al.* (1989) have described complete protection by dizocilpine (1 mg/kg) against damage induced in neonatal (10 day old) rat brain by exposure to hypobaric ischaemia. In these experiments care was taken to maintain constant body temperature, in order to avoid the possibility that the neuroprotective effects of dizocilpine could be due to drug-induced hypothermia.

Focal ischaemia

Dizocilpine has been assessed in a variety of animal models of focal ischaemia (Table 20.3) (for review see McCulloch *et al.* 1992). Most of these studies involved surgical occlusion of the middle cerebral artery, followed by histological assessment of the resulting cerebral infarct after survival times ranging from 4 h to 7 days. In control animals this procedure leads to a massive involvement of cortical tissue, with up to half of the total cerebral cortex in the affected hemisphere showing signs of ischaemic damage. Dizocilpine given either 30 min before or up to 2 h after the ischaemic insult provided a remarkable degree of neuroprotection, with the volume of cortical tissue damage in cat, mouse, and rat reduced by approximately half. In caudate nucleus, where there is no possibility of alternative blood supply from collateral vessels, dizocilpine was unable to offer any significant degree of neuroprotection. The ED_{50} of dizocilpine for neuroprotection is comparable to that required for anticonvulsant effect in seizure models, and is in the range 0.2–2.0 mg/kg (i.p.). When an infusion regime was used to maintain a constant plasma level of dizocilpine, the concentration in plasma required for neuroprotection corresponded to that which blocks the NMDA receptor *in vitro* (Gill *et al.* 1991a). Other less potent non-competitive NMDA antagonists reported to be effective in

Table 20.3 The effects of non-competitive NMDA antagonists in focal cerebral ischaemia models

Species	Model	Agent	Pretreatment/ post-treatment	Magnitude of cortical neuroprotection	Reference
Cat	MCA	dizocilpine	pre and post	-50%	Oyzurt et al. (1988); Park et al. (1988a)
	MCA (temp.)	dizocilpine	post	-30%	Dezsi et al. (1992)
	MCA	ifenprodil/SL82-0715	post	-42%	Gotti et al. (1988)
Baboon	ACA/CC (temp.)	dizocilpine	post	-65%	Zabramski et al. (1991)
Mouse	MCA	dizocilpine/SL82-0715	post	-63%	Benavides et al. (1989)
Rat	MCA	dizocilpine	pre and post	-41%	Park et al. (1988b)
	MCA	dizocilpine	pre	-40%	Tamura et al. (1988)
	MCA	dizocilpine	pre	-54%	Bielenberg (1989)
	MCA/CC/SHR	dizocilpine	pre	-23%	Dirnagl et al. (1990)
	MCA	dizocilpine	pre	-45%	Lythgoe et al. (1989)
	MCA	TCP	pre	-27%	Gotti et al. (1988)
	MCA	SL82-715	post	-48%	Gotti et al. (1988)
	MCA	kynurenate	pre and post	-56%	Germano et al. (1987)
	MCA/SHR	kynurenate	pre	-2% (n.s.)	Roussel et al. (1989)
	MCA/CC	dextrorphan	post	-53%	Kent et al. (1989)
	MCA	dizocilpine	post	-60%	Gill et al. (1991a)
	MCA	dizocilpine	post	-50%	Hatfield et al. (1992)
	MCA	dizocilpine	pre	-73%	Buchan et al. (1992)
	MCA	(+) cis-β-methyl HA-966 (L-687,414)	post	-41%	Gill et al. (1991b)

The experimental models were MCA = permanent middle cerebral artery occlusion, MCA/CC = tandem occlusion of the middle cerebral and carotid arteries, ACA/CC temp. = temporary occlusion of anterior cerebral and carotid arteries. In all investigations, there was a statistically significant reduction in ischaemic damage with drug treatment with the exception of the two studies marked (n.s.), which were not significantly different from controls.

focal ischaemia models include dextrorphan, dextromethorphan, PCP, ifenprodil and the related compound SL82.0715 (eliprodil), and the glycine site blockers kynurenate and (+)*cis*-β-methyl HA-966 (L-687,414) (Table 20.3). The consistently positive results obtained in these animal models suggest that the use of NMDA antagonists may be valuable in focal ischaemia, including human stroke. The mechanism is likely to involve the rescue of tissue in the 'penumbra' region of an infarct by protecting against damage caused by excess activation of glutamate mechanisms.

In an alternative multi-infarct model of focal cerebral ischaemia, irreversible occlusion of small cerebral blood vessels in rabbit brain was induced by injecting 50 μm diameter plastic microsphere into the internal carotid artery (Gill *et al.* 1991*a*). The results showed that dizocilpine (0.5 mg/kg i.p.) was effective in reducing CNS damage when given at the time of or shortly after the onset of ischaemic injury in this model.

Other neuroprotection models

A role for NMDA receptors mediating spinal cord damage was suggested by reports that dizocilpine offered significant protection against both ischaemia- and mechanical injury-induced spinal deficits (Faden and Simon 1988; Kochhar *et al.* 1988).

Dizocilpine (3 mg/kg) was also able to protect against striatal damage caused by insulin-induced hypoglycaemia in rat brain (Westerberg *et al.* 1988), suggesting that this too is a condition in which excitotoxic mechanisms are involved.

Some other properties of dizocilpine

Dizocilpine has been tested in many animal models, as a prototype NMDA antagonist with high potency and free CNS penetration. It has a number of unexpected properties, e.g. in delaying or preventing the development of morphine tolerance and dependence (Trujillo and Akil 1991), blocking the development of behavioural sensitization to cocaine and to amphetamine (Karler *et al.* 1989), and inhibiting alcohol withdrawal signs (Morrisett *et al.* 1990). The ability of dizocilpine to block the neurotoxic effects of the HIV viral coat protein gp120 *in vitro* (Lipton *et al.* 1991) and to prevent measles virus-induced neurodegeneration *in vivo* (Andersson *et al.* 1990) suggests the possible involvement of NMDA receptor mechanisms in the spread of these neurotrophic viruses. The PCP-like neurochemical and behavioural effects of dizocilpine (Koek *et al.* 1988; Piercey *et al.* 1988; Tricklebank *et al.* 1989), together with the ability to induce transient vacuolization in neurones in certain limbic cortical areas (Olney *et al.* 1989; Allen and Iversen 1990) have, however, given cause for concern. The finding that HA-966 and the related cis-β-methyl analogue (L-687,414) do not cross-generalize to PCP or cause neuronal vacuolization at neuroprotective doses, however, suggests that these are not insurmountable problems (Singh *et al.* 1990*b*; Hargreaves *et al.* 1991).

Conclusions

The results obtained in neuroprotection experiments with dizocilpine and other NMDA antagonists support the hypothesis that NMDA receptors play an important role in ischaemia-induced neuronal degeneration. The ability of peripherally administered antagonists to prevent neuronal loss even when given some hours after the ischaemia episode suggests potential uses of these compounds in the treatment of human ischaemia neuropathologies. The results also indicate that the process of neuronal degeneration triggered by the initial ischaemic insult develops over a relatively long time course, and involves excess activation of NMDA receptors. Dizocilpine, and related non-competitive NMDA antagonists, have many effects on CNS function, at high doses acting as sedatives and anaesthetics, while at lower doses causing behavioural effects and metabolic activation like those of PCP. It remains to be seen whether such compounds can be safely tolerated in clinical use, and clinical trials with at least one such agent (CNS 1102) are currently in progress.

References

Allen, H. L. and Iversen, L. L. (1990). Phencyclidine, dizocilpine and cerebrocortical neurons. *Science*, **245**, 221.

Andersson, T., Schultzberg, M., Schwarcz, R., Love, A., Wickman, C., and Kristensson, K. (1990). NMDA-receptor antagonist prevents measles virus-induced neurodegeneration. *European Journal of Neuroscience*, **3**, 66–71.

Beal, M. F., Kowall, N. W., Swatz, K. J., Ferrante, R. J., and Martin, J. B. (1988). Systemic approaches to modifying quinolinic acid striatal lesions in rats. *Journal of Neuroscience*, **8**, 3901–8.

Benavides, J., Cornu, P., Dubois, A., Gotti, B., MacKenzie, E. T., and Scatton, B. (1989). ω_3 Binding sites as a tool for the detection and quantification of brain lesions: application to the evaluation of neuroprotective agents. In *Pharmacology of cerebral ischaemia 1988*, (ed J. Krieglstein), pp. 187–96. CRC Press, Inc., Boca Raton, FL.

Bielenberg, G. W. (1989). Pre- or postischemic treatment with NMDA antagonists reduces infarct size after MCA occlusion in rat. *Journal of Cerebral Blood Flow and Metabolism*, **9**, S298.

Bowery, N. G., Wong, E. H. F., and Hudson, A. L. (1988). Quantitative autoradiography of MK-801-binding sites in mammalian brain. *British Journal of Pharmacology*, **93**, 944–54.

Buchan, A. and Pulsinelli, W. A. (1990). Hypothermia but not the *N*-methyl-D-aspartate antagonist, MK-801, attenuates neuronal damage in gerbils subjected to transient global ischemia. *Journal of Neuroscience*, **10**, 311–16.

Buchan, A., Li, H., and Pulsinelli, W. A. (1991). The *N*-methyl-D-aspartate antagonist, MK-801, fails to protect against neuronal damage caused by transient, severe forebrain ischemia in adult rats. *Journal of Neuroscience*, **11**, 1049–56.

Buchan, A. M., Slivka, A., and Zue, D. (1992). The effect of the NMDA receptor antagonist MK-801 on cerebral blood flow and infarct volume in experimental focal stroke. *Brain Research*, **574**, 171–7.

Carter, C., Rivy, J.-P., and Scatton, B. (1989). Ifenprodil and SL 82.0715 are antagonists at the polyamine site of the *N*-methyl-D-aspartate (NMDA) receptor. *European Journal of Pharmacology*, **164**, 611–12.

Choi, D. W. (1991). Excitoxicity. In *Excitatory amino acid antagonists*, (ed. B. Meldrum), pp. 216–36. Blackwell Scientific, Oxford.

Choi, D. W., Peters, S., and Visekul, V. (1987). Dextrorphan and Levorphanol selectively block *N*-methyl-D-aspartate receptor-mediated neurotoxicity on cortical neurons. *Journal of Pharmacology and Experimental Therapeutics*, **242**, 713–17.

Church, J., Zeman, S., and Lodge, D. (1988). The neuroprotective action of ketamine and MK-801 after transient cerebral ischemia in rats. *Anesthesiology*, **69**, 702–9.

Clineschmidt, B. V., Martin, G. E., and Buntin, P. R. (1982*a*). Anticonvulsant activity of dextro-5 methyl-10,11 dihydro-5H dibenzo-A D-cyclohepten-5,10-imine MK-801, a substance with potent anticonvulsant central sympathomimetic and apparent anxiolytic properties. *Drug Development Research*, **2**, 123–34.

Clineschmidt, B. V., Martin, G. E., Buntin, P. R., and Papp, N. L. (1982*b*). Central sympathomimetic activity of dextro-5 methyl-10,11 dihydro-5H dibenzo-A D-cyclohepten-5 10-imine MK-801, a substance with potent anticonvulsant central sympathomimetic and apparent anxiolytic properties. *Drug Development Research*, **2**, 135–45.

Corbett, D., Evans, S., Thomas, C., Wang, D., and Jonas, R. A. (1990). MK-801 reduced cerebral ischemic injury by inducing hypothermia. *Brain Research*, **514**, 300–4.

Dezsi, L., Greenberg, J. H., Hamor, J., Sladky, J., Karp, A., and Reivich, M. (1992). Acute improvement in histological outcome by MK-801 following focal cerebral ischemia and reperfusion in the cat independent of blood flow changes. *Journal of Cerebral Blood Flow and Metabolism*, **12**, 390–9.

Dirnagl, U., Tanabe, J., and Pulsinelli, W. (1990). Pre- and post-treatment with MK-801 but not pretreatment alone reduces neocortical damage after focal cerebral ischemia in the rat. *Brain Research*, **527**, 62–8.

Erdö, S. L. and Schäfer, M. (1991). Memantine is highly potent in protecting cortical cultures against excitotoxic cell death evoked by glutamate and *N*-methyl-D-aspartate. *European Journal of Pharmacology*, **198**, 215–17.

Faden, A. I. and Simon, R. P. (1988). A potential role for excitotoxins in the pathophysiology of spinal cord injury. *Annals of Neurology*, **23**, 623–6.

Fleischer, J. E., Tateislin, A., Drummond, J. C., Schetler, M. S., Zornow, M. H., Crafe, M. R., Shearman, G. T., and Shapiro, H. M. (1988). MK-801, an excitatory amino antagonist, does not improve neurologic outcome following cardiac arrest in cats. *Anesthesiology Reviews*, **15**, 102–3.

Fletcher, E. J. and Lodge, D. (1988). Glycine reverses antagonism of *N*-methyl-D-aspartate (NMDA) by 1-hydroxy-3-aminopyrrolidone-2 (HA-966) but not by D-2-amino-5-phosphonovalerate (D-AP5) on rat cortical slices. *European Journal of Pharmacology*, **151**, 161–2.

Ford, L. M., Sanberg, P. R., Norman, A. B., and Fogelson, M. H. (1989). MK-801 prevents hippocampal neurodegeneration in neonatal hypoxic-ischemic rats. *Archives of Neurology*, 1090–6.

Foster, A. C. and Kemp, J. A. (1989). HA-966 antagonizes *N*-methyl-D-aspartate receptors through a selective interaction with the glycine modulatory site. *Journal of Neuroscience*, **9**, 2191–6.

Foster, A. C. and Wong, E. H. F. (1987). The novel anticonvulsant MK-801 binds to the activated state of the *N*-methyl-D-aspartate receptor in rat brain. *British Journal of Pharmacology*, **91**, 403–9.

Foster, A. C., Gill, R., Kemp, J. A., and Woodruff, G. N. (1987). Systemic administration of MK-801 prevents *N*-methyl-D-aspartate-induced neuronal degeneration in rat brain. *Neuroscience Letters*, **76**, 307–11.

Foster, A. C., Gill, R., and Woodruff, G. N. (1988). Neuroprotective effects of MK-801 *in vivo*: selectivity and evidence for delayed degeneration mediated by NMDA receptor activation. *Journal of Neuroscience*, **8**, 4745–54.

Foster, A. C., Kemp, J. A., Leeson, P. D., Grimwood, S., Donald, A. E., Marshall, G. R., Priestley, T., Smith, J. D., and Carling, R. W. (1992). Kynurenic acid analogues with improved affinity and selectivity for the glycine site on the *N*-methyl-D-aspartate receptor from rat brain. *Molecular Pharmacology*, **41**, 914–22.

Fuller, T. A., Lawrence, J. J., and Olney, J. W. (1987). Blockade of *N*-methyl-aspartate-induced arcuate nucleus damage by PCP, MK-801 and related compounds. *Society of Neuroscience Abstracts*, **13**, 412.11.

Germano, I. M., Pitts, L. H., Meldrum, B. S., Bartkowski, H. M., and Simon, R. P. (1987). Kynurenate inhibition of cell excitation decreases stroke size and deficits. *Annals of Neurology*, **22**, 730–4.

Gill, R. and Woodruff, G. N. (1990). The neuroprotective actions of kynurenic acid and MK-801 in gerbils are synergistic and not related to hypothermia. *European Journal of Pharmacology*, **176**, 143–49.

Gill, R., Foster, A. C., and Woodruff, G. N. (1987a). Systemic administration of MK-801 protects against ischaemia-induced hippocampal neurodegeneration in the gerbil. *Journal of Neuroscience*, **7**, 3343–9.

Gill, R., Foster, A. C., and Woodruff, G. N. (1987b). Systemic administration of MK-801 protects against ischaemic neuropathology in rats. *British Journal of Pharmacology*, **91**, 311P.

Gill, R., Foster, A. C., and Woodruff, G. N. (1988). MK-801 is neuroprotective in gerbils when administered during the post-ischaemic period. *Journal of Neuroscience*, **25**, 847–55.

Gill, R., Brazell, G., Woodruff, G. N., and Kemp, J. A. (1991a). The neuroprotective action of dizocilpine (MK-801) in the rat middle cerebral artery occlusion model of focal ischaemia. *British Journal of Pharmacology*, **103**, 2030–6.

Gill, R., Hargreaves, R., and Kemp, J. A. (1991b). Neuroprotective effects of the glycine site antagonist (+)*cis*-4-methyl-HA-966 (L-687,414) in a rat focal ischaemia model. *Journal of Cerebral Blood Flow and Metabolism*, **11**, S304.

Goldberg, M. P., Viskul, V., and Choi, D. W. (1988). Phencyclidine receptor ligands attenuate cortical neuronal injury after *N*-methyl-D-aspartate exposure or hypoxia. *Journal of Pharmacology and Experimental Therapeutics*, **245**, 1081–92.

Gotti, B., Duverger, D., Bertin, J., Carter, C., Dupont, R., Frost, J., Gaudilliere, B., MacKenzie, E. T., Rousseau, J., Scatton, B., and Wick, A. (1988). Ifenprodil and SL82.0715 as cerebral anti-ischemic agents. I. Evidence for efficacy in models of focal cerebral ischemia. *Journal of Pharmacology and Experimental Therapeutics*, **247**, 1211–21.

Hahn, J. S., Aizenman, E., and Lipton, S. A. (1988). Central mammalian neurons normally resistant to glutamate toxicity are made sensitive by elevated extracellular Ca^{2+}: toxicity is blocked by the *N*-methyl-D-aspartate antagonist MK-801. *Proceedings of the National Academy of Science, USA*, **85**, 6556–60.

Hargreaves R. J., Hill R. G., and Iversen, L. L. (1994). Neuroprotective NMDA antagonists: the controversy over their potential for adverse effects on cortical neuronal morphology. *Acta Neurochir.* [Suppl] **60**: 15–19.

Hatfield, R. H., Gill, R., and Brazell, C. (1992). The dose–response relationship and therapeutic window for dizocilpine (MK-801) in a rat focal ischaemia model. *European Journal of Pharmacology*, **216**, 1–7.

Hattori, H. and Wasterlain, C. G. (1991). Hypothermia does not explain MK-801 neuroprotection in a rat model of neonatal hypoxic-ischemic encephalopathy. *Neurology*, **41**, 330.

Hattori, H., Morin, A. M., Schwartz, P. H., Fujikawa, D. G., and Wasterlain, C. G. (1989). Posthypoxic treatment with MK-801 reduces hypoxic-ischemic damage in the neonatal rat. *Neurology*, **39**, 713–18.

Honey, C. R., Miljkovic, Z., and MacDonald, J. F. (1985). Ketamine and phencyclidine cause a voltage-dependent block of responses to L-aspartic acid. *Neuroscience Letters*, **61**, 135–9.

Huettner, J. E. and Bean, B. P. (1988). Block of *N*-methyl-D-aspartate-activated current by the anticonvulsant MK-801: selective binding to open channels. *Proceedings of the National Academy of Science, USA*, **85**, 1307–11.

Johnson, J. W. and Ascher, P. (1987). Glycine potentiates the NMDA response in cultured mouse brain neurons. *Nature*, **325**, 329–31.

Karler, R., Calder, L. D., Chaudhry, L. A., and Turkanis, S. A. (1989). Blockade of 'reverse tolerance' to cocaine and amphetamine by MK-801. *Life Science*, **45**, 599–606.

Kato, H., Araki, T., and Kogure, K. (1990). Role of the excitotoxic mechanism in the development of neuronal damage following repeated brief cerebral ischemia in the gerbil: protective effects of MK-801 and pentobarbital. *Brain Research*, **516**, 175–9.

Keana, J. F. W., McBurney, R. N., Scherz, M. W., Fischer, J. B., Hamilton, P. N., Smith, S. M., Seneer, A. C., Finkbeiner, S., Stevenss, C. F., Jahr, C., and Weber, E. (1989). Synthesis and characterization of a series of diarylguanidines that are noncompetitive *N*-methyl-D-aspartate receptor antagonists with neuroprotective properties. *Proceedings of the National Academy of Science, USA*, **86**, 5631–5.

Kemp, J. A., Foster, A. C., Leeson, P. D., Priestley, T., Tridgett, R., Iversen, L. L., and Woodruff, G. N. (1988). 7-Chlorokynurenic acid is a selective antagonist at the glycine modulatory site of the *N*-methyl-D-aspartate receptor complex. *Proceedings of the National Academy of Science, USA*, **85**, 6547–50.

Kemp, J. A., Marshall, G. R., and Priestley, T. (1991). A comparison of the agonist-dependency of the block produced by uncompetitive NMDA receptor antagonists on rat cortical slices. *Molecular Pharmacology*, **1**, 65–70.

Kemp, J. A., Priestley, T., Marshall, G. R., Leeson, P. D., and Williams, B. J. (1991b). Functional assessment of the actions of 4-methyl derivatives of HA-966 at the glycine site of the *N*-methyl-D-aspartate receptor. *British Journal of Pharmacology*, **102** (Proc. Suppl.), 65P.

Kent, T. A., Eisenberg, H., Quast, M., Anderson, A., Hillman, G., and Campbell, G. J. (1989). Dextrorphan reduces infarct volume after middle cerebral occlusion in rats: a magnetic resonance imaging and histopathology study. *Journal of Cerebral Blood Flow and Metabolism*, **9**, S153.

Kochhar, A., Zivin, J., Lyden, P., and Mazzarella, V. (1988). Glutamate antagonist therapy reduces neurologic deficits produced by focal central nervous system ischemia. *Archives of Neurology*, **45**, 148–53.

Koek, W., Woods, J. H., and Winger, G. D. (1988). MK-801, a proposed non-competitive antagonist of excitatory amino acid neurotransmission, produces phencyclidine-like behavioral effects in pigeons, rats and rhesus monkeys. *Journal of Pharmacology and Experimental Therapeutics*, **245**, 969–74.

Lanier, W. L., Perkins, W. J., Karlsson, B. R., Milde, J. H., Scheithauer, B. W., Shearman, G. T., and Michenfelder, J. D. (1990). The effects of dizocilpine maleate (MK-801), an antagonist of the N-methyl-D-aspartate receptor, on neurologic recovery and histopathology following complete cerebral ischemia in primates. *Journal of Cerebral Blood Flow and Metabolism*, **10**, 252–61.

Lawrence, J. J., Fuller, T. A., and Olney, J. W. (1987). MK-801 and PCP protect against ischemic neuronal degeneration in the gerbil hippocampus. *Society of Neuroscience Abstracts*, **13**, 300.12.

Legendre, P. and Westbrook, G. L. (1991). Ifenprodil blocks N-methyl-D-aspartate receptors by a two-component mechanism. *Molecular Pharmacology*, **40**, 289–98.

Lehmann, A. and Jönsson, T. (1992). MK-801 selectively protects mouse arcuate neurons *in vivo* against glutamate toxicity. *NeuroReport*, **3**, 421–4.

Levy, D. I. and Lipton, S. A. (1990). Comparison of delayed administration of competitive and uncompetitive antagonists in preventing NMDA receptor-mediated neuronal death. *Neurology*, **40**, 852–5.

Lewis, S. J., Barres, C., Jacob, H. J., Ohta, H., and Brody, M. T. (1989). Cardiovascular effects of the N-methyl-D-aspartate receptor antagonist MK-801 in conscious rats. *Hypertension*, **13**, 759–65.

Lipton, S. A., Sucher, N. J., Kaiser, P. K., and Dreyer, E. B. (1991). Synergistic effects of HIV coat protein and NMDA receptor-mediated neurotoxicity. *Neuron*, **7**, 111–18.

Lythgoe, D., McCarthy, H. D., O-Shaugnessy, C. T., and Steward, M. C. (1989). Effects of dimethylthiourea and dizocilpine on infarct size following middle cerebral artery occlusion in the rat. *British Journal of Pharmacology*, **98**, 903P.

McBurney, R. N., Reddy, N. L., Hamilton, P. N., Taylor, E. M., Cotter, R. E., Fischer, J. B., Goldin, S. M., Keana, J. F. W., Wolcott, T. J., and Kirk, C. J. (1991). Neuroprotective efficacy of CNS 1102, a novel non-competitive NMDA antagonist. *Journal of Cerebral Blood Flow and Metabolism*, **11** Suppl. 2, S219.

McCulloch, J. (1992). Excitatory amino acid antagonists and their potential for the treatment of ischaemic brain damage in man. *British Journal of Clinical Pharmacology*, **34**, 106–14.

McCulloch, J., Bullock, R., and Teasdale, G. M. (1992). Stroke and other causes of the ischaemic brain damage in man. In *Excitatory amino acid antagonists*, (ed. B. Meldrum), pp. 287–326. Blackwell Scientific, Oxford.

MacDermott, A. B., Mayer, M. L., Westbrook, G. L., Smith S. J., and Barker, J. L. (1986). NMDA-receptor activation increases cytoplasmic calcium concentration in cultured spinal cord neurones. *Nature*, **321**, 519–22.

McDonald, J. W., Silverstein, F. S., and Johnston, M. V. (1987). MK-801 protects the neonatal brain from hypoxic-ischemic damage. *European Journal of Pharmacology*, **140**, 359–61.

McDonald, J. W., Roeser, N. F., Silverstein, F. S., and Johnson, M. V. (1989*a*). Quantitative assessment of neuroprotection against NMDA-induced brain injury. *Experimental Neurology*, **106**, 289–96.

McDonald, J. W., Silverstein, F. S., and Johnston, M. V. (1989*b*). Neuro-protective effects of MK-801, TCP, PCP and CPP against *N*-methyl-D-aspartate induced neurotoxicity in an *in vivo* perinatal rat model. *Brain Research*, **490**, 33–40.

Michenfelder, J. D., Lanier, W. L., Scheithauer, B. W., Perkins, W. J., Shearman, G. T., and Milde, J. H. (1989). Evaluation of the glutamate antagonist dizocilpine maleate (MK-801) on neurologic outcome in a canine model of complete cerebral ischemia: correlation with hippocampal histopathology. *Brain Research*, **481**, 228–34.

Moroni, F., Alesiani, M., Facci, L., Fadda, E., Skaper, S. D., Galli, A., Lombardi, G., Mori, F., Ciuffi, M., Natalini, B., and Pellicciari, R. (1992). Thiokynuren-ates prevent excitotoxic neuronal death *in vitro* and *in vivo* by acting as glycine antagonists and as inhibitors of lipid peroxidation. *European Journal of Pharma-cology*, **218**, 145–51.

Morrisett, R. A., Rezvani, A. H., Overstreet, D., Janowsky, D. S., Wilson, W. A., and Swartzwelder, H. S. (1990). MK-801 potently inhibits alcohol with-drawal seizures in rats. *European Journal of Pharmacology*, **176**, 103–5.

Nellgård, B., Gustafson, I., and Wieloch, T. (1991). Lack of protection by the *N*-methyl-D-aspartate receptor blocker dizocilpine (MK-801) after transient severe cerebral ischemia in the rat. *Anesthesiology*, **75**, 279–87.

Olney, J. W., Price, M. T., Salles, K. S., Labruyere, J. and Frierdich, G. (1987). Anti-parkinsonian agents are phencyclidine agonists and *N*-methyl-D-aspartate antagonists. *European Journal of Pharmacology*, **141**, 357–61.

Olney, J. W., Ikonomidou, C., Mosinger, J. L., and Frierdich, G. (1989*a*). MK-801 prevents hypobaric-ischemic neuronal degeneration in infant rat brain. *Jour-nal of Neuroscience*, **9**, 1701–4.

Olney, J. W., Labruyere, J., and Price, M. T. (1989*b*). Pathological changes induced in cerebrocortical neurons by phencyclidine and related drugs. *Science*, **244**, 1360–2.

Oyzurt, E., Graham, D. I., Woodruff, G. N., and McCulloch, J. (1988). Protective effect of the glutamate antagonist, MK-801, in focal cerebral ischemia in the cat. *Journal of Cerebral Blood Flow and Metabolism*, **8**, 138–43.

Park, C. K., Nehls, D. G., Graham, D. I., Teasdale, G. M., and McCulloch, J. (1988*a*). Focal cerebral ischaemia in the cat: treatment with the glutamate antagonist MK-801 after induction of ischaemia. *Journal of Cerebral Blood Flow and Metabolism*, **8**, 762–7.

Park, C., Nehls, D. G., Graham, D. I., and McCulloch, J. (1988*b*). The glutamate antagonist MK-801 reduces focal ischaemic brain damage in the rat. *Annals of Neurology*, **24**, 543–51.

Park, C. K., McCulloch, J., McBurney, R. N., Kang, J. K., and Choi, C. R. (1991). Respiratory depression alternates the anti-ischaemic effects of the NMDA ion channel blocker CNS 1102. *Journal of Cerebral Blood Flow and Metabolism*, **11** Suppl. 2, S220.

Peterson, C., Neal, J. H., and Cotman, C. W. (1989). Development of *N*-methyl-D-aspartate excitotoxicity in cultured hippocampal neurons. *Developmental Brain Research*, **48**, 187–95.

Piercey, M. F., Hoffmann, W. E., and Kaczkofsky, P. (1988). Functional evidence for PCP-like effects in the anti-stroke candidate MK-801. *Psychopharmacology*, **96**, 561–2.

Priestley, T., Horne, A. L., McKernan, R. M., and Kemp, J. A. (1990). The effect of NMDA receptor glycine site antagonists on hypoxia-induced neurodegeneration of rat cortical cell cultures. *Brain Research*, **531**, 183–8.

Prince, D. A. and Feeser, H. R. (1988). Dextromethorphan protects against cerebral infarction in a rat model of hypoxia-ischaemia. *Neuroscience Letters*, **85**, 291–6.

Rod, M. R. and Auer, R. N. (1989). Pre- and post-ischemic administration of dizocilpine (MK-801) reduces cerebral necrosis in the rat. *Canadian Journal of Neurological Science*, **16**, 340–4.

Roussel, S., Pinard, E., Peres, M., and Seylaz, J. (1984). Kynurenate and R-Pia do not improve the histopathological consequences of MCA-occlusion in spontaneously hypertensive rats. In *Neurotransmission and cerebrovascular function*, (ed. J. Seylas and E. T. MacKenzie), pp. 453–6. Elsevier, Amsterdam.

Saywell, K., Singh, L., Oles, R. J., Vass, C., Leeson, P. D., Williams, B. J., and Tricklebank, M. D. (1991). The anticonvulsant properties in the mouse of the glycine/NMDA receptor antagonist, L-687,414. *British Journal of Pharmacology*, **102** (Proc. Suppl.) 66P.

Schanne, F. A., Kane, A. B., Young, E. E., and Farber, J. L. (1979). Calcium dependence of toxic cell death: a final common pathway. *Science*, **206**, 700–2.

Schwarcz, R. and Meldrum, B. S. (1985). Excitatory aminoacid antagonists provide a therapeutic approach to neurological disorders. *Lancet*, **ii**, 140–3.

Shoemaker, H., Allen, J., and Langer, S. Z. (1990). Binding of [^{3}H]ifenprodil, a novel NMDA antagonist, to a polyamine-sensitive site in the rat cerebral cortex. *European Journal of Pharmacology*, **176**, 249–50.

Singh, L., Donald, A. E., Foster, A. C., Hutson, P. H., Iversen, L. L., Iversen, S. D., Kemp, J. A., Leeson, P. D., Marshall, G. R., Oles, R. J., Priestley, T., Thorn, L., Tricklebank, M. D., Vass, C. A., and Williams, B. J. (1990a). Enantiomers of HA-966 (3-amino-1-hydroxypyrrolid-2-one) exhibit distinct central nervous system effects: (+)-HA-966 is a selective glycine/*N*-methyl-D-aspartate receptor antagonist, but (−)-HA-966 is a potent gamma-butyrolactone-like sedative. *Proceedings of the National Academy of Science, USA*, **87**, 347–51.

Singh, L., Menzies, R., and Tricklebank, M. D. (1990b). The discriminative stimulus properties of (+)-HA-966, an antagonist at the glycine/*N*-methyl-D-aspartate receptor. *European Journal of Pharmacology*, **186**, 129–32.

Sterz, F., Leonov, Y., Safter, P., Radovsky, A., Stezoski, W., Reich, H., Shearman, G. T., and Greber, T. F. (1989). Effect of excitatory amino acid receptor blocker MK-801 on overall neurologic, and morphologic outcome after prolonged cardiac arrest in dogs. *Anesthesiology*, **71**, 907–18.

Swan, J. H. and Meldrum, B. S. (1990). Protection by NMDA antagonists against selective cell loss following transient ischemia. *Journal of Cerebral Blood Flow and Metabolism*, **10**, 343–51.

Tamura, A., Kirino, T., Sano, K., Tomukai, N., Hirakawa, M., and Narita, K. (1988). Effect of blocker of excitatory amino acid neurotransmitter on focal cerebral ischemia. *Journal of Clinical and Experimental Medicine*, **146**, 131–2.

Tricklebank, M. D., Singh, L., Oles, R. J., Preston, C., and Iversen, S. D. (1989). The behavioural effects of MK-801: a comparison with antagonists acting non-competitively and competitively at the NMDA receptor. *European Journal of Pharmacology*, **167**, 127–35.

Trujillo, K. A. and Akil, H. (1991). Inhibition of morphine tolerance and dependence by the NMDA receptor antagonist MK-801. *Science*, **251**, 85–7.

Watson, G. B., Hood, W. F., Monahan, J. B., and Lanthorn, T. H. (1988). Kynurenate antagonizes actions of *N*-methyl-D-aspartate through a glycine-sensitive receptor. *Neuroscience Research Communications*, **2**, 169–74.

Westerberg, E., Kehr, J., Ungerstedt, U., and Weiloch, T. (1988). The NMDA-antagonist MK-801 reduces extracellular amino acid levels during hypoglycemia and prevents striatal damage. *Neuroscience Research Communications*, **3**, 151–8.

Wong, E. H. F., Kemp, J. A., Priestley, T., Knight, A. R., Woodruff, G. N., and Iversen, L. L. (1986). The anticonvulsant MK-801 is a potent *N*-methyl-D-aspartate antagonist. *Proceedings of the National Academy of Science, USA*, **83**, 7104–8.

Zabramski, J. M., Spetzler, R. F., and Lee, K. S. (1991). Protective effect of *N*-methyl-D-aspartate antagonists after focal cerebral ischemia in rabbits. *Journal of Cerebral Blood Flow and Metabolism*, **11**, S290.

Index

ACBD
  nomenclature for cis and trans isomers
    44, 66
  cis, in binding studies 44
  trans
    in binding studies 44
    in molecular modelling studies 75–80
    as an NMDA receptor agonist 6, 66,
      67
    structure 3, 45
    as a template in molecular modelling
      studies 75, 77
absence seizures, see epilepsy
acetylcholine,
  effect on LTP in neocortex 322
  effect on ocular dominance plasticity
    319–20, 331
ACPD
  nomenclature for cis and trans isomers
    44, 66
  cis(±), in ligand binding studies 44
  trans(±), in ligand binding studies 44
  (1R,3R) isomer
    in molecular modelling studies 76, 78
    as NMDA receptor agonist 66
    specific NMDA receptor agonist 6
    structure 45
  (1S,3S) isomer
    as mGluR agonist 6
    in molecular modelling studies 78
  (1R,3S) isomer
    in molecular modelling studies 78
  (1S,3R) isomer
    as an inducer of LTP 303–6
    as mGluR agonist 6, 258–9
    in molecular modelling studies 78
ADCI
  as an anticonvulsant 400, 413
α₂-adrenoceptor
  agonists as synaptic depressants 271
agatoxin
  as an EAA receptor antagonist 112
ageing 380–1
AIDS 380, 464
alanine
  D-, as a glycine site agonist 114, 115
  L-, as a glycine site agonist 137–8
alcohol, see ethanol
allosteric interactions
  between glycine and NMDA agonists
    195–7
ALS, see amyotrophic lateral sclerosis

Alzheimer's disease 120, 379
α-aminoadipate
  affinity for ligand binding sites 46
  dissociation rate 209–11
  as NMDA receptor antagonist, historical
    10
  structure 10
  as a synaptic depressant 209–11
1-aminocyclobutane-1, 3-dicarboxylate, see
    ACBD
1-aminocyclopentane-1, 3-dicarboxylate, see
    ACPD
α-amino-6,7-dichloro-3-(phosphonomethyl)-
    2-quinoxalinepropionic acid
  in binding studies 61
  as an NMDA receptor antagonist 32, 74
  in molecular modelling studies 74
  structure 33, 61
α-amino-3-hydroxy-5-methyl-4-
    isoxazolepropionate, see AMPA
3-amino-1-hydroxypyrrolidone-2, see HA-
    966
2-amino-4-phosphonobutanoate, see AP4
α-amino-ω-phosphonocarboxylates
  as NMDA receptor antagonists 13, 14
  in receptor binding studies 46–65
2-amino-7-phosphonoheptanoate, see AP7
2-amino-6-phosphonohexanoate, see AP6
2-amino-5-phosphonopentanoate, see AP5
2-amino-3-phosphonopropanoate, see AP3
2-amino-5-phosphonovalerate, see AP5
α-aminopimelate
  binding site affinity 46
  as an NMDA receptor antagonist 10
  structure 10
α-aminosuberate
  binding site affinity 46
  as an NMDA receptor antagonist 10
  structure 10
amitriptyline, as an EAA receptor
    antagonist 9
AMMA
  in binding studies 44
  in molecular modelling studies 76, 77
  as NMDA receptor agonist 43, 66
  structure 45
amnesia, see learning and memory
AMPA
  as selective agonist for receptor sub-type
    6, 11
  locomotion 283
  structure 3

AMPA receptors, 3
  agonists for 132–3
  antagonists for 16
  as EAA receptor subtype 6, 8
  general distribution 8
  in LTP 295, 308, 322
  role in neurotransmission
    in hippocampus 296–7
    in various brain regions 246–59
amygdala
  distribution of NMDA receptor subunits
    159–64
  fear conditioning in 355–65
  LTP in 355
amyotrophic lateral sclerosis 379, 457
anaesthesia 383
analgesia 383, 463–4
anticonvulsants
  NMDA receptor antagonists as 32, 34,
    120, 376–7, 399–400, 413–18
antiepileptogenic agents 32, 400–3,
    407–10, 460
anti-inflammatory drugs 271
antispastic activity of NMDA receptor
    antagonists 383
anxiety 382, 457, 464
AP3
  effect on induction of LTP 306
  as mGluR antagonist 6
  as an NMDA receptor antagonist 40
AP4
  D-, as an NMDA receptor antagonist
    36, 40
  D-, in receptor binding studies 46
  distribution following intra-hippocampal
    injection 345–6
  effect on induction of LTP 306
  L-, as mGluR agonist 6
AP4 receptors, *see* mGluRs
AP5
  as a blocker of LTP induction 296–7,
    342–3
  as a synaptic depressant
    in cerebellum 248–53
    in hippocampus 206–7, 296–300,
      340–51
    in neocortex 253–6, 320, 326–7
    in red nucleus 248–53
    in spinal cord 246–8
    in thalamus 248–53
  as an anticonvulsant 32, 400–1, 411,
    417, 458–61
  as an antiepileptogenic agent 407–10
  as an NMDA receptor antagonist 6, 12,
    32, 36, 244
  effect on
    epileptiform activity 397, 401–2
    imprinting in chicks 367

learning and memory 340–51, 353–60,
    367
  neurite outgrowth 431–2
  ocular dominance plasticity 320
  in molecular modelling studies 81, 83,
    84, 87
  kinetics of action 137–9, 206–8
  in receptor binding studies 36, 46
  structure 13, 33, 143, 458
  structure–activity studies 139–41
AP6
  in molecular modelling studies 83, 84, 90
  as an NMDA receptor antagonist 36
  in receptor binding studies 46
AP7
  as an anticonvulsant 32, 405–6, 458–60
  as an NMDA receptor antagonist
    138–41, 244
  effect of pH 141–42
  in molecular modelling studies 83, 84
  kinetics of action 138–41
  in receptor binding studies 36, 46
  as a neuroprotective agent 378, 462
  as a synaptic depressant
    in neocortex 253–6
    in red nucleus 248–53
    in striatum 248–53
  structure 13, 33, 458
  structure-activity studies 139–41
APB, *see* AP4
APH, *see* AP7
APPA
  as an NMDA receptor antagonist
    139–41
  structure-activity studies 139–41
APV, *see* AP5
arachidonate
  NMDA receptors and 117
  role in neurodegeneration 446
argiotoxin 636, as an EAA receptor
    antagonist 112
ASP-AMP
  as an NMDA receptor antagonist 12, 36
  in receptor binding studies 47
  structure 13
asparagine
  role in permeation through NMDA
    receptor 149–53, 179, 183–4, 188
aspartate
  excitatory action 1
  in binding studies 40
  as an NMDA receptor agonist 133–6,
    211–15
  L-, as neurotransmitter candidate 18–19
  structure 1
β-aspartylaminomethylphosphonate, *see*
    ASP–AMP
associativity *see* LTP

ataxia 464–5
auditory cortex, *see* neocortex
autoradiographic studies
  distribution of NMDA receptor
    antagonists 345–6
  distribution of NMDA receptor subtypes
    164–9
  distribution of NMDA receptor subunits
    154–5, 159–64
autoreceptors
  role in induction of LTP 301–2

baclofen
  as a synaptic depressant 271, 286–8
barbiturates 413–14
basal ganglia
  distribution of NMDA receptor subunits
    159–64
  distribution of NMDA receptor subtypes
    165–72
behavioural studies 110–11, 120–2,
    277–80, 340–68, 385
benzodiazepines
  as synaptic depressants 271–2
benz(f)isoquinolines
  as NMDA receptor antagonists 109
benzomorphans as NMDA receptor
    antagonists 109, 110
binding studies
  α-amino-6,7-dichloro-3-
    (phosphonomethyl)-2-
    quinoxalinepropionic acid in 61
  CPP in, 165–9, 459
  D-AP5 in, 134–135
  in development 428
  in epilepsy 402, 412
  isoquinoline derivatives in 49–51, 60
  L-glutamate in, 165–9
  MK-801 in, 165–9
  NMDA receptor agonists in 134–5, 165–8
  phenylalanine and phenylglycine
    derivatives in 52, 64
binding techniques
  use in structure/activity studies 31–74
blood-brain-barrier
  NMDA receptor antagonists and 20,
    121, 458
blood pressure
  NMDA receptor antagonists and 119
BMAA, neurotoxic action of 379–80
BOAA, *see* ODAP
bradykinin 269
brain
  distribution of NMDA receptor subunits
    159–64
  distribution of NMDA receptor subtypes
    164–72

1-(4-bromobenzoyl)piperazine 2,
    3-dicarboxylate
  as EAA receptor antagonist 16
brain stem
  distribution of NMDA receptor subunits
    159–64
burst activity, *see* epilepsy

Ca²⁺, *see* calcium ions
cadmium ion, as an NMDA receptor
    antagonist 107
calcium channels
  role in LTD in neocortex 325–30
  role in LTP in neocortex 325–30
  role in spinal cord 287
calcium ions
  enzyme activation by 444–8
  permeability of
    AMPA receptors 152, 430
    expressed NMDA receptor subunits
      151–3
    native NMDA receptors 178–180
  role in
    epilepsy 397, 401–2, 406, 411–12
    excitotoxic neuronal death 442–8
    locomotion 279–83
    LTD 324
    LTP 306–7, 321–2
    neurodegeneration 442–8
    NMDA receptor activation 11–12, 20,
      107, 151–3, 279–83, 306–7, 319–30,
      442–8
    NMDA receptor desensitization 197
    ocular dominance plasticity 319–21
    rhythmic activity 279–83
calpain
  role in neurodegeneration 446–7
capsaicin 268–9
carbamazepine 413–4
carboxylate
  effect of pH 141–2
  importance in NMDA receptor
    antagonists 139–41
4-carboxyphenylglycine, *see* CPG
4-carboxy-3-hydroxyphenylglycine, *see*
    4C3HPG
α-(carboxycyclopropyl)glycine, *see* CCG
trans-2-carboxy-3-pyrrolidine acetic acid,
    see CPAA
cardiac arrest 378, 457, 462–3
catalepsy
  caused by PCP receptor ligands 110
caudate nucleus, *see* striatum
*p*CB-PzDA
  as EAA receptor antagonist 16, 244
  as synaptic depressant
    in red nucleus 248–53

catalepsy (*contd.*)
  as synpatic depressant (*contd.*)
    in spinal cord 246–8
    in thalamus 250
  structure 16
CCG
  (2S,3S,4S) isomer (L-CCG-I)
    as mGluR agonist 6
  (2S,3R,4S) isomer (L-CCG-IV)
    in ligand binding studies 44
    in molecular modelling studies 76, 78
    as an NMDA receptor agonist 6, 66
    structure 3, 45
  (2R,3S,4R) isomer (D-CCG-IV)
    in ligand binding studies 44
    in molecular modelling studies 76, 78
    as an NMDA receptor agonist 66
    structure 45
  (2R,3S,4S) isomer (D-CCG-II)
    in ligand binding studies 44
    in molecular modelling studies 76
    as an NMDA receptor agonist 6,
      66
    structure 3, 45
4C3HPG
  as an mGluR antagonist 257–9
  as a synaptic depressant 257–9
cell death, *see* neurodegeneration *and*
    neurotoxicity
central pattern generators
  role of EAA receptors in 277–89
cerebellar granule cells
  NMDA receptor subtypes 165–7,
    169–70
  NMDA receptor subunits 159–64
  sensitivity to EAAs during development
    430–3
  synaptic activation of 234–7, 250, 253,
    433–5
  synaptic NMDA receptor channel
    properties of 234–7
cerebellar Purkinje cells
  blockade of synaptic excitation of 250,
    253, 434
  sensitivity to EAAs during development
    430, 432–3
cerebellum, 428–48
  development *see* development
  distribution of NMDA receptor subtypes
    165–7, 169–70
  distribution of NMDA receptor subunits
    159–64
  EAA pathways in 250, 253, 429, 433–5
  EAA receptors in 428–48
  excitatory synapses in 135
  morphogenesis, *see* development
  neurodegeneration, *see*
    neurodegeneration

neurotoxicity 439–48
synaptic depression in, by
  AP5 250, 253, 433–5
  CNQX 250, 433–5
  CPP 250
  DGG 250
  kynurenate 250
  magnesium ions 433–5
trophic effects, *see* development
cerebral cortex, *see* neocortex
cerebroprotection, *see* neuroprotection
CGP 35348
  effect on induction of LTP 301–2
CGP 37849
  as anticonvulsant 34, 417, 459–61
  as NMDA receptor antagonist 13, 34, 70
  structure 14, 33
  structure-activity studies 139–141
CGP 39551
  as anticonvulsant 34, 417, 459–61
  as NMDA receptor antagonist 13, 34
  structure 14, 55
CGP 39653
  as NMDA receptor antagonist 34
  in binding studies 55, 168
  structure 33
CGP 40116
  as an anticonvulsant 458–9
  as an NMDA receptor antagonist 34
  in binding studies 55
  in molecular modelling studies 84, 86–9
  structure 33, 458
CGP 43487
  as an anticonvulsant 458–9
  structure 458
CGP 55845
  effect on induction of LTP 301
CGS 19755
  as anticonvulsant 458–9
  clinical trials 463
  conformational analysis 81, 82
  in molecular modelling studies 81–3,
    86–90
  as NMDA receptor antagonist 6, 13, 33,
    70, 71
  structure 14, 33, 143, 458
  structure-activity studies 139–41
  as a neuroprotective agent 462
  as a template in molecular modelling
    studies 87
channels
  NMDA receptor channel kinetics 151–2,
    177–201, 208–9, 219–38
1-(*p*-chlorobenzoyl)piperazine-2,3-
    dicarboxylate *see* *p*CB-PzDA
7-chloro-5-iodokynurenate
  as a glycine site antagonist 471
  structure 471

7-chlorokynurenate
  as antagonist at glycine site 6, 15, 113,
    115, 193–5
  as an anticonvulsant 400
  blocker of LTP induction 297
  kinetics of action 137–8
  as a neuroprotective agent 473
  structure 15
chlorpromazine, as EAA receptor
    antagonist 9
climbing fibres
  synaptic transmission in cerebellum 250,
    253, 434
clinical studies 376–86, 460, 463
close-time distribution, *see* shut-time
    distribution
clusters and super-clusters 225–30
CMP
  kinetics of action 139–41
  as an NMDA receptor antagonist
    139–41
CNQX
  in learning and memory studies 360–2
  as an antagonist at glycine site 15, 113,
    115
  as an anti-epileptiform agent 397
  as an EAA receptor antagonist 6, 244
  as a synaptic depressant in
    cerebellum 248–53
    hippocampus 246
    in neocortex 253–6
    in spinal cord 246–8, 286–7
    in thalamus 248–53
  structure 16
CNS 1102
  as a neuroprotective agent 470–1
  as an NMDA receptor antagonist 470–1
  structure 470
cobalt ion, as an NMDA receptor
    antagonist 10, 107
cognition enhancers 383–4
colliculus, *see* superior colliculus *and*
    inferior colliculus
concentration jump experiments 132–46,
    190–200, 206–15, 219, 227–30
conditioned fear, *see* fear conditioning
conditioned freezing, *see* fear conditioning
conductance properties
  of expressed NMDA receptor subunits
    151–3
  of native NMDA receptors 177–201
confusion 465
contingency matching, *see* ocular
    dominance plasticity
co-operativity
  effect on ocular dominance plasticity 320
  in LTP 295
cortex, *see* neocortex

CPAA
  in binding studies 44
  as an NMDA receptor agonist 67
CPC
  kinetics of action 139–41
  as an NMDA receptor antagonist
    139–41
CPC-ene
  kinetics of action 139–41
  as an NMDA receptor antagonist
    139–41
CPG
  as mGluR antagonist 6
CPP
  as an anticonvulsant 399–400, 405, 411,
    458–9
  dissociation rate 209–11
  in binding site studies 35–7, 70–71,
    165–9
  in learning and memory 359
  as a ligand in autoradiographic studies
    164–72
  in molecular modelling studies 86, 90
  as a neuroprotective agent 378
  as an NMDA receptor antagonist 6, 13,
    32, 244
    in spinal cord 246–8
  as a synaptic depressant 209–11
    in cerebellum 248–53
    in neocortex 253–6
    in red nucleus 248–53
    in thalamus 248–63
  structure 14, 33, 458
  structure-activity studies 139–41
CPP analogues
  in NMDA receptor studies 32, 33 70–71
CPP-ene
  as an anticonvulsant 399, 458–61
  in binding studies 169–71
  clinical trials 460
  as a neuroprotective agent 462
  in molecular modelling studies 86
  as an NMDA receptor antagonist 13,
    32
  structure 14, 33, 458
  structure-activity studies 139–41
CPPP, *see* LY 257883
critical period 314–15, 365–7
6-cyano-7-nitroquinoxaline-2,3-dione, *see*
    CNQX
cyclases, NMDA receptor antagonists and
    117
cyclazocine
  as a neuroprotective agent 473
  as an NMDA receptor antagonist 108,
    473
  structure 109
cyclic GMP 448

cycloleucine
  as a glycine site antagonist 114
cyclopropaneaminocarboxylate
  as a glycine site agonist 114, 115
cyclopropylglutamate, *see* CCG
cycloserine
  as a cognitive enhancer 384
  as a glycine site agonist 384
cysteate
  as an AMPA receptor agonist 135–6
  as an NMDA receptor agonist 133–6,
    211–15
cysteine derivatives,
  in binding studies 40
  nomenclature of enantiomers 40
cysteine sulphinate
  in binding studies 40, 41
  as neurotransmitter candidate 19
  as an NMDA receptor agonist 133–6

D-AP4, *see* AP4
D-AP5, *see* AP5
D-AP7, *see* AP7
D-APV, *see* AP5
DEDTC 350
delayed matching to spatial sample 348–9
dependence 382
depotentiation 308
desensitization 151, 197–200, 212–15, 221–2
  effects of calcium 197
  effects of glycine 114–6, 195–7
  of EPSC 212–15
  of expressed NMDA receptor subunits
    151
  glycine-insensitive 197–200
desmethylimipramine
  effect of MK–801 binding 117
development, 415–18, 428–39
  acquisition of receptors in 431
  changes in NMDA receptor properties
    during 398–9, 434–6
  changes in NMDA receptor sensitivity
    during 428–9, 433–5
  differentiation of neurones 432
  distribution of NMDA receptor subtypes
    168–9, 324,
  distribution of NMDA receptor subunits
    436
  of expression of NMDA receptor
    subunits 154–5
  imprinting 365–7
  migration of neurones 431–2
  morphogenesis 429–30, 438–9
  plasticity in visual cortex 313–32
  stabilization of synaptic connections
    438–9

of susceptibility to LTP 322–4
of susceptibility to seizures 398–9,
    415–18
synaptic potentials in spinal cord 268
synaptogenesis 465
trophic effects of NMDA receptor
    activation 429–32, 437–8
dexoxadrol
  as an NMDA receptor antagonist 108
dextromethorphan
  effect on focal ischaemia 478
  as an NMDA receptor antagonist 108
  structure 109, 470
dextrorphan
  effect on focal ischaemia 477–8
  as a neuroprotective agent 473
  as an NMDA receptor antagonist 108
  structure 109
DGG
  in binding site studies 47
  as an EAA receptor antagonist 16, 244
  as a neuroprotective agent 378
  as a synaptic depressant
    in cerebellum 248–53
    in hippocampus 296–7
    in neocortex 253–6
    in spinal cord 246–8
    in thalamus 248–53
  structure 16
diaminopimelate
  as an NMDA receptor antagonist 10
  structure 10
diazepam, as a synaptic depressant 271–2
5,7-dichlorokynurenate
  as antagonist at glycine site 115
  tritiated, in binding studies 115
differential reinforcement of low rates of
    response 346
digger wasp venom
  extract of as an EAA receptor
    antagonist 112
6,7-dinitroquinoxaline-2,3-dione, *see*
    DNQX
discrimination
  studies with PCP receptor ligands
    110–11, 120–1
dissociative anaesthetics (*see also* PCP,
    ketamine, *etc*)
  in binding studies 110
  as NMDA receptor antagonists 108, 470
dizocilpine, *see* MK–801
DMCM 459
DNQX
  as AMPA/kainate receptor antagonist 6,
    244
  as glycine antagonist 15
  as synaptic depressant in neocortex 253–6
  structure 16

dopamine, role in central pattern
generation 287–9
dorsal horn, *see* spinal cord
drug abuse 382

EAA
antagonists, historical development 9–11
general structure 5
in NMDA receptor site structure/activity
studies 37–95
EAA receptors
classification table 6
general characteristics 8
historical development 9–11
role in synaptic plasticity in
amygdala 351–65
cerebellum 438
hippocampus 294–309, 340–51, 401–3
IMHV 365–8
neocortex 313–32
role in synaptic transmission in
cerebellum 234–7, 250, 253, 433–5
hippocampus 206–15, 246, 288–309,
406–11
historical 17–19
neocortex 253–6, 313–32
red nucleus 249–52
spinal cord 246–8, 266–73, 277–89
thalamus 248–52, 257–9
sub-types 6, 9–11
electrographic seizures, *see* epilepsy
eliprodil
effect on focal ischaemia 477–8
as an NMDA receptor antagonist 470
emesis 457
endocrinology 382–3
endothelium-derived relaxing factor *see*
nitric oxide
entorhinal cortex, *see* neocortex
epilepsy 120, 395–418, 457–61
alcohol withdrawal seizures 412–3
absence seizures 406
burst activity 397, 410–11
clinical trials 460
electrographic seizures 407–11
epileptiform activity 396–8
epileptogenesis 395–6
human tissue studies in 411–12
genetic models 405–6
kindling 401–3, 460, 464–5
limbic seizures 460
paroxysmal depolarizing shift 396–7
photosensitive baboons 460–1
seizures 395–406, 460
status epilepticus 418, 457, 465
epileptiform activity, *see* epilepsy

epileptogenesis, *see* epilepsy
EPSC
in cerebellum 234–7, 250, 253
desensitization of NMDA receptor-
mediated 212–15
in hippocampus 206–15, 299, 309
in neocortex 254–6
in spinal cord 272–3
time-course of AMPA receptor-
mediated 235
time-course of NMDA receptor-
mediated 206–15, 219–20, 227–38
EPSP
in cerebellum 250, 253
dual component 246, 279–81
in hippocampus 295–300, 403–5
in neocortex 326–7, 253–6, 321–30
in red nucleus 249–52
in spinal cord 246–8, 267–9, 278–87
in thalamus 248–51, 256–7
ethanol 412–13
etoxadrol, as an NMDA receptor
antagonist 108
excitatory amino acids, *see* EAA
excitatory post-synaptic current, *see* EPSC
excitatory post-synaptic potential, *see* EPSP
excitotoxicity 469, *see also*
neurodegeneration *and* neurotoxicity
exclusion volume, at the competitive
NMDA receptor antagonist site 82,
85, 87, 91
extinction 362–5
eye-blink conditioning 351

fear conditioning 351–65
fear-potentiated startle 357–8
fictive locomotion, *see* motor activity
filial imprinting, *see* imprinting
first latency, *see* kinetics
flumazenil 272
focal ischaemia, *see* ischaemia
four-vessel occlusion 462, 474–6
free radicals, role in neurodegeneration
448
freezing, *see* fear conditioning

GABA
in cerebellar pathways 429
role in epilepsy 402–3, 410
role in LTP 297–302, 321
role in spinal transmission 286–8
GABA$_A$ receptors
role in LTP 297–8

GABA$_B$ receptors
  role in LTP 301–2
  role in spinal transmission 271, 286–8
GAMS
  in binding studies 36
  as EAA receptor antagonist 6, 244
  as synaptic depressant,
    in red nucleus 248–53
    in spinal cord 246–8
    in thalamus 248–53
  structure 16
GDEE, as an EAA receptor antagonist
    9
genetic models of epilepsy, *see* epilepsy
geniculate nucleus
  distribution of NMDA receptor subtypes
    165–7, 169–70
  distribution of NMDA receptor subunits
    159–64
global ischaemia, *see* ischaemia
glutamate
  and analogues in binding studies 39–44
  excitatory action of 1, 133–7, 150–3,
    208–14, 217–37
  in epilepsy 395, 412
  kinetics of action 132–46, 208–14,
    217–37
  as a ligand in autoradiographic studies
    37, 164–72
  as a ligand in membrane binding studies
    35, 37, 366
  in molecular modelling studies 76–7,
    79–80
  as a neurotransmitter 19
  structure 1
  as a trophic factor 431–2
glutamate diethylester, *see* GDEE
glutamate dehydrogenase
  as a glutamate scavenger in
    autoradiographic experiments 37
glutaminase, stimulation of activity by
    NMDA 432
γ-D-glutamylaminomethylphosphonate
  as NMDA receptor antagonist 13
  structure 13
γ-D-glutamylaminomethylsulphonate, *see*
    GAMS
γ-D-glutamylglycine, *see* DGG
γ-D-glutamyltaurine
  as EAA receptor antagonist 16
  structure 16
glycine
  binding studies 113, 115
  effect on desensitization of native
    NMDA receptors 114–16, 137–8,
    195–7
  effects on recombinant NMDA
    receptors 190, 196–7

effects on synaptic transmission 268
  extracellular levels of glycine 190
  glycine-insensitive desensitization
    197–200
  kinetics of action 137, 189–200
  and NMDA receptors 6, 12, 112–13,
    189–200
  nucleated patch clamp recordings
    198–200
  role in
    learning 351
    LTP 297
  structure 15
glycine site of NMDA receptor
  agonists 113–5, 268, 471–2
  antagonists 6, 14–15, 112–16, 137,
    193–5, 268, 297, 471–2, 477–8
  partial agonists 193–5, 212, 471–2
  therapeutic potential of drugs active at
    20, 119–22, 472, 476–8
granule cells, *see* cerebellar granule cells
grease-gap recording
  in cerebellum 433–5
  in hippocampus 303–4, 398, 402
  in spinal cord 266–273
growth-hormone 382–3
GYKI 52466, as AMPA receptor
    antagonist 6

HA-966
  as an anticonvulsant 400
  as EAA receptor antagonist, historical
    10
  as a neuroprotective agent 473
  as partial agonist at glycine site 6, 15,
    113, 115, 193–5, 212–13, 471–2
  structure 15, 471
head injury, *see* trauma
Hebbian synapse, 295, 331
hepatic encephalopathy 379
high pressure neurological syndrome 377,
    399
hippocampus
  AP5 as a synaptic depressant in 296–300
  CNQX as a synaptic depressant in 246
  DGG as a synaptic depressant in 296–7
  distribution of NMDA receptor subunits
    153–5, 159–64
  epileptiform activity 395–418
  kindling 401–3
  kinetics of synaptic transmission in
    206–15, 298–9
  learning and memory 294–5
  LTP in 294–309
  NMDA receptor channel properties
    220–34

neuroprotection 474–8
neurotoxicity in 441
seizures 395–418
historical development of the NMDA
    receptor concept 1–30, 108–12
homocysteate
    in binding studies 40
    as an AMPA receptor agonist 135–136
    as an NMDA receptor agonist 133–36
    kinetics of action 132–5
    as a neurotransmitter candidate 19
homocysteine sulphinate
    in binding studies 40
    as a neurotransmitter candidate 19
    as an NMDA receptor agonist 133–6
homoquinolinate,
    in binding studies 169–71
    in molecular modelling studies 76, 77
    affinity for NMDA receptors 44
    as an NMDA receptor agonist 133–6
    structure 45
hormonal disturbances, *see* endocrinology
5-HT
    effect on ocular dominance plasticity 319
    effects in spinal cord 287
    modulation of NMDA responses 271
    role in central pattern generation 287–9
Huntington's disease 120, 379, 457
1-hydroxy-3-amino-pyrrolidone-2, *see* HA-
    966
6-hydroxydopamine
    effect on ocular dominance plasticity
    318–19
5-hydroxytryptamine, *see* 5–HT
hypoglycaemia, *see* ischaemia
hypothalamus, distribution of NMDA
    receptor subunits 159–64
hypoxia *see* ischaemia

ibotenic acid
    as agonist at mGluRs 6
    in NMDA receptor binding studies 44
    structure 45
ictal-like activity, *see* epilepsy
ifenprodil
    in binding studies 168–9
    developmental changes in sensitivity to
    168–9
    effect on focal ischaemia 477–8
    as an NMDA receptor antagonist 472
IMHV, role in learning and memory
    366–7
indole derivatives, as glycine site
    antagonists 116
imprinting 365–7
inferior colliculus, distribution of NMDA
    receptor subunits 159–64

inhibitory avoidance 359–60
inhibitory postsynaptic current, *see* IPSC
inhibitory postsynaptic potential, *see* IPSP
interictal-like activity, *see* epilepsy
intermediate extent of the hyperstriatum
    ventrale, *see* IMHV
5-iodo-7-chlorokynurenic acid
    as antagonist at glycine site 193
    structure 116
in situ hybridization 154–5, 160–4, 430
INTERVOL 75
IP$_3$
    effect on NMDA responses 322
    role in induction of LTP 306–7
IPSC
    in hippocampus 301–2
IPSP
    in hippocampus 295, 297–302
    in neocortex 321
    role in LTP 295, 297–302
ischaemia, 120, 378 457, 460–3, 474–8
    effect of MK-801 on global ischaemia
    474–6
    effect on focal ischaemia of
    dextromethorphan 478
    dextrophan 477–8
    eliprodil 477–8
    ifenprodil 477–8
    kynurenate 477–8
    L-687, 414 477–8
    MK-801 476–8
    PCP 478
    TCP 477–8
isoquinoline derivatives
    in binding studies 49–51, 60
    as NMDA receptor antagonists 33, 71–2

K-252b
    effect on induction of LTP 304
    effect on NMDA responses 303–4
kainate
    as an epileptiform agent 403–5, 415–7
    as an excitant in spinal cord 3
    kinetics of action 132–3
    locomotion 279–80
    neurotoxicity of 439–43
    role in receptor classification 5–8
    structure 3
ketamine
    agonist-dependency 111, 470
    as a synaptic depressant
        in red nucleus 248–53
        in neocortex 253–6
        in spinal cord 246–8
    as an NMDA receptor antagonist 6, 14,
        108, 244, 246–8, 470

ketamine (*contd.*)
  effect on LTP in hippocampus 297
  structure 109, 470
  voltage dependency 111, 470
kindling, *see* epilepsy
kinetics
  analysis of NMDA receptor agonists
    132–6, 208–15, 219–38
  analysis of NMDA receptor antagonists
    137–9, 180–3, 194–7, 206–15
  of expressed NMDA receptor subunits
    150–3
  of glycine binding to NMDA receptors
    190–2
  of magnesium block of native NMDA
    receptors 189–90
kynurenate
  as an EAA receptor antagonist 244
  effect on focal ischaemia 477–8
  effect on neurite outgrowth 431–2
  in epilepsy 417
  as a glycine site antagonist 15, 113, 115,
    193–5, 471
  structure 16
  synaptic depressant
    in cerebellum 248–53
    in neocortex 253–6
    in spinal cord 246–8
    in striatum 248–53
    in thalamus 248–53

L-687,414
  as an anticonvulsant 472
  effect on focal ischaemia 477–8
  as a glycine site antagonist 471–2
  structure 471
L-689,560
  as a glycine site antagonist 471–2
  structure 471
lamotrigine 414
lamprey, synaptic mechanisms in 278–89
L-AP3, *see* AP3
L-AP4, *see* AP4
L-AP5, *see* AP5
L-689560, as antagonist at glycine site 115,
  193
lateral geniculate nucleus, *see* thalamus
lathyrism 379–380
learning 313–14, 414–15
  role of NMDA receptors in 119,
    340–368, 385
levorphanol
  as a neuroprotective agent 473
  as an NMDA receptor antagonist 108
limbic seizures, *see* epilepsy
locomotion, *see* motor activity

long-term depression, *see* LTD
long-term potentiation, *see* LTP
LTD
  in hippocampus 308
  in neocortex 321–31
  role in learning and memory 348
LTP
  in amygdala 355
  associativity 295
  co-operativity 295
  effect of acetylcholine 322
  effect of noradrenaline 322
  expression mechanisms 308–9
  Hebbian synapse 295
  in hippocampus 294–309, 341–51
  induction mechanisms of 296–308,
    321–2, 324
  in Mg^{2+}-free solutions 307
  input specificity 295
  in neocortex 321–31
  priming 297, 301–2, 348
  role of AMPA receptors 308, 322
  role of calcium 321–2
  role of IPSPs 297–301, 321
  role in learning and memory 294–5,
    341–52
  role of mGluRs 301–7
  role of second messengers 301–7, 322
  theta rhythm 295, 301
luteinizing hormone 382–3
LY 202157
  as an NMDA receptor antagonist
    139–43
  structure 143
  structure-activity studies 139–41
LY 221501,
  effect of pH 141–2
  as an NMDA receptor antagonist
    139–41
  structure-activity studies 139–41
LY 233053
  as an anticonvulsant 458–9
  in binding studies 48
  as an NMDA receptor antagonist 33,
    70–1, 139–41
  structure-activity studies 139–41
  structure 33, 143, 458
LY 233536
  as an anticonvulsant 458–9
  in binding studies 166–7
  structure 458
LY 235959
  in molecular modelling studies 87, 92
  as an NMDA receptor antagonist 33–34,
    68, 72, 139–41
  structure 33, 143
  structure-activity studies 139–41
  unusual stereospecificity of action 68, 72

LY 257883
  conformational analysis 82
  kinetics of action 138–9
  in molecular modelling studies 82, 86
  as an NMDA receptor antagonist 33,
    139–41
  structure 33, 48, 86
  structure-activity studies 139–41
LY 274614
  as an anticonvulsant 458–9
  structure 458

magnesium ions
  effect on induction of LTP 297–300,
    307–8
  effect on synaptic transmission 245,
    256–7
    in cerebellum 434–5
    in hippocampus 297–300, 307–8
    in neocortex 253–4
    in spinal cord 266
  extracellular, blockade by 180–5
  intracellular, blockade by 185–9, 395
  kinetics of action 180–3, 206–8
  mechanism of action at NMDA
    receptors 106–7, 180–9, 206–8
  as an NMDA receptor antagonist,
    historical 10–11, 19
  permeability to
    of expressed NMDA receptor subunits
      152–3
  role in
    epilepsy 395
    locomotion 279–83
    rhythm generation 279–83
  voltage-dependent block 180–9,
    297–300, 436
manganese ion
  as an NMDA receptor antagonist 10,
    107
Markov assumptions 225, 232–3
maximal electroshock seizures 399–400,
    459
MCA, *see* middle cerebral artery occlusion
MCPG
  as antagonist at mGluRs 6
  effect on induction of LTP 306–7
MDL 100, 453
  derivatives in binding studies 55, 59
  as an NMDA receptor antagonist 34, 68,
    70
  structure 33
MDL 100, 925
  derivatives in binding studies 48, 60–1
  as an NMDA receptor antagonist 33, 71
  structure 33

2-MDP
  as an NMDA receptor antagonist 109
  structure 109
measles 380
memantine
  as a neuroprotective agent 473
  as an NMDA receptor antagonist 109
  structure 470
memory
  role of NMDA receptors in 340–68
MEPSCs, NMDA receptor mediated
    235–6
MES, *see* maximal electroshock seizures
metabotropic EAA receptors, *see* mGluRs
metabotropic glutamate receptors, *see*
    mGluRs
metaphit, as an NMDA receptor
    antagonist 111
cis-methanoglutamate, *see* ACBD
α-methyl-4-carboxyphenylglycine, *see*
    MCPG
β-methylaminoalanine, *see* BMAA
methyldiphenylpropanolamines, as NMDA
    receptor antagonists 109
(+)-4-methyl-HA-966
  action at glycine site 114
  structure 116
mGluRs 6, 8, 11
  in cerebellar pathways 429
  in LTP 301–7, 328–9
  in synaptic transmission 257–9
midbrain
  distribution of NMDA receptor subtypes
    165–7, 169–70
  distribution of NMDA receptor subunits
    159–64
middle cerebral artery occlusion 462,
    476–8
migraine 383
migration, *see* development
mitochondria, role in neurodegeneration
    444–5
Mg²⁺ *see* magnesium ions
MK-801
  agonist dependency 470
  as an anticonvulsant 400–1, 406, 411–13,
    470
  as an antiepileptogenic agent 401,
    415–17
  as an anxiolytic 470
  in binding studies 166–9, 470
  as a central sympathomimetic 470
  as a dissociative anaesthetic 470
  effect on focal ischaemia 476–8
  effect on global ischaemia 474–6
  effect on kindling 401
  effect on LTP induction 297
  effect on morphogenesis 438–9

MK-801 (*contd.*)
  as a neuroprotective agent 378, 469–79
  as an NMDA receptor antagonist 6, 14,
    109, 469–71
  regional distribution of binding sites 166–7
  side effects 469
  structure 109, 470
  voltage dependency 470
mnemonic processes, *see* learning *and*
    memory
molecular biology 147–55, 158–73, 179,
    183–4, 190, 193, 195–7
molecular modelling,17, 74–95
  binding site in 75–95
  excitotoxic pocket in binding site 43, 78
  hydrophobic pocket in binding site 34,
    74, 91–3
  pharmacophore 77, 80
(R)-MNT 950A
  in binding studies 44
  in molecular modelling studies 76, 77
  as NMDA receptor agonist 43, 66
  structure 45
MNQX, as glycine antagonist 15, 115, 116
monocular deprivation, *see* ocular
    dominance plasticity
morphinans, as NMDA receptor
    antagonists 108–9
morphogenesis *see* development
mossy fibres
  LTP in 297
  synaptic tranmission in,
    cerebellum 433–5
    hippocampus 297
motoneurone disease, *see* amyotrophic
    lateral sclerosis
motor activity, role of EAA receptors in
    119, 277–89
motor cortex, *see* neocortex
MPTP 463
mRNA 154–5, 160–4
muscle relaxants 383–4
muscle weakness 464
mussel poisoning, *see* shellfish poisoning
MULTIFIT (module of SYBYL computer
    software) 76, 80, 83, 84, 86, 88, 89
mutagenesis of expressed NMDA receptor
    subunits 152–3

NAAG, affinity for NMDA receptors 44
N-acetylaspartylglutamate, *see* NAAG
naloxone, effects on PCP and sigma
    receptor ligands 108
NBQX
  as an AMPA receptor antagonist 6, 244
  as a synaptic depressant in red nucleus
    248–53

N-allylnormetazocine, *see* SKF 10, 047
neocortex
  distribution of NMDA receptor subtypes
    165–7, 169–70
  distribution of NMDA receptor subunits
    159–64
  EPSPs 253–7
  LTP 321–32
  ocular dominance plasticity 314–21
  PCP receptor ligands as NMDA receptor
    antagonist in 110
  synaptic depression in, by
    AP5 253–6
    AP7 257
    CNQX 253–6
    DNQX 253–6
    CPP 253–6
    DGG 253–6
    ketamine 253–6
    kynurenate 253–6
    PDA 253–6
neural rhythmicity 107, 279–84
neurite outgrowth, *see* development
neurodegeneration, *see also* neurotoxicity
    120, 428, 439–48
  developmental susceptibility to 440–42
  differential vulnerability of neurones to
    440–42
  protection from by NMDA receptor
    antagonists 377–81, 460–4, 472–8
  as therapeutic targets 457, 464
neurokinin receptor, *see* NK receptor
neuronal development, *see* development
neuronal survival, *see* development
neuropeptides 268–71
neuroprotection 32, 377–81, 460–4, 472–9
neurotoxicity, *see also* neurodegeneration
  of NMDA receptor antagonists 414
  role of calcium ions in 442–8
neurotransmitter
  concentration at synaptic receptors
    209–11
  identification at NMDA receptors
    18–19, 211–12
  time course of binding to NMDA
    receptors 206–15
nickel ion, as an NMDA receptor
    antagonist 107
nitric oxide
  NMDA receptor antagonists and 117
  role in neurodegeneration 447–8
NK receptor 270–1
NMDA
  action 2–4
  structure 1
  synthesis 2
  uptake and 4
NO, *see* nitric oxide

nociception, role of NMDA receptors in 268–71
non-competitive NMDA receptor antagonists 105–131, 469–79 *see also* magnesium ions *and* glycine site of NMDA receptor *and* MK-801 etc.
non-NMDA receptors, *see also* AMPA receptors *and* kainate
  antagonists 16
  classification 6
  concept, historical 9–11
  synaptic pathways utilizing 243–59
noradrenaline
  effect on LTP in visual cortex 331–2
  effect on ocular dominance plasticity 318–20
  role in central pattern generation 289
norepinephrine, *see* noradrenaline
NPC 17742
  in binding studies 62
  as an NMDA receptor antagonist 34, 73
  structure 33
NR1
  gene 148–9, 158–62
  splice variants 148–9, 158–62
  structure 148–9, 158–62
  subunit 147–55, 158–62, 169–72, 179, 183–4
NR2
  gene 149–50, 162–4
  structure 150, 162–4
  sub-units 147–55, 162–4, 169–72, 179, 183–4
β-N-oxalylamino-L-alanine (BOAA), *see* ODAP
β-N-oxalyl-α,β-diaminopropionate, *see* ODAP
N-site, *see* asparagine
nucleus of the diagonal band, distribution of NMDA receptor subunits 159–64
nucleotide cyclases, NMDA receptors and 117
nucleus accumbens, distribution of NMDA receptor subunits 159–64
neural rhythmicity 279–84

ocular dominance plasticity 314–21
ODAP
  affinity for NMDA receptors 47
  neurotoxic action of 379–80
6-OHDA, *see* 6-hydroxydopamine
olfactory bulb, distribution of NMDA receptor subunits 159–64
olfactory cortex, *see* neocortex
olfactory system, synaptic transmission in 255

olivo-cerebellar-positive atrophy 120
ontogeny, *see* development
open time distributions of NMDA receptor channels 222–7
opiate receptors
  effects of PCP and sigma receptor ligands 108–9
  as synaptic depressants 271
ornithine decarboxylase, activity in relation to NMDA receptors 117
β-N-oxalylamino-L-alanine *see* ODAP

pain 246–8, 258–9, 268–72, 383, 457
parallel fibre pathway, synaptic transmission in 250, 253, 434
Parkinson's disease 379, 457, 463
paroxysmal depolarizing shift, *see* epilepsy
patch-clamp, *see* voltage clamp studies
Pavlovian fear conditioning, *see* fear conditioning
pCB-PzDA (*indexed under* C)
PCMP, as an NMDA receptor antagonist 110
PCP
  agonist dependency 111, 470
  as an anticonvulsant 120, 400
  as an antiepileptic agent 415–17
  behavioural studies 110–111, 120–1
  binding to membranes 110
  channel blocking action of 111, 470
  effect on focal ischaemia 478
  as an NMDA receptor antagonist 6, 14, 108, 469–70, 473
  as a neuroprotective agent 473
  other actions 120–1
  psychotomimetic effects 120
  relation to MK–801 470
  schizophrenia 121
  structure 109, 470
  voltage-dependency 470
2,3-PDA
  cis(±)
    as an EAA receptor antagonist 244
    in binding studies 44
    as early NMDA receptor antagonist 16
    structure 45
    synaptic depressant action of
      in neocortex 253–6
      in spinal cord 246–8
  trans(±)
    in binding studies 44
    structure 45
  cis(2R,3S) isomer
    in binding studies 44
    in molecular modelling studies 79
    as an NMDA receptor agonist 66–7

2,3-PDA (*contd.*)
  cis(2S,3R) isomer
    in binding studies 44
    as an NMDA receptor agonist 66–67
2,4-PDA
  cis(±)
    in binding studies 44
    as an NMDA receptor agonist 66–7
    structure 45
  trans(±)
    in binding studies 44
    in molecular modelling studies 79
    as an NMDA receptor agonist 66–7
    structure 45
pentazocine
  as a neuroprotective agent 473
  as an NMDA receptor antagonist 108, 473
  structure 109
pentobarbitone, as EAA receptor antagonist 9
pentylenetetrazol 459
peptides, *see* neuropeptides
perforant path 295
  LTP in 294–7
perinatal asphyxia 457
peripheral effects of EAAs 384
periqueductal grey
  distribution of NMDA receptor subtypes 165–7, 169–70
  distribution of NMDA receptor subunits 159–64
pH, and NMDA receptor sensitivity 118, 237
phencyclidine, *see* PCP
phenobarbitone 413–14
phenylalanine derivatives
  in binding studies 52–53, 64
  as NMDA receptor antagonists 34, 73–4
phenylglycine derivatives
  in binding studies 52–3, 64
  as mGluR antagonists 257–9, 306
  as NMDA receptor antagonists 73–4
4-trans-phenylurea, *see* L–689,560
phenytoin 413–14
philanthotoxin, as an EAA receptor antagonist 112
phospholipases
  NMDA receptor antagonists and 117
  role in LTP 304–7
  role in neurodegeneration 446
phosphoinositide hydrolysis
  in epilepsy 402
  role in LTP 304–7
ω-phosphono group
  effect of pH 141–42
  importance in NMDA receptor antagonists 12–14, 68–9, 139–41

phosphorylation
  role in NMDA channel regulation 183–5
photosensitive baboons *see* epilepsy
PI, *see* phosphoinositide hydrolysis
pilocarpine, as an epileptiform agent 403
pineal, distribution of NMDA receptor subunits 159–64
piperazine derivatives
  in binding studies 48, 56, 60, 63
  as NMDA receptor antagonists 6, 13, 16, 70–1
  in synaptic blockade 246–52
  structure 14, 16, 33, 47, 48, 56, 60, 63
piperidine dicarboxylate, *see* PDA
PKC, *see* protein kinase C
P$_{open}$, *see* kinetics
polyamines, action at modulatory site on NMDA receptors 16, 118
pontine nuclei, distribution of NMDA receptor subunits 159–64
potassium conductance, role in rhthymic activity 282–3
presynaptic inhibition 286–8
primary afferents, *see also* spinal cord
  magnesium ions 266
  synaptic transmission mediated by 246–8, 266–73
priming, *see* LTP
prostaglandins 271
protein kinase C
  effect on magnesium block of NMDA receptors 184, 436
  effect in neurite outgrowth 432
  in LTP 303–4
  NMDA receptors and 117, 284–5, 303
  role in neurodegeneration 447
psychiatric disorders 381
psychotomimetic effects
  of PCP and other agents 120–1, 384–5
Purkinje cells, *see* cerebellar Purkinje cells
PzDA, *see* pCB-PzDA (*indexed under* C)

quinolinate
  as EAA receptor agonist 38
  as an NMDA receptor agonist 133–6, 473
  in molecular modelling studies 76, 77
  as a possible neurotransmitter 19
  receptor binding by 44
  role in neurodegenerative disease 378–9
  structure 45
quinoxaline derivatives (*see also* CNQX, DNQX, NBQX)
  in binding studies 61
  as EAA receptor antagonists 6
  as NMDA receptor glycine site antagonists 15, 34, 74, 115, 116
  structures 16

quisqualate
    as activator of metabotropic receptor 6
    as EAA receptor agonist 2
    kinetics of action 132–3
    neurotoxicity of 441
    structure 3
quisqualate receptors, *see* AMPA receptors

radiolabelled ligands for the NMDA
        receptor 35–7
recognition memory 347
recombinant NMDA receptors 147–55,
        179, 183–4, 190, 193, 195–7, 237–8,
        436
red nucleus
    blockade of synaptic transmission in
        249–52
    distribution of NMDA receptor subunits
        159–64
redox state of NMDA receptors 118
retention, *see* memory
reverse suture, *see* ocular dominance
        plasticity
rhythmic neuronal activity, *see* neural
        rhythmicity

Schaffer-collateral-commissural pathway
    blockade of synaptic transmission in
        294–309
    LTP in 294–309
schizophrenia 121, 381–2
SDZ EAB 515
    derivatives, in binding studies 52
    in molecular modelling studies 91, 92
    as an NMDA receptor antagonist 68, 73
    structure of triphenyl analogue 33
SEARCH, conformational searching
        module of SYBYL software 83,
        88–90
second messenger systems, NMDA
        receptors and 117, 445–8
second order conditioning 362–3
sedation 464–5
seizures, *see* epilepsy
sensory systems 246–8, 258–9, 385
septum, distribution of NMDA receptor
        subunits 159–64
serine, D-, as glycine site agonist 6,
        112–13, 115, 268–9
serine-*O*-sulphate, as an NMDA receptor
        agonist 133–6
serotonin, *see* 5-HT
shell-fish poisoning 380
short-term potentiation, *see* STP

shut time distribution 220–7
sigma receptor, effect of PCP receptor
        ligands 108–12
single channels, *see* channels
SKF 10,047
    as a neuroprotective agent 473
    as an NMDA receptor antagonist
        108–10, 470, 473
    structure 470
SL82.0715 *see* eliprodil
solvent effects, in molecular mechanics
        calculations 85, 94
somatosensory cortex, *see* neocortex
spasticity 383, 457
spatial learning, *see* learning
spermidine, action at NMDA receptors
        118
spider toxins, as EAA receptor antagonists
        112
spinal cord
    analgesic drugs 271–2
    benzodiazepines 271–2
    glycine co-agonist site in 268–9
    myorelaxant drugs 271–2
    role of EAA receptors in synaptic
        transmission in 277–88
    role of neuropeptides 268–71
    synaptic depression in, by
        AP5 246–8, 267–73, 279–81
        pCB-PzDA 246–8
        CNQX 246–8, 268–73, 286–7
        CPP 246–8
        DGG 246–8
        DNQX 279–81
        GAMS 246–8
        ketamine 246–8
        kynurenate 246–8
        magnesium ions 266, 278
        PDA 246–8
    trauma, NMDA receptor antagonist
        therapy of 463, 478
spinal reflexes, *see* spinal cord
status epilepticus, *see* epilepsy
staurosporine
    effect on induction of LTP 304
    effect on NMDA responses 303–4
step-down inhibitory avoidance 360
stereotypies 464
STP 306
striate cortex, *see* neocortex
striatum
    blockade of synaptic transmission in
        248–52
    distribution of NMDA receptor subtypes
        165–7, 169–70
    distribution of NMDA receptor subunits
        159–64
stroke 457, 462–3

structure-activity studies
  of EAA receptor agonists, historical 1–4
  of EAA receptor antagonists, historical
    10, 12–16
  of NMDA receptor agonists 39–45,
    66–7, 132–46
  of NMDA receptor antagonists
    competitive 32–35, 68–74, 132–46
    non-competitive 110–16
strychnine-insensitive glycine site, *see*
    glycine site of NMDA receptor
substance P 270
substantia nigra
  distribution of NMDA receptor subunits
    159–64
  MPP$^+$ toxicity in 379
subtypes of NMDA receptor 38, 158–73
subunits of NMDA receptor 17, 147–55,
    158–73
sulpho-L-cysteine, as an EAA receptor
    agonist 133–6
ω-sulphino group, effect on receptor
    binding 39–41
ω-sulpho group, effect on receptor binding
    39–41
sulphur-containing amino acids
  as neurotransmitter candidates 19
  as NMDA receptor agonists 6, 133–5,
    211–15
superior colliculus, distribution of NMDA
    receptor subunits 159–64
super clusters, *see* clusters
superoxide ions, role in neurodegeneration
    446–8
suprachiasmatic nucleus, distribution of
    NMDA receptor subunits 159–64
supraoptic nucleus, distribution of NMDA
    receptor subunits 159–64
surface potential, effect on calcium
    permeability of NMDA receptors
    179–80
swimming, *see* motor activity
SYBYL, molecular modelling computer
    software 76, 86, 88, 89
synaptic current, *see* EPSC
synaptic integration 277–89
synaptic pathways (*see also individual*
    regions, and synaptic transmission)
  EAA receptors and 243–59
  NMDA receptor role in, historical
    17–18
synaptic plasticity
  epileptogenesis 395–6
  fear conditioning 351–65
  imprinting 365–7
  kindling 401–3, 460, 464–5
  learning and memory 119, 313–14,
    340–68, 385, 414–15

LTD 308, 321–31, 348
LTP 294–309, 321–31, 341–52, 355
  ocular dominance plasticity 314–21
  wind-up 268
synaptic transmission in
  cerebellum 234–7, 250, 253, 433–5
  hippocampus 206–15, 294–309, 404–11
  neocortex 253–6, 321–30
  red nucleus 249–53
  spinal cord 246–8, 266–73, 277–89
  striatum 249–52
  thalamus 248–50, 256–9

tachykinins 268–71
TCP
  effect on focal ischaemia 477–8
  as an NMDA receptor antagonist 110
tetrahydroisoquinoline derivatives, as
    NMDA receptor antagonists 116
ω-tetrazole group
  effect on NMDA receptor agonist
    activity 43
  effect on NMDA receptor antagonist
    activity 34, 68–9, 71, 139–41
  effect of pH on 141–2
tetrazolylglycine, ((RS)-Tet-Gly)
  in binding studies 44
  as potent NMDA receptor agonist 2, 43
  structure 3, 45
thalamus
  distribution of NMDA receptor subtypes
    165–7, 169–70
  distribution of NMDA receptor subunits
    159–64, 170–2
  blockade of synaptic transmission in
    248–50, 256–9
thapsigargin
  effect on induction of LTP 304
  effect on NMDA responses 303–4
therapeutic applications 119–22, 376–86,
    457–65, 469–79
theta rhythm 348 *see also* LTP
thienylcyclohexylpiperidine, *see* TCP
thiokynurenates, as neuroprotective agents
    473
tiletamine, as an NMDA receptor
    antagonist 108
tinnitus 383, 465
tolerance 382
trans-APPA, *see* APPA
trauma 378, 457, 463, 478
  effect of
    CGS 197.55 463
    CPP 463
    MK-801 478
tricyclic antidepressants 117

trophic effects, *see* development
two-vessel occlusion 460, 474–6

uncompetitive NMDA receptor antagonists
  see non-competitive NMDA receptor
    antagonists

valproate 413, 417
ventral horn, *see* spinal cord
ventral root potential, *see* VRP
ventral midbrain, *see* midbrain
vertebrate locomotor output 277
vestibular nuclei
  distribution of NMDA receptor subunits
    159–64
viral infection 380, 478
visual cortex, *see* neocortex
visual discrimination 342–4
voltage-clamp studies
  NMDA receptor agonists 133–46,
    150–2, 177–8, 219–38
  NMDA receptor antagonists 133–46,
    152–3, 180–9, 193–5, 206–13

of synaptic transmission 272–3, 297–9,
    301–2, 306–9
voltage-gated calcium channels, *see* calcium
  channels
VRP 266–73

water maze 342–51
willardiine derivatives
  affinity for NMDA receptors 44
  as AMPA and kainate receptor agonists 6
wind-up, role of NMDA receptors in 268
withdrawal 382, 417

Xenopus embryo 278–9, 283–4

zinc
  modulation of NMDA receptor subunits
    148
  modulatory site on NMDA receptor 16
  as an NMDA receptor antagonist 107,
    116–17